VACCINE DEVELOPMENT AND MANUFACTURING

Wiley Series in

BIOTECHNOLOGY AND BIOENGINEERING

Significant advancements in the fields of biology, chemistry, and related disciplines have led to a barrage of major accomplishments in the field of biotechnology. The Wiley Series in Biotechnology and Bioengineering will focus on showcasing these advances in the form of timely, cutting-edge textbooks and reference books that provide a thorough treatment of each respective topic.

Topics of interest to this series include, but are not limited to, protein expression and processing; nanotechnology; molecular engineering and computational biology; environmental sciences; food biotechnology, genomics, proteomics, and metabolomics; large-scale manufacturing and commercialization of human therapeutics; biomaterials and biosensors; and regenerative medicine. We expect these publications to be of significant interest to practitioners both in academia and industry. Authors and editors were carefully selected for their recognized expertise and their contributions to the various and far-reaching fields of biotechnology.

The upcoming volumes will attest to the importance and quality of books in this series. I would like to acknowledge the fellow co-editors and authors of these books for their agreement to participate in this endeavor. Lastly. I would like to thank Ms. Anita Lekhwani, Senior Acquisitions Editor at John Wiley & Sons, Inc. for approaching me to develop such a series. Together, we are confident that these books will be useful additions to the literature that will not only serve the biotechnology community with sound scientific knowledge, but also with inspiration as they further chart the course in this exciting field.

Anurag S. Rathore
Amgen Inc.
Thousand Oaks, CA, USA

Titles in series

Quality by Design for Biopharmaceuticals: Principles and Case Studies / Edited by Anurag S. Rathore and Rohin Mhatre

Emerging Cancer Therapy: Microbial Approaches and Biotechnological Tools / Edited by Arsenio Fialho and Ananda Chakrabarty

Risk Management Applications in Pharmaceutical and Biopharmaceutical Products Manufacturing / Edited by A. Hamid Mollah, Mike Long, and Harold Baseman

Vaccine Development and Manufacturing / Edited by Emily P. Wen, Ronald Ellis, Narahari S. Pujar

VACCINE DEVELOPMENT AND MANUFACTURING

Edited by

EMILY P. WEN
RONALD ELLIS
NARAHARI S. PUJAR

Wiley Series in Biotechnology and Bioengineering

WILEY

Published by John Wiley & Sons, Inc., Hoboken, New Jersey
Published simultaneously in Canada

Library of Congress Cataloging-in-Publication Data:

Vaccine development and manufacturing / edited by Emily P. Wen, Ronald Ellis, Narahari S. Pujar.
pages cm. – (Wiley series in biotechnology and bioengineering)
Includes index.
ISBN 978-0-470-26194-1 (cloth)
1. Vaccines–Laboratory manuals. I. Wen, Emily P. II. Ellis, Ronald III. Pujar, Narahari S.
QR189.V2512 2015
615.3′72–dc23

2015028866

MIX
Paper from responsible sources
FSC® C013604

CONTENTS

ACKNOWLEDGMENTS

During the preparation of this book, one of our authors, Dr. Stanley Lawrence Hem passed away on 23 January 2011. Dr. Hem led a distinguished career at Purdue for more than forty years where he was a gifted and dedicated teacher. He was a recognized leader in vaccine adjuvants and he served as the major professor for 40 Ph.D. students. Also, CTJ would like to acknowledge with gratitude the many helpful discussions and exchanges that Stan provided over the past 20 years.

PREFACE

The advent of vaccine development has increased lifespan and improved quality of life. Measles was once an epidemic in the United States, with more than 55,000 cases and 120 deaths as recently as 1989–1991. Today, it is no longer circulating in the United States with the introduction of the measles vaccine. Rubella is no longer endemic in the United States; however in the 1960s, many people witnessed first-hand the terrible effects of the rubella virus. During an epidemic between 1964 and 1965, about 20,000 infants were born with deafness, blindness, heart disease, mental retardation, or other birth defects because the rubella virus infected their pregnant mothers. The same is true for other diseases such as polio, hepatitis A and B, peumococcal, and invasive Hib diseases, whereas the introduction of vaccines greatly diminishes the disease incidence, morbidity, and mortality.

Vaccines work by presenting a foreign antigen to the immune system in order to evoke an immune response. A vaccine can be in the form of inactivated virus particles, attenuated virus, virus-like particles, subunit vaccine, DNA vaccine, and recombinant particles. Vaccine containing inactivated virus particles is grown in culture, purified, and then killed with heat, formaldehyde, or other methods. The inactivated virus particles cannot replicate, but the intact particle can elicit an immune response. Attenuated vaccines contain low virulent particles, whereas virus-like particle vaccines are derived from the structural proteins of a virus and lack viral nucleic acids for reproduction. A subunit vaccine, as the name suggests, consists only a part of a virulent strain, such as polysaccharides on the surface of bacterial cells.

Since the introduction of penicillin, antibiotics have been effective against most bacterial diseases. However, with an increase in antibiotic resistance and newer bacterial diseases, antibiotics have shown diminished efficacy, and vaccines are needed for prevention of diseases. New-generation vaccines are also being developed not only to prevent diseases, but also to cure ailments such as cancer. The development of a vaccine is a complex process, requiring multiple clinical trials to demonstrate the product's safety, efficacy, purity, potency, and consistency in manufacturing. Unlike the manufacturing of small molecules, vaccines are usually derived from highly variable living sources and cannot be easily characterized or analyzed completely. Changes in manufacturing process can have a large impact on the final vaccine product and may require additional clinical testing. The same can be said of generic vaccines because the production process generally defined the product, and regulators still require follow-on biologics and vaccines to complete a new filing and perform clinical trials. The production process of vaccines thus plays an important role in defining the end product.

The process of vaccine production comprises fermentation, purification, formulation, and analytics. In recent years, there have been tremendous advances in all aspects of vaccine manufacturing. Improved technology and growth media have been developed for the production of cell culture with high cell density or fermentation. Advances in expression systems help lower some manufacturing costs and minimize problems seen in older manufacturing processes, such as contamination frequently observed in the manufacturing of influenza vaccines. Improvements in large-scale purification equipment have enabled the efficient processing of large biomasses. Novel adjuvants discovered in the past few years have shown great promises in human clinical trials by helping to elicit stronger immune response and provide long-lasting memory effects. New concepts in facility designs have allowed for multiple use of the same facility.

This book is written with the aim to provide comprehensive information on the various fields involved in the production of vaccines, from fermentation, purification, and formulation to regulatory filing and facility designs. The book can be divided into five sections. First is a review of the history of vaccines development (Chapter 1). The second section comprises new advances in fermentation technology, such as the use of recombinant DNA technology (Chapter 2), different fungal expression systems (Chapter 3), and novel expression systems using host plant systems (Chapter 4). The third section focuses on different purification technology on viral vaccines, protein subunit vaccines, and conjugate vaccines (Chapters 5–7). The next section discusses advances in formulation technology, starting with a general summary on how to stabilize a vaccine via formulation (Chapter 8), followed by specifics such as freeze drying, production of heat-stable vaccine, and the use of aluminum-containing adjuvants (Chapters 9–11). The last section covers other topics that are very important in vaccine production, including regulatory filing, facility design, and production economics (Chapters 12–15).

We hope this book will be useful to a broad cross section of biotechnology professionals, medical and biomedical scientists, health care professional, and anyone who is interested in the making of vaccines.

Emily P. Wen
Ronald Ellis
Narahari S. Pujar

CONTRIBUTORS

Michel Chartrain, Merck & Co., Inc., Kenilworth, NJ, USA

Sudha Chennasamudram, Laboratory of Bacterial Polysaccharides, Office of Vaccine Research and Review, Center for Biologics Evaluations and Research, Bethesda, MD, USA

Tony D'Amore, Sanofi Pasteur, Toronto, Ontario, Canada

Anand Ekambaram, Merck & Co., Inc., West Point, PA, USA

Stanley L. Hem, Purdue University, West Lafayette, IN, USA

Zbigniew Janowicz, Dynavax Europe/Rhein Biotech GmbH, Düsseldorf, Germany

Volker Jenzelewski, Dynavax Europe/Rhein Biotech GmbH, Düsseldorf, Germany

Cliff T. Johnston, Purdue University, West Lafayette, IN, USA

Peter Latham, Latham Biopharm Group, Maynard, MA, USA

David Lechuga-Ballesteros, Aridis Pharmaceuticals LLC, San Jose, CA, USA

Ann L. Lee, Genentech, South San Francisco, CA, USA

Karl Melber, Dynavax Europe/Rhein Biotech GmbH, Düsseldorf, Germany

C. Russell Middaugh, Department of Pharmaceutical Chemistry, University of Kansas, Lawrence, KS, USA

Satoshi Ohtake, Aridis Pharmaceuticals LLC, San Jose, CA, USA

Eric J. Patzer, Aridis Pharmaceuticals LLC, San Jose, CA, USA

Bret R. Phillips, Merck & Co., Inc. West Point, PA, USA

Timothy S. Priddy, Department of Pharmaceutical Chemistry, University of Kansas, Lawrence, KS, USA

Narahari S. Pujar, Merck & Co., Inc. West Point, PA, USA

Shailaja Rabindran, US Department of Agriculture Animal and Plant Health Inspection Service, Riverdale, MD, USA

Udo Reichl, Max Planck Institute for Dynamics of Complex Technical Systems, Bioprocess Engineering, Magdeburg, Germany; Otto-von-Guericke University, Magdeburg, Germany

R.S. Robin Robinett, Merck & Co., Inc., West Point, PA, USA

Sangeetha L. Sagar, Merck & Co., Inc. West Point, PA, USA

Ranjit Sarpal, Amgen, Thousand Oaks, CA, USA

Abraham Shamir, Shamir Biologics LLC, Ft. Washington PA, USA

Andrew Sinclair, Biopharm Services US, Maynard, MA, USA.

Vu Truong-Le, Aridis Pharmaceuticals LLC, San Jose, CA, USA

Willie F. Vann, Laboratory of Bacterial Polysaccharides, Office of Vaccine Research and Review, Center for Biologics Evaluations and Research, Bethesda, MD, USA

Alexis Wasserman, Merck & Co., Inc. West Point, PA, USA

Roland Weyhenmeyer, Dynavax Europe/Rhein Biotech GmbH, Düsseldorf, Germany

Yan-ping Yang, Sanofi Pasteur, Toronto, Ontario, Canada

Vidadi Yusibov, Fraunhofer USA Center for Molecular Biotechnology, Newark, DE, USA

Bernd Kalbfuss-Zimmermann, Novartis Pharma AG, Basel, Switzerland

1

HISTORY OF VACCINE PROCESS DEVELOPMENT

NARAHARI S. PUJAR AND SANGEETHA L. SAGAR
Merck & Co., Inc. West Point, PA, USA
ANN L. LEE*
Genentech, South San Francisco, CA, USA

1.1 INTRODUCTION

The goal of vaccine process development is to develop a manufacturing process that can consistently produce a vaccine that is safe and efficacious. During vaccine discovery, the etiologic agent is identified, the immunogen, adjuvant (if applicable), and administration regimens are developed in animal models such that the vaccine candidate produces a prophylactic immune response that is safe and effective. A requirement of the manufacturing process is to preserve the immunological properties innate to the molecular/biological architecture defined in vaccine discovery and enable production of the vaccine in increasingly larger quantities for use in human clinical studies and later commercial supplies. These activities of vaccine discovery and process development must be well integrated, require collaborative efforts and iterative refinements. The safety and efficacy of the vaccine gets proven though phases of clinical studies with increasing number of subjects. The final process developed and used to produce the vaccine for pivotal clinical trials becomes the manufacturing process which is licensed by regulatory authorities for full-scale production to supply the market.

*Previous affiliation—*Merck & Co., Inc, West Point, PA, USA*

Vaccine Development and Manufacturing, First Edition.
Edited by Emily P. Wen, Ronald Ellis, and Narahari S. Pujar.

Unlike for many other pharmaceutical drugs, the manufacturing process used to produce the vaccine is still frequently tied to the definition of the product. While many modern vaccines are highly purified biomolecules, others are complex preparations, such as live viral vaccines or multivalent conjugate vaccines, consisting of the antigen, trace levels of cellular and process residuals, excipients, as well as adjuvants. For some types of vaccines the "product-is-the-process" interdependence can be greatly alleviated by modern process and analytical technology. This approach is built upon much greater scientific understanding of the process and product characteristics which allows greater process control and performance.

Generally speaking, the immunogen is generated via a cultivation process (also referred to as *the upstream process*) and is characterized by an appropriate choice of cell substrate, growth media and a fermentation or cell culture conditions that reproducibly produce the antigen in large quantities (note that in the rest of the chapter, the word *antigen* is used as a synonym for immunogen). The vaccine purification process (also referred to as *the downstream process*) maybe designed to remove host cell impurities, as well as process additives and yields a bulk vaccine (drug substance). The bulk vaccine is converted into a final vaccine product (drug product) in the formulation, fill, and finish processes. Through this stage, the vaccine is formulated into a final composition that imparts long-term stability, whether in liquid or lyophilized form, and then presented in an appropriate final container, such as vials or prefilled syringes. An adjuvant may or may not be used as part of the drug product depending on the type of the vaccine.

This chapter outlines the history of vaccine manufacturing from a bioprocess development perspective. With the maturation of the biotechnology industry, vaccine manufacturing has evolved significantly over the years. An understanding of the evolution of vaccine manufacturing processes can be instructive in the development of future generations of vaccines. There have been previous reviews on various aspects of vaccine bioprocessing. An excellent review on viral vaccine production is presented by Aunins (2000, 2009). Other viral vaccine production reviews have been written by Shevitz et al. (1990), Ellis (2001), Bailey (2007), and Genzel and Reichl (2007a; 2007b), which also include production of viral vectors. Bacterial vaccine production has been reviewed by Liljeqvist and Stahl (1999a; 1999b) and Ellis (2001). Broader reviews of vaccine bioprocessing include those by Aunins et al., (2010), Dekleva (1999a; 1999b), and Josefsberg and Buckland (2012). This chapter encompasses a broad range of vaccine bioprocesses including whole-viral and -bacterial vaccines, as well as subunit and conjugate vaccines. This chapter is focused on drug substance processes; the area of drug product manufacturing processes, including the topic of adjuvants, is quite rich in its own right, but is beyond the scope of this chapter.

1.2 VACCINES BIOPROCESS EVOLUTION

Vaccines and vaccine candidates have been directed at infectious (bacteria, viruses, and fungi), parasitic, and non-infectious diseases, such as cancer and Alzheimer's disease. They can be largely classified as either live, attenuated, inactivated (or killed), or subunit. Production can be in the native organism or in a heterologous host. Recombinant vaccines have been in the form of protein subunit vaccines and modern live viral vaccines (Nkolola and Hanke, 2004; Polo and Dubensky, 2002; Ellis; 2003). Genetic and peptide vaccines are some other categories, which could be considered subcategories of the aforementioned broad categories. Genetic vaccines are those where the immunogen is delivered in the form of a gene via a naked DNA or a viral vector. The evolution in vaccinology has taken vaccines from complex preparation of undefined contents to whole organisms to highly purified whole organisms and subunit components. This evolution of vaccines is directly related to the development of bioprocess technologies. At the outset, identification of the etiologic agent requires bioprocessing, albeit at a much smaller scale and without the worry of scalability or manufacturability. Although the long-held goal of vaccine innovation would not include any whole organisms (live, attenuated, or inactivated) it is not currently possible nor necessary, particularly in the case of some viral vaccines. Further simplification via reverse vaccinology (Hilleman, 2002; Rappuoli, 2007) leading to genetic or peptide-based vaccines is certainly an attractive goal from the bioprocess technology perspective. If these approaches can be established, they will represent a powerful step change not only in vaccinology, but also in the ease of vaccine bioprocessing because they can consistently be based on well-defined platform technologies.

Although contemporary vaccine history is known to start with Edward Jenner, who developed the small pox vaccine in 1796 using the pus of patients with cowpox with a predecessor, variolation, was known to have been practiced much earlier in China, India, Turkey, Persia, and Africa (Behbehani, 1893). Nevertheless, Jenner is credited for initiating this safer approach in vaccine development, as well as coining the term *vaccine* from *vacca* (Latin for cow). This early history has been reviewed quite extensively (e.g., Galambos, 1999; Hilleman, 2000; Plotkin and Plotkin, 1999; Lederberg, 2000; Plotkin, 2009). Since the days of Jenner, vaccinology has proven to be a tremendous benefit to all mankind. In particular, vaccines have had a significant impact on increasing life expectancy since dawn of the twentieth century. With modern molecular techniques, the molecular architecture of the etiologic agent and the antigen continues to be better defined, and consequently, vaccine manufacturing processes are more capable of producing better defined antigens, in many cases rivaling the production of therapeutic proteins where the concept of a "well-characterized" biologic is well established.

1.3 LIVE ATTENUATED AND INACTIVATED VIRUS VACCINES

The earliest vaccines were live attenuated organisms – e.g. smallpox vaccine by Jenner and rabies vaccine by Pasteur. Live vaccines have complex upstream cultivation processes and undergo minimal downstream processing. Because they are live, the degree of attenuation and genetic stability is particularly important, as it relates to the reversal of virulence. Furthermore, the choice of the host can have an impact on vaccine safety and reactogenicity because of potential host cell residuals, growth media components, as well as the potential for adventitious agents. The production system, in the case of Jenner's smallpox vaccine was patients with cowpox. Pasteur used rabbits as the bioreactor to produce the immunogen for the rabies vaccine. This type of *in vivo* production is still in use for the production of a Japanese encephalitis (JE) vaccine. JE-VAX®, licensed in 1954 in Japan and in 1992 in the United States, was derived from mouse brain (in this case, the vaccine is administered as an inactivated virus) and was being supplied in the United States until it was discontinued in 2007. Other mouse-brain-derived JE vaccines are still being manufactured in South Korea, Taiwan, Thailand, and Vietnam but are slowly being replaced by cell-culture derived vaccines. (www.path.org, JE vaccines at a glance; Zanin et al., 2003). *In vivo* production continues to be widely used in veterinary vaccines (Aunins, 2000).

In 1931, Ernest Goodpasture discovered that a hen's egg was an ideal sterile production system for fowl pox virus, and a whole new, enduring bioreactor system was born (Woodruff and Goodpasture, 1931). This led to the licensure of the first influenza vaccine in 1945 (Salk and Francis, 1946). Also, in the 1930s, a yellow fever vaccine based on the 17D strain was developed (Vainio and Cutts, 1998). *In ovo* production is still widely practiced today for the production of both of these vaccines. Scale-up of vaccine production is accomplished by scale-out, that is, simply increasing the number of eggs used with automation to facilitate processing (Hickling and D'Hondt, 2006). At 1–3 flu vaccine doses yielded per egg (Blyden and Watler, 2010), millions of eggs need to be processed each year. *In vivo* or *in ovo* cultivation of viruses is not optimally suited for the industrialization of vaccine production (although it has been practiced for a very long time owing to the slow implementation of alternatives; to be discussed in the following sections) because of the need for sufficient quantities of controlled live animals (e.g., pathogen-free) at the very outset, difficulties of process control during production and inability to scale-up, as well as the very long cycle time for vaccine production.

A major breakthrough in the use of *in vitro* cultivation was the success in propagation of polio virus by Enders (Enders et al., 1949) in primary cells. The cell substrate used was non-neural human cells. Soon thereafter, the inactivated polio Salk vaccine was licensed and produced in primary monkey kidney cells related to the now widely used Vero continuous cell line (Barrett et al., 2009). The significance of this breakthrough is still playing out, with viral vaccines previously prepared in animals or eggs being transitioned to more industrially suitable cell-culture-based production systems. The advantages of this transition are many, including ease of scale-up, rapid response to potential pandemics, as well as a way to address the problem of egg-related allergies. In addition, cell culture allows for the direct monitoring and control of the cell and virus culturing processes. The choice of cell substrates is one of the most critical factors in the manufacture of viral vaccines. This is a topic that has garnered a lot of attention in the literature (Hayflick, 2001; Aunins, 2009; Lubiniecki and Petricciani, 2001; Petricciani and Sheets, 2008) and is of continued interest. Workshops held by the World Health Organization (http://www.who.int) and the International Association of Biological Standardization (http://www.iabs.org) continue to advance the field, particularly in the establishment of standards.

This transition from *in vivo* to *in vitro* production came about with the use of primary cells, where cells from specific organ of an animal was used for virus propagation. Primary monkey kidney cells were used by polio vaccine manufacturers but later discontinued in the United States and Europe. Vaccines still produced in primary cells include measles, mumps, and rabies (e.g., chick embryo fibroblasts for M-M-R® II and RabAvert®). However, they suffer from many of the same drawbacks as *in vivo* and *in ovo* productions, such as the need to maintain captive herds (Aunins, 2000). Hence, the field transitioned to the use of human diploid cells. There are two popular cell lines—WI-38 developed in the Wistar Institute in the United States and subsequently MRC-5 in the United Kingdom, both derived from human lung cell from distinct sources. Cell banking was initiated with this transition and is now a standard feature of any biomanufacturing activity. Cell banking allows the use of a consistent, stable, and well-tested substrate for each batch of vaccine production. These cells are used for the production of rubella, varicella, hepatitis A, polio, and rabies (e.g., WI-38 for rubella in M-M-R II, MRC-5 for Varivax®, Vaqta®, Havrix®, Imovax®, Poliovax®; FRhL-2 for Rotashield®, a rotavirus vaccine from Wyeth, now withdrawn, after reports of intussusception).

Human diploid cell lines have had a long and excellent safety record. However, they do suffer from the limitation of senescence, the need for surface adherence and requirement for bovine serum during cell culture. Senescence is the ceasing of cell division after a certain number of cell divisions and is characterized by the Hayflick limit (Hayflick and Moorhead, 1961). Continuous cell lines overcome many of the disadvantages presented by human diploid cells. Being theoretically immortal, they differ from human diploid cell lines primarily in their capacity to replicate. Prominent examples include Vero cells from African Green Monkey and Madin-Darby canine kidney (MDCK) cells. The use of continuous cell lines drove the need for an explicit purification target on the final product residual DNA level to address potential safety concerns related to oncogenicity of the host cell DNA or infectivity by adventitious agent(s). This level has evolved over time as the assessment of oncogenicity and adventitious agent risk has been better understood and is now recommended to be less than 10 ng host cell DNA/dose (WHO, 2010). The exact level may need to be adjusted if cells with specific concerns (e.g., tumorigenic phenotype) are used. In addition, mitigation of the aforementioned risks also calls for reducing the length of DNA to less than that of a functional gene, which is thought to be approximately 200 base pairs (FDA, 2010). Continuous cell lines are used for flu, JE, rotavirus, and polio vaccines (e.g., Vero for Ixiaro®, Imojev®, Ipol® and Rotateq®, Rotarix®; MDCK for Optaflu®, Celtura®, Flucelvax®).

The aforementioned cell lines require adherent surfaces for growth. As such, bioreactor systems such as roller bottles, T-flasks, cell cubes, and cell factories are widely used for the production of vaccines at the industrial scale. However, these suffer from many limitations driven primarily by the need to scale-up by increasing the surface area (Ozturk, 2006). The use of microcarriers provides a more scalable solution for vaccine production in attachment-dependent cell lines. This technology is employed for the production of polio and rabies vaccines, primarily with Vero cells. Vero cells have also been adapted to serum-free media (e.g., Gould et al., 1999; Butler et al.,

2000; Merten, 2002; Rourou et al., 2007; Bergener and Butler, 2006; Rourou et al., 2009; Toriniwa and Komiya, 2008; Chen and Chen, 2009) and ultimately for suspension (Paillet et al., 2009). Scalable microcarrier technology is now the convention for newer vaccines in development using adherent cell lines such as the one for chikungunya (Tiwari et al., 2009). Similar advances have been made with MDCK cells (Genzel et al., 2006a; Genzel et al., 2006b; Chu et al., 2009). Corresponding changes to downstream processing have also been made to match the advances to upstream processing, such as the use of more conventional harvest technologies along with column chromatography to achieve a high level of purification (Wolff and Reichl, 2008).

The evolution in the commercial production for flu and JE vaccines nicely illustrates the advances in upstream bioprocess technology for viral vaccines. Starting with *in vivo* or *in ovo* production, these vaccines have transitioned to continuous cell lines in adherent culture and finally to fully suspension cultures with the recent licensure of Optaflu®, Celtura®, and Flucelvax® in MDCK cells (Genzel and Reichl, 2007a; Genzel and Reichl, 2007b; Doroshenko and Halperin, 2009; Genzel and Reichl, 2009). A cell-culture-based JE vaccine is now approved (Ixiaro®) in the United States as is a serum-free cell-culture-based JE vaccine (Imojev®) in Thailand and Australia (Zanin et al., 2003). The scale of flu vaccine manufacture has reached multiple thousands of liters. As examples, Baxter has a 6000 l facility in the Czech Republic for production of flu vaccine in Vero cells on microcarriers (capacity of 20 MM doses/year) (Kistner, 2005), Novartis has a 2500 l scale facility in Marburg, Germany for flu in MDCK cells in suspension, and a 5000 l scale facility (reported to produce 150 MM doses/year) in Holly Springs, United States. The scale of these operations rival those used for animal viral vaccine production. A recent review on the scale-up of viral vaccine production has been published (Whitford and Fairbank, 2011).

Recombinant or designer cell lines such as PER.C6®, AGE1.CR®, CAP®, and EB66® are now being used in the development of various vaccines (Fallaux et al., 1998; Altaras et al., 2005; Jordan et al., 2009; Olivier et al., 2010; Tintrup, 2011). In these cases, normal human or animal cells are transformed by viral or cellular oncogenes or by immortalizing cellular genes, to render them practically immortal. These cell lines are also amenable to serum-free suspension cell culture. No vaccine has been licensed to date in these cell lines.

1.4 LIVE OR WHOLE-KILLED BACTERIAL VACCINES

Although currently less prevalent compared to the live viral vaccines, there is still a rich history of live bacterial vaccines, and it may be experiencing renewed interest (Lindberg, 1995, Detmer and Glenting, 2006). The use of live attenuated bacteria started with Louis Pasteur's discovery of attenuation and immunogenicity of a chicken cholera culture in 1879 (Plotkin and Plotkin, 1999). The Bacille Calmette-Guerin (BCG) vaccine for tuberculosis, as well as vaccines for typhoid and plague, were developed around the same time (Plotkin and Plotkin, 1999). Live and whole-killed bacteria have comparatively the simplest manufacturing bioprocesses of all vaccines. Production generally involves cultivation of the bacteria, harvesting, and then inactivation if applicable, followed sometimes by lyophilization. Akin to cell culture technology, microbial fermentation technology has evolved significantly over time. Microbial cultivation technology has evolved from static cultures using complex medium with animal-derived components in bottles to the contemporary use of fed-batch fermentation with chemically defined medium in stirred tank fermentors using aeration for aerobic cultures with state-of-the-art process monitoring and control (Aunins et al., 2010). The literature is rich – with historical aspects (Scott, 2004; El-Mansi et al., 2007; Junker, 2005; Shiloach and Fass, 2005) as well as advances in microbial fermentation technology (Junker, 2004; Choi et al., 2005; Schmidt, 2005; Hewitt and Nienow, 2007).

Live bacterial vaccines are of special significance in bacterial enteric diseases, where the live bacteria mimic the route of infection and provide immunity. Cholera and typhoid fever caused by enteric pathogens *Vibrio cholerae* and *Salmonella typhi*, respectively, are key examples (Dietrich et al., 2008). Cholera vaccines have been produced in either live or whole-killed forms. Oral live cholera vaccines contain the *V. cholerae* bacteria attenuated by removal of genes encoding subunits of the cholera enterotoxin (Chaudhuri and Chatterjee, 2009). Dukoral® made by Crucell in the SBL Vaccin AB facility in Solna, Sweden, is a multivalent oral cholera vaccine consisting of three different strains of *V. cholera*. The bacteria are inactivated by heat and/or formalin treatment, and then combined with a recombinantly produced and purified cholera toxin B (which is really a strain of *V. cholerae* lacking the toxin A gene). The production of this vaccine is by traditional microbial fermentation in a stirred tank (EMEA, 2005) and leverages the advances made in classical fermentation processes, such as those for *Escherichia coli* (de Mare et al., 2003). Shanchol™ from Shanta Biotechnics (now a division of Sanofi-Pasteur) is another vaccine for cholera, and Crucell's Vivotif® is an oral, live bacterial vaccine for typhoid. The bacteria are grown using standard fermentation technology. They are then lyophilized and formulated into a solid dosage form to resist the low pH environment in the stomach. The bioprocessing for the manufacture of BCG vaccine is also quite simple and involves propagation of the chosen strain, and then harvest, which is followed by formulation for lyophilization. In contrast to the vaccines previously mentioned, BCG is administered intradermally. Advances in molecular biology have enabled the development of nonvirulent and nonreverting strains of these and other pathogenic bacteria as delivery vehicles of heterologous antigens, although the bioprocess aspects are not much different than these two traditional vaccines.

An important parenteral whole-bacterial vaccine is the one against pertussis. *Bordetella pertussis* is a small gram-negative bacterium that causes whooping cough. The vaccine, first licensed in 1918, was a suspension of whole-killed bacteria. The fermentation culture is harvested, inactivated by heat, and the suspension is formulated with formaldehyde (Aunins et al., 2010; Plotkin and Ornstein, 1999). The whole-cell pertussis vaccine was combined with the subunit vaccines for diphtheria and tetanus in the combination vaccine – DTwP. The whole-cell pertussis vaccine was eventually replaced in the 1990s with the acellular subunit vaccine in many developed countries to address reactogenicity of the whole-cell vaccine (more on acellular subunit vaccine to be discussed in the following section). The production for both vaccines has now reached large industrial scale fermentors up to 15,000 l (FDA, 1992; Njamkepo et al., 2002). In addition, there have been significant advances in the understanding and control of the toxin production during fermentation (Bogdan et al., 2001; van de Waterbeemd et al., 2009; Streefland et al., 2009). Techniques for enhanced process control such as process analytical technology (PAT) and Quality by Design (QbD) (Streefland et al., 2007; Streefland et al., 2009) are now employed. PAT is "*a system for designing, analyzing, and controlling manufacturing through timely measurements (i.e., during processing) of critical quality and performance attributes of raw and in-process materials and processes with the goal of ensuring final product quality*," as defined by the FDA (http://www.fda.gov). This is now employed across most modern biomanufacturing operations.

It is important to mention a few words on lyophilization, particularly within the realm of live vaccines. Lyophilization was introduced as a process step as early as in the 1930s and represented a true bioprocess advance (Adams, 2003) enabling the delivery of live bacteria and viruses in a stable form for administration. Lyophilization also allows some vaccines such as typhoid vaccine to be delivered in a solid dosage form. Lyophilization needs to be carefully considered, since it can cause loss of potency during processing and in extreme cases, can render the vaccine ineffective (Levine et al, 1976). This technology continues to be a key focus of process development for the enhancement of thermostability of vaccines (Rexroad et al., 2002a; Rexroad et al., 2002b).

1.5 CLASSICAL SUBUNIT VACCINES

Classical subunit vaccines are a natural evolution to the killed bacterial vaccines analogous to the pertussis vaccine described previously. Diphtheria and tetanus vaccines were the first subunit vaccines to be developed in the 1930s (Plotkin and Plotkin, 1999). The diphtheria toxin is also the first protein purified for active immunization. The toxin is produced by the bacterium that causes the disease *Corynebacterium diphtheriae*. The early fermentations were performed using a beef digest medium and the toxin was secreted into the medium. The medium was harvested via centrifugation and/or filtration, and the toxin was inactivated using formaldehyde (Rappouli and Pizza, 1989). The toxoiding process, namely the conversion of the toxin into an inactive vaccine antigen using formalin was a result of a serendipitous bioprocess experiment (Glenny and Hopkins, 1923) where residual formalin in "cleaned" containers was found to have weakened the toxin. Contemporary processes for the production of diphtheria vaccine include more extensive protein purification steps such as ammonium sulfate precipitation and chromatography and membrane filtration to isolate the toxin from cellular impurities (Rappouli and Pizza, 1989; Relyveld et al., 1998). The fermentation process has also evolved in a manner similar to that described previously for pertussis. Beef digest medium has been replaced by a semisynthetic medium made up of an alternate protein source, such as casein (Tchorbanov, et al., 2004; WHO, 2012).

Analogous to diphtheria and pertussis, the tetanus vaccine is produced by the fermentation of *Clostridium tetani*. Its process evolution is also similar where early fermentations were performed with media containing animal components such as brain–heart infusion broth, followed by a shift to dairy sources such as casein digest. More recently, the complete removal of animal-derived components has been demonstrated (Demain et al., 2005; Fratelli et al., 2005; Demain et al., 2007). Similar to diphtheria toxin purification, tetanus toxoid purification has advanced from employing precipitation and low resolution chromatography (Surian and Richter, 1954; Schwick et al., 1967) to using modern tangential flow membranes, facilitating large scale manufacturing (Vancetto et al., 1997; Ravetkar et al., 2001).

Besides the diphtheria and tetanus protein vaccines, another important class of subunit vaccines is the capsular polysaccharide vaccines. For example, an alternative to the live oral typhoid vaccine is a capsular polysaccharide subunit vaccine, Typhim Vi®. This involves a lot more bioprocessing, including purification of the bacterial capsular polysaccharide via precipitation using CTAB (Sanofi-Pasteur, 2005). The most prominent vaccines in this class are the pneumococcal and meningococcal polysaccharide vaccines. The pneumococcal polysaccharide vaccine, was first licensed as a 14-valent vaccine in the 1970s but then grew to a – 23-valent vaccine in the 1980s to form the broadest valency vaccine to-date (e.g., Pneumovax®23). The fermentation processes used for these capsular polysaccharide vaccine have evolved similarly to the processes mentioned previously – transitioning away from animal-derived components. Furthermore, as with the aforementioned microbial fermentations, the application of fermentation process design principles evolved significantly (Baart et al., 2007). Fermentation processes for these pathogenic microorganisms are generally of the batch type owing to the desire to minimize intrusions into the fermentor, and are conducted in specially designed facilities to address biocontainment. The biodefense vaccine for anthrax such as BioThrax® also falls in this classical subunit vaccines category, where the strain of *Bacillus anthracis* used is avirulent and nonencapsulated (FDA, 2012).

All of these subunit vaccines undergo downstream processing designed to remove cellular components and process residuals. The extent of purification depends on the particular vaccine, although most modern vaccines are designed to be highly purified. Downstream processing is discussed further below.

Most inactivated and subunit vaccines are formulated with adjuvants to enhance the immunogenicity of the vaccines either in magnitude of the immune response or in its persistence. The field of adjuvants is quite vast and is getting more attention with the recent advances in the understanding of innate immunity. Vaccines that contain adjuvants make the manufacturing process more complex. Although adjuvants such as aluminum salts were relegated to being simply an added excipient in the early days of their use, greater understanding of the physicochemical properties of the adjuvant (Hem and HogenEsch, 2007) and the impact of the interactions between the antigen and the adjuvant on immunogenicity is emerging. For example, the strength of adsorption of hepatitis B surface antigen on aluminum adjuvant has an impact on the immune response (Hansen et al., 2009). As stated previously, the area of adjuvants in a rich one and a more in-depth discussion is beyond the scope of this chapter.

1.6 RECOMBINANT SUBUNIT VACCINES

The classical examples described in the previous section, where the cell substrate is a strain of the microorganism that is closely related to the one that causes disease, constitute the vast majority of "cell substrates" used for producing subunit vaccines. Recombivax HB®, a hepatitis B vaccine, was the first recombinant vaccine for human use licensed in the United States in 1986. Cloning of the hepatitis B surface antigen into Saccharomyces cerevisia commenced the use of rDNA technology in the vaccine industry and has been followed by significant activity in heterologous production of vaccine antigens over the last 30 years (Burnette, 1991; Burnette, 1992). Many reviews on the production of recombinant subunit vaccines exist (e.g., Liljeqvist and Stahl, 1999; Hansson et al., 2000; Clark and Cassidy-Hanley, 2005; Soler and Houdebine, 2007). Furthermore, owing to the significant growth in the therapeutic protein and monoclonal antibody industry, there have been significant technological advancements in the production of recombinant proteins that extend to vaccine antigen production. These advances have been cataloged extensively for *E. coli* (Chou 2007, Ni and Chen, 2009, Kolai et al., 2009, de Marco, 2009), CHO (Butler, 2005, Butler, 2006, Butler, 2007, Jayapal et al., 2007, Kwaks and Otte, 2006, Durocher and Butler, 2009, Grillberger et al., 2009, Kantardjieff et al., 2019), and yeast (Galao et al., 2007, Hamilton and Gerngross, 2007, Marasugi, 2008, Takegawa et al., 2009, Curran and Bugeja, 2009, Graf et al., 2009, Potgieter et al., 2009).

Needless to say, the etiology of disease, specifically the correct identification and cloning of a protective immunogen, is critical to such an approach. At the same time, the pitfalls of pushing the envelope of reductionism are noted (Van Regenmortel, 2001). Generally, antigen presentation – either in the form of virus-like particles (VLPs) (in the case of viral subunit vaccines) and/or with the use of adjuvants – is an important attribute owing to the lower inherent immunogenicity of these kinds of vaccines relative to their classical counterparts (Perrie et al., 2008; Reed et al., 2009). Recombivax HB is a 22-nm VLP consisting of the recombinant Hepatitis B surface antigen (rHBsAg) associated with lipids and was first produced in *Saccharomyces cervesiae* (Elliott et al., 1994; Dekleva et al., 1999; Zhou et al., 2006). Since then, the same host has been used to produce Engerix®, another hepatitis B vaccine, and Gardasil®, human papillomavirus (HPV) vaccine. Another HPV vaccine, Cerverix®, is made using a recombinant baculovirus system in Hi-5 cells derived from Trichoplusia ni (a type of moth). In addition, a seasonal influenza vaccine made in insect cells, Flublok®, was recently approved. *E. coli* was used to produce Lymerix®, although the vaccine was later withdrawn. Besides these host systems, Chinese hamster ovary cells, *Pichia pastoris* and *Hensenula polymorpha*, have also been used, mostly for the production of Hepatitis B vaccine. Lysogenic *Corynebacterium diphtheria* (Rappuoli, 1983; Srivastava and Deb, 2005) has been used for the production of the carrier protein CRM197, used in polysaccharide conjugate vaccines. *E. coli* is also used as the recombinant host for the production of three of the four antigens in Bexsero® (Serruto et al., 2012), the only meningococcal serogroup B vaccine to be approved to date.

For vaccines in development, a variety of expression systems are being used (or have been used), including the ones described previously. In addition to the workhorse *E. coli*, novel microbial hosts being evaluated in vaccine development include *Pseudomonas fluorescens* and *Lactococcus lactis* (Bahey-El-Din, 2012; Chen, 2012; Unnikrishnan et al., 2012). Baculovirus expression in insect cells is increasingly being used for the production of glycoprotein antigens (Hu et al 2008; Dalemans, 2006; van Oers, 2006). Mammalian cell lines have also been used for the development of glycoprotein-based subunit vaccines. The HIV vaccine candidate gp120 protein was produced in CHO cell line (Billich, 2004). Other examples include HCV vaccine candidates from Chiron (Choo et al., 1994), HSV-2 (Langenberg et al., 1995, Corey et al., 1999), EBV subunit vaccines (Jackman et al., 1999), CMV (Spaete, 1991), and HSV (Lasky, 1990). Finally, plants have garnered a lot of interest recently as recombinant hosts for vaccines (Yusibov et al, 2011). Plants had seen a similar surge in interest in the past decade for the production of monoclonal antibodies, until improvements in more conventional mammalian methods made their use less attractive.

Principles developed for choosing an expression host for therapeutic proteins naturally translate to the production of vaccine antigens. There are many resources for providing guidance to choose a host (Andersen and Krummen, 2002; Makrides and Prentice, 2003, Graumann and Premstaller, 2006, Giuliani et al 2007, Choi et al., 2005, Demain and Vaishnav, 2009, Ferrer-Miralles et al., 2009, Chen, 2012). In general, however, the antigen productivity burden on the manufacturing process for vaccines is far less than that for therapeutic proteins, particularly monoclonal antibodies, because of the low dosage, although cost of goods pressure on vaccines is much more severe than for therapeutic proteins. Finally, as with the classical subunit vaccines, downstream purification is critical for the production of consistent and characterized recombinant vaccines, which is discussed further below.

1.7 CONJUGATE VACCINES

Conjugate vaccines are another interesting class of vaccines. They are complex vaccines, because they are comprised of two subunit components—a hapten and a carrier protein, covalently joined by chemical conjugation. Conjugation to the carrier protein to the hapten helps to elicit a T-cell-dependent immune response, which is particularly important in humans with a less developed immune system, such as infants. As such, conjugate vaccines have become an integral part of infant immunization. The first conjugate vaccine was a *Haemophilus influenzae* type b (Hib) conjugate vaccine, ProHibit®, licensed in the United States in 1987. ProHibit was a PRP-diphtheria toxoid conjugate vaccine, but was quickly superceded by more improved Hib vaccines conjugated to CRM197 (nontoxic mutant diphtheria toxin),

OMPC (the outer membrane protein carrier from *Neisseria meningitidis*) and tetanus toxoid. Menjugate®, a meningococcal C conjugate vaccine, was licensed in 2000 as was Prevnar®, a pneumococcal conjugate vaccine. Prevnar®, consists of seven different polysaccharide-CRM197 conjugates and has had a significant impact on the burden of pneumococcal disease in the pediatric population. The vaccine won the Discovers Award from PhRMA in 2005. The 7-valent vaccine has now been exceeded by Prevnar-13®, where six additional polysaccharide-CRM197 conjugates have been added, making it the world's most complex biological product ever produced (Frasch, 2009; Emini, 2010). This tour de force vaccine won the Prix Galien award in 2011. Analogous to the pneumococcal conjugate vaccine, a quadrivalent meninogococcal conjugate vaccine, Meactra®, was first licensed in 2005. Menafrivac®, a meningococcal A conjugate vaccine, was licensed for the developing world in 2010 in a unique collaboration between the developed and developing world partners (Frasch et al., 2012), with vaccine manufacturing expertise at large scale and low production cost supplied by Serum Institute of India.

In order to facilitate conjugation, chemistry is performed on one or both of the biomolecules to prepare them suitable for the conjugation reaction. It is critical to maintain antigenic fidelity of the hapten, while also optimizing the extent of reaction and process yields for both the antigen and the carrier protein, because both are high value intermediates. Minimizing the many side reactions including degradation of one or more of the components involved is also important. Several different chemistries have been used, each with its own pros and cons (Frasch, 2009). Process control and scale-up of such conjugation operations are more akin to chemical processing, where control of the relative rates of reaction and fluid transport is very relevant. The bioprocess steps used subsequent to conjugation, are similar to those of subunit vaccine purification, where the unreacted components are removed from the conjugate. Removal of the unreacted polysaccharide from the conjugate is one separation challenge, especially if only size-based methods are employed (Meacle et al., 1999; Wen et al., 2005).

Until recently, conjugate vaccines were manufactured at a relatively modest scale owing to the small number of doses sold. However, with the advent of the GAVI Alliance, Hib vaccines and now pneumococcal vaccines are slated for near-universal global infant immunization, thus needing large-scale production of these conjugate vaccines (http://www.gavialliance.org/funding/pneumococcal-amc/). Scale-up of these vaccines is nontrivial because of the issues listed previously and is further complicated by the multivalent composition of these vaccines.

1.8 DOWNSTREAM PROCESSING

Downstream processing has received relatively less attention in vaccine bioprocessing relative to upstream production. This is probably due to the dominance of whole-organism vaccines for most of vaccine history. Owing to the lack of complete knowledge of the etiology of disease and the molecular basis of immune protection, the conservative approach had been to keep the preparation rather crude.

As illustrated by the pertussis vaccine (La Montagne, 1997), reactogenicity concerns with whole-organism vaccines have led to the development and proliferation of subunit vaccines (Ellis 1996; Lattanzi et al., 2004), thus increasing the need and relevance of downstream processing. Even for whole-viral vaccines, the removal of residual DNA is of particular concern when produced in continuous cell lines (Sheng-Fowler et al., 2009). The manufacturing requirements of subunit vaccines today rivals those of therapeutic proteins. Although the dose of a vaccine is much lower relative to monoclonal antibodies, the safety requirements for vaccines are much greater, since they are administered prophylactically to a healthy population including infants.

The first recombinant vaccine—Recombivax-HB® used many contemporary bioseparation techniques. The vaccine consists of a highly hydrophobic protein–lipid particles of 22 nm. As a result, the manufacture of this vaccine is quite challenging, analogous to the expression and purification of membrane proteins. In fact this is a common feature of many subunit vaccine candidates because many are bacterial or viral surface protein antigens. The downstream process of Recombivax-HB® also involves a thiocyanate treatment step which results in reforming the disulfide bonds in the virus-like particle (VLP), thus adding to the complexity. Purification of the HBSAg was initially performed using density gradient ultracentrifugation. This is a common feature of historical processes where the scale-up methodology had been to scale-up laboratory techniques, or simply scale-out. Modern processes use unit operations that are designed to be scaleable. Density gradient ultracentrifugation has been replaced by chromatographic adsorption steps (Sitrin and Kubek, 1992), which have further evolved in sophistication with regard to the configuration of the binding surface to enable adsorption and transport of the large macromolecular sizes of these particles, such as with the use of membrane chromatography or monoliths. The Hepatitis A vaccine, Vaqta® is an excellent example of the use of modern bioseparation techniques for the manufacture of a highly purified complete inactivated virus (Junker et al., 1994; Hagen et al., 1996; Hennessey et al., 1999). The manufacturing process for Vaqta® was awarded the 1998 ACS Industrial Biotechnology Award. The same award was garnered in 2006 for the process to manufacture an HPV vaccine (Gardasil®), which incorporates not only modern bioseparation techniques, but also a highly sophisticated well-controlled virus-like particle disassembly/re-assembly step. The structural protein of the virus when expressed in *Saccharomyces cerevesiae* spontaneously assembles into VLPs inside the cell. After purification of the VLPs, they are disassembled and then reassembled in a controlled manner to produce highly uniform and stable VLPs (Shi et al., 2007). Gardasil® also received the Prix Galien Award in 2007 and the PhRMA Discovers Award in 2009. Purification processes for the capsular polysaccharide vaccines include the use of selective precipitation steps, facilitated by the development of newer analytical methods to analyze and quantify the product, host cell impurities, and process residuals (Abeygunawardana et al., 2000; Pujar et al., 2005). Conjugate vaccines have additional purification challenges that were outlined above. Two other examples, although for vaccine development candidates which were not commercialized, have also contributed to the state of the art of vaccine purification.

An industrial-scale purification of plasmid DNA vaccines was developed using controlled and continuous heat lysis of cell paste, and nonchromatographic methods to overcome the low binding capacity of plasmid DNA to conventional wide-pore chromatographic resins (Lee and Sagar 2001; Murphy et al., 2006). Large scale live adenovirus suitable for human use was accomplished by developing a novel selective precipitation step for cellular DNA among other steps (Goerke et al., 2005; Konz et al, 2008). Overall the downstream purification processes for such diverse entities such as a fully intact virus, a protein–lipid complex virus-like particles, multimeric protein complex, and plasmid DNA represent significant bioseparation process technology advances, significantly enabling the development of modern vaccines and vaccine candidates.

Key issues for downstream processing can be summed up as follows: removal of cellular impurities including proteins, DNA, RNA, and lipids; removal of process residuals; preservation of the structure of the antigen; and formulation of the antigen in an environment that keeps it stable for at least 2 years in a refrigerated state. Vaccines are diverse, complex biomolecules, often multivalent, and, consequently, the bioseparation challenges are manifold and vaccine specific. This can be contrasted with the purification of monoclonal antibodies where a platform process using protein A chromatography followed by typically two additional chromatography steps is commonly used across the industrial landscape. Despite these challenges, modern analytical techniques enable a deep understanding and control of both upstream and downstream operations, increasing yielding well-characterized vaccines, a feature nicely illustrated by Gardasil®.

1.9 VACCINES FOR THE DEVELOPING WORLD: LARGE VOLUME, LOW COST, AND THERMOSTABLE

Vaccine technology that has largely originated in the United States and Europe is fast proliferating to the developing world because of the combined efforts of developing country vaccine manufacturers, nongovernmental organizations such as GAVI and Bill and Melinda Gates Foundation, and technology developers in the developed world (Jadhav et al., 2008; Pagliusi et al., 2013). The vaccines that are of most relevance in this case are the pediatric vaccines, where the large birth cohort in countries such as India and China dominates vaccine needs. Hence, large volume production at low cost, with sufficient thermostablilty to address cold chain issues, is very important (Chen and Zehrung, 2012). The biomanufacturing challenges of accomplishing these goals have been well articulated (Rexroad et al., 2002a; Rexroad et al., 2002b; Milstien et al., 2009). Bioprocess advances in making vaccine manufacturing processes robust, productive, and portable will be necessary for achieving greater access to a much larger population; this need is particularly acute for live viral vaccines.

1.10 SUMMARY

Vaccine manufacturing processes have come a long way since Edward Jenner's cow pox vaccine. The evolution in the biomanufacturing of influenza and JE vaccines truly captures the transformation of upstream processes technology—from production *in vivo* to *in ovo*, to microcarriers, and finally to suspension cell culture, as well as the evolution from a whole virus to a subunit vaccine. Downstream processing has evolved significantly as well, from simple filtration or lyophilization of the upstream feedstock to highly selective purification unit operations as well as operations involving chemical reactions. This is uniquely illustrated by Prevnar-13®, which consists of 14 distinct fermentation and purification processes as well as 39 different chemical reactions. The modern vaccine manufacturing processes of today are already producing consistent, well-defined and highly purified antigens, with a high level understanding of the vaccine critical quality attributes. However opportunities exist to extend these advances for the more complex vaccines, as well as in the production of all vaccines at desired quantities and cost. Only then would bioprocess science and engineering fully deliver on its promise.

ACKNOWLEDGMENTS

The authors acknowledge Drs. John Aunins, and Barry Buckland for helpful discussions in the preparation of this manuscript.

REFERENCES

www.path.org, JE vaccines at a glance. 2001.

Abeygunawardana C, Williams TC, Sumner JS, Hennessey JP Jr., Development and validation of an NMR-based identity assay for bacterial polysaccharides. Anal Biochem 2000;279: 226–240.

Adams GDJ. Lyophilization of vaccines. In: Robinson AT, Hudson MJ, Cranage MP, editors. *Methods in Molecular Medicine*. Vaccine Protocols. 2nd ed. Vol. 87. Totowa, NJ: Humana Press Inc; 2003. p 223–243.

Altaras NE, Aunins JG, Evans RK, Kamen A, Konz JO, Wolf JJ. Production and formulation of adenovirus vectors. Adv Biochem Eng Biotechnol 2005;99:193–260.

Andersen DC, Krummen L. Recombinant protein expression for therapeutic applications. Curr Opin Biotechnol 2002;13:117–123.

Aunins JG. Viral vaccine production in cell culture. In: Spier RE, Griffiths JB, editors. *The Encyclopedia of Cell Technology*. New York: Wiley & Sons; 2000. p 1182–1217.

Aunins JG. Viral vaccine production in cell culture. In Flickinger MC, editor. *Encyclopedia of Industrial Biotechnology*. Hoboken: John Wiley & Sons; 2010. p 4789–4840.

Baart GJE, de Jong G, Philippi M, van't RK, van der Pol LA, Beuvery EC, Tramper J, Martens DE. Scale-up for bulk production of vaccine against meningococcal disease. Vaccine 2007;25:6399–6408.

Bahey-El-Din M. Lactococcus lactis-based vaccines from laboratory bench to human use: an overview. Vaccine 2012;30:685–690.

Bailey A. The manufacture of gene therapy products and viral vaccines. In: Subramanian, editor. *Bioseparation and Bioprocessing*. 2nd ed. Vol. 2. Weinhein, Germany: Wiley-VCH Verlag GmbH & Co. KGaA; 2007. p 575–600.

Barrett PN, Mundt W, Kistner O, Howard MK. Vero cell platform in vaccine production: moving towards cell culture-based viral vaccines. Expert Rev Vaccines 2009;8:607–618.

Behbehani AM. The small pox story: life and death of an old disease. Microbiol Rev 1893;47:455–509.

Billich A. AIDSVAX. Curr Opin Investig Drugs 2004;5:214–221.

Blyden ER, Watler PK. New approaches to improved vaccine manufacturing in embryonated eggs. BioPharm Int Jan 2010.

Bogdan JA, Nazario-Larrieu J, Sarwar J, Alexander P, Blake MS. *Bordetella pertusis* autoregulates pertusis toxin production through the metabolism of cysteine. Infect Immun 2001;69: 6823–6830.

Burgener A, Butler M. Medium development. In: Ozrutk S, Hu WS, editors. *Cell Culture Technology for Pharmaceutical and Cell-Based Therapies*. Boca Raton, FL: CRC Press; 2006. p 41–79.

Burnette WN. Recombinant subunit vaccines. Curr Opin Biotechnol 1991;2:882–892.

Burnette WN. Recombinant subunit vaccines. Curr Biol 1992;2:102.

Butler M. Animal cell cultures: recent achievements and perspectives in the production of biopharmaceuticals. Appl Microbiol Biotechnol 2005;68:283–291.

Butler M. Optimisation of the cellular metabolism of glycosylation for recombinant proteins produced by mammalian cell systems. Cytotechnology 2006;50:57–76.

Butler M. Cell line development and culture strategies: future prospects to improve yields. In: Butler A, editor. *Cell Culture and Upstream Processing*. New York: Taylor and Francis; 2007. p 3–15.

Butler M, Burgener A, Patrick M, Berry M, Moffatt D, Huzel N, Barnabe N, Coombs K. Application of a serum-free medium for the growth of vero cells and the production of reovirus. Biotechnol Prog 2000;16:854–858.

Chaudhuri K, Chatterjee SN. *Cholera Toxins*. Springer; 2009.

Chen T, Chen K. Investigation and application progress of Vero cell serum-free culture. Int J Biol 2009;1:41–47.

Chen R. Bacterial expression systems for recombinant protein production: *E. coli* and beyond. Biotechnol Adv 2012;30:1102–1107.

Chen D, Zehrung D. Desirable attributes of vaccines for deployment in low-resource settings. J Pharm Sci 2012;102:29–33.

Choi JH, Keum KC, Lee SY. Production of recombinant proteins by high cell density culture of *Escherichia coli*. Chem Eng Sci 2005a;61:876–885.

Choo QL, Kuo G, Ralston R, Weiner A, Chien D, Van Nest G, Han J, Berger K, Thudium K, Kuo C. Vaccination of chimpanzees against infection by the *hepatitis C virus*. Proc Natl Acad Sci 1994;91:1294–1298.

Chou CP. Engineering cell physiology to enhance recombinant protein production in *Escherichia coli*. Appl Microbiol Biotechnol 2007;76:521–532.

Chu C, Lugovtsev V, Golding H, Betenbaugh M, Shiloach J. Conversion of MDCK cell line to suspension culture by transfecting with human siat7e gene and its application for influenza virus production. Proc Natl Acad Sci U S A 2009;106:14802–14807.

Clark TG, Cassidy-Hanley D. Recombinant subunit vaccines: potentials and constraints. Dev Biol 2005;121:153–163.

Corey L, Langenberg AGM, Ashley R, Sekulovich RE, Izu AE, Douglas JM Jr, Handsfield HH, Warren T, Marr L, Tyring S, et al. Recombinant glycoprotein vaccine for the prevention of genital HSV-2 infection: two randomized controlled trials. JAMA 1999;282:331–340.

Curran BPG, Bugeja VC. The biotechnology and molecular biology of yeast. In: *Molecular Biology and Biotechnology*. 5th ed. 2009. p 159–195.

Dalemans W. Insect cells as a new substrate for vaccine production. Dev Biol 2006;123:235–241.

De Mare L, Andersson L, Hagander P. Probing control of glucose feeding in Vibrio cholerae cultivations. Bioprocess Biosyst Eng 2003;25:221–228.

Dekleva ML. Vaccine technology. In: Flickinger MC, Drew SW, editors. *Encyclopedia of Bioprocess Technology*. New York: John Wiley & Sons; 1999a. p 2611–2622.

Dekleva ML. Vaccine technology. In: Flickinger MC, Drew SW, editors. *Encyclopedia of Bioprocess Technology*. New York: John Wiley & Sons; 1999b. p 2611–2622.

Demain AL, Vaishnav P. Production of recombinant proteins by microbes and higher organisms. Biotechnol Adv 2009;27:297–306.

Demain AL, Gerson DF, Fang A. Effective levels of tetanus toxin can be made in a production medium totally lacking both animal (e.g., brain heart infusion) and dairy proteins or digests (e.g., casein hydrolysates). Vaccine 2005;23:5420–5423.

Demain AL, George S, Kole M, Gerson DF, Fang A. Tetanus toxin production in soy-based medium: nutritional studies and scale-up into small fermentors. Lett Appl Microbiol 2007;45:635–638.

Detmer A, Glenting J. Live bacterial vaccines—a review and identification of potential hazards. Microb Cell Fact 2006;5:23–34.

Dietrich G, Collioud A, Rothen SA. Developing and manufacturing attenuated live bacterial vaccines. BioPharm Int 2008;(Oct Suppl):6–14.

Doroshenko A, Halperin SA. Trivalent MDCK cell culture-derived influenza vaccine Optaflu. Expert Rev Vaccines 2009;8:679–688.

Durocher Y, Butler M. Expression systems for therapeutic glycoprotein production. Curr Opin Biotechnol 2009;20:700–707.

Elliott AY, Morges W, Olson MG. Experience in manufacturing, testing, and licensing a hepatitis B vaccine produced by recombinant technology. In: Lubiniecki AS, Vargo SA. *Regulatory Practice for Biopharmaceutical Production*. (1994) p 255–269.

Ellis RW. The new generation of recombinant viral subunit vaccines. Curr Opin Biotechnol 1996;7:646–652.

Ellis RW. Viral vaccines. In: Austen KF, Burakoff SF, Rosen FS, Strom TB, editors. *Therapeutic Immunology*. 2nd ed. Oxford: Wiley-Blackwell; 2001. p 413–429.

Ellis RW. New technologies for bacterial vaccines. In: Ellis RW, Brodeur BR, editors. *New Bacterial Vaccines*. New York: Kluwer Academic/Plenum Publishers; 2003. p 80–92.

El-Mansi EMT, Bryce CFA, Hartley BS. Fermentation microbiology and biotechnology: an historical perspective. In: El-Mansi EMT, Bryce CFA, editors. *Fermentation Microbiology and Biotechnology*. 2nd ed. London, UK: Taylor & Francis; 2007. p 1–9.

EMA Dukoral EPAR Scientific Discussion. 2005.

Emini E. FDA approves a new form of Prevnar vaccine, the pediatric drug, developed before Pfizer acquired Wyeth, is said to offer wider protection. The Philadelphia Inquirer. 2010.

Enders JF, Weller TH, Robbins FC. Cultivation of the Lansing strain of the poliomyelitis virus in cultures of various embryonic tissues. Science 1949;109:85–87.

Fallaux FJ, Bout A, van der Velde I, van den Wollenberg DJ, Hehir KM, Keegan J, Auger C, Cramer SJ, van Ormondt H, van der Eb AJ. New helper cells and matched early region 1-deleted adenovirus vectors prevent generation of replication-competent adenoviruses. Hum Gene Ther 1998;9:1909–1917.

FDA. FDA summary basis of approval for TripediaTM. Reference No. 90–0353. 1992.

FDA. FDA Guidance for Industry. Characterization and qualification of cell substrates and other biological materials used in the production of viral vaccines for infectious disease indications; 2010.

FDA. Summary Basis of Regulatory Action for Biothrax®. 2012.

Ferrer-Miralles N, Domingo-Espin J, Corchero JL, Vazquez E, Villaverde A. Microbial factories for recombinant pharmaceuticals. Microb Cell Fact 2009;8:17.

Frasch CE. Preparation of bacterial polysaccharide-protein conjugates: analytical and manufacturing challenges. Vaccine 2009;27:6468–6470.

Frasch C, Preziosi M-P, La Force M. Development of a group A meningococcal conjugate vaccine, MenAfriVac. Hum Vaccine Immunother 2012;8:715–724.

Fratelli F, Siquini TJ, Prado SMA, Higashi HG, Converti A, Monteiro de Carvalho JC. Effect of medium composition on the production of tetanus toxin by *Clostridium tetani*. Biotechnol Prog 2005;21:756–761.

Galambos L. A century of innovation in vaccines. Vaccine 1999;17(Suppl 3):S7–S10.

Galao RP, Scheller N, Alves-Rodrigues I, Breinig T, Meyerhans A, Diez J. *Saccharomyces cerevisiae*: a versatile eukaryotic system in virology. Microb Cell Fact 2007;6:32–41.

Genzel Y, Reichl U. Vaccine production: state of the art and future needs in upstream processing. Meth Biotechnol 2007a;24:457–473.

Genzel Y, Reichl U. Vaccine production: state of the art and future needs in upstream processing. Meth Biotechnol 2007b;24:457–473.

Genzel Y, Reichl U. Continuous cell lines as a production system for influenza vaccines. Exp Rev Vaccines 2009;8:1681–1692.

Genzel Y, Fischer M, Reichl U. Serum-free influenza virus production avoiding washing steps and medium exchange in large-scale microcarrier culture. Vaccine 2006a;24:3261–3272.

Genzel Y, Olmer RM, Schaefer B, Reichl U. Wave microcarrier cultivation of MDCK cells for influenza virus production in serum containing and serum-free media. Vaccine 2006b;24:6074–6087.

Giuliani SE, Landorf EV, Collart FR. Protein production for biotechnology. In: *Nature Encyclopedia of Life Sciences*. Vol. 2. New York: John Wiley & Sons; 2007. p 931–936.

Glenny AT, Hopkins BE. Diphtheria toxoid as an immunising agent. Br J Exp Pathol 1923;4:283–288.

Goerke AR, To BCS, Lee AL, Sagar SL, Konz JO. Development of a novel adenovirus purification process utilizing selective precipitation of cellular DNA. Biotechnol Bioeng 2005;91:12–21.

Gould SL, Distefano DJ, Robinson DK, Seamans TC. 1999. Serum-free, low-protein media for rotavirus vaccine production. PCT Int. Appl. WO 9921969 A1 19990506.

Graf A, Dragosits M, Gasser B, Mattanovich D. Yeast systems biotechnology for the production of heterologous proteins. FEMS Yeast Res 2009;9:335–348.

Graumann K, Premstaller A. Manufacturing of recombinant therapeutic proteins in microbial systems. Biotechnol J 2006;1:164–186.

Grillberger L, Kreil TR, Nasr S, Reiter M. Emerging trends in plasma-free manufacturing of recombinant protein therapeutics expressed in mammalian cells. Biotechnol J 2009;4:186–201.

Hagen AL, Oliver CJ, Sitrin R. Optimization of Poly(ethylene glycol) Precipitation of Hepatitis A Virus Used To Prepare VAQTA, a Highly Purified Inactivated Vaccine. Biotech Progress 1996;12:406–412.

Hamilton SR, Gerngross TU. Glycosylation engineering in yeast: the advent of fully humanized yeast. Curr Opin Biotechnol 2007;18:387–392.

Hansen B, Belfast M, Soung G, Song L, Egan PM, Capen R, HogenEsch H, Mancinelli R, Hem SL. Effect of the strength of adsorption of hepatitis B surface antigen to aluminum hydroxide adjuvant on the immune response. Vaccine 2009;27:888–892.

Hansson M, Nygren PA, Stefan S. Design and production of recombinant subunit vaccines. Biotechnol Appl Biochem 2000;32:95–107.

Hayflick L. A brief history of cell substrates used for the preparation of human biologicals. Dev Biol 2001;106:5–24.

Hayflick L, Moorhead PS. The serial cultivation of human diploid cell strains. Exp Cell Res 1961;25:585–621.

Hem SL, HogenEsch H. Relationship between physical and chemical properties of aluminum-containing adjuvants and immunopotentiation. Expert Rev Vaccines 2007;6: 685–698.

Hennessey JP Jr, Oswald CB, Dong Z, Lewis JA, Sitrin RD. Evaluation of the purity of a purified, inactivated hepatitis A vaccine (VAQTA). Vaccine 1999;17:2830–2835.

Hewitt CJ, Nienow AW. The scale-up of microbial batch and fed-batch fermentation processes. Adv Appl Microbiol 2007;62:105–135.

Hickling J and D'Hondt E. A review of production technologies for influenza virus vaccines and their suitability for deployment in developing countries for influenza pandemic preparedness. Geneva: World Health Organization. Initiative for Vaccine Research; 2006.

Hilleman MR. Overview of vaccinology with special reference to papillomavirus vaccines. J Clin Virol 2000;19:79–90.

Hilleman MR. Overview of the needs and realities for developing new and improved vaccines in the 21st century. Intervirology 2002;45:199–211.

Hu YC, Yao K, Wu TY. Baculovirus as an expression and/or delivery vehicle for vaccine antigens. Expert Rev Vaccines 2008;7:363–371.

Jackman WT, Mann KA, Hoffmann HJ, Spaete RR. Expression of Epstein-Barr virus gp350 as a single chain glycoprotein for an EBV subunit vaccine. Vaccine 1999;17:660–668.

Jadhav S, Datla M, Kreeftenberg H, Hendriks J. The Developing Countries Vaccine Manufacturers' Network (DCVMN) is a critical constituency to ensure access to vaccines in developing countries. Vaccine 2008;26:1611–1615.

Jayapal KP, Wlaschin KF, Hu WS, Yap MGS. Recombinant protein therapeutics from CHO cells—20 years and counting. Chem Eng Prog 2007;103:40–47.

Jordan I, Vos A, Beilfuss S, Neubert A, Breul S, Sandig V. An avian cell line designed for production of highly attenuated viruses. Vaccine 2009;27:748–756.

Josefsberg JO, Buckland B. Vaccine process technology. Biotechnol Bioeng 2012;109: 1443–1460.

Junker BH. Scale-up methodologies for *Escherichia coli* and yeast fermentation processes. J Biosci Bioeng 2004;97:347–364.

Junker B. Fermentation. In: Seidel A, editor. *Kirk-Othmer Encyclopedia of Chemical Technology*. 5th ed. Hoboken, NJ: John Wiley & Sons, Inc; 2005. p 1–55.

Junker B, Lewis JA, Oliver CN, Orella CJ, Sitrin RD, Aboud RA, Aunins JG, Buckland BC, Dephillips PA. Biotechnological process for hepatitis A virus vaccine manufacture. European Patent Application EP 583142 A2 19940216. . 1994.

Kantardjieff A, Nissom PM, Chuah SH, Yusufi F, Jacob NM, Mulukutla BC, Yap M, Hu WS. Developing genomic platforms for Chinese hamster ovary cells. Biotechnol Adv 2009;27:1028–1035.

Kistner O. Baxter H5N1 vaccine. Development and evaluation. WHO Meeting on Development and Evaluation of Influenza Pandemic Vaccines. 2005 Nov 2–3; Geneva; 2005

Kolaj O, Spada S, Robin S, Wall JG. Use of folding modulators to improve heterologous protein production in *Escherichia coli*. Microb Cell Fact 2009;8:9.

Konz JO, Pitts LR, Sagar SL. Scaleable purification of adenovirus vectors. Methods Mol Biol 2008;434:13–23.

Kwaks THJ, Otte AP. Employing epigenetics to augment the expression of therapeutic proteins in mammalian cells. Trends Biotechnol 2006;24:137–142.

La Montagne JR. The United States research strategy on pertussis. Dev Biol Stand 1997;89: 25–28.

Langenberg AG, Burke RL, Adair SF, Sekulovich R, Tigges M, Dekker CL, Corey L. A recombinant glycoprotein vaccine for herpes simplex virus type 2. Ann Intern Med 1995;122: 889–898.

Lasky LA. 1990. From virus to vaccine: recombinant mammalian cell lines as substrates for the production of herpes simplex virus vaccines. J Med Virol 31:59–61.

Lattanzi M, Del Giudice G, Rappuoli R. Subunit vaccines and toxoids. In: Kaufmann SHE, editor. *Novel Vaccination Strategies*. Weinheim: Wiley-VCH Verlag Gmbh & Co., KGaA; 2004. p 243–263.

Lederberg J. Pathways of discovery: infectious history. Science 2000;288:287–293.

Lee AL and Sagar S. Method for large scale plasmid purification. US Patent 06197553. 2001.

Levine MM, DuPont HL, Hornick RB, Snyder MJ, Woodward W, Gilman RH, Libonati JP. Attenuated, streptomycin-dependent *Salmonella typhi* oral vaccine: potential deleterious effects of lyophilization. J Infect Dis 1976;133:424–429.

Liljeqvist S, Stahl S. Production of recombinant subunit vaccines: protein immunogens, live delivery systems and nucleic acid vaccines. J Biotechnol 1999a;73:1–33.

Liljeqvist S, Stahl S. Production of recombinant subunit vaccines: protein immunogens, live delivery systems and nucleic acid vaccines. J Biotechnol 1999b;73:1–33.

Lindberg AA. The history of live bacterial vaccines. Dev Biol Stand 1995;84:211–219.

Lubiniecki AS, Petricciani JC. Recent trends in cell substrate considerations for continuous cell lines. Curr Opin Biotechnol 2001;12:317–319.

Makrides SC, Prentice HL. Why choose mammalian cells for protein production? New Compr Biochem 2003;38:1–8.

de Marco A. Strategies for successful recombinant expression of disulfide bond-dependent proteins in *Escherichia coli*. Microb Cell Fact 2009;8:26.

Meacle F, Aunins A, Thornton R, Lee A. Optimization of the membrane purification of a polysaccharide-protein conjugate vaccine using backpulsing. J Membrane Sci 1999;161: 171–184.

Merten OW. Development of serum-free media for cell growth and production of viruses/viral vaccines—safety issues of animal products used in serum-free media. Dev Biol 2002; 111:233–257.

Milstien J, Costa A, Jadhav S, Dhere R. Reaching international GMP standards for vaccine production: challenges for developing countries. Expert Rev Vaccines 2009;8:559–566.

Murasugi A. Optimized productions of recombinant human proteins in fermentor cultures of the yeast, *Pichia pastoris*. Curr Top Biotechnol 2008;4:101–108.

Murphy JC, Winters MA, Sagar SL. Large-scale nonchromatographic purification of plasmid DNA. In: *DNA Vaccines*. Methods in Molecular Medicine. 2nd ed. Vol. 127. 2006. p 351–362.

Ni Y, Chen R. Extracellular recombinant protein production from *Escherichia coli*. Biotechnol Lett 2009;31:1661–1670.

Njamkepo E, Rimlinger F, Thiberge S, Guiso N. Thirty-five years' experience with the whole-cell pertussis vaccine in France: Vaccine strains analysis and immunogenicity. Vaccine 2002;20:1290–1294.

Nkolola JP, Hanke T. Engineering virus vectors for subunit vaccines. In: Kaufmann SHE, editor. *Novel Vaccination Strategies*. Wiley-VCH Verlag GmbH & Co. KGaA: Weinheim; 2004. p 265–287.

van Oers MM. Vaccines for viral and parasitic diseases produced with baculovirus vectors. Adv Virus Res 2006;68:193–253.

Olivier S, Jacoby M, Brillon C, Bouletreau S, Mollet T, Nerriere O, Angel A, Danet S, Souttou B, Guehenneux F. EB66 cell line, a duck embryonic stem cell-derived substrate for the industrial production of therapeutic monoclonal antibodies with enhanced ADCC activity. MAbs 2010;2:405–415.

Ozturk SS. In: Ozturk SS, Hu W-S, editors. *Cell Culture Technology—An Overview in Cell Culture Technology for Pharmaceutical and Cell-Based Therapies*. Boca Raton, FL: CRC Press Taylor and Francis Group; 2006.

Pagliusi S, Leite LCC, Datla M, Makhoana M, Gao Y, Suhardono M, Jadhav S, Harshavardhan GVJA, Homma A. Developing countries vaccine manufacturers network: doing good by making high-quality vaccines affordable for all. Vaccine 2013;31:B176–B183.

Paillet C, Forno G, Kratje R, Etcheverrigaray M. Suspension-Vero cell cultures as a platform for viral vaccine production. Vaccine 2009;27:6464–6467.

Perrie Y, Mohammed AR, Kirby DJ, McNeil SE, Bramwell VW. Vaccine adjuvant systems: enhancing the efficacy of sub-unit protein antigens. Int J Pharm 2008;364:272–280.

Petricciani J, Sheets R. An overview of animal cell substrates for biological products. Biologicals 2008;36:359–362.

Plotkin S. Vaccines: the fourth century. Clin Vaccine Immunol 2009;16:1709–1719.

Plotkin SL, Plotkin SA. A short history of vaccination. In: Plotkin SL, Orenstein WA, editors. *Vaccines*. 3rd ed. Philadelphia: WB Saunders Company; 1999. p 1–10.

Polo JM, Dubensky TW. Virus-based vectors for human vaccine applications. Drug Discov Today 2002;7:719–727.

Potgieter TI, Cukan M, Drummond JE, Houston-Cummings NR, Jiang Y, Li F, Lynaugh H, Mallem M, McKelvey TW, Mitchell T, Nylen A, Rittenhour A, Stadheim TA, Zha D, d'Anjou M. Production of monoclonal antibodies by glycoengineered *Pichia pastoris*. J Biotechnol 2009;139:318–325.

Pujar NS, Gayton MG, Herber WK, Abeygunawardana C, Dekleva ML, Yegneswaran PK, Lee AL. 2005. Process validation of multivalent bacterial vaccine: a novel matrix approach. *Process Validation in Manufacturing of Biopharmaceuticals Biotechnology and Bioprocessing*. Volume 29; p 523–544.

Rappuoli R, Pizza M. In: Perlman P, Wiazell H, editors. *Vaccines*. Springer; 1989.

Rappuoli R. Isolation and characterization of *Corynebacterium diphtheriae* nontandem double lysogens hyperproducing CRM197. Appl Environ Microbiol 1983;46:560–564.

Rappuoli R. Bridging the knowledge gaps in vaccine design. Nat Biotech 2007;25:1361–1366.

Ravetkar SD, Rahalkar SB, Kulkarni CG. Large scale processing of tetanus toxin from fermentation broth. J Sci Ind Res 2001;60:773–778.

Reed SG, Bertholet S, Coler RN, Friede M. New horizons in adjuvants for vaccine development. Trends Immunol 2009;30:23–32.

Relyveld EH, Bizzini B, Gupta RK. Rational approaches to reduce adverse reactions in man to vaccines containing tetanus and diphtheria toxoids. Vaccine 1998;16:1016–1023.

Rexroad J, Wiethoff CM, Jones LS, Middaugh CR. Lyophilization and the thermostability of vaccines. Cell Preserv Technol 2002a;1:91–104.

Rexroad J, Wiethoff CM, Jones SL, Middaugh CR. Lyophilization and the thermostability of vaccines. Cell Preserv Technol 2002b;1:91–104.

Rourou S, van der Ark A, van der Velden T, Kallel H. A microcarrier cell culture process for propagating rabies virus in Vero cells grown in a stirred bioreactor under fully animal component free conditions. Vaccine 2007;25:3879–3889.

Rourou S, van der Ark A, van der Velden T, Kallel H. Development of an animal-component free medium for vero cells culture. Biotechnol Prog 2009;25:1752–1761.

Salk JE, Francis T Jr. Immunization against influenza. Ann Intern Med 1946;25:443–452.

Schmidt FR. Optimization and scale up of industrial fermentation processes. Appl Microbiol Biotechnol 2005;68:425–435.

Schwick HG, Biel H, Schmidtberger R. Purification of tetanus toxoid by a combined Rivanol-ammonium sulfate procedure. Symposia Series Immunobiol Stand 1967;3: 143–148.

Scott C. Microbial fermentation: the oldest form of biotechnology. BioProcess Int 2004;2(Suppl 2):8–20.

Serruto D, Bottomley MJ, Ram S, Giuliani MM, Rappuoli R. The new multicomponent vaccine against meningococcal serogroup B, 4CMenB: immunological, functional and structural characterization of the antigens. Vaccine 2012;30(Suppl 2):B87–B97.

Sheng-Fowler L, Lewis AM Jr, Peden K. Issues associated with residual cell-substrate DNA in viral vaccines. Biologicals 2009;37:190–195.

Shevitz J, LaPorte TL, Stinnett TE. Production of viral vaccines in stirred bioreactors. Adv Biotechnol Processes 1990;14:1–35.

Shi L, Sings HL, Bryan JT, Wang B, Wang Y, Mach H, Kosinski M, Washabaugh MW, Sitrin R, Barr E. GARDASIL: prophylactic human papillomavirus vaccine development—from bench top to bed-side. Clin Pharmacol Ther 2007;81:259–264.

Shiloach J, Fass R. Growing *E. coli* to high cell density—a historical perspective on method development. Biotechnol Adv 2005;23:345–357.

Sitrin RD, Kubek DJ. Purification of hepatitis B virus surface proteins from transgenic host cells with wide-pore silica. US Patent 5102989A. 1992.

Soler E, Houdebine L. Preparation of recombinant vaccines. Biotechnol Annu Rev 2007;13: 65–94.

Spaete RR. A recombinant subunit vaccine approach to HCMV vaccine development. Transplant Proc 1991;23:90–96.

Srivastava P, Deb JK. Gene expression systems in corynebacteria. Protein Expr Purif 2005;40: 221–229.

Streefland M, van de Waterbeemd B, Happe H, van der Pol LA, Beuvery EC, Tramper J, Martens DE. PAT for vaccines: the first stage of PAT implementation for development of a well-defined whole-cell vaccine against whooping cough disease. Vaccine 2007;25:2994–3000.

Streefland M, van Herpen PFG, van de Waterbeemd B, van der Pol LA, Beuvery EC, Tramper J, Martens DE, Toft M. A practical approach for exploration and modeling of the design space of a bacterial vaccine cultivation process. Biotechnol Bioeng 2009;104:492–504.

Surjan M, Richter P. Purification of diphtheria and tetanus toxoids by trichloroacetic acid. I. Purification of diphtheria toxoid. Acta Microbiol Acad Sci Hung 1954;1:339–344.

Takegawa K, Tohda H, Sasaki M, Idiris A, Ohashi T, Mukaiyama H, Giga-Hama Y, Kumagai H. Production of heterologous proteins using the fission-yeast (*Schizosaccharomyces pombe*) expression system. Biotechnol Appl Biochem 2009;53:227–235.

Tchorbanov AI, Dimitrov JD, Vassilev TL. Optimization of casein-based semisynthetic medium for growing of toxigenic *Corynebacterium diphtheriae* in a fermentor. Can J Microbiol 2004;50:821–826.

Tintrup H. CAP-technology: production of biopharmaceuticals in human amniocytes. Abstracts of Papers, 241st ACS National Meeting & Exposition; 2011 Mar 27–31; Anaheim, CA. BIOT-156; 2011.

Tiwari M, Parida M, Santhosh SR, Khan M, Dash PK, Rao PVL. Assessment of immunogenic potential of Vero adapted formalin inactivated vaccine derived from novel ECSA genotype of Chikungunya virus. Vaccine 2009;27:2513–2522.

Toriniwa H, Komiya T. Long-term stability of Vero cell-derived inactivated Japanese encephalitis vaccine prepared using serum-free medium. Vaccine 2008;26:3680–3689.

TYPHIM Vi® . TYPHIM Vi® Prescribing information. Sanofi-Pasteur, 2005.

Unnikrishnan M, Rappuoli R, Serruto D. Recombinant bacterial vaccines. Curr Opin Immunol 2012;24:337–342.

Vainio J, Cutts F. *Yellow Fever*. Geneva: World Health Organization; 1998.

Van Regenmortel MHV. Pitfalls of reductionism in the design of peptide-based vaccines. Vaccine 2001;19:2369–2374.

Vancetto MDC, de Oliveira JM, Prado SMA, Fratelli F, Higashi HG. Tetanus toxoid purification: a case study. Nat Biotechnol 1997;15:807–808.

van de Waterbeemd B, Streefland M, van der Pol L, Coen B, Tramper J, Martens D. Gene-expression-based quality scores indicate optimal harvest point in *Bordetella pertusis* cultivation for vaccine production. Biotechnol Bioeng 2009;103:900–908.

Wen E, Cinelli LD, Murray D, Lander RJ, Sagar SL, Lee AL. Purification of a polysaccharide conjugate vaccine using microfiltration membranes in backpulsing mode. J Membr Sci 2005;258:23–34.

Whitford WG and Fairbank A. 2011. Considerations in scale-up of viral vaccine production. BioProcess Int. 2011;9s:16–28.

WHO. WHO Technical Report Series 978. Recommendations for the evaluation of animal cell cultures as substrates for the manufacture of biological medicinal products and for the characterization of cell banks. Annex 3; 2010.

WHO. Recommendations to assure the quality, safety and efficacy of diphtheria vaccines. 2012.

Wolff MW, Reichl U. Downstream processing: from egg to cell culture-derived influenza virus particles. Chem Eng Technol 2008;31:846–857.

Woodruff AM, Goodpasture EW. The susceptibility of the chorio-allantoic membrane of chick embryos to infection with the fowl-pox virus. Am J Pathol 1931;7:209–222.

Yusibov V, Streatfield SJ, Kushnir N. Clinical development of plant-produced recombinant pharmaceuticals: vaccines, antibodies and beyond. Hum Vaccin 2011;7:313–321.

Zanin MP, Webster DE, Martin JL, Wesselingh SL. Japanese encephalitis vaccines: moving away from the mouse brain. Expert Rev Vaccines 2003;2:407–416.

Zhou Q, Wang Y, Freed D, Fu T, Gimenez JA, Sitrin R, Washabaugh MW. Maturation of recombinant hepatitis B surface antigen particles. Hum Vaccin 2006;2:174–180.

2

THE PRODUCTION OF PLASMID DNA VACCINE IN *Escherichia coli*: A NOVEL BACTERIAL-BASED VACCINE PRODUCTION PLATFORM

MICHEL CHARTRAIN
Merck & Co. Inc., Kenilworth, NJ, USA

2.1 INTRODUCTION: *E. coli* IN VACCINE PRODUCTION

Although it is one of the most metabolically and genetically studied microorganisms (Neidhardt, 1996), as of today there is yet an *Escherichia coli*-manufactured vaccine intended for humans to reach registration with the FDA (Ulmer et al. 2006). There are, however, multiple *E. coli*-based vaccines that are undergoing human clinical evaluation. The biochemical repertoire of *E. coli* restricts the use of this microbe as a vaccine production platform for simple nonglycosylated proteins or for the production of plasmid DNA vaccines (Walsh, 2006). Moreover, even for the production of nonglycosylated proteins, *E. coli* presents some drawbacks, as the overproduced protein tends to aggregate and form inclusion bodies. Since only those proteins presenting a native epitope can be used to trigger a protective immune response, complex and costly refolding step(s) needed to refold the protein correctly must be implemented (Gnoth et al., 2008). Partially alleviating these issues, the implementation of secretory systems has met with success in delivering correctly folded proteins to the periplasmic space (Baneyx and Mujacic, 2004; Sorensen and Mortensen, 2005). Although these improvements are likely to help *E. coli* increase its role as a protein vaccine production platform in the future, we believe that the prime example of the

Vaccine Development and Manufacturing, First Edition.
Edited by Emily P. Wen, Ronald Ellis, and Narahari S. Pujar.

perfect marriage between *E. coli* and vaccine production resides in the manufacture of DNA plasmid vaccine.

Indeed, *E. coli* is perfectly positioned for this task because for several decades it has been genetically manipulated using plasmids whose design and replication processes are well understood and easily manipulated. This vast amount of know-how and experience uniquely positions this microorganism at the top of the list for the industrial production of plasmid DNA vaccine.

The development of an industrial plasmid DNA vaccine production process may not be as trivial as expected because, unlike most vaccines, DNA vaccine dosages are large, on the order of several milligrams per dose (Babuik et al., 2000; Donnelly, 2003), and therefore are likely to require extensive production efforts. As for other vaccines (Buckland, 2005), to support positive economics, the production of large amounts of plasmid will require that the entire host/plasmid selection, cultivation, purification, and formulation processes be efficient and consistent while containing operating costs.

In this chapter, after a brief review of the mode of action of DNA vaccines, the upstream portion of the process is reviewed, which will address the design and selection of the plasmid backbone and host cells and the design and scale-up of high yielding cultivation processes.

2.2 BRIEF OVERVIEW OF DNA VACCINES: MECHANISMS AND METHODS OF VACCINATIONS

DNA vaccination, a recently introduced vaccination method (Wolf et al., 1990; Danko and Wolff, 1994), has the potential to elicit both cellular and humoral immune responses. This novel vaccination approach rapidly moved from discovery to its first clinical trial in less than 10 years (MacGregor et al., 1998) and is currently under evaluation for multiple indications ranging from protection against intracellular pathogens to gene therapy and cancer treatment (http://www.wiley.co.uk/genetherapy/clinical/). Plasmids encoding a specific protein antigen are transformed into the bacterial host *E. coli* and mass produced. The plasmids are designed to replicate in *E. coli* and usually contain an antibiotic resistance selection gene. The other portion of the plasmid is designed for expression of the *trans* gene and production of the antigen once injected into the recipient cell.

Once purified and formulated, the plasmids are injected into the muscle of patients, where they are believed to reach a subpopulation of antigen-presenting cells (APCs), such as dendritic cells residing in the Langerhans islands, as well as muscle cells. The plasmids reach the nucleus via endosomal trafficking, where the *trans* gene will eventually be transcribed using the available nuclear transcription equipment. It has been shown that the plasmid(s) remains episomal and transcriptionally active for lengthy periods that can extend up to several months (Wolf et al., 1990; Ledwith et al., 2000; Manam et al., 2000). On mRNA reaching the endoplasmic reticulum, the antigen protein is synthesized. It is now widely believed that a complete immune response is triggered, involving MHC-I and MHC-II pathways.

2.3 CURRENT STATUS OF DNA VACCINES

Several compelling examples of viral challenges in animal models are testimony to their efficacy. Although the concept of vaccination with DNA is only about 15 years old, its application has already clearly met with the success of three veterinary vaccines that have so far been approved or conditionally approved. One DNA vaccine, approved for commercial use in Canada, is aimed at protecting salmons against the infectious hematopoetic necrosis virus, which can completely devastate an entire fish-farm population (Anderson and Leong, 2000; Lorenzen and LaPatra, 2005; Salonius et al., 2007). The second approved DNA vaccine is directed at protecting horses against West Nile virus infections that cause serious and potentially deadly encephalomyelitis (Davis et al., 2001; Powell 2004). A third vaccine, aimed at treating melanomas in dogs, has been granted a conditional approval by the FDA (Bergman et al., 2006; Itd 2007). With a cancer treatment application, this last approval is of importance, as it clearly highlights the far-reaching potential of a DNA vaccine that can extend beyond the "classical" anti-infective vaccine applications. In addition to the three veterinary DNA vaccines discussed previously, a DNA vaccine directed at protecting horses and dogs against rabies appears extremely promising (Lodmell et al., 2002; Fischer et al., 2003), as exemplified by the challenge data in dogs showing 100% protection after single-dose vaccination with 50 μg of DNA (Lodmell et al., 2002). A large number of publications pertaining to the testing of DNA vaccines in animals for either development purposes or veterinary applications can be easily found in the literature.

Applications to humans are still at the experimental stage, targeting every major infectious disease such as HIV (Mascola and Nabel, 2001), enteric infections (Hermann 2006), malaria (Doolan and Hoffman, 2001), tuberculosis (Lowrie, 2006), cancers (Lowe et al., 2006), and the novel application of gene therapy (including novel approaches to introduce the potential for host-based production of therapeutic protein) (Baumgartner et al., 1998; Losordo et al., 1998; Gaffney et al., 2007; Mahvi et al., 2007). Although many have progressed to the clinic, their commercial implementation still appears challenging. The elicitation of a clear immune response with protective potential will likely require a better understanding of the fundamental peculiarities of the human immune system before being successfully applied widely. This key issue seems especially challenging because robust immune responses are achieved in animals at doses that are approximately 10- to 50-folds lower that those tested in humans.

In response to these challenges, the development of various adjuvants and the implementation of novel vaccination technologies are viewed as potentially helpful. These approaches range from the development of cationic surfactants aimed at facilitating the delivery and transport of plasmid DNA (Perrie et al., 2001; Singh et al., 2002; Locher et al., 2003; Meng and Butterfield, 2005) to the coinjection of not only adjuvants such as the classical alum (Wang et al., 2000), but also cytokines (Wassef and Plaeger, 2002). Greater sophistication can be achieved either by adding a gene coding for the coexpression of specific cytokines onto the plasmid (Kim et al.,

2001) or by designing the plasmid back bone for recognition by APCs toll-like receptors (TLR) (discussed later in the chapter) (Lemieux 2002; Krieg 2003). Recently described, the TLR-independent positive role of TANK-binding kinase 1 (TNK1) in stimulating the immune response may offer additional avenues to boost DNA vaccines immunogenicity (Ishii et al., 2008). Finally, needle injection seems to be the least favored and has been replaced by high velocity vaccination employing microparticles coated with DNA or when combined with electroporation (Yoshida et al., 2000; Bachy et al., 2001; Aguiar et al., 2002; Babiuk et al., 2004; Hannaman et al., 2008; Pokorna et al., 2008; Wang et al., 2008; Yuan, 2008). Combinations and better understanding of these technologies are likely to yield DNA vaccination methods that will result in adequate immune responses in humans.

2.4 REQUIRED PHYSICAL PROPERTIES OF PLASMID DNA VACCINES

Plasmid construction is an important step in the design of a DNA plasmid vaccine. Basically, a few required key elements need to be present in the plasmid to ensure both its appropriate replication in the *E. coli* host and the effective transcription of the encoded foreign gene by the transfected mammalian cell. The introduction of patterns recognized by the innate immune system is believed to help in increasing immunogenicity. It is also important to select carefully and insert restriction sites and *trans* gene cassette insertion sites in order to facilitate all construction steps.

In addition, it is important to ensure that the plasmid DNA will be safe. To avoid replication in the mammalian host, only microbial-specific replication origins are used. To avoid integration in the host genome, only circular and mostly supercoiled plasmids should be used, and the sequence needs to be carefully verified in order to prevent any unintended homologies with the host genome. Several regulatory texts outline these requirements and check points (discussed later in the chapter). Finally, the size of the plasmid should be kept to a minimum, as a large plasmid tends to be more mechanically fragile and may generate unwanted open forms and fragments.

Salient plasmid construction points are briefly reviewed in the following section.

2.4.1 Plasmid Source and Origin of Replication

A large diversity of *E. coli*-compatible plasmid features exists to choose from. However, one of the key aspects is to ensure appropriate and effective replication in the host *E. coli* at high copy numbers so that vaccine production can be as efficient and cost effective as possible. For this reason, the well-studied, modified ColE1-type vectors, which only require host-encoded proteins for their replication and which replicate independently of the bacterial "chromosome," provide an excellent source for the replication cassette (Balbás et al., 1986). Historically, advances in the molecular biology involved in the regulation of plasmid replication have helped in understanding the mechanisms involved and yielded better design of the replication elements, resulting in the accumulation of several hundred copies per cell.

The replication of the ColE1 plasmid and its derivatives is a very well understood and genetically easy-to-manipulate entity. Replication of the plasmid is regulated by two interconnected mechanisms that are plasmid encoded. DNA replication at the origin of replication (ori) is under the control of two short RNA transcripts known as *RNAI* and *RNAII*, which are transcribed in opposite directions from the same DNA strand. RNAII acts as the preprimer for DNA replication, which on processing by ribonuclease RNase H binds to its complementary DNA sequence on the plasmid and in conjunction with host-encoded DNA polymerase allows for replication. RNAI encodes for an antisense strand complementary to a small region of RNAII. On formation of the RNAI–RNAII complex, the processing of RNAII by RNase H is prevented, therefore disallowing plasmid replication.

Moreover, the interaction between RNAI and RNAII is enhanced by a plasmid-encoded protein, first called *Rop* and later renamed *Rom*. This short protein encoded by the plasmid was first thought to act a repressor of the primer (Rop), but its role was then clarified as acting as a stabilizing partner of the RNAI–RNAII complex (RNA one modulator or Rom), thereby negatively controlling plasmid replication (reviewed in Davison, 1984; Balbás et al., 1986).

As expected from the mechanism described, mutations affecting the Rop/Rom protein or the interaction of RNAI/RNAII can result in a modified plasmid copy number. At first, higher copy numbers of a pBR322 plasmid were linked with a defective Rop/Rom (Lin-Chao et al., 1992). More recently, additional increase in copy number was traced to a single point mutation affecting the coding region of the RNAII and resulting in a change in the RNAI–RNAII complex binding affinity in a temperature-dependent manner. In a Rop/Rom-deficient background, this effect is fully achieved when cultivating the cells at a higher temperature (42°C), where the association of the RNAI/RNAII is weakened, thus resulting in high plasmid copy numbers (Lahijani et al., 1996). This point mutation combined with a Rop/Rom deficient background in pBR322-derived constructs has been successfully employed to improve the yield of plasmid DNA for DNA vaccine purposes and is likely to remain the standard for most plasmid DNA vaccines.

2.4.2 Selectable Markers

A second feature required for the production of plasmids in *E. coli* is the inclusion of a selectable marker that should support the selection of bacterial transformants that harbor the desired plasmid. Mostly because of the ease of use and the vast pre-existing know-how, the insertion of genes coding for antibiotic resistance has been employed in order to support rapid and effective plasmid-containing clone selection. The choice of antibiotic resistance is, however, of importance. Beta-lactams, for example, are undesirable because they can trigger allergic reactions to the staff involved in the production, and any residual traces could potentially exhibit toxicities on injection into the human host. Instead, the use of the aminoglycosides neomycin or kanamycin is preferred because they present a higher safety profile (European Agency for the Evaluation of Medicinal Products, 1998). In addition, because the mechanism of resistance codes for an enzyme that deactivates these antibiotics, the likelihood of residual amounts in the final drug substance is practically null. The two features just described, namely the efficient replication machinery and the presence of a selectable marker, are the *sine qua non* requirements for efficient selection and replication in the *E. coli* bacterial host.

2.4.3 Eukaryotic Expression of the Antigen

To ensure correct expression of the *trans* gene in the eukaryotic host, at minimum, a eukaryotic promoter, a transcription termination, and a polyadenylation signal are required (Feltquate, 1998; Gurunathan et al., 2000a; Gurunathan et al., 2000b; Montgomery and Jones Prather, 2006). Of the multiple well-described promoters available for recombinant gene expression in mammalian cells, the human cytomegalovirus/immediate-early gene (CMVIE), simian virus/early (SV40), human elongation factor-1 α (EF-1 α), and human ubiquitin C (UbC) are most often encountered. The CMVIE promoter, especially when combined with intron A, is believed to be the most effective (Davis and Huang, 1988; Chapman et al., 1991), with this combination most frequently used in DNA vaccine applications (Garapin et al., 2001). The added advantage of placing the *trans* gene under the control of a mammalian promoter is the lack of antigen synthesis in the microbial host, resulting in a lower metabolic burden to the cells during plasmid amplification or even in avoiding the production of a protein toxic to the microbe. Finally, transcription terminators and polyadenylation signals are both required, with those from bovine growth hormone (BGH), SV40, and human beta-globin being the most frequently used (Jones Prather et al., 2003; Montgomery and Jones Prather et al., 2006).

2.4.4 Plasmid Backbone: Immunostimulatory and *trans* Gene Expression Enhancements

It is now well established that cells of the mammalian immune system can detect pathogen-associated molecular patterns via receptors known as *toll-like receptors*. These receptors, expressed on dendritic and B-cells, for example, activate cytokine secretion, which modulates the immune response. Unlike mammalian DNA, bacterial DNA presents specific unmethylated CpG motifs that have been shown specifically to activate the TLR 9-associated pathway (Krieg, 2003; Krieg, 2006). The deliberate inclusion of CpG motifs in the back bone of the plasmid is a common feature of many DNA plasmid vaccines that is believed to add immunostimulatory properties to the vaccine (Krieg et al., 1998; Krieg, 1999; Van Uden and Raz, 2000; Herve et al., 2001; Bergmann-Leitner and Leitner 2004). Studies have also shown that the flanking sequences can influence the effectiveness of the CpG motif (Krieg, 2006). For proper expression in the eukaryotic host, if required, the insertion of a "Kozak" sequence and codon optimization will facilitate translation and lead to higher efficacy (Garmory et al., 2003). Figure 2.1 presents a typical DNA plasmid vaccine construct and highlights the salient features briefly reviewed in this chapter.

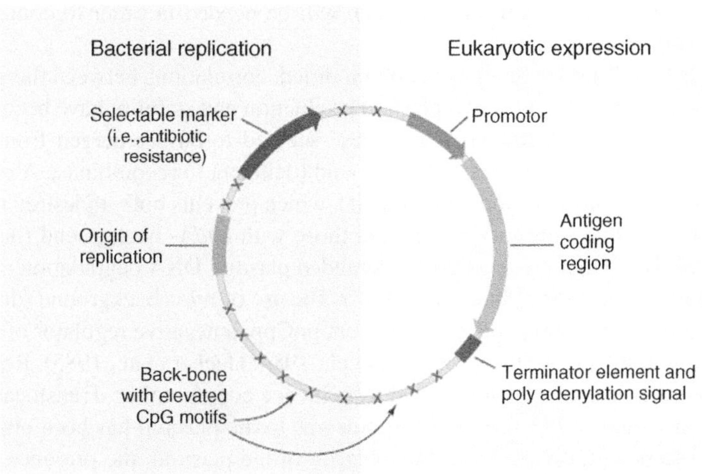

Figure 2.1 Pictogram of a typical DNA vaccine plasmid vector.

2.4.5 Influence of Insert

In addition to excluding any potential sequence that could trigger integration into the host genome, the physical quality of the DNA is of importance. Z-DNA structures, which may originate from the cloned antigen sequence, should be avoided, as they are unstable in *E. coli* (Cooke et al., 2004). Nicked DNA is likely to be more prone to either integration or degradation. The degree of supercoiling seems to dictate vaccine efficacy partially, as correlation between high supercoil content and greater vaccine efficacy have been reported (Cupillard et al., 2005; Pillai et al., 2008).

The *trans* gene insert may also influence the level of productivity, as the result from two studies seem to indicate (Listner et al., 2007; Rozkov et al., 2007). However, as discussed later in the chapter, these differences may also simply be the result of clonal variation, as the evaluation of a large number of clones is not routine.

2.5 CHOICE OF *E. coli* HOST STRAIN

As of now, various strains of *E. coli* (e.g., DH5, BL21) have been used with success in the production of plasmid DNA vaccine, as exemplified by the information available from the literature. A recent publication that compared 17 common *E. coli* strains suggests that certain strains may be better hosts (Yau et al., 2008). Depending on the strain employed, specific and volumetric production varied over a 10-fold range, with a BL21 derivative and DH5α strains giving some of the highest yields and percentages of supercoiled plasmids. The authors suggest that several strains be tested before embarking into scale-up activities. Further work, employing bioreactors and fed-batch conditions that closely mimic large-scale production conditions (described later in this chapter), will be needed in order to confirm the capabilities of the best strains.

Since all *E. coli* strains are genetically modified, correlations between the genetic background of the *E. coli* host and plasmid production and stability have been established over the years. A few general "rules" seemed to have emerged from these studies. *E. coli* strains with a *recA*- background (deficient in recombinase A enzyme activity that is responsible for dsDNA repair), which prevents both undesired recombination and plasmid multimerization, and those with *endA*- background (deficient in Endonuclease 1) that prevents double stranded plasmid DNA degradation are preferred (Balbás et al., 1986; Phue et al., 2008). The use of *relA*- background (deficient in ppGpp synthase) ensures that on starvation, ppGpp, a negative regulator of ColE1 replication, will not be produced (Hecker et al., 1983; Hecker et al., 1985). Recently, the host genome has also been reported to influence copy number. Translocation of the insertion sequence IS1 from the chromosome to the plasmid has been observed. In addition to potentially affecting the integrity of the plasmid, the presence of IS1 on the plasmid has been linked with low plasmid copy numbers (Jones Prather et al., 2006).

Host strain engineering aimed at reaching either greater productivity or higher quality (% supercoiling, lack of genomic DNA and RNA in the final product) has been recently reported. One study engineered the host background to express a plasmid-safe nuclease that helps in the removal of contaminating genomic DNA during purification (Hodgson and Williams, 2006). A second recent study showed that BL21, a very robust and easy-to-cultivate strain, could be engineered to support very high plasmid production once its background was made *recA*- and *endA*- (Phue et al., 2008).

2.6 FACTORS INFLUENCING PLASMID STABILITY

Segregational plasmid instability is often observed and can result from stress caused by nutritional limitation and metabolic burden imposed to the cells by the replicating plasmid (Jones et al., 1980; Zabriskie et al., 1987; Summers 1991; Bentley and Quiroga, 1993; Wróbel and Wegrzyn, 1998; Wegrzyn 1999; Wang et al., 2006). Under these circumstances and in the absence of selective pressure, the cells that lose plasmids will reduce their metabolic burden and gain a competitive advantage, mostly through a higher growth rate (Ow et al., 2006). These losses can, however, be mitigated by process design, especially through the careful balancing of the nutritional environment. Traditionally, plasmid stability is usually controlled by maintaining the selective pressure through the addition of antibiotic to the cultivation medium. However, a recent study (Rozkov et al., 2004) pointed out that in addition to the burden of plasmid DNA synthesis, the production of the enzyme coding for antibiotic resistance can add a substantial metabolic burden: in the study, enzyme synthesis represented about 18% of the total cell protein.

The presence of a non-beta-lactam antibiotic in the cultivation medium is not truly problematic because its clearance or that of its inactivated form is usually readily achieved during the downstream steps (Swartz, 2001). Because the mechanisms of resistance encoded by the plasmid usually involve either deactivation or degradation of the antibiotic, selective pressure diminishes with time in liquid culture as deactivation of the antibiotic occurs (Dennis et al., 1985; Bech Jensen and Carlsen, 1990). It is therefore important to keep in mind that although an antibiotic has been added, the potential for plasmid loss exists because of its inactivation. Selective pressure must be maintained during all cloning, cell banking, and inoculum expansion steps. When factoring dilution and deactivation, the final product is highly unlikely to contain any remaining traces. It has been demonstrated that antibiotic selective pressure can be removed during the last step of the cultivation process (production stage) without undesirable effects (Listner et al., 2007).

2.7 TRANSFORMATION, SELECTION OF PRODUCING CLONES, AND CELL BANKING

2.7.1 Transformation and Clone Selection

Introduction of the plasmid into the naïve *E. coli* host cells is usually performed using standard electroporation protocols, employing cells that have been made electrocompetent. After transformation, the cells are first allowed to recover before being plated on an antibiotic-containing selective solid medium. On growth, transformants are picked and tested for presence of the desired plasmid DNA. This is usually performed employing agarose gel analysis of a small post-cultivation sample. To ensure clonality, it is usually advisable to perform a second step of cloning on the same solid selective medium.

Further selection of robustly producing clones is usually based on selecting a few clones cultivated on selective medium and evaluating the amount of plasmid DNA produced either by assessing the intensity of the plasmid DNA band on an agarose gel or by measuring its actual concentration by either photospectrometry or HPLC analyses. Published information on this topic is very scarce, but it is likely accurate to postulate that the evaluation of as many clones as possible under conditions that mimic actual process conditions will help in selecting the best producing clone (Chartrain et al., 2005). In order to establish a pre-Master Cell Bank (MCB), a colony picked from the selective solid medium is used to inoculate a small flask whose content on growth of the cells will be mixed with a cryopreservant such as glycerol. The resulting mixture is allocated in small cryovials that are stored at −70°C. On selection and banking of the desired producing clone, several quality steps need to be performed before engaging in the Good Manufacturing Practices (GMP) cell banking steps. Establishing the purity and identity of the cells, verifying the integrity of the plasmid, and confirming the sequence of the *trans* gene by sequence analysis are keys in this quality assurance exercise.

Of prime importance is the maintenance of a very thorough documentation of all these steps, as they eventually lead to the selection of a clone that will be used to generate a GMP set of cell banks.

2.7.2 Production of Cell Banks

MCB and Working Cell Banks (WCBs) need to be produced in accordance to the regulatory texts. Traditionally, microbial cell banks are reasonably simple to produce, and *E. coli* fits very well in this category. Keys to producing a high viable and reliable cell bank are the need to maintain selective pressure during expansion in order to ensure that no plasmid losses will occur, and second, to use cells that are actively growing (midexponential). To produce the (MCB, cells from the pre-MCB are cultivated in flasks of increasing volume until the targeted amount is obtained. Mixing the cells with an equal volume of 20–30% glycerol solution and dispensing the mixture into cryovials (volumes ranging from 1 to 5 ml) are sufficient to create a cell bank. The vials are kept at −70°C, and *E. coli* is well known to maintain high viability on storage under these conditions for extended periods (Listner et al., 2006). The production of the WCB is performed according to the same protocol by expanding cells from the MCB. It is advisable to prepare several hundred vials of MCB so that it will never need to be remade. Since their usage is more intensive, it is acceptable to remake WCB cell banks occasionally during the life span of a vaccine. A reasonably large number of vials should be earmarked for tests that are required for ensuring quality of the cell banks. In general, the regulatory guidance texts are self-explanatory in terms of expectations for GMP cell banks and should be reviewed before producing the banks. Of importance is ensuring that all equipment, raw ingredients, and facilities be tested as required. Personnel should be adequately trained not only in both microbiological techniques, but also in performing operations under stringent conditions required by GMP, such as gowning and environmental testing.

Although rarely mentioned, the preparation of cell banks for industrial purposes is a crucial step that should be executed in the most accurate manner because every batch that will be produced during the entire commercial life of the vaccine originates from this stock of cells. Preservation in the case of disasters is a must, as unplanned events can lead to variation in the temperature storage of both MCB and WCB.

Figure 2.2 presents a pictorial of the various steps leading to the preparation of MCB and WCBs.

2.8 PRODUCTION PROCESS

Efficient and economic large-scale plasmid production from *E. coli* requires that elevated plasmid copy number (specific yield) and biomass concentration be achieved, thereby yielding high volumetric plasmid production. Achieving elevated specific yields is particularly important, as it positively impacts downstream processing and, ultimately, purification yields. Reviewed in this chapter are the impacts of process inputs followed by specific examples of clinical DNA vaccine production.

E. coli is a nonfastidious microorganism that grows well in rich complex organic media usually containing plant hydrolysates, yeast extract, and metabolized sugars such as glucose. *E. coli* can also be cultivated in salt-based chemically defined media, provided that a source of organic carbon is provided. As can be expected, the type

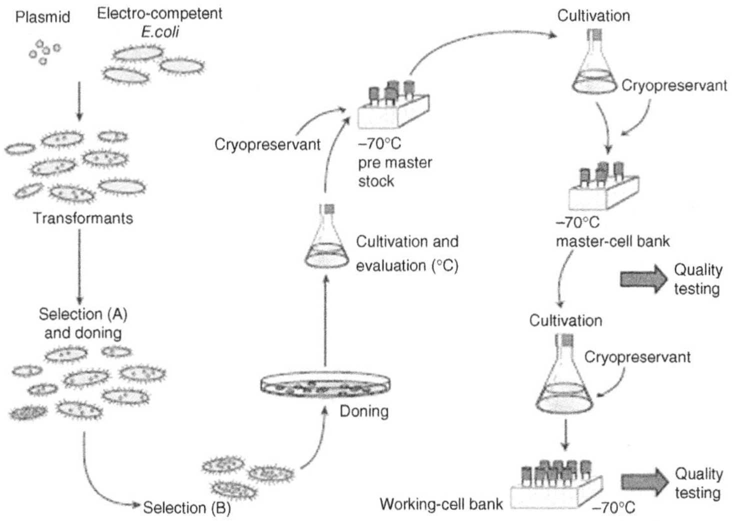

Figure 2.2 Selection of producing clone and cell bank construction logistics.

and concentration of the key ingredients used in the cultivation medium formulation directly impact the amount of biomass produced. However, as presented in the following sections, it also can influence the level of plasmid content. Since many complex interactions take place between the nutritive and the physicochemical environment, it is difficult to totally uncouple the influence of each of these process inputs. For this reason, both are discussed in the following section using pertinent examples.

2.8.1 Processes Based on Complex Cultivation Media

These processes are presented in two sections that correlate: first with the production of very small amounts of plasmids using laboratory equipment and second with the scale-up of these protocols in small- to medium-scale bioreactors.

2.8.1.1 Small-Scale Production Protocols Using Complex Media Complex cultivation media suitable for the cultivation of *E. coli* can either be purchased or be prepared according to formulations easily obtainable in the literature (Prather-Jones et al., 2003). They provide a nutritional base that will rapidly allow for the cultivation of the desired *E. coli* clone. Hence, most laboratory-scale DNA vaccine production schemes rely on the use of cultivation media such as Luria Bertrani (LB) or brain heart infusion (BHI), which are made up of complex ingredients. Well suited for small-scale cultivation, these cultivation media invariably support low cell mass yields that in turn support very modest volumetric plasmid yields. Slightly better yields can be achieved by boosting the strength of the cultivation medium either by supplementing with additional nutrients, by increasing the overall strength, or by affecting the balance of key nutrients delivering carbon and nitrogen. Interestingly,

TABLE 2.1 Plasmid DNA Processes and Associated Productivities

Preparatory scale
Shake flask scale: 5.2–74 mg/l (Diogo et al., 2000; O'Kennedy et al., 2000)
Shake flask scale (GMP grade material): estimated 25–30 mg/l (Przybylowski et al., 2007)
Laboratory scale fermentations (<100-l scale)
Batch (complex media): 4–60 mg/l (Reinikainen et al., 1989a; Reinikainen et al., 1989b; Horn et al., 1995; Lahijani et al., 1996; Diogo et al., 2001; Wang et al., 2001)
Fed-batch (complex media): 55–1900 mg/l (Lahijani et al., 1996; Chen et al., 1997; Schmidt et al., 2001; Carnes, 2005; Listner et al., 2006; Rozkov et al., 2006; O'Mahony et al., 2007; Phue et al. 2008)
Fed-batch (defined medium): 296 mg/l (Rozkov et al., 2004)
Pilot/production scale
Fed-batch (complex media): 70–225 mg/l (Chen, 1999; Schmidt et al., 2001)
Fed-batch (complex media GMP grade material): 1000 mg/l (Urthaler et al., 2005)
Fed-batch (defined medium GMP grade material, 2000-l scale): 1000–1600 mg/l (Listner et al., 2007)

these strategies tend to boost the overall biomass production and volumetric plasmid yields, whereas specific yields are largely unaffected. Although most of these processes are intended for the production of laboratory grade supplies, a recent publication outlines the use of a small-scale process on the basis of the cultivation of the *E. coli* host in shake flask, using LB medium (Przybylowski et al., 2007). This process was implemented under GMP conditions and produced DNA intended for human vaccination and provides an excellent example for the small-scale production of high quality vaccines. Table 2.1 presents a few representative yields that have been reported in the literature.

2.8.1.2 Bioreactor-Based Production Protocols Using Complex Media In addition to small volume capacity, the major limitations of shake flask cultivation are that it rapidly becomes very difficult to deliver enough oxygen to the cells in order to support vigorous aerobic growth. Oxygen limitation is quickly reached, causing the *E. coli* cells to switch to fermentative metabolism. This results in the accumulation of acidic by-products and, correlatively, a lower biomass yield from carbon. The accumulation of acid by-products presents a secondary negative effect because it can lead to lowering pH value to a point at which the cells can no longer grow. By delivering higher rates of oxygen transfer and offering pH control capabilities, the use of well-instrumented bioreactors partly alleviates these issues (Cherrington et al., 1990; Luli and Strohl, 1990). In addition, the implementation of fed-batch technology that delivers nutrients over an extended period allows the control of nutrient availability to a level compatible with the oxygen transfer capacities of the bioreactor. The feeding of nutrients, usually glucose or a mixture of glucose and nitrogen-containing substrates, has been extensively developed and encompasses various approaches ranging from simple constant delivery rates to the use of highly elaborate algorithms aimed at maintaining a desired growth rate. Generally, fed-batch technology yields high biomass accumulation that, depending on the specific combination of construct and clone, can reach anywhere from 60 to 120 g dry cell/l (Riesenberg 1991; Yee and Blanch, 1992; Lee 1996).

In addition to supporting the high biomass production, fed-batch technology offers control of growth rate, which in turn is known to control plasmid copy number.

Relationships between growth rate and plasmid copy number have been established using continuous, fed-batch, and batch cultivations (Seo and Bailey, 1986; Reinikainen, et al. 1989a; Reinikainen et al., 1989b; Reinikainen and Virkajärvi 1989; Rozkov et al., 2006). It is quite clear that for each construct, an optimal growth rate window with respect to plasmid accumulation exists. Very high growth rates likely do not allow for timely accumulation of plasmid because rapid cell division "dilutes" the plasmids. Very low growth rates on the other end probably reach a point at which the amount of energy and nutrients diverted to maintenance essentially competes with plasmid replication. In addition to the main body of data obtained in continuous fed-batch cultures, the increase in plasmid copy number during both the late exponential and early stationary phases of growth has also been reported and correlates well with this theory. Basically, high plasmid content achieved under reduced growth rate conditions is attributed both to higher plasmid stability (owing to effectively equivalent growth rates of plasmid-free and plasmid-bearing cells) and to privileged plasmid synthesis over other biochemical pathways. It is an operating zone that needs to be refined for each construct when developing a process (Prather-Jones et al., 2003).

A simple process developed by our group has proven to be a very easily scalable method for the production of small to medium quantities of plasmid DNA. It has been fully described in a previous publication and is summarized in this section (Listner et al., 2006). The use of large volume (300 ml) frozen working seed banks allows for direct inoculation of a medium size fermentor and thereby eliminates the shake flask stage in the inoculum development. This implementation reduces the number of manipulation with "open containers" and increases overall control of the process. On inoculation, the conditions in the bioreactors are controlled to maintain a growth-conducive environment (pH is maintained at 7.1, and dissolved oxygen is maintained at 30–40% of initial saturation via the automated control of the agitation). Once mid-exponential growth is reached (measured on-line via carbon evolution rate or off-line by optical density determination), the feeding of a nutrient solution, made up of yeast extract and glucose, is initiated. The nutrient delivery rate is controlled to maintain a reduced growth rate conducive to plasmid amplification. At all times during this phase, pH and DO are maintained to initial set-points. Figure 2.3 shows a representative pictogram of the operations involved, while Figures 2.4 provides representative kinetics of this process and clearly shows that plasmid amplification takes place during the feeding phase of the process.

Overall, the examples summarized in Table 2.1 show that a clear benefit can be obtained from using fed-batch technology in bioreactors when employing a complex cultivation medium. Although perhaps not optimal, complex medium-based

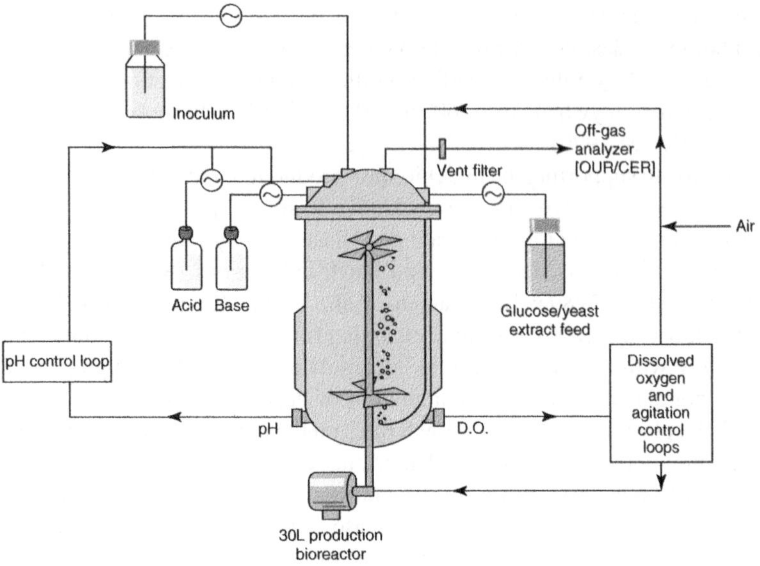

Figure 2.3 Overview of a typical set up for the production of small/medium quantities of plasmid DNA.

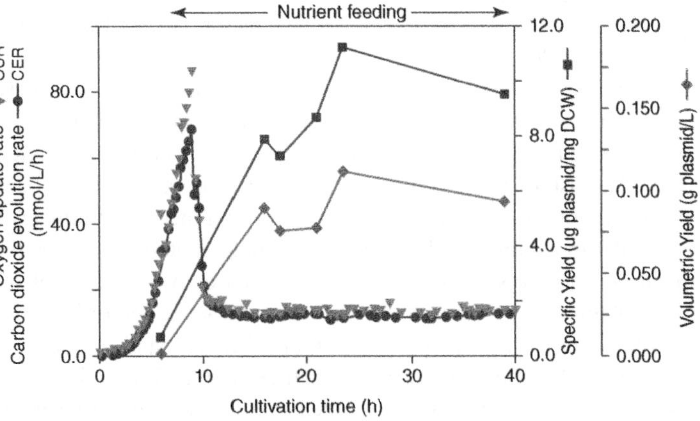

Figure 2.4 Typical kinetics of plasmid DNA production in fed-batch.

fed-batch technology has generally been successfully applied for the production of plasmid DNA for clinical investigations.

2.8.2 Fed-Batch Technology Based on Defined Cultivation Media

The development of a well-controlled process based on a specifically designed chemically defined cultivation medium is very likely to lead to the reproducible production of high quality plasmid DNA vaccines. Chemically defined formulations offer multiple advantages. First, by eliminating any complex ingredient from their formulation, they avoid the well-documented lot-to-lot variability that complex ingredients inherently have. Second, defined media offer the ability to perform extensive analytical investigations and, in return, help in establishing a clear understanding of the metabolism of the microorganism and serve in establishing quality by design into the process (Zhang and Greasham, 1999). However, even defined media can present some variability, as trace contaminants in the raw ingredients may influence the performance of the fermentation. A rational investigative approach usually leads to the control and mitigation of these issues fairly rapidly (Kizer-Bentley et al., 2005).

Nutritional requirements and cellular composition of *E. coli* are well defined, and this information can be advantageously used in the design of cultivation media formulations (Bolivar et al., 1977; Harris and Adams, 1979; Reiling et al., 1985; Fieschko and Ritch, 1986; Paalme et al., 1990; Riesenberg et al., 1990). Employing this approach, investigators reported the rational design of a defined medium optimized for plasmid production by a JM-109 *E. coli* strain. After carefully balancing the amino acids and nucleotides contents, they designed a cultivation medium that supported plasmid DNA-specific yields of about 17.1 μg plasmid/mg dry cell weight (Wang et al., 2001).

Using a slightly different approach, we first developed a simple defined medium based on salts and glycerol (Listner et al., 2007). The advantage of employing glycerol as a carbon source is the low to nil production of acetic acid. This medium is very simple, easy to prepare, and sterilize even in large quantities. For reference, the composition is described in Table 2.2.

The process itself revolves around the basic principles described previously. The pH is controlled, and the oxygen supply is always kept in excess. In addition, we implemented a well-controlled inoculum strategy that allows for the simplest process, with respect to the size of the operations, process. Using large frozen inocula preserved in bags, the process can be reduced to a one-stage (production stage) process for up to several thousand liters. For very high foot print facilities, an additional stage (inoculum) needs to be inserted, in order to manage both the size of the frozen inoculum bags and the duration of the apparent lag phase. If desired, the algorithm developed will adjust the selection on the basis of the volume of the available equipment and the growth rate of the specific clone used (Okonkowski et al., 2004).

In this process, the cells are first allowed to grow rapidly during the first part of the cultivation. On reaching mid-exponential, the feeding of glycerol is implemented at a rate that supports a reduced growth rate, and thereby maximum plasmid amplification. The source of nitrogen needed for maintaining balanced metabolism is supplied from ammonium hydroxide used in the pH control. Under the conditions selected and glycerol feed rate employed, the fermentation is carbon but not nitrogen limited. By the end of the feeding period, a high biomass has accumulated (~40 g dry cell weight per liter), and high plasmid volumetric (1–1.6 g/l) and specific productivities (20–28 μg plasmid DNA/mg dry cell weight) are achieved. Kinetics data clearly highlight that

TABLE 2.2 Composition of a Defined Medium Used for the cGMP Production of Vaccine Plasmid DNA at Industrial Scale[a]

Ingredient concentration[b]
KH_2PO_4: 7.0 g/l
K_2HPO_4: 7.0 g/l
$(NH_4)_2SO_4$: 6.0 g/l
Glycerol: 15.0 g/l
Sodium chloride: 0.1 g/l
Thiamine hydrochloride: 0.6 g/l
$MgSO_4$.7H2O: 2.0 g/l
Trace elements 1.0 ml/l
Composition of trace element solution
$FeCl_3$ $6H_2O$ 27 g/l
$ZnCl_2$ 2 g/l
$CoCl_2$ $6H_2O$ 2 g/l
Na2MoO4, $2H_2O$ 2 g/l
$CaCl_2$ $2H_2O$ 1 g/l
$CuCl_2$ $2H_2O$ 1.27 g/l
H_3BO_3 0.5 g/l
1.2 N HCl QS

[a]From Listner et al., 2007.
[b]These components form the basal medium. They are dissolved in water, and the pH is adjusted to 7.2 with 50% NaOH.

plasmid accumulation (or amplification) takes place during the phase of slow growth. This process supported the preparation of clinical supplies for several DNA plasmid vaccines, while exhibiting excellent scalability to the 2000-l scale. Figure 2.5 presents an overview of the production process.

2.9 REQUIREMENTS FOR CLINICAL SUPPLIES

When preparing clinical supplies, all applicable regulatory guidelines should be applied. The guidance pertaining to the cultivation of the microbial host, *E. coli*, is similar to that in place for the production of recombinant proteins and is captured in the FDA current GMP (cGMP) for vaccine production documents (United States, 1999). The guidelines are designed to ensure the quality, potency, and consistency of each lot and require that all operations be consistent with current revisions. Cultivation must be performed under controlled conditions so as to reproducibly yield a product of high quality. Although an antibiotic can be used for maintaining selective pressure, it should be well understood that its use is not intended to prevent contamination in replacement of proper sterile techniques (European Agency for the Evaluation of Medicinal Products, 1998). In addition, the quality of the plasmid DNA must be carefully controlled (Smith 1994; FDA 1996; WHO, 1998; Cichutek

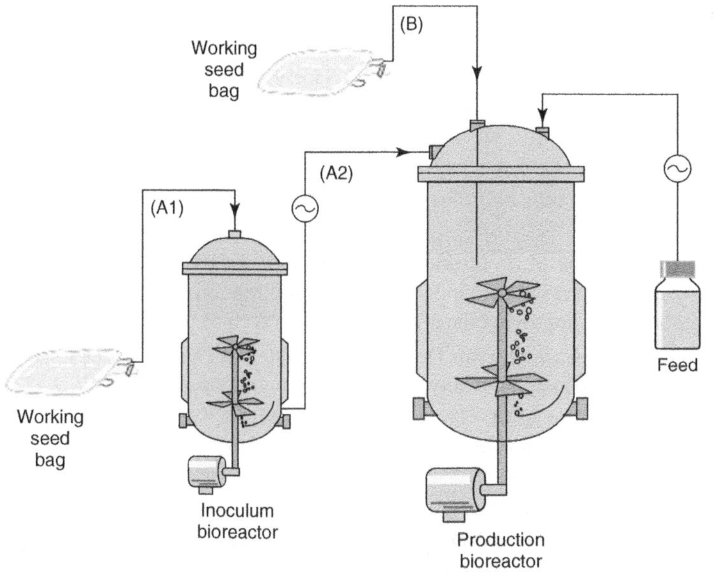

Figure 2.5 Overview of a typical set up for large-scale production of plasmid DNA vaccine.

2000; Robertson and Cichutek, 2000; Smith 2000; Falk and Ball, 2001; Smith and Klinman, 2001).

2.10 CONCLUSIONS

It is probable that a plasmid DNA intended for human applications will eventually reach the registration stage in the next 10 years. The production of high quality, inexpensive vaccines will need to be in place, in order to ensure lasting success. One of the keys to this future success is the implementation of a highly reproducible, scalable, simple, and productive fermentation process.

The use of a stable, high plasmid-producing *E. coli* clone cultivated under plasmid DNA amplification-permissive conditions is essential. A defined cultivation medium will be of help, as it supports higher process reproducibility and facilitates regulatory compliance. Briefly, a two-phase strategy, namely a phase of biomass buildup where the cells grow exponentially, followed by a phase of slow growth achieved via fed-batch technology in which plasmid amplification takes place, is likely to be the method of choice.

The platform-like features employed, from a predesigned plasmid backbone where the antigen-coding sequence is inserted, to the selection and efficient cultivation of a well-producing clone, and finally an efficient purification and formulation of the final product give this vaccine technology the potential to rapidly support the production of large amounts of life-saving vaccines (Forde 2005; Hoare et al., 2005).

REFERENCES

Aguiar J, Hedstrom R, Rogers W, Charoenvit Y, Sacci J, Lanar D, Majam V, Stout R, Hoffman S. Enhancement of the immune response in rabbits to a malaria DNA vaccine by immunization with a needle-free jet device. Vaccine 2002;20:275–280.

Anderson, E., and Leong J-A (2000). *Development of DNA Vaccine for Salmonid Fish. DNA Vaccines: Methods and Protocols.* In: Lowrie R.W.D. Totowa, NJ: Humana Press; p 105–121.

Babiuk S, Baca-Estrada M, Foldvari M, Middleton D, Rabussay D, Widera G, Babiuk L. Increased gene expression and inflammatory cell infiltration caused by electroporation are both important for improving the efficacy of DNA vaccines. J Biotechnol 2004;110:1–10.

Babuik L, Babiuk S, Loehr B, van Drunnen Littel-van den Hurk S. Nucleic acid vaccines: research tool or commercial reality. Vet Immunol Immunopathol 2000;76:1–23.

Bachy M, Boudet F, Bureau M, Girerd-Chambaz Y, Wils P, Scherman D, Meric C. Electric pulses increase the immunogenicity of an influenza DNA vaccine injected intramuscularly in the mouse. Vaccine 2001;19:1688–1693.

Balbás P, Soberón X, Merino E, Zurita M, Lomeli H, Valle F, Flores N, Bolivar F. Plasmid vector pBR322 and its special-purpose derivatives—a review. Gene 1986;50:3–40.

Banchereau J, Briere F, Caux C, Davoust J, lebecque S, Liu Y-J, Pulendran B, Paluka K. Immunobiology of dendritic cells. Annu Rev Immunol 2000;18:767–811.

Baneyx F, Mujacic M. Recombinant protein folding and misfolding in *Escherichia coli.* Nat Biotechnol 2004;22:1399–1408.

Baumgartner I, Pieczek A, Manor O, Blair R, Kearney M, Walsh K, Isner J. Constitutive expression of phVEGF165 after intramuscular gene transfer promotes collateral vessel development in patients with critical limb ischemia. Circulation 1998;97:1114–1123.

Bech Jensen E, Carlsen S. Production of recombinant human growth hormone in *Escherichia coli*: expression of different precursors and physiological effects of glucose, acetate and salts. Biotechnol Bioeng 1990;36:1–11.

Bentley W, Quiroga O. Investigation of subpopulation heterogeneity and plasmid stability in recombinant *Escherichia coli* via a simple segregated model. Biotechnol Bioeng 1993;42:222–234.

Bergman P, Camps-Palau M, McKnigh J, Leibmabn N, Craft D, Leung C, Liao J, Riviere I, Sadelain M, Hohenhaus A, Gregor P, Houghton A, Perales M, Wolchok J. Development of a xenogenic DNA vaccine program for canine malignant melanoma at the Animal Medical Center. Vaccine 2006;24:4582–4585.

Bergmann-Leitner ES, Leitner WW. Danger, death and DNA vaccines. Microbes Infect 2004;6(3):319–327.

Bolivar F, Rodriguez R, Betlach M, Boyer H. Construction and characterization of new cloning vehicles: I. Ampicillin-resistant derivatives of the plasmid pMB9. Gene 1977;2:75–93.

Buckland B. The process development challenge for a new vaccine. Nat Med 2005; 11(Suppl):S16–S19.

Carnes A. Fermentation design for the manufacture of therapeutic plasmid DNA. BioProcess Int 2005:36–44.

Chapman B, Thayer R, Vincent K, Haigwood N. Effect of intron A from human cytomegalovirus (Towne) immediate-early gene on heterologous expression in mammalian cells. Nucleic Acids Res 1991;19(14):3979–3986.

Chartrain, M., L. Bentley, B. Krulewitcz, K. Listner, W-J. Sun, and C. Lee. Process for large scale production of plasmid DNA by *E. coli* fermentation. WO/2005/078115. (2005).

Chen, W. Automated high yield fermentation of plasmid DNA in *Escherichia coli*. US patent 5,955,323, American Home Product Corp. 1999.

Chen W, Graham C, Ciccarelli RB. Automated fed-batch fermentation with feed-back controls based on dissolved oxygen (DO) and pH for production of DNA vaccines. J Ind Microbiol Biotechnol 1997;18:43–48.

Cherrington C, Hinton M, Chopra I. Effect of short-chain organic acids on macromolecular synthesis in *Escherichia coli*. J Bacteriol 1990;68:69–74.

Cichutek K. DNA vaccines: development, standardization and regulation. Intervirology 2000;43:331–338.

Cooke J, McKie E, Ward J, Keshavarz-Moore E. Impact of intrinsic structure on processing of plasmids for gene therapy and DNA vaccines. J Biotechnol 2004;114:239–254.

Cupillard L, Juillard V, Latour S, Colombet G, Cachet N, Richard S, Blanchard S, Fisher L. Impact of plasmid supercoiling on the efficacy of a rabies DNA vaccine to protect cats. Vaccine 2005;23:1910–1916.

Danko I, Wolff J. Direct gene transfer into muscle. Vaccine 1994;12:149–1502.

Davis BS, Chang GJ, Cropp B, Roehrig JT, Martin DA, Mitchell CJ, Bowen R, Bunning ML. West Nile virus recombinant DNA vaccine protects mouse and horse from virus challenge and expresses in vitro a noninfectious recombinant antigen that can be used in enzyme-linked immunosorbent assays. J Virol 2001;75(9):4040–4047.

Davis M, Huang E. Transfer and expression of plasmids containing human cytomegalovirus immediate-early gene 1 promoter-enhancer sequences in eukaryotic and prokaryotic cells. Biotechnol Appl Biochem 1988;10:6–12.

Davison J. Mechanism of control of DNA replication and incompatibility in ColE1-type plasmids—a review. Gene 1984;28:1–15.

Dennis K, Srienc F, Bailey J. Ampicillin effects on five recombinant *Escherichia coli* strains: implications for selection pressure design. Biotechnol Bioeng 1985;27:1490–1494.

Diogo M, Queiroz J, Monteiro G, Martins S, Ferreira G, Prazeres D. Purification of a cystic fibrosis plasmid vector for gene therapy using hydrophobic interaction chromatography. Biotechnol Bioeng 2000;68(5):576–583.

Diogo M, Ribeiro S, Queiroz J, Montiero G, Tordo N, Perrin P, Prazeres D. Production, purification and analysis of an experimental DNA vaccine against rabies. J Gene Med 2001;3:577–584.

Donnelly J, Berry K, Ulmer J. Technical and regulatory hurdles for DNA vaccines. Int J Parasitol 2003;33:457–467.

Doolan D, Hoffman S. DNA-based vaccines against malaria: status and promises of the multi-stage malaria DNA vaccine operation. Int J Parasitol 2001;31:753–762.

European Agency for the Evaluation of Medicinal Products. Note on guidance on pharmaceutical and biological aspects of combined vaccines. 1998.

Falk L, Ball L. Current status and future trends in vaccine regulation—USA. Vaccine 2001;19:1567–1572.

FDA. Points to consider on plasmid DNA vaccines for preventive infectious diseases. Docket No 96N-0400. 1996.

Feltquate D. DNA vaccines: vector design, delivery, and antigen presentation. J Cell Biochem 1998;S30/31:304–311.

Fieschko J, Ritch T. Production of human alpha consensus interferon in recombinant *Escherichia coli*. Chem Eng Commun 1986;45:229–240.

Fischer L, Minke J, Dufay N, Baudu P, Audonnet J-C. Rabies DNA vaccine in the horse: strategies to improve serological responses. Vaccine 2003;21:4593–4596.

Forde G. Rapid-response vaccines-does DNA offer a solution? Nat Biotechnol 2005;23:1059–1062.

Gaffney M, Hynes S, Barry F, O'Brien T. Cardiovascular gene therapy: current status and therapeutic potential. Br J Pharmacol 2007;152:175–188.

Garapin A, Ma L, Pescher P, Lagranderie M, Marchal G. Mixed immune response induced in rodents by two naked DNA genes coding for mycobacterial glycosylated proteins. Vaccine 2001;19:2830–2841.

Garmory H, Brown K, Titball R. DNA vaccines: improving expression of antigens. Genet Vaccines and Ther 2003;1:1–5.

Gnoth S, Jenzsch M, Simutis R, Lubbert A. Product formation kinetics in genetically modified *E coli* bacteria: inclusion body formation. Bioprocess Biosyst Eng 2008;31:41–46.

Hannaman D, Bernard R, Alas M d l. Delivery technology reenergizes DNA drug development. BioProcess 2008;May 2008:44–52.

Harris R, Adams S. Determination of the carbon-bound electron composition of microbial cells and metabolites by dichromate oxidation. Appl Environ Microbiol 1979;37:237–243.

Hecker M, Schroeter A, Mach F. Replication of pBR322 DNA in stringent and relaxed strains of *Escherichia coli*. Mol Gen Genet 1983;190:355–357.

Hecker M, Schroeter A, Mach F. *Escherichia coli* relA strains as hosts for amplification of pBR322 plasmid DNA. FEMS Microbiol Lett 1985;29:331–334.

Herrmann J. DNA vaccines against enteric infections. Vaccine 2006;24:3705–3708.

Herve M, Dupre L, Ban E, Schacht A-M, Capron A, Riveau G. Features of the antibody response attributable to plasmid backbone adjuvancy after DNA immunization. Vaccine 2001;19:4549–4556.

Hoare M, Levy S, Bracewell D, Doig S, Kim S, Titchener-Hooker N, Ward J, Dunnill P. Bioprocess engineering issues that would be faced in producing a DNA vaccine at up to 100 m^3 fermentation scale for an influenza pandemic. Biotechnol Prog 2005;21:1577–1592.

Hodgson, C., and J. Williams. Improved strains of *E. coli* for plasmid DNA production. WIPO. WO 2006/026125 A2. 2006.

Horn N, Meek J, Budahazi G, Marquet M. Cancer gene therapy using plasmid DNA: purification of DNA for human clinical trials. Hum Gene Ther 1995;6:565–573.

Ishii KJ, Kawagoe T, Koyama S, Matsui K, Kumar H, Kawai T, Uematsu S, Takeuchi O, Takeshita F, Coban C, Akira S. TANK-binding kinase-1 delineates innate and adaptive immune responses to DNA vaccines. Nature 2008;451(7179):725–729.

ltd M USDA grants conditional approval for first therapeutic vaccine to treat cancer: Merial's new vaccine treats deadly cancer in dogs. Press release. 2007.

Jones I, Primrose S, Robinson A, Ellwood D. Maintenance of some ColE1-type plasmids in chemostat culture. Mol Gen Genet 1980;180:579–584.

Jones Prather K, Edmonds MC, Herod J. Identification and characterization of IS1 transposition in plasmid amplification mutants of *E coli* clones producing DNA vaccines. Appl Microbiol Biotechnol 2006;73:815–826.

Jones Prather K, Sagar S, Murphy J, Chartrain M. Industrial scale production of plasmid DNA for vaccine and gene therapy: plasmid design, production and purification. Enzyme Microbiol Technol 2003;33:865–883.

Kim J, Yang J, Manson K, Weiner D. Modulation of antigen-specific cellular immune responses to DNA vaccination in rhesus macaques through the use of IL-2, IFN-g. or IL-4 gene adjuvants. Vaccine 2001;19:2496–2505.

Kizer-Bentley L, Sweeney J, Krulewicz B, Lee C, Tsai P-K, Chartrain M. The effect of monosodium glutamate lot to lot variability on the process performance of a recombinant *E. coli*. BioProcess Int 2005. Forthcoming.

Krieg A. Direct immunologic activities of CpG DNA and implications for gene therapy. J Gene Med 1999;1:56–63.

Krieg A. CpG motifs: the active ingredient in bacterial extracts? Nat Med 2003;9:831–835.

Krieg AM, Yi AK, Schorr J, Davis HL. The role of CpG dinucleotides in DNA vaccines. Trends Microbiol 1998;6(1):23–27.

Krieg AM. Therapeutic potential of Toll-like receptor 9 activation. Nat Rev Drug Discov 2006;5(6):471–484.

Lahijani R, Hulley G, Soriano G, Horn N, Marquet M. High-yield production of pBR322-derived plasmids intended for human gene therapy by employing a temperature controllable point mutation. Hum Gene Ther 1996;7:1971–1980.

Ledwith B, Manam S, Trolo P, Barnum A, Pauley C, Griffiths T, Harper L, Beare C, Bagdon W, Nichols W. Plasmid DNA vaccines: investigation of integration into host cellular DNA following intramuscular injection in mice. Intervirology 2000;43:258–272.

Lee SY. High cell density culture of *Escherichia coli*. Trends Biotechnol 1996;14:98–105.

Lemieux P. Technological advances to increase immunogenicity of DNA vaccines. Expert Rev Vaccines 2002;1:85–93.

Lin-Chao S, Chen W, Wong T. High copy number of the pUC plasmid results from a Rom/Rop-suppressible point mutation in RNA II. Mol Microbiol 1992;6(22):3385–3393.

Listner, K., L. Bentley, and M. Chartrain (2006). *A Simple Method for the Production of Plasmid DNA in Bioreactors. DNA Vaccines: Methods and Protocols*. In: Saltzman W, Shen H, and Brandsma J. Totowa, NJ: Humana Press; p 295–310.

Listner K, Bentley L, Okonkowski J, Kistler C, Wnek R, Caparoni A, Junker B, Robinson D, Salmon P, Chartrain M. Development of a highly productive and scalable plasmid DNA production platform. Biotechnol Prog 2007;22:1335–1345.

Locher C, Putnam D, Langer R, Witt S, Ashlock B, Levy J. Enhancement of a human immunodeficiency virus end DNA vaccine using a novel polycationic nanoparticle formulation. Immnunol Lett 2003;90:67–70.

Lodmell DL, Parnell MJ, Bailey JR, Ewalt LC, Hanlon CA. One-time gene gun or intramuscular rabies DNA vaccination of non-human primates: comparison of neutralizing antibody responses and protection against rabies virus 1 year after vaccination. Vaccine 2002;20:838–844.

Lorenzen N, LaPatra S. DNA vaccines for aquacultured fish. Rev Sci Technol 2005;24:201–213.

Losordo, D., P. Vale, J. Symes, C. Dunnington, D. Esakof, M. Maysky, A. Ashare, K, Lathi, and J. Isner (1998). Gene therapy for myocardial angiogenensis. Circulation 98: 2800–2804.

Lowrie D. DNA vaccines for therapy of tuberculosis: where are we now? Vaccine 2006;24:1983–1989.

Lowe D, Shearer M, Kennedy R. DNA vaccines: successes and limitations in cancer and infectious diseases. J Cell Biochem 2006;98:235–242.

Luli G, Strohl W. Comparison of growth, acetate production, and acetate inhibition of *Escherichia coli* strains in batch and fed-batch fermentations. Appl Environ Microbiol 1990;56:1004–1011.

MacGregor RR, Boyer JD, Ugen KE, Lacy KE, Gluckman SJ, Bagarazzi ML, Chattergoon MA, Baine Y, Higgins TJ, Ciccarelli RB, Coney LR, Ginsberg RS, Weiner DB. First human trial of a DNA-based vaccine for treatment of human immunodeficiency virus type 1 infection: safety and host response. J Infect Dis 1998;178:92–100.

Mahvi, D. M. H., M. Albertini, S. Weber, K.Meredith, H. Schalch, A. Rekhmilevich, J. Hank, and P. Sondel (2007). Intratumoral injection of IL-12 plasmid DNA-results of a phase I/IB clinical trial. Cancer Gene Ther 14: 717–723.

Manam S, Ledwith B, Barnum A, Troilo P, Pauley C, Harper L, Griffiths T, Niu Z, Denisova L, Follmer T, Pacchione S, Wang Z, Beare C, Bagdon W, Michols W. Plasmid DNA vaccines: tissue distribution and effects of DNA sequence, adjuvants, and delivery method on integration into host DNA. Intervirology 2000;43:273–281.

Mascola J, Nabel G. Vaccines for the prevention of HIV-1 disease. Curr Opin Immunol 2001;13:489–495.

Meng W, Butterfield L. Activation of antigen-presenting cells by DNA delivery vectors. Expert Opin Biol Ther 2005;5:1019–1028.

Montgomery, D., and K. Jones Prather (2006). *Design of Plasmid DNA Constructs for Vaccines. DNA Vaccines, Methods and Protocols.* In: W. Saltzman, H. Shen, and J. Brandsma. Totowa,NJ: Humana Press; p 11–22.

Neidhardt F. *Escherichia coli* and *Salmonella.* Washington DC, USA: ASM press; 1996.

O'Kennedy R, Baldwin C, Keshavarz-Moore E. Effects of growth medium selection on plasmid DNA production and initial processing steps. J Biotechnol 2000;76:175–183.

Okonkowski J, Kizer-Bentley L, Listner K, Robinson D, Chartrain M. Development of a robust, versatile, and scaleable inoculum train for the production of a DNA vaccine. Biotechnol Prog 2004;21:1038–1047.

O'Mahony RF, Hilbrig F, Muller P, Schumacher I. Strategies for high titre plasmid DNA production in *Escherichia coli* DH5a. Process Biochem 2007;42:1039–1049.

Ow D, Morin-Nissom P, Philp R, Oh S, Yap M. Global transcriptional analysis of metabolic burden due to plasmid maintenance in *Escherichia coli* DH5a during batch fermentation. Enzyme Microbial Technol 2006;39:391–398.

Paalme T, Tiisma K, Kahru A, Vanatalu K, Vilu R. Glucose-limited fed-batch cultivation of *Escherichia coli* with computer-controlled fixed growth rate. Biotechnol Bioeng 1990;35:312–319.

Perrie Y, Frederik P, Gregoriadis G. Liposome mediated DNA vaccination: the effect of vesicle composition. Vaccine 2001;19(3301–3310).

Phue J-N, Lee S, Trinh L, Shiloach J. Modified *Escherichia coli* B (BL21), a superior producer of plasmid DNA compared with *Escherichia coli* K (DH5 a). Biotechnol Bioeng 2008. Forthcoming.

Pillai V, Hellerstein M, Yu T, Amara R, Robinson H. Comparative studies on *in vitro* expression and *in vivo* immunogenicity of supercoiled and open circular forms of plasmid DNA. Vaccine 2008;26:1136–1141.

Pokorna D, Rubio I, Muller M. DNA-vaccination via tattooing induces stronger humoral and cellular immune responses than intramuscular delivery supported by molecular adjuvants. Genetic Vaccines and Therapy 2008;6:1–8.

Powell K. DNA vaccines-back in the saddle again? Nat Biotechnol 2004;22:799–801.

Prather-Jones K, Sagar S, Murphy J, Chartrain M. Industrial scale production of plasmid DNA for vaccine and gene therapy: plasmid design, production, and purification. Enzyme Microb Technol 2003;33(7):865–883.

Przybylowski M, Bartido S, Borquez-Ojeda O, Sadelain M, Riviere I. Production of clinical-grade plasmid DNA for human Phase I clinical trials and large animal clinical studies. Vaccine 2007;25:5013–5025.

Reiling H, Laurila H, Fiechter A. Mass culture of *Escherichia coli*: medium development for low and high density cultivation of *Escherichia coli* B/r in minimal and complex media. J Biotechnol 1985;2:191–206.

Reinikainen P, Korpela K, Nissinen V, Olkku J, Soderlund H, Markkanen P. (a) *Escherichia coli* plasmid production in fermentor. Biotechnol Bioeng 1989a;33:386–393.

Reinikainen P, Korpela K, Nissinen V, Olkku J, Söderlund H, Markkanen P. *Escherichia coli* production in fermentor. Biotechnol and Bioeng 1989b;33:386–393.

Reinikainen P, Virkajärvi I. *Escherichia coli* growth and plasmid copy numbers in continuous cultivations. Biotechnol Lett 1989;11(4):222–230.

Riesenberg D. High-cell density cultivation of *Escherichia coli*. Curr Opin Biotechnol 1991;2:380–384.

Riesenberg D, Menzel K, Schultz V, Schumann K, Veith G, Zuber G, Knorre W. High cell density fermentation of recombinant *Escherichia coli* expressing human interferon alpha 1. Appl Microbiol Biotechnol 1990;34:77–82.

Robertson J, Cichutek K. European union guidance on the quality, safety and efficacy of DNA vaccines and regulatory requirements. Dev Biol 2000;104:53–56.

Rozkov A, Avignone-Rossa A, Erlt P, Jones P, O'Kennedy R, Smith J, Dale J, Bushell M. Characterization of the metabolic burden on *Escherichia coli* DH1 cells imposed by the presence of a plasmid containing a gene therapy sequence. Biotechnol Bioeng 2004;88: 909–915.

Rozkov A, Avignone-Rossa C, Erlt P, Jones P, O'Kennedy R, Smith J, Dale J, Bushell M. Fed-batch culture with declining specific growth rate for high-yielding production of a plasmid containing a gene therapy sequence in *Escherichia coli* DH1. Enz Microbiol Technol 2006;39:47–50.

Rozkov A, Larsson B, Gillstrom S, Bjornestedt R, Schmidt S. Large-scale production of endotoxin-free plasmids for transient expression in mammalian cell culture. Biotechnol Bioeng 2007;99:557–566.

Salonius K, Simard N, Harland R, Ulmer J. The road to licensure of a DNA vaccine. Curr Opin Invest Drugs 2007;8:635–641.

Schmidt T, Friehs K, Schleef M, Voss C, Flaschel E. In-process analysis of plasmid copy number for fermentation control. Pacesetter 2001;5(1):4–6.

Seo J, Bailey J. Continuous cultivation of recombinant *Escherichia coli*: existence of an optimum dilution rate for maximum plasmid and gene product concentration. Biotechnol Bioeng 1986;28:1590–1594.

Singh M, Vajdy M, Gardner J, Briones M, O'Hagan D. Mucosal immunization with HIV-1 gag DNA on cationic microparticules prolongs gene expression and enhances local and systemic immunity. Vaccine 2002;20:594–602.

Smith H. Regulatory considerations for nucleic acid vaccines. Vaccine 1994;12:1515–1528.

Smith H. Regulation and review of DNA vaccine products. Dev Biol 2000;104:57–62.

Smith H, Klinman D. The regulation of DNA vaccines. Curr Opin Biotechnol 2001;12:299–303.

Sorensen H, Mortensen K. Advanced genetic strategies for recombinant protein expression in *Escherichia coli.* J Biotechnol 2005;115:113–128.

Summers DK. The kinetics of plasmid loss. Trends Biotechnol 1991;9:273–278.

Swartz J. Advances in *Escherichia coli* production of therapeutic proteins. Curr Opin Biotechnol 2001;12:195–201.

Ulmer J, Valley U, Pappupoli R. Vaccine manufacturing: challenges and solutions. Nat Biotechnol 2006;24:1377–1383.

United States. Title 21 part 601.25(d)(4). Code of Federal Regulations. Washington DC: US Government Printing Office; 1999.

Urthaler J, Buchinger W, Necina R. Industrial scale cGMP purification of pharmaceutical grade plasmid DNA. Chem Eng Commun 2005;28:1408–1420.

Van Uden, J., and E. Raz (2000). *Immunostimulatory DNA Sequences: An Overview. DNA Vaccines. Methods and Protocols.* In: R.W. Lowrie. Totowa, NJ: Humana Press; p 145–172.

Walsh G. Biopharmaceutical benchmarks 2006. Nat Biotechnol 2006;24(7):769–776.

Wang S, Zhang C, Zhang L, Li J, Huang Z, Lu S. The relative immunogenicity of DNA vaccines delivered by the intramuscular needle injection, electroporation, and gene gun methods. Vaccine 2008;26:2100–2110.

Wang S, Liu X, Fisher K, Smith J, Chen F, Tobery T, Ulmer J, Evans R, Caulfield M. Enhanced type I immune response to a hepatitis B DNA vaccine by formulation with calcium- or aluminum phosphate. Vaccine 2000;18:1227–1235.

Wang Z, Le G, Shi Y, Wegrzyn G. Medium design for plasmid DNA production based on stoichiometric model. Process Biochem 2001;36:1085–1093.

Wang Z, Xiang L, Shao J, Wegrzyn A, Wegrzyn G. Effect of the presence of ColE1 plasmid DNA in *Escherichia coli* on the host cell metabolism. Microbial Cell Fact 2006;5:34–52.

Wassef N, Plaeger S. Cytokines as adjuvants for HIV DNA vaccines. Clin Appl Immunol Rev 2002;2:229–240.

Wegrzyn G. Replication of plasmids during bacterial response to amino acid starvation. Plasmid 1999;41:1–16.

WHO. WHO guidelines for assuring the quality of DNA vaccines. Biologicals 1998;26:205–212.

Wolf J, Malone R, Williams P, Chong W, Acsadi G, Jani A, Felgner P. Direct gene transfer into mouse muscle in vitro. Science 1990;247:1465–1468.

Wróbel B, Wegrzyn G. Replication regulation of ColE1-like plasmids in amino acid-starved *Escherichia coli.* Plasmid 1998;39:48–62.

Yau S, Keshavartz-Moore E, Ward J. Host strain influences on supercoiled plasmid DNA production in *Escherichia coli*: implications for efficient design of large-scale processes. Biotechnol Bioeng 2008. Forthcoming.

Yee L, Blanch H. Recombinant protein expression in high cell density fed-batch cultures of *Escherichia coli.* Biotechnology 1992;10:1550–1556.

Yoshida A, Nagata T, Uchijima M, Higashi T, Koide Y. Advantage of gene gun-mediated over intramuscular inoculation of plasmid DNA vaccine in reproducible induction of specific immune responses. Vaccine 2000;18:1725–1729.

Yuan T-F. Vaccine submission with muscle electroporation. Vaccine 2008;26:1805–1806.

Zabriskie D, Wareheim D, Polanski M. Effects of fermentation feeding strategies prior to induction of expression of a recombinant malaria antigen in *Escherichia coli*. J Indus Microbiol 1987;2:87–95.

Zhang J, Greasham R. Chemically defined media for commercial fermentations. Appl Microbiol Biotechnol 1999;51:407–421.

3

FUNGAL EXPRESSION SYSTEMS FOR VACCINE PRODUCTION

Karl Melber, Volker Jenzelewski, Roland Weyhenmeyer, and Zbigniew Janowicz
Dynavax Europe/Rhein Biotech GmbH, Düsseldorf, Germany

3.1 INTRODUCTION

Vaccines are typically developed and produced by either of two basic strategies. Live vaccines are based on nonpathogenic attenuated viruses or bacteria. In contrast, killed vaccines consist of inactivated microbes. A special form of this class represents the subunit vaccines, which contain only isolated antigens of the pathogenic microorganism. With the advent of recombinant DNA technology, it has become possible to synthesize microbial antigens independently of the pathogen's availability for vaccine development. Fungal or, to be precise, yeast expression systems have occupied a prominent role in the production of recombinant subunit vaccines against infectious diseases. This chapter gives an overview of the development of yeast-based vaccines, current production processes, regulatory requirements, and economical aspects.

Yeast-based vaccine production is essentially the success story of the recombinant hepatitis B vaccine, which was the first ever vaccine developed as a recombinant subunit vaccine. This prototype became one of the biotechnology industry's blockbuster products and in the last two decades has enabled tremendous achievement in reducing hepatitis B virus (HBV) infections worldwide. Until the recent introduction of a novel vaccine against human papillomavirus (HPV) infections, however, this remained the only yeast-based vaccine. The underlying reasons are discussed, and arguments for the further use of yeast expression technology in the field of vaccine development are summarized.

Vaccine Development and Manufacturing, First Edition.
Edited by Emily P. Wen, Ronald Ellis, and Narahari S. Pujar.

3.2 HEPATITIS B VACCINES

Hepatitis B is a blood-borne, highly contagious infection of the liver and represents one of the major human infectious diseases. Approximately 2 billion people have been infected with the HBV at some point in their lifetime (Lavanchy, 2005). A striking feature of HBV is that infection can take either an acute or a chronic course. Acute infection is typically self-limiting, although approximately 2% of acute infections lead to fulminant hepatitis, which is often fatal. Chronic infection is initially asymptomatic but after a long latency period can develop into chronic liver disease and eventually into liver cirrhosis and primary hepatocellular carcinoma (Ganem and Prince, 2004). Worldwide, more than 350 million people are chronically infected with HBV. It is estimated that the mortality because of HBV is between 500,000 and 1,000,000 per year (Lavanchy, 2005).

HBV was identified as the causative agent of serum hepatitis in the 1960s after the discovery of the Australia antigen (Blumberg et al., 1967), which turned out to be the viral envelope protein. This immediately spurred efforts to develop a protective vaccine. HBV is a small enveloped DNA virus belonging to the hepadnaviridae. The envelope of HBV consists of three hepatitis B surface antigens that are embedded into a host cell-derived lipid membrane: the major S antigen (HBsAg), which comprises 226 amino acids, and two less abundant antigens M(iddle)- and L(arge)-HBsAg, which share the C-terminal 226 amino acids with the major S antigen (Fig. 3.1). In the virion, all three surface antigens are present in a glycosylated and a nonglycosylated form. A special feature of HBV is that in infected patients not only the mature virus particles are found, but also noninfectious, subviral particles (with a diameter of 22 nm), which essentially consist of the major S antigen and lipids.

HBV could not be grown (and still is difficult to propagate) in cell culture, which represented a formidable barrier to vaccine development. Nevertheless, a first hepatitis B vaccine could be developed from the noninfectious, subviral particles abundantly

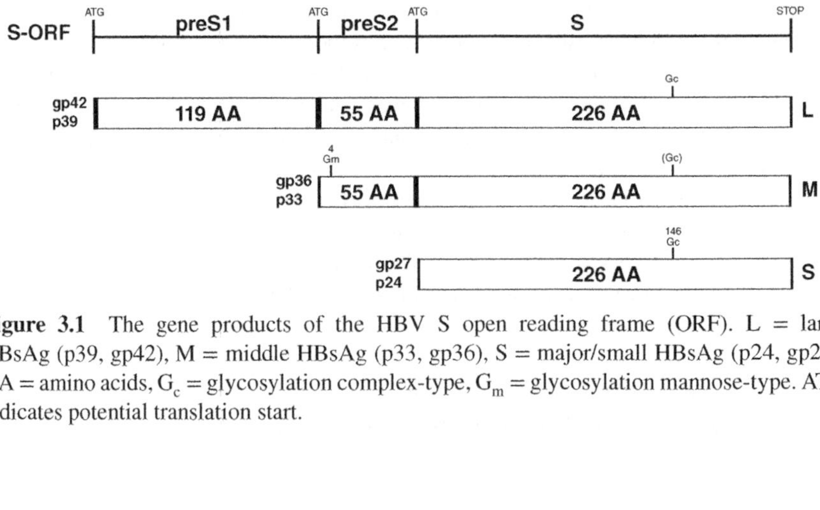

Figure 3.1 The gene products of the HBV S open reading frame (ORF). L = large HBsAg (p39, gp42), M = middle HBsAg (p33, gp36), S = major/small HBsAg (p24, gp24), AA = amino acids, G_c = glycosylation complex-type, G_m = glycosylation mannose-type. ATG indicates potential translation start.

present (>100 mg/l) in the plasma of HBV chronic carriers. The plasma-derived subviral particles were purified, and after several inactivation steps, the antigen was adsorbed to alum salt as an adjuvant. The resulting vaccine was found to be protective and safe in humans (Hilleman, 1993). The vaccine was available preferably to persons with high risk for infection. It was soon realized that the supply of suitable plasma from chronic HBV carriers would not be sufficient to meet the production needs for extended vaccination against HBV infection. Although great care was applied to inactivate adventitious viruses, the discovery of HIV at that time also raised concerns about the safety of blood-derived products. These considerations gave rise to efforts for developing a second generation vaccine using recombinant DNA technology.

HBV was cloned, and its open reading frames were expressed in *Escherichia coli* (Burrell et al., 1979; Sninsky et al., 1979). However, the expression of the S antigen proved to be difficult in this host, and only poor yields of immunogenic antigen were obtained (Burrell et al., 1979; Edman et al., 1981; MacKay et al, 1981). The assembly of S antigen into lipoprotein particles does not occur in bacterial cells, and thus, attempts to produce immunogenic HBsAg in *E. coli* have not been successful. A breakthrough in expression was achieved by demonstrating that the yeast, *Saccharomyces cerevisiae*, genetically engineered with a plasmid encoding the HBsAg gene, was not only able to synthesize the polypeptide but was also able to assemble it into lipoprotein particles that have the same morphology as those isolated from the plasma of infected patients (Valenzuela et al., 1982).

3.2.1 *Saccharomyces cerevisiae* Yeast Expression System

The baker's yeast, *S. cerevisiae*, was an obvious choice as a host organism for recombinant gene expression owing to the broad knowledge of its genetics and to the experience in industrial use. The production of foreign proteins in *S. cerevisiae* became possible by the availability of techniques for the introduction of exogenous DNA into yeast cells (Hinnen et al., 1978). The most commonly used procedure for yeast transformation is by introducing a plasmid DNA vector encoding the foreign gene of interest with suitable genetic elements guiding its expression and securing replication and segregation of the plasmid during cell proliferation. The ability to detect the successful uptake of exogenous DNA and its stable maintenance depends on the presence of a selection marker, for example, complementation of host cell auxotrophy. For expression in yeast, the HBsAg coding sequence was flanked at the 5′-terminus by a promoter derived from the yeast alcohol dehydrogenase 1 (*ADH1*) gene and at the 3′-terminus by a transcription termination/polyadenylation signal from the same gene. Proper promoter and termination signals are essential for efficient transcription in yeast (Kingsman et al., 1985). Transcription is directed by the yeast promoter, as the viral transcription initiation signal is not functional in yeast (Valenzuela et al., 1982). The resulting HBsAg expression cassette was inserted into a yeast 2-μm plasmid, which allows extrachromosomal replication and segregation during cell proliferation. This basic yeast vector further harbored the yeast *LEU2* gene as a selection marker

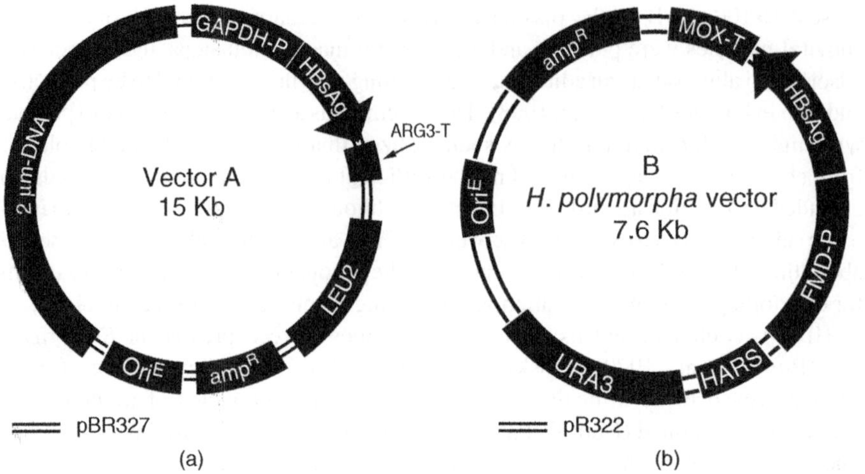

Figure 3.2 Schematic representation of yeast expression plasmids. (a) *S. cerevisiae* vector (adapted from Harford et al., 1987). (b) *H. polymorpha* vector pFPMT-Sadw2. GAPDH-P = glyceraldehyde-3′-phosphate dehydrogenase gene promoter, ARG3-T = *ARG3* gene transcription termination signal, *leu2*, *ura 3* = yeast selection markers, FMD-P = FMD-Promoter, MOX-T = *MOX* transcription termination signal, *HARS* = *Hansenula* autonomous replication sequence, amp^R = ampicillin resistance gene, ori^E = *E. coli* origin of replication.

(complementing leucine auxotrophy of the host strain) and sequences encoding a bacterial origin of replication and an antibiotic resistance marker (Valenzuela et al., 1982). Such yeast/*E. coli* shuttle vectors allow to perform the plasmid construction work in *E. coli* and heterologous gene expression in *S. cerevisiae* (Fig. 3.2a).

Similar expression constructs for HBsAg were described by other groups (Hitzeman et al., 1983; Miyanohara et al., 1983; Harford et al., 1983). The final expression vector was subsequently introduced into a leu^- host strain (carrying a mutation in the *leu2* gene). Transformants were selected in medium without leucine. Single colonies from a transformation experiment were isolated, cultured at small scale, and analyzed for the production of HBsAg. In yeast, the recombinant HBsAg was localized intracellularly (Valenzuela et al., 1982). This was in contrast to the situation in HBV-infected hepatocytes where 20-nm HBsAg particles are secreted. It was hypothesized that the yeast cell wall represents a natural barrier for secretion of HBsAg particles. However, the finding that the enzymatic removal of the cell wall and gentle lysis of HBsAg-expressing yeast cells did not release measurable amounts of HBsAg particles into the culture medium (Hitzeman et al., 1983) led to the speculation that the particles are formed *ex vivo* during disruption and homogenization of the cells. More recent studies using immunoelectron microscopy indicate that particle formation occurs in the yeast endoplasmatic reticulum and that the transport of particles along the secretion pathway is blocked (Biemans et al., 1992). All commercial production processes for HBsAg are based on intracellular expression, so far. Therefore, recovery and purification of the yeast-derived HBsAg require disruption of the cells.

The level of HBsAg expression achieved in *S. cerevisiae* was about 1–2% of the total cell protein (Burnette et al., 1985; Harford et al., 1987). The amount of total antigen synthesized correlates with the number of gene copies per cell. Plasmids of 2 μm can reach up to 100 copies per cell (Kingsman et al., 1985). In strains used for large-scale production of HBsAg, an average number of 30–40 plasmid copies per cell have been described (Harford et al., 1987). In addition, there is a direct correlation of the total amount of heterologous protein with the generated biomass. In later production strains, the *ADH1* promoter was substituted by the promoter of the glyceraldehyde-3′-dehydrogenase (*GAPDH*) gene. Both *ADH1* and *GAPDH* are constitutively expressed in yeast; however, the *GAPDH* promoter seems to be more efficient for the expression of HBsAg than the *ADH1* promoter (Valenzuela et al., 1985).

The yield of HBsAg particles from yeast also seems to depend on the conditions of cell disruption. Initially, it was found that only 2–5% of the totally generated (monomeric) HBsAg was present in the form of particles in the crude cell extract (Hitzeman et al., 1983). The recombinant HBsAg could be purified from the crude extract in form of spherical particles (containing yeast-derived lipids), with a diameter ranging from 18 to 24 nm and a buoyant density of approximately 1.2 g/mL. These particles are morphologically similar to those isolated from human plasma (Valenzuela et al., 1982; McAleer et al., 1984; Emini et al., 1986; Petre et al., 1987). SDS/PAGE (sodium dedecyl sulfate/polyacrylgelelectrophoresis) of yeast-derived HBsAg under reducing conditions revealed a major band at a molecular weight of 24 kDa corresponding to the nonglycosylated major S antigen. The yeast-derived lipids consisted mainly of phospholipids (Petre et al., 1987). In radioimmunoassays, yeast-derived HBsAg showed a reactivity of 20–50% compared to the reference antigen derived from human plasma. Immunogenicity studies in mice and chimpanzees, however, showed that the yeast-HBsAg elicited equal or even higher antibody responses compared to the licensed plasma vaccine. Most decisively, chimpanzees vaccinated with the yeast vaccine were fully protected against a challenge with the virus (McAleer et al., 1984).

The achieved expression levels in *S. cerevisiae* enabled the development of large-scale production processes. Highly purified HBsAg from yeast crude extract was obtained by various industry groups by performing a sequence of precipitation, filtration, centrifugation, and chromatography steps. Some purification schemes also include rate zonal sedimentation and/or isopycnic density gradient centrifugation.

3.2.2 Methylotrophic Yeasts

Soon after employing *S. cerevisiae* as the expression host for recombinant protein production, some general limitations of this yeast became obvious, which were not restricted to the case of HBsAg (for review see Gellissen and Hollenberg, 1997). The promoters typically used (e.g., *GAPDH* promoter) were derived from genes of the glycolytic pathway and enabled constitutive expression. A constitutive expression mode exerts negative selection pressure on cells during fermentation because of product accumulation. Plasmid loss occurs even in selective medium, resulting in instability of expression strains and product yield (Srienc et al., 1986). Alternative inducible promoters such as the one of the acid phosphatase gene (*PHO5*) that requires low phosphate levels for activity are difficult to control at a larger scale (Miyanohara et al., 1983). Those from galactose utilization genes need high amounts of expensive carbon sources for induction (McCarty et al., 1989).

These limitations and the quest for higher yields prompted the search for alternative yeasts and filamentous fungi as novel expression hosts for recombinant protein production. A focus, among others, was the presence of strong inducible promoters in such organisms, which brought the methylotrophic yeasts into the limelight. A number of yeasts belonging to the genera *Pichia*, *Hansenula*, *Candida*, and *Torulopsis* are able to grow on methanol as the sole carbon and energy source (Gleeson and Sudbery, 1988). Of these, *Hansenula polymorpha* and *Pichia pastoris* have been developed as high yield expression systems (Gellissen and Hollenberg, 1997; Cereghino and Cregg, 2000).

Both *H. polymorpha* and *P. pastoris* are taxonomically related to *S. cerevisiae* and are amenable to the genetic, biochemical, and molecular biology techniques that have been developed for *S. cerevisiae* with little or no modification. However, heterologous expression yields are often higher as demonstrated for a range of recombinant proteins (Buckholz and Gleeson, 1991). Of equal importance is the feature that both methlyotrophic yeast species easily allow integration of expression cassettes into the genome, yielding production strains that are mitotically stable under nonselective growth conditions.

3.2.2.1 Hansenula polymorpha Expression System *H. polymorpha* is a ubiquitous yeast naturally occurring in soil, the gut of various insects, spoiled orange juice, and maize meal. Besides its capability to grow on methanol, it has attracted attention because of its heat tolerance, permitting growth at temperatures until 49 C (Middelhoven 2002). It was developed as a high yield recombinant expression system and has been established for a number of industrial applications because of its high productivity, stability, and favorable fermentation characteristics (Gellissen et al., 1995).

The methanol utilization pathway is essentially similar in all methylotrophic yeasts. In *H. polymorpha*, in the first step, methanol is converted by methanol oxidase (MOX) to formaldehyde. The formaldehyde either enters the assimilatory pathway to increase biomass or is oxidized to CO_2 by a sequence of two dehydrogenase reactions to, the last step being catalyzed by formate dehydrogenase (FMD) (for a review of methanol metabolism see Yurimoto et al., 2002). In methanol-grown cultures of *H. polymorpha*, the key enzymes of the methanol metabolism are found in abundance: MOX 20–30% and FMD 10–20% of total cell protein, respectively (Gellissen et al., 1995). Significant levels of MOX and FMD are also present in glycerol-grown cells but are absent when the culture medium contains measurable amounts of glucose. This reflects a repression/derepression/induction mechanism, which depends on the carbon source available (repression on glucose, derepression on glycerol, and induction on methanol).

The production of the enzymes of the methanol utilization pathway is regulated at the transcriptional level. *MOX* and *FMD* genes have been cloned (Janowicz et al., 1985; Ledeboer et al., 1985), and their promoters were employed for the expression of heterologous proteins. For the production of HBsAg in *H. polymorpha*, a vector was constructed by positioning the DNA fragment encoding HBsAg between the *MOX* (or *FMD*) promoter and the *MOX* transcription termination signal. This expression cassette was inserted into an *E. coli*/yeast shuttle vector carrying an antibiotic resistance marker for propagation in *E. coli*, HARS1 (*Hansenula* autonomous replicating sequence) from *H. polymorpha*, and the *URA3* gene from *S. cerevisiae* as auxotrophic selection marker (Fig. 3.2b). Transformation of *H. polymorpha* with this vector and subsequent selection in culture medium lacking uracil generated strains carrying one to multiple copies integrated into the yeast genome (Janowicz et al., 1991). Integration of multiple copies (between 30 and 50) of an expression vector into the genome occurs with high frequency and is a special characteristic of *H. polymorpha*. Strains carrying high copy numbers of the expression cassette in integrated form were remarkably stable. Once selected, these strains can be grown in nonselective medium without loss of the foreign gene construct. The unusually high mitotic stability of a strain expressing HBsAg was demonstrated by Southern blot analysis after cultivation in nonselective medium for 600 generation doublings, which by far exceeds the estimated number of doublings in a production cycle from master cell bank (MCB) to cell harvest (Fig. 3.3).

Recombinant strains carrying up to 50 integrated copies of an HBsAg expression cassette were grown in a medium containing glucose, glycerol, or glycerol/methanol as the sole carbon source, and the expression level of antigen was determined.

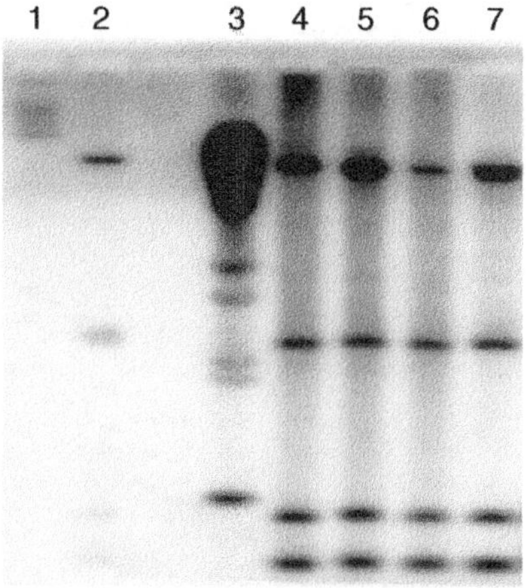

Figure 3.3 Southern blot analysis of *H. polymorpha* strain expressing HBsAg at various cultivation time points. Lane 1: expression vector, undigested; lane 2: expression vector, Asp718/SalI-digested; lane 3: molecular weight marker; lane 4: Asp718/SalI-digested DNA of *H. polymorpha* strain master seed; lane 5: Asp718/SalI-DNA at 200 generations; lane 6: Asp718/SalI-DNA at 400 generations; lane 7: Asp718/SalI-DNA at 600 generations.

When grown on glycerol and induced by methanol, HBsAg constituted between 2 and 4% of the total extracted cell protein. When grown on glycerol, only 30% of the HBsAg level compared to methanol induction is obtained. HBsAg expression could not be detected at all in glucose-grown cells, indicating that heterologous gene expression under the *MOX* (or *FMD*) promoter was controlled as expected from its repression/derepression/ induction mode. Expression studies using both *MOX* and *FMD* promoters have shown that HBsAg is produced at comparable levels (Janowicz et al., 1991). As with other heterologous genes, a copy dosage effect was observed for HBsAg expression (Janowicz et al 1991). Multicopy production strains for HBsAg of different genotype have been established and characterized. The mechanism of integration was originally thought to be a random event, but more recent studies benefiting from the availability of the complete *H. polymorpha* genome sequence indicate that integration occurs at a few specific sites (U. Dahlems, M. Suckow, Z. Janowicz; unpublished results). Owing to the mechanism of integration, the *MOX* or *FMD* genes stay intact, and their functionality is conserved.

As in *S. cerevisiae*, the major S antigen is expressed intracellularly in *H. polymorpha*, and the antigen analyzed from crude cell extracts shows the same features: high reactivity in the AUSZYME® assay indicative of conformational epitopes and formation of lipoprotein particles with a density of 1.17–1.20 g/cm^3. Electron microscopy demonstrated the presence of 20-nm particles (diameter ranging from 16 to 26 nm; Fig. 3.4).

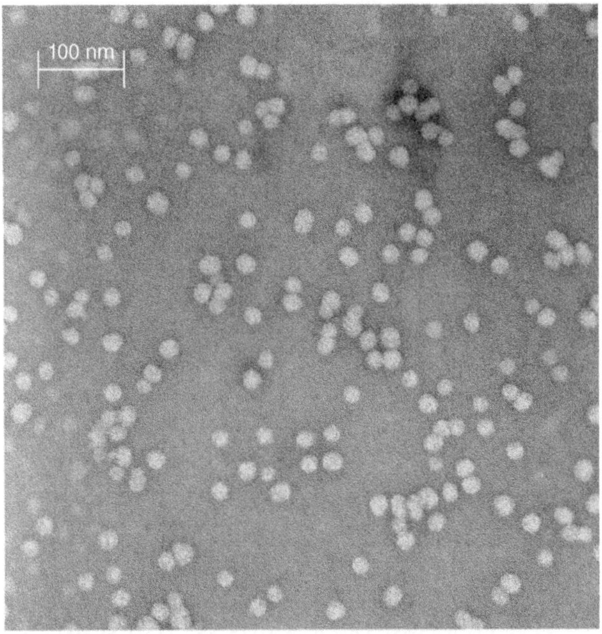

Figure 3.4 Electron microscopy of *H. polymorpha*-derived HBsAg particles.

The S antigen is synthesized as a nonglycosylated protein, with an apparent molecular weight of 24 kDa. The amino acid composition of the purified protein has been determined and was identical to that deduced from the coding gene sequence. The overall amount and composition of the *H. polymorpha*-derived lipids in the HBsAg particles closely resembled those derived from *S. cerevisiae* (Petre et al., 1987; Diminsky et al., 1997). Lipids represent roughly 30–50% of the total particle weight, and phospholipids are the main lipid component. In contrast to plasma- or mammalian cell (CHO)-derived particles, the yeast-derived HBsAg particles contain ergosterol instead of cholesterol.

The high HBsAg expression levels achieved in *H. polymorpha* may be attributable not only to the use of very strong promoter signals, but also to phenomena involving peroxisomal and membrane proliferation associated with conditions of methanol induction (Rattray and Hambleton, 1980). *H. polymorpha*-derived HBsAg shows a high degree of intramolecular and intermolecular disulfide bridging as demonstrated by determination of free thiol groups and the low amount of yeast antigen migrating at the apparent molecular weight in nonreducing SDS/PAGE (Diminsky et al., 1997). Intramolecular and intermolecular disulfide bonds appear to play a major role in the tertiary and quaternary structures of HBsAg and are crucial for antigen stability and proper epitope conformation (Dreesman et al., 1972).

3.2.2.2 ***Pichia pastoris Expression System*** Another methylotrophic yeast applied in biotechnology is *P. pastoris*. Originally, it was developed as a protein source for animal feed produced from methanol. In continuous fermentation, yields up to 130 g dry cell weight per liter can be achieved. Nowadays, it is widely used for the expression of recombinant proteins (Cereghino and Cregg, 2000). The expression and production of HBsAg have been described in this system (Cregg et al., 1987). For this purpose, an expression vector was constructed comprising the following elements: an expression cassette in which the major S antigen coding sequence was placed between the *AOX1* (alcohol oxidase 1) promoter and the transcription termination signal of the same gene; a sequence from the $3'$-downstream region of the *AOX1* termination site to enable *AOX1* gene replacement; a *Pichia* autonomous replicating sequence; *HIS4* (histidinol dehydrogenase) gene as a selectable marker for transformation of a his^- host strain; and pBR322 sequences for propagation of the construct in *E. coli*. After transformation, the expression cassette was integrated into the host genome (*AOX1* locus) via homologous recombination. This insertion led to the deletion of the *AOX1* gene. Nevertheless, slow growth on methanol was still possible because of the presence of a second *AOX2* gene. His^+ strains with impaired ability to use methanol (mut^s) were isolated and tested for HBsAg expression. In these transformants, typically one copy of the expression cassette was stably integrated into the yeast genome. Thus, in *P. pastoris* as in *H. Polymorpha*, there is no danger of plasmid loss during cultivation. The *AOX1* promoter is tightly regulated by methanol induction. Cultivation of the *P. pastoris* strain expressing HBsAg is performed as a two-step process: first, the cells are grown on a repressing carbon source (glucose or glycerol) to generate biomass; second, when the desired biomass is reached, the cells are allowed to deplete the repressing carbon source, and methanol is added to "switch on" the *AOX 1* promoter. For high level expression of HBsAg, the cells were first fermented on glycerol, and subsequently on depletion of glycerol, methanol was added continuously at 0.5% (w/v) for 200 h (Cregg et al., 1987). In contrast to the situation in *H. polymorpha*, in *P. pastoris*, growth on glycerol as the sole carbon source does not derepress *AOX1* promoter-regulated expression. In this fermentation, a final dry cell weight of 59 g/l and a productivity of 0.4 g HBsAg per liter were described. HBsAg was reported to constitute 3–4% of the total soluble protein and 2–3% of total soluble protein assembled into 20-nm particles (Cregg et al., 1987). It was argued that the slow growth rate in methanol because of the poor efficiency of the *AOX2* gene may account for the higher rate of particle formation. However, the experience with *H. polymorpha* with its much shorter fermentation/induction time schedule contradicts that point (see Large-scale manufacturing). The Pichia system has proven to be a powerful tool for the expression of antigens and proteins in general. The requirement of large amounts of methanol for induction, however, poses a technical challenge for up-scaling of the fermentation process.

3.2.3 Large-Scale Production of HBsAg in Yeast and Regulatory Aspects

HBsAg is produced for commercial vaccines in both *S. cerevisiae* and *H. polymorpha* for worldwide markets. Manufacturing is also established with *P. pastoris* for local markets. The various production processes have many similarities owing to the use of yeast as the common production host. The general outline is described in the following section, with some differences in notable details addressed.

3.2.4 Cell Bank System

For pharmaceutical manufacturing of HBsAg using yeast, a cell bank system is used (Stephenne, 1990; Elliott et al., 1994). Cell banks represent a collection of vials with well-defined and uniform composition. On the basis of the characteristics of individual transformed colonies, a clone with high expression level is chosen for large-scale production. From this clone, a MCB is prepared after expansion in liquid culture by aliquoting the cell suspension in vials that are stored at temperatures of −60 C or below. All the components used for establishing the MCB must be documented in detail: cell substrate (expression vector, source, lineage and characterization of the yeast host strain, procedures for transformation, and propagation), culture medium, containers, and storage conditions. Cryoprotectants such as glycerol (10–50% final concentration) are used to minimize freeze-thaw stress to the cells and to increase the recovery of viable cells from the cell bank. For characterization of the MCB viability of the cell substrate, presence and functionality of the expression construct, genetic stability (copy number of integrated expression cassettes for methylotrophic yeasts or plasmid copy number for *S. cerevisiae*, respectively), and microbial purity are determined. Characterization is to be performed according to documented and established procedures. Since the MCB is considered to be the crucial biological starting material for manufacturing, maintenance of its integrity is of utmost importance during the life cycle of the vaccine product. Typically, one vial of the MCB is subsequently expanded in liquid culture, aliquoted into individual vials, and stored frozen to provide a working cell bank (WCB). This WCB is characterized in terms of identity, purity, and content (i.e., cell viability), with a subset of methods employed for the MCB. Regulatory authorities request production of the WCB under Good Manufacturing Practice (GMP) as well as a strict documentation of the use, location, and disposition of all cell bank supplies. A cell bank system has to assure the availability and consistency of the starting material for manufacturing of the product during its entire life cycle. As mentioned previously, yeast strains with expression constructs stably integrated into their genome may offer an advantage over episomal expression vectors. It should be noted that loss or damage to the MCB will require preparation of a new cell bank. This may necessitate repetition of at least part of the clinical development for the product.

3.2.5 Cultivation/Fermentation

S. cerevisiae. The biomass required for one production cycle is generated from one or a few vials of the WCB. The yeast cells are grown in a shake-flask culture or a small fermenter, and cultivation proceeds in fermenters (typically, stirred-tank bioreactors) with increasing volumes 5- to 20-fold at each step depending on the scale of the production fermenter ("fermentation train"). For a commercial production process in *S. cerevisiae*, 20- and 300-l seed fermenters and a 1500-l production fermenter have been described (Stephenne, 1990). The total propagation of the cell substrate including the 1500-l fermentation takes 1 week. Fermentation is accomplished using a defined medium (lacking leucine to maintain selective pressure in the leu^- host strain) and operated in a fed-batch mode, that is, nutrients are fed to the culture in a way ensuring steady cell growth and antigen production. In the fed-batch fermentation mode, high cell densities of 50–60 g/l were described (Schulman et al., 1991). As the promoters typically used in *S. cerevisiae* are derived from constitutive glycolytic genes, the fermentation process is straightforward in that the expression of HBsAg simply parallels the utilization of glucose, and the increase of biomass. *S. cerevisiae*-based expression relies on episomal plasmids and, therefore, bears the risk of plasmid loss especially under conditions of high cell density fermentation. Excessive plasmid loss can lead to low expression yields and problems in downstream processing. In order to minimize this risk, in-process controls are performed for monitoring plasmid retention. In addition, the identity of the host strain (presence of auxotrophic marker) is confirmed. The final harvest of the fermentation culture is also tested for microbial purity. It has been described that such assays can detect <100 contaminating organisms per milliliter of fermentation culture (Elliott et al., 1994). Yeast-based production systems inherently do not bear the risk of contamination with human or animal viruses, and thus, do not require specific testing in this respect.

H. polymorpha/P. pastoris. The fermentation process for the methylotrophic yeasts is dependent on efficient methanol induction. Both *H. polymorpha* and *P. pastoris* strains can be cultivated in defined synthetic medium under nonselective conditions using glycerol as carbon source for the initial build-up of biomass. For *H. polymorpha*-based production, a 5-l seed and a 50-l production fermenter are commercially used (Schaefer et al., 2002). Another manufacturing process proceeds from shake-flask cultivation to a 30-l seed and 300-l production fermenter. The seed fermentation is performed within 2 days in a batch mode without oxygen limitation. The production fermentation is conducted in a two-carbon-source mode (Fig. 3.5). Cultivation is started with glycerol in fed-batch mode followed by semicontinuous glycerol feeding controlled by dissolved oxygen level. Thus, low glycerol concentrations are maintained, allowing for derepression of the *MOX* (or *FMD*) promoter. For the short (overnight) induction period, methanol is added batch wise (at 5–10 g/l final concentration), which substantially increases HBsAg expression level. In this production, fermentation 100 g dry cell weight and 0.4 g HBsAg/ll are generated after less than 70 h (Schaefer et al., 2002). During fermentation, pH, temperature, dissolved oxygen level, and aeration are monitored and controlled. Microscopic examination, turbidity measurements, and dry cell weight determinations are carried out off-line as in-process controls. In addition, microbial purity is tested in the end of production cells. For establishing a commercial production process, the stability of the integrated expression construct in the *H. polymorpha* strain had to be demonstrated. Analysis of end of production cells showed that the integrated expression construct (structural arrangement, copy number) was not changed compared to the master seed. Thus, *H. polymorpha* strains are well suited for robust large-scale fermentation.

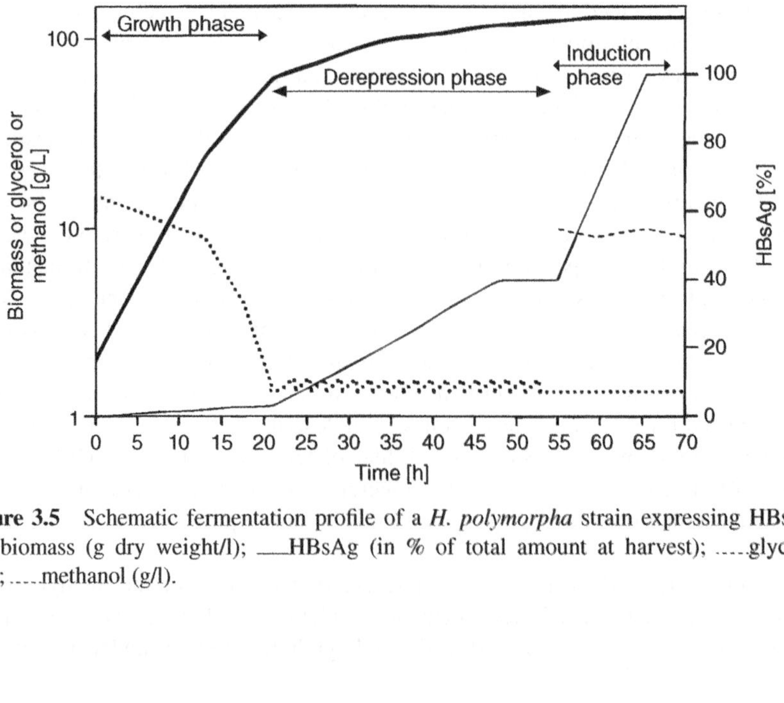

Figure 3.5 Schematic fermentation profile of a *H. polymorpha* strain expressing HBsAg. ___ biomass (g dry weight/l); ___HBsAg (in % of total amount at harvest); .....glycerol (g/l); .....methanol (g/l).

For *P. pastoris* a two-step fermentation process at a 200-l scale has been described for prototype production of HBsAg (Cregg et al., 1987). In a fed-batch system using glycerol as a carbon source, the desired cell density was achieved. On complete depletion of glycerol, the fermentation culture is shifted to methanol as the sole carbon source. Owing to the low growth rate of the strain under these conditions, 200 h of continuous methanol feeding was required to achieve maximum expression rate. A production process at a 3000-l scale has been described (Hardy et al., 2000) using a strain, which also expressed HBsAg under control of the *AOX1* promoter. Dry cell weights of 75–88 g/l and HBsAg expression levels of 1.5% of total cell protein were achieved.

3.2.6 Purification of HBsAg/Downstream Processing

Cell Harvest. The yeast cells are harvested from the fermentation culture, medium components removed from the cells, and exchanged against a buffer appropriate for cell breakage. For large-scale purposes, continuous centrifugation or tangential flow filtration are the preferred methods used.

Cell Disruption. The yeast cell wall, especially that of cells cultivated in methanol, is very robust (much more than the bacterial cell wall), and, hence, breaking of this structure is a critical step for satisfactory product recovery. Two mechanical methods are applied for yeast cell disruption: grinding in a glass bead-mill (Stephenne, 1990; Hardy et al., 2000) and high pressure homogenization (Schaefer et al., 2002). Owing to the considerable energy input for cell disruption, efficient temperature control of the cell suspension/crude extract is necessary. Although both techniques result in a crude extract suitable for further HBsAg purification and are being used for large-scale commercial production, the use of high pressure homogenization offers some advantage compared to grinding. First, the amount of product released per gram of dry cells can be substantially higher using a homogenizer compared to grinding (M. Weniger, V. Jenzelewski, Z. Janowicz; unpublished data). Pressures of >1000 bars for homogenization are efficient for yeast. Second, the effectiveness of the grinding process depends strongly on the quality of the glass beads. In addition, heat dissipation gets difficult with increasing volume size of the grinding chamber. For any of the disruption methods used, the buffer system may be supplemented with inhibitors to block intracellular proteases, which are released together with the product. Also, the addition of a mild, nonionic detergent facilitates the release of 20-nm lipoprotein particles in the crude cell extract.

Purification. The development of a technical scale purification scheme yielding pharmaceutical quality HBsAg particles from yeast extract is challenging because of the lipoprotein nature of HBsAg particles and the diverse constituents of the crude cell extract. Cell disruption generates a crude extract that is highly heterogeneous in composition: a low percentage of more or less intact cells, a mass of cell debris of varying shapes and sizes as well as dissolved proteins, carbohydrates, lipids, and

DNA. For purification, the unique physicochemical properties of the HBsAg particles (size, buoyant density, charge, hydrophobicity, and affinity interaction) are used.

S. cerevisiae. For commercial vaccines based on *S. cerevisiae* as the expression host, HBsAg purification processes have been described in some detail. One of these purification schedules starts with disruption of the yeast cells and antigen extraction in the presence of a detergent followed by two precipitation steps to eliminate cell debris and the bulk of impurities. After centrifugation and ultrafiltration of the supernatant, the process volume is sufficiently reduced to allow the subsequent steps at a convenient volume (10-l scale). This purification cascade uses gel filtration and anion exchange chromatography. The eluate is further subjected to isopycnic ultracentrifugation in cesium chloride gradients (Petre et al., 1987; Stephenne, 1990). The HBsAg particles band at a density of approximately 1.2 g/cm^3. This band is harvested, desalted, and sterile filtered. The complete purification process takes 1 week. Another commercial process follows a slightly different scheme using nonimmune affinity chromatography, hydrophobic interaction chromatography (butyl agarose), and gel filtration (the latter is omitted in a more recent process design) for purification (Emini et al., 1986; Elliott et al., 1994). As a notable difference compared to the process described previously, the purified antigen is chemically disassembled and reassembled using thiocyanate (Wampler et al., 1985; Elliott et al. 1994). In this instance, the HBsAg particles are present in the crude extract in a form in which the antigen is linked only to a low degree by disulfide bonds. The reassembly step maximizes the intramolecular and intermolecular disulfide bonds of HBsAg within the lipoprotein particle. These HBsAg particles show improved stability and immunogenicity compared to the untreated antigen. Other manufacturers do not use a disassembly/reassembly strategy but, nevertheless, obtain stable and highly immunogenic HBsAg particles. Some manufacturers subject the purified antigen to mild formalin treatment (Emini et al., 1986; Elliott et al., 1994). This is not aimed at inactivation of contaminating microbes but rather to introduce further cross-linking of HBsAg, which may improve stability.

H. polymorpha. For *H. polymorpha*-based production, a purification process has been described on the basis of a 50-l fermentation scale (Fig. 3.6; Schaefer et al., 2002). After high pressure homogenization of the yeast cells, the crude cell extract is subjected to polyethylene glycol precipitation. Solid–liquid phase separation is facilitated by the use of a continuous high speed centrifuge with automated solid harvest, allowing for closed operation throughout the complete purification process. This clarification step results in a drastic reduction of cell debris and yeast host cell protein. The cleared supernatant is subsequently adsorbed to a silica gel matrix, washed, and desorbed by pH and temperature shifts. This is followed by anion exchange chromatography in order to remove further host cell and process-derived impurities. After volume reduction by ultrafiltration, the product is subjected to isopycnic cesium chloride ultracentrifugation. The HBsAg band is harvested from the gradients manually or using an automatic device. Finally, the cesium chloride

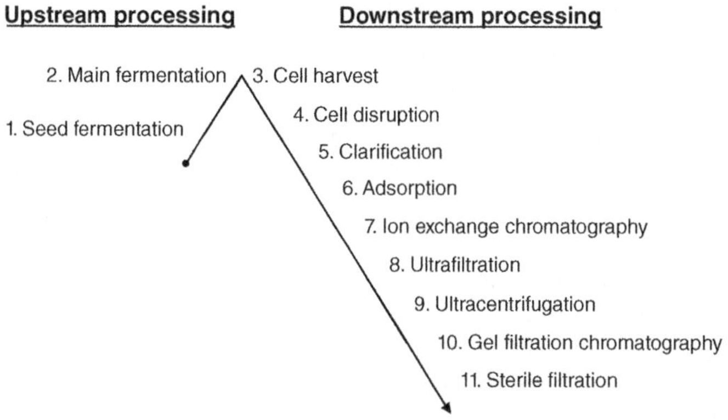

Figure 3.6 Production process for recombinant HBsAg in *H. polymorpha*.

is removed by gel filtration, and the HBsAg particles are diluted with buffer to a concentration that is suitable for storage.

P. pastoris. Large-scale purification of HBsAg has been described for a *P. pastoris*-based process at a 3000-l fermentation scale (Hardy et al., 2000). After disruption of the cells in a glass bead-mill, the crude extract was supplemented with thiocyanate-containing buffer (probably to increase HBsAg disulfide linkage for better immunogenicity) and subjected to acid precipitation by shifting the pH from 8 to 4.5. The precipitate was removed by centrifugation, and the clarified supernatant was subjected to batch adsorption at acidic pH onto diacetameceous earth matrix. The adsorbed HBsAg is eluted from the matrix at low ionic strength and basic pH. Further purification of the HBsAg was performed by subsequent immunoaffinity (using a monoclonal anti-HBs antibody), ion-exchange, and size-exclusion chromatographies.

In summary, the various processes described often employ similar purification modules, albeit in different sequence and combination. All processes aim at a purification strategy employing orthogonal purification methodology to ensure an efficient and robust purification of the antigen from the complex matrix of the crude extract. The design and implementation of individual large-scale purification schemes essentially depend on the following:

- productivity of the expression host (amount of HBsAg expressed per cell);
- production scale (i.e., number of antigen doses per production run).

More specific parameters are the following:

- the efficiency of yeast cell disruption;
- the efficiency of HBsAg extraction;

- the degree of HBsAg disulfide linkage;
- step recovery of purification methods used;
- presence of host cell-derived impurities copurifying with HBsAg;
- necessity to remove process-derived impurities (e.g., detergents, polyethylene glycol, thiocyanate, protease inhibitors, formaldehyde, chromatography matrix compounds, antibodies).

For registration and licensing of the vaccine, the respective regulations of current GMP (cGMP) must be met. A prerequisite for GMP compliant manufacturing is a properly designed, qualified, and maintained manufacturing facility. For production of recombinant antigens, the facility design and operation are following the same scheme as typically applied for pharmaceutical recombinant proteins. Manufacturing of recombinant subunit vaccines can be divided into two main parts: (1) manufacturing of the antigen bulk that represents the active pharmaceutical ingredient of the vaccine and (2) manufacturing of the formulated vaccine bulk (drug substance) and filling/packaging of the final vaccine for marketing (drug product). The complete manufacturing process has to be validated, as it is performed according to written procedures in established and qualified facilities. As a prerequisite for registration of the vaccine product, it is crucial to demonstrate lot-to-lot consistency of the established production process at the final stage for at least three production runs.

3.2.7 Quality Control and Analytical Methods

Ph. Eur. requires that HBsAg is characterized by amino acid composition, partial amino acid sequencing, peptide mapping, lipid and carbohydrate structure, electron microscopy, buoyant density, and epitope characterization. Routinely, individual antigen batches have to be tested for the following:

- protein content;
- antigenicity;
- identity (Western blot);
- protein purity (SDS/PAGE or (high-performance liquid chromatography) HPLC; not less than 95%; larger than or equal to 95% of total protein should consist of HBsAg);
- lipid content;
- carbohydrate content;
- cesium (if used during the purification process); and
- sterility.

SDS-PAGE analysis of recombinant purified final bulk antigen using reducing conditions shows the major S antigen band of 24 kDa and minor bands representing dimeric and trimeric forms of HBsAg as well as higher mobility forms. It was demonstrated that these higher mobility forms are also present in plasma-derived

HBsAg (Elliott et al. 1994). Specific impurity testing may be required depending on the purification process used. For example, one manufacturer has described copurification of a 60-kDa *S. cerevisiae* protein together with HBsAg, which is measured by size-exclusion HPLC (Elliott et al., 1994). The safety profile of the yeast-derived antigen is perceived superior compared to the plasma-derived antigen, and tedious validation of removal and inactivation of adventitious viruses and other pathogens is not needed (Elliott et al., 1994). The common specifications and quality criteria for yeast-derived HBsAg for use in humans in addition to Ph. Eur. are outlined in WHO Technical Report Series 786 (WHO Expert Committee on Biological Standardization, 1989).

3.2.8 Formulation

HBsAg is formulated with an adjuvant for use as a hepatitis B vaccine. For this purpose, the HBsAg may be adsorbed to aluminum salts, for example, aluminum hydroxide (recently, aluminum has been supplemented or replaced by novel, more potent adjuvants; see Outlook on HBV vaccines). Care must be taken to ensure that all antigens are completely bound to the surface of the aluminum hydroxide. The adsorption process is influenced by the source of the aluminum salt and the buffer system used. The amount of antigen for a single human (adult) dose is typically 20 μg (Engerix-B®, Hepavax-Gene®, AgB®, Gene-Vac B®), except for Recombivax HB®, which uses 10 μg per adult dose. The respective dosages were independently established in clinical studies (Zajac et al., 1986; Ellis, 1993; André, 1989).

Until recently, a preservative (thimerosal) was added to the vaccine formulation. However, improvements in aseptic manufacturing have enabled the major suppliers of hepatitis B vaccines to omit mercury-containing preservatives, which are a health concern particularly for use in newborns (points to consider on the reduction, elimination, or substitution of thimerosal in vaccines; EMEA CPMP 2517/00; April 26, 2001).

3.2.9 Quality Control for Final Vaccine

For the formulated vaccine protein and aluminum content, pyrogenicity, and *in vivo* potency are determined. For some vaccines, strong binding of the antigen to aluminum does not allow its identification by SDS-PAGE, Western blot, or ELISA. Here, *in vivo* potency may also serve as an identity test. Potency is determined as ED_{50} (vaccine dilution, which yields an anti-HBsAg antibody response in 50% of immunized animals as determined by anti-HBsAg immunoassay) relative to a reference standard. Recently, efforts were made to replace the *in vivo* assay by *in vitro* methods (antigenicity by ELISA), if the antigen can be reliably dissociated from aluminum. For substitution of the *in vivo* assay, a convincing correlation between both assays has to be shown (I. Collaborative Study for the Establishment of Biological Reference Preparations for rDNA Hepatitis B Vaccine. *Pharm Eur* Special Issue, BIO 97–2, p3–18). If used for production, free formaldehyde and thimerosal have to be quantified. These tests are complemented by the general assays required for parenteral vaccines such as appearance, pH, and sterility.

3.2.10 Clinical Experience and Vaccine Products

In clinical studies, the yeast-derived vaccines were demonstrated to be safe and well tolerated. Analogous to the plasma-derived vaccine, the recombinant vaccine was administered in three doses at 0, 1, and 6 months and found to be highly immunogenic with seroprotection rates ranging from 90 to 100% in adults, adolescents, and children (Ellis, 1993; Assad and Francis, 1999). Initially, there was a theoretical concern regarding the potential for allergenic reactions because of residual *S. cerevisiae* impurities. Such yeast-associated effects could have been enhanced because of the adsorption to alum adjuvant. This potential was assessed during clinical trials by determining the increase or de-novo induction of yeast-specific antibodies in vaccines and correlation with any reported hypersensitivity reaction. No relationship or adverse events because of yeast-associated contaminants were found (Petre et al., 1987; Elliott et al., 1994).

S. cerevisiae-derived vaccines Recombivax HB and Engerix-B were licensed in 1986 and subsequently registered and marketed worldwide. In Japan, Bimmugen®, another *S. cerevisiae*-derived vaccine, was licensed. In the following, *H. polymorpha*-based vaccines have been developed. Clinical studies were performed comparing the *H. polymorpha*-derived vaccines with previously licensed vaccines produced in *S. cerevisiae* (Hieu et al, 2002). These studies demonstrated that the *H. polymorpha*-derived vaccines were well tolerated and as immunogenic as the standard vaccines demonstrating that human vaccines can be produced safely in this yeast species. Several *H. polymorpha*-derived vaccines are now manufactured in Korea (Hepavax-Gene, licensed in >90 countries in Europe, Asia, and Latin America), Argentina (AgB), and India (Gene Vac-B®). Hepatitis B vaccines derived from *P. pastoris* have been developed in Cuba (Heberbiovac®) and India (Shanvac™) for local markets.

3.2.11 PreS-HBsAg-Containing Vaccine Candidates

The envelope of HBV contains three related surface antigens: the major HBsAg (S), middle (M) HBsAg (preS2 + S), and large (L) HBsAg (preS2 + preS2 + S) (Fig. 3.1). The preS domain containing antigens attracted considerable interest owing to their strong immunogenic properties and putative role in resolution of acute HBV infection (Budkowska et al., 1986; Milich et al., 1986; Itoh et al., 1986; Neurath et al., 1989). Although the vaccines containing only the major S antigen induced protective immune responses in the vast majority of vaccinated individuals, nonresponsiveness to the licensed vaccine was reported for a few percent in the general population (Craven et al., 1986) and considerably higher in certain specific populations, for example, hemodialysis patients (Jilg et al., 1986) and elderly people (Cook et al., 1987). Therefore, M and L antigens were expressed in mammalian cells, insect cells, and yeast used to develop an improved vaccine for these target groups.

3.2.12 Expression of M- and L-HBsAg Separately

For expression of M and L antigens in *S. cerevisiae*, the respective coding sequences were initially placed under control of the constitutive *GAPDH* promoter (Valenzuela et al., 1985; Imamura et al., 1987; Langley et al., 1988). This approach typically resulted in a single primary translation product confirming that in yeast only the ATG codon adjacent to the promoter region is recognized within an open reading frame. Although the M antigen was assembled into 20-nm particles, which were similar to those obtained with the major S antigen, a number of problems were encountered. The yeast M antigen was hyperglycosylated at amino acid Asn 4 of the preS2 region, which raised concerns about potential detrimental effects in humans. In addition, the M antigen was highly sensitive to proteolytic degradation. Purified M antigen particles elicited antibodies against the preS2 domain in animals; however, overall immunogenicity was low compared to the major S antigen (Petre et al., 1992). Efforts were taken to adapt the yeast expression system to improve the quality of the expressed M antigen. In order to minimize proteolytic degradation, M antigen was expressed in a protease-deficient *S. cerevisiae* strain yielding better recovery of full-length protein (Langley et al., 1988). In order to avoid hyperglycosylation, a mutant *S. cerevisiae* strain (*mnn9*) was used (Ip et al., 1992). A drawback for industrial application of such mutant yeast strains, however, is their impaired growth characteristic.

Expression of L-HBsAg was difficult to achieve under constitutive conditions because of a deleterious effect of the antigen to the *S. cerevisiae* host cell (Kniskern et al., 1988). Therefore, regulable promoters such as *PHO5* (Dehoux et al., 1986) and *ADH2* (active in the absence of glucose) were used (Kniskern et al., 1988). These efforts improved growth rates of the transformed yeast cells and resulted in the expression of a nonglycosylated 39-kDa protein. Although antigenic reactivity for preS1, preS2, and S domains could be detected in crude extracts, the L antigen did not form typical 20-nm particles, and recovery was low.

3.2.13 Simultaneous Expression of Mixed S/M, S/L, and S/M/L Particles

Attempts were made to generate mixed particles composed of S + M, S + L, or S + M + L antigens. The feasibility of such an approach could be demonstrated by the generation of mixed particles in *S. cerevisiae* based on Ty1(yeast transposon 1) integrative vectors carrying the respective coding sequences under control of the *GAPDH* promoter. The formation of S/L and S/M/L particles was detected in cell lysates of respective strains as indicated by cobanding of pre-S1, preS2, and S-specific antibody reactivity in density gradient fractions of approximately 1.2 g/cm^3 (Jacobs et al., 1989). These mixed particles were detectable only when the antigens were expressed simultaneously in the same cell, but not when cell lysates from strains expressing S, M, or L antigen separately were mixed. However, owing to the high frequency of homologous recombination in *S. cerevisiae,* strains harboring integrated multicopy expression cassettes have not been practical for production purposes. A technical solution was offered by the use of the methylotrophic yeast, *H. polymorpha*, in which coexpression of two foreign gene products based on integrated multicopy gene constructs has been demonstrated for industrial use (Gellissen and Hollenberg, 1997). *H. polymorpha* strains expressing L or L/S antigens (under control of *MOX* and/or *FMD* promoters) were generated (Janowicz et al.; 1991). Mixed L + S particles were formed when L antigen was coexpressed with the major S antigen, but not when L antigen was expressed alone. The unique mitotic stability and the possibility of integrating multiple copies (until 50) of different expression cassettes into the genome offered a means to select strains, which synthesize HBsAg particles with defined ratio of L and S antigens.

In an alternative approach, the L antigen was modified by removing specific sequences (glycosylation and protease cleavage sites, and sequences suspected to be immunosuppressive), whereas retaining sequences assumed to be key for immunogenicity (B- and T-cell epitopes). The selected preS1 and preS2 regions were fused to the major S antigen, generating a coding sequence designated L* (Petre et al., 1992). L* was coexpressed with the major S antigen in *S. cerevisiae*. Mixed particles were formed containing about 25% of L* and 75% of S antigen. These S,L* particles were highly immunogenic and induced anti-S and anti-preS antibodies in animals. S,L* particles are currently tested in clinical trials in combination with novel adjuvant systems for eliciting more potent cellular and humoral immune responses compared to the licensed vaccines (Vandepapelière et al., 2005).

3.2.14 Outlook on HBV Vaccines

Hepatitis B vaccination has dramatically reduced the number of new HBV infections in countries with implemented pediatric vaccination programs. Twenty-five years after the first licensing of a hepatitis B vaccine, its impact is best evidenced by the significant decline of HBV-associated liver cancer (Huang and Lin, 2000). Thus, the hepatitis B vaccine was also the first prophylactic vaccine against cancer. Nevertheless, owing to the chronic nature of HBV infection, continuing vaccination efforts are required worldwide to prevent HBV infection and its sequelae.

Efforts to improve on current hepatitis B vaccines are ongoing. Mammalian cell-derived vaccines containing preS antigens have been developed and tested in the clinic. Novel vaccines including L, M, and S antigens showed superior immunogenicity in terms of faster induction of protective antibody titers and higher response rate and allowed for shorter, two-dose vaccination schedule (Raz et al., 2001; Zuckerman et al., 2001). However, their large-scale production and stability remain challenging. As the market price for mammalian cell-derived vaccines would be significantly higher, the yeast-derived HBV vaccines are still preferred for vaccination programs worldwide. Recently, pediatric pentavalent and hexavalent combination vaccines, which rely on the yeast-derived HBsAg, were developed and licensed (Mallet et al., 2004; Zepp et al., 2004).

Considerable progress in vaccine development came from the availability of novel adjuvants (e.g., toll-like receptor [TLR] agonists). Many of these have been tested together with HBsAg as a vaccine antigen. Novel hepatitis B vaccines containing monophosphoryl lipid A (an agonist of TLR4) or immunostimulatory CpG-motif oligonucleotides (TLR9 agonist) were demonstrated to provide faster protection in general and improved efficacy in dialysis patients and older people (Tong et al., 2005; Dupont et al., 2006; Higgins et al., 2007).

3.3 HUMAN PAPILLOMAVIRUS VACCINE

HPVs are a major cause of sexually transmitted infections worldwide (Trottier and Franco, 2006). Although the vast majority of genital HPV infections is without symptoms and is self-limiting, persistent infection can cause cervical cancer in women and other types of anogenital cancers and genital warts in both men and women. Of the approximately 100 different HPV types known, more than 40 infect the genital area. These are classified according to their epidemiological association with cervical cancer. While low risk types (e.g., HPV6 and 11) cause benign genital warts, the high risk types (e.g., HPV16 and 18) are responsible for cervical and anogenital cancer. Infection with HPV is shielded from the host immune response because of restriction to the epithelium. Humoral and cellular immune responses against HPVs can be detected, but no correlates of protective immunity have been established (Stanley et al., 2006). HPVs are nonenveloped, double-stranded DNA viruses. Their shell is composed of a major L1 and a minor L2 capsid protein. As HPVs cannot be propagated in cell culture, vaccine development had to rely on recombinant DNA technology. However, owing to the absence of cross-reactivity of the major L1 capsid between the various HPV types, the development of a protective subunit vaccine seemed challenging.

Expression studies in yeast, insect, and plant cells demonstrated that L1 protein self-assembles into virus-like particles (VLPs) (Kirnbauer et al., 1993). The availability of VLPs (of HPV and animal papillomaviruses) enabled studies that revealed that L1-based VLPs might act as a protective antigen in humans. As the number of L1 antigens in a vaccine should be kept within a practical range, the vaccine composition was designed to protect against the predominant HPV types. Epidemiological data showed that approximately 70% of cervical cancers are associated with HPV types 16 and 18 and that the majority of genital warts is caused by types 6 and 11. Therefore, a quadrivalent vaccine design was adopted as having the greatest impact on HPV-related disease. *S. cerevisiae* was selected as the expression system for large-scale production. Expression vectors were constructed to allow regulated expression of L1 protein by galactose induction (*GAL1* promoter) (Hofmann et al., 1995). This choice was certainly favored by the previous experience of the developing company with *S. cerevisiae* in large-scale fermentation and production of HBsAg particles. It also shows that the obstacles of *S. cerevisiae* in terms of using episomal vectors can be satisfactorily handled, whereas the use of a regulated promoter element is a clear asset for process design. Using four plasmids encoding L1 of HPV types 6, 11, 16, and 18, individual *S. cerevisiae* production strains were obtained. Fermentation is performed in a chemically defined culture medium. L1 protein is expressed by galactose induction on glucose depletion. The L1-VLPs are formed intracellularly, released by cell disruption, and purified by a series of chemical and physical methods. Purification includes a VLP disassembly/reassembly step for HPV 6, 11, and 16 types, which is achieved by altering salt concentrations. Polysorbate 80 and high salt concentration are employed for long-term VLP stabilization in solution and to prevent aggregation. The four different L1-VLPs are adsorbed to amorphous aluminum hydroxyphosphate sulfate as an adjuvant and combined for the final quadrivalent vaccine (Bryan, 2007). A major hurdle in development of a prophylactic HPV vaccine was the clinical trial design. A combination of antibody immunoassays and histological assessment of cervical biopsies was employed for evaluating vaccine efficacy. When administered at three doses (at 0, 2, and 6 months) in young women, 100% efficacy (absence of persistent infection) was demonstrated against the vaccine HPV types 6,11, 16, and 18 (Bryan, 2007). The vaccine (Gardasil®) was licensed in 2006 and contains 20 μg HPV 6 L1, 40 μg HPV11 L1, 40 μg HPV16 L1, and 20 μg HPV18 L1 protein per dose. HPV vaccines are essentially viewed as a prophylaxis against cervical cancer and are expected to significantly reduce the HPV-related disease burden. This HPV vaccine not only is another example for the feasibility of recombinant subunit vaccines, but also confirms that yeast is a robust and efficient production system for complex biochemical structures such as VLPs.

3.4 MALARIA VACCINE CANDIDATES

Malaria, a parasitic infection caused by several species of *Plasmodium*, is a major cause for mortality in the tropic world regions. Owing to the complexity of the parasite and its life cycle, the development of a vaccine for malaria prevention is a major challenge. A number of candidate antigens from *Plasmodium falciparum*, which cause most of malaria mortality, were identified that represent targets of different stages of the life cycle. All these candidate antigens were successfully expressed in various expression systems including yeasts.

The most advanced malaria vaccine candidate so far is RTS,S produced in *S. cerevisiae* (Ballou et al., 2004). This vaccine candidate is based on parts of the circumsporozoit protein (CSP) of *P. falciparum*. The protein's tetrapeptide repeat motif and the carboxyl-terminal region are combined and fused to HBsAg. This hybrid fusion protein is coexpressed together with HBsAg in the same way as described previously for preS-containing hepatitis B vaccines. HBsAg particles were previously established as a potent vaccine antigen with proven safety and have been propagated as antigen carrier for heterologous vaccines. Coexpression in the same yeast cell leads to the formation of composite particles containing both hybrid RTS and unfused S antigen. RTS,S shows much better immunogenicity as the recombinant CSP alone. The hybrid RTS,S antigen was complemented by a potent adjuvant, AS02 (oil-in-water emulsion containing MPL® and QS21 immunostimulants). RTS,S/AS02 was demonstrated to be safe and immunogenic in several clinical trials. Vaccine efficacy, that is, protection from infection, is estimated to be approximately 70% during the first 9 weeks after vaccination but wanes subsequently. Nevertheless, in the malaria field, this is considered a remarkable achievement and spurs hopes that finally a fully protective vaccine can be developed.

3.5 HIV VACCINE CANDIDATES

A number of HIV gene products, primarily those encoded by the env and gag genes, have been successfully expressed in the yeast *S. cerevisiae* as potential components of an HIV vaccine (Barr et al., 1987; Vlasuk et al., 1989). However, similar to the instance of gp120, antigens produced in mammalian cells were preferred for use in human clinical trials. Others such as yeast-derived p55 did not elicit protective immunity in primate models (Emini et al., 1990) and were not pursued further. Another approach was based on HIV-1 p17/p24:Ty VLPs produced in *S. cerevisiae*. The yeast retrotransposon Ty encodes a capsid protein, which forms VLPs. This vaccine candidate contained parts of the HIV gag sequence (carboxy-terminal p17 and amino-terminal p24) fused to the Ty capsid protein which was assembled into VLPs for improved antigen presentation. Although this therapeutic vaccine candidate induced anti-p24 antibodies and proliferative T-cell responses in HIV-negative individuals, no anti-p24 antibodies were elicited in HIV-positive volunteers, and no therapeutic effect was observed (Lindenburg et al., 2002). This drawback is definitely owed to the inherent problems of vaccine development against HIV rather than a failure of the yeast-derived VLP antigen. The fact that the yeast-derived VLPs were highly immunogenic in healthy individuals is just another example demonstrating the merits of yeast as a host organism when it comes to expression and production of complex antigens.

3.6 VETERINARY VACCINES

The veterinary field offers a creative setting for vaccine research, and a number of recombinant vaccine products have been developed. One of these is manufactured in yeast: a vaccine against cattle tick (*Boophilus microplus*). The vaccine antigen Bm86 (a membrane glycoprotein from tick gut endothelial cells) is expressed intracellularly in *P. pastoris* in glycosylated form at levels of 1.5–2.0 g/l (Rodriguez et al., 1994). After cell disruption, rBm86 is denatured and solubilized with urea and, after refolding, purified in a particulate form by a sequence of precipitation and filtration steps. A large-scale production process has been established (Canales et al., 1997). Vaccines for veterinary use are subject to stringent cost considerations in terms of productivity, capital investment, and operating costs. Therefore, for the development of this vaccine (Gavac®), the *P. pastoris* system was compared with *E.coli* and the fungal expression system, *Aspergillus nidulans*. The fact that *P. pastoris* was selected for production demonstrates the suitability of a yeast-based production system under an economic point of view. rBm86 when adjuvanted with an oil emulsion elicited antibodies in immunized cattle. These antibodies are to destroy the tick's digestive cells on blood feeding and, thus, should lead to reduction of tick infestation in vaccinated herds. Gavac has been reported to be effective in controlling *B. microplus* infections under field conditions and is currently licensed in several countries in Latin America.

3.7 PERSPECTIVES

In a recent approach, genetically engineered *S. cerevisiae* expressing hepatitis C virus (HCV) NS3 and core proteins is heat-killed and administered as a whole-cell vaccine. As yeast cells per se are effective inducers of innate and adaptive cellular immunity, this yeast whole-cell vaccine induced HCV-specific cytotoxic T-cells and Th1-type cytokines in mice (Haller et al., 2007). In this case, the recombinant yeast not only provides for the target antigens, but also serves as a potent adjuvant. A candidate therapeutic vaccine against chronic HCV infection is currently in phase I clinical testing.

3.8 CONCLUDING REMARKS

Yeasts have proven to be efficient and robust host organisms for the production of vaccine antigens. Yeast expression systems combine the ease of using a bacterial expression system with features typical for eukaryotic gene expression, protein modification, and secretion. Large-scale production has been established for two major vaccine indications (hepatitis B and HPV), and the resulting experience will serve as a basis for the future use of yeast in the production of vaccine antigens. The most critical issue for the choice of yeast as the production organism seems to depend on the success of initial expression studies. Once the feasibility of expressing an immunogenic antigen in yeast has been demonstrated, there are many well-defined parameters to optimize expression and upstream/downstream processing to allow the set-up of a robust manufacturing process.

ACKNOWLEDGMENTS

The authors are grateful to U. Dahlems and M. Suckow for discussion and critical reading of the manuscript. The assistance of U. Kullmann for the preparation of the figures and help with the manuscript is appreciated.

REFERENCES

André FE. Summary of safety and efficacy data on yeast-derived hepatitis B vaccine. Am J Med 1989;87:S14–S20.

Assad S, Francis A. Over a decade of experience with a yeast recombinant hepatitis B vaccine. Vaccine 1999;18:57–67.

Ballou WR, Arevalo-Herrera M, Carucci D, Richie T, Corradin G, Diggs C, Druilhe P, Giersing BK, Saul A, Heppner DG, Kester KE, Lanar DE, Lyon J, Hill AVS, Pan W, Cohen JD. Update on the clinical development of candidate malaria vaccines. Am J Trop Mol Hyg 2004;71(S2):239–247.

Barr PJ, Steimer KS, Sabin EA, Parkes D, George-Nascimento C, Stephans JC, Powers MA, Gyenes A, Van Nest GA, Miller ET, et al. Antigenicity and immunogenicity of domains of the human immunodeficiency virus envelope polypeptide expressed in the yeast *Saccharomyces cerevisiae*. Vaccine 1987;5:90–101.

Biemans R, Thines D, Petre-Parent B, de Wilde M, Rutgers T, Cabezon T. Immunoelectron microscopic detection of the hepatitis B virus major surface protein in dilated perinuclear membranes of yeast cells. DNA Cell Biol 1992;11:621–626.

Blumberg BS, Gerstley BJS, Hungerford DA, London WT, Sutnick AI. A serum antigen (Australia antigen) in Down's syndrome, leukemia, and hepatitis. Ann Intern Med 1967;66:924–931.

Bryan JT. Developing an HPV vaccine to prevent cervical cancer and genital warts. Vaccine 2007;25:3001–3006.

Buckholz RG, Gleeson MA. Yeast systems for the commercial production of heterologous proteins. Biotechnology 1991;9:1067–1072.

Budkowska A, Dubreuil P, Capel F, Pillot J. Hepatitis B virus preS gene-encoded antigenic specificity and anti-preS antibody: relationship between anti-preS response and recovery. Hepatology 1986;6:360–368.

Burnette WN, Samal B, Browne J, Ritter GA. Properties and relative immunogenicity of various preparations of recombinant DNA-derived hepatitis B surface antigen. Dev Biol Stan 1985;59:113–120.

Burrell CJ, Mackay P, Greenaway PJ, Hofschneider PH, Murray K. Expression in *Escherichia coli* of hepatitis B virus DNA sequences cloned in plasmid pBR322. Nature 1979;279:43–47.

Canales M, Enriquez A, Ramos E, Cabrera D, Dandie H, Soto A, Falcón V, Rodriguez M, de la Fuente J. Large-scale production in *Pichia pastoris* of the recombinant vaccine Gavac® against cattle tick. Vaccine 1997;15:414–422.

Cereghino JL, Cregg JM. Heterologous protein expression in the methylotrophic yeast *Pichia pastoris*. FEMS Microbiol Rev 2000;24:45–66.

Cook JM, Gualde N, Hessel L, Mounier M, Michel JP, Denis F, Ratinaud MH. Alterations in the human immune response to the hepatitis B vaccine among the elderly. Cell Immunol 1987;109:89–96.

Craven DE, Awdeh ZL, Kunches LM, Yunis EJ, Dienstag JL, Werner BG, Polk BF, Syndman DR, Platt R, Crumpacker CS, et al. Non-responsiveness to hepatitis B vaccine in health care workers. Ann Intern Med 1986;105:356–360.

Cregg JM, Tschopp JF, Stillman C, Siegel R, Akong M, Craig WS, Buckholz KR, Madden KR, Kellaris PA, Davis GR, Smiley BL, Cruze J, Torregrossa R, Velicelebi G, Thill GP. High-level expression and efficient assembly of hepatitis B surface antigen in the methylotrophic yeast, *Pichia pastoris*. Biotechnology 1987;5:479–485.

Dehoux P, Ribes V, Sobczak E, Streeck RE. Expression of the hepatitis B virus large envelope protein in *Saccharomyces cerevisiae*. Gene 1986;48:155–163.

Diminsky D, Schirmbeck R, Reimann J, Barenholz Y. Comparison between hepatitis B surface antigen particles derived form mammalian (CHO) and yeast cells (*Hansenula polymorpha*): composition, structure and immunogenicity. Vaccine 1997;15:637–647.

Dreesman GR, Hollinger FB, Suriano JR, Fujioka RS, Brunschwig JP, Melnick JL. Biophysical and biochemical heterogeneity of purified hepatitis B antigen. J Virol 1972;10:469–476.

Dupont J, Altclas J, Lepetic A, Lombardo M, Vázquez V, Salgueira C, Seigelchifer M, Arndtz N, Antunez E, von Eschen K, Janowicz Z. A controlled clinical trial comparing the safety and immunogenicity of a new adjuvanted hepatitis B vaccine with a standard hepatitis B vaccine. Vaccine 2006;24:7167–7174.

Edman JC, Hallewell RA, Valenzuela P, Goodman HM, Rutter WJ. Synthesis of hepatitis B surface and core antigens in *E. coli*. Nature 1981;291:503–506.

Elliott AY, Morges W, Olson MG. Experience in manufacturing, testing, and licensing a hepatitis B vaccine produced by recombinant technology. In: Lubiniecki AS, Vargo SA, editors. *Regulatory Practice for Biopharmaceutical Production*. New York: Wiley-Liss; 1994. p 255–269.

Ellis RW, editor. *Hepatitis B Vaccine in Clinical Practice*. New York: Marcel Dekker; 1993.

Emini EA, Ellis RW, Miller WJ, McAleer WJ, Scolnick EM, Gerety RJ. Production and immunological analysis of recombinant hepatitis B vaccine. J Infect 1986;13:3–9.

Emini EA, Schleif WA, Quintero JC, Pg C, Eichberg JW, Vlasuk GP, Lehman ED, Polokoff MA, Schaeffer TF, Schultz LD, et al. Yeast-expressed p55 precursor core protein of human immunodeficiency virus type 1 does not elicit protective immunity in chimpanzees. AIDS Res Hum Retroviruses 1990;6:1247–1250.

Ganem D, Prince AM. Hepatitis B infection—natural history and clinical consequences. N Engl J Med 2004;350:1118–1129.

Gellissen G, Hollenberg CP. Application of yeasts in gene expression studies: a comparison of *Saccharomyces cerevisiae*, *Hansenula polymorpha* and *Kluyveromyces lactis*—a review. Gene 1997;190:87–97.

Gellissen G, Hollenberg CP, Janowicz Z. Gene expression in methylotrophic yeasts. In: Smith A, editor. *Gene Expression in Recombinant Microorganisms*. New York: Marcel Dekker; 1995. p 195–239.

Gleeson M, Sudbery P. The methylotrophic yeasts. Yeast 1988;4:1–15.

Haller AA, Lauer GM, King TH, Kemmler C, Fiolkowski V, Lu Y, Bellgrau D, Rodell TC, Apelian D, Franzusoff A, Duke RC. Whole recombinant yeast-based immunotherapy induces potent T cell responses targeting HCV NS3 and core proteins. Vaccine 2007;25: 1452–1463.

Hardy E, Martinez E, Diago D, Diàz R, Gonzàlez D, Herrera L. Large-scale production of recombinant hepatitis B surface antigen from *Pichia pastoris*. J Biotechnol 2000;77: 157–167.

Harford N, Cabezon T, Colau B, Delisse AM, Rutgers T, De Wilde M. Construction and characterization of a *Saccharomyces cerevisiae* strain (RIT4376) expressing hepatitis B surface antigen. Postgrad Med J 1987;63:65–70.

Harford N, Cabezon T, Crabeel M, Simoen E, Rutgers T, De Wilde M. Expression of hepatitis B surface antigen in yeast. Dev Biol Stan 1983;54:125–130.

Hieu TH, Kim KH, Janowicz Z, Timmermans I. Comparative efficacy, safety and immunogenicity of Hepavax-Gene and Engerix-B, recombinant hepatitis B vaccines, in infants born to HBsAg and HBeAg positive mothers in Vietnam: an assessment at 2 years. Vaccine 2002;20:1803–1808.

Higgins D, Marshall JD, Traquina P, Van Nest G, Livingston BD. Immunostimulatory DNA as a vaccine adjuvant. Expert Rev Vaccines 2007;6:747–759.

Hilleman MR. Plasma-derived hepatitis B vaccine: a breakthrough in preventive medicine. In: Ellis R, editor. *Hepatitis B vaccines in Clinical Practice*. New York: Marcel Dekker; 1993. p 17–39.

Hinnen A, Hicks JB, Fink GB. Transformation of yeast. Proc Natl Acad Sci U S A 1978;75: 1929–1933.

Hitzeman RA, Chen CY, Hagie FE, Patzer EJ, Liu CC, Estell DA, Miller JV, Yaffe A, Kleid DG, Levinson AD, Oppermann H. Expression of hepatitis B surface antigen in yeast. Nucl Acids Res 1983;11:2745–2763.

Hofmann KJ, Cook JC, Joyce JG, Brown DR, Schultz LD, George HA, Rosolowsky M, Fife KH, Jansen KU. Sequence determination of human papillomavirus type 6a and assembly of virus-like particles in *Saccharomyces cerevisiae*. Virlogy 1995;209:506–518.

Huang K, Lin S. Nationwide vaccination: a success story in Taiwan. Vaccine 2000;18: S35–S38.

Imamura T, Araki M, Miyanohara A, Nakao J, Yonemura H, Ohtomo N, Matsubara K. Expression of hepatitis B virus middle and large surface antigen genes in *Saccharomyces cerevisiae*. J Virol 1987;61:3543–3549.

Ip CCY, Miller WJ, Kubek DJ, Strang AM, van Halbeek H, Piesecki SJ, Alhadef JA. Structural characterization of the N-glycans of recombinant hepatitis B surface antigen derived from yeast. Biochemistry 1992;31:285–295.

Itoh Y, Takai E, Ohnuma H, Kitajama K, Tsuda F, Machida A, Mishiro S, Nakamura T, Miyakama Y, Mayumi M. A synthetic peptide vaccine involving the product of the preS2 region of hepatitis B virus DNA: protective efficacy in chimpanzees. Proc Natl Acad Sci U S A 1986;83:9174–9178.

Jacobs E, Rutgers T, Voet P, Dewerchin M, Cabezon T, de Wilde M. Simultaneous synthesis of various hepatitis B surface proteins in *Saccharomyces cerevisiae*. Gene 1989;80: 279–291.

Janowicz ZA, Eckart MR, Drewke C, Roggenkamp RO, Hollenberg CP, Maat J, Ledeboer AM, Visser C, Verrips CT. Cloning and characterization of the DAS gene encoding the major methanol assimilatory enzyme from the methylotrophic yeast *Hansenula polymorpha*. Nucl Acid Res 1985;13:3043–3062.

Janowicz ZA, Melber K, Merckelbach A, Jacobs E, Harford N, Comberbach M, Hollenberg CP. Simultaneous expression of the S and L surface antigens of hepatitis B, and formation of mixed particles in the methylotrophic yeast, *Hansenula polymorpha*. Yeast 1991;7:431–443.

Jilg W, Schmidt M, Weinel B, Küttler T, Brass H, Bommer J, Müller R, Schulte B, Schwarzbeck A, Deinhardt F. Immunogenicity of recombinant hepatitis B vaccine in dialysis patients. J Hepatol 1986;3:190–195.

Kingsman S, Kingsman AJ, Dobson MJ, Mellor J, Roberts NA. Heterologous gene expression in *Saccharomyces cerevisiae*. Biotechnol Genet Eng Rev 1985;3:377–416.

Kirnbauer R, Taub J, Greenstone H, Rogen R, Dürst M, Gissmann L, Lowy DR, Schiller JT. Efficient self-assembly of human papillomavirus type 16 L1 and L1-L2 into virus-like particles. J Virol 1993;67:6929–6936.

Kniskern PJ, Hagopian A, Burke P, Dunn N, Emini E, Miller WJ, Yamazaki S, Ellis RW. A candidate vaccine for hepatitis B containing the complete viral surface antigen. Hepatology 1988;8:82–87.

Langley KE, Egan KM, Barendt JM, Parker CG, Bitter GA. Characterization of purified hepatitis B surface antigen containing pre-S2 epitopes expressed in *Saccharomyces cerevisiae*. Gene 1988;67:229–245.

Lavanchy D. Worldwide epidemiology of HBV infection, disease burden, and vaccine prevention. J Clin Virol 2005;34:S1–S3.

Ledeboer AM, Edens L, Maat J, Visser C, Bos JW, Verrips CT, Janowicz ZA, Eckart M, Roggenkamp R, Hollenberg CP. Molecular cloning and characterization of a gene coding for methanol oxidase in *Hansenula polymorpha*. Nucl Acid Res 1985;13:3063–3082.

Lindenburg CEA, Stolte I, Langendam MW, Miedema F, Williams IG, Colebunders WJN, Fisher M, Coutinho RA. Long-term follow-up: no effect of therapeutic vaccination with HIV-1 p17/p24:Ty virus-like particles on HIV-1 disease progression. Vaccine 2002;20: 2343–3247.

MacKay P, Pasek M, Magazin M, Kovacic RT, Allet B, Stahl S, Gilbert W, Schaller H, Bruce SA, Murray K. Production of immunologically active surface antigens of hepatitis B virus by *Escherichia coli*. Proc Natl Acad Sci U S A 1981;78:4510–4514.

Mallet E, Behloradsky BH, Lagos R, Gothefors L, Camier P, Carrière JP, Kanra G, Hoffenbach A, Langue J, Undreiner F, Roussel F, Reinert P, Flodmark CE, Stojanov S, Liese J, Levine MM, Munoz A, Schödel F, Hessel L; Hexavalent Vaccine Trial Study Group. A liquid hexavalent combined vaccine against diphtheria, tetanus, pertussis, poliomyelitis, *Haemophilus influenzae* type B and hepatitis B: review of immunogenicity and safety. Vaccine 2004;22:1343–1357.

McAleer WJ, Buynak EB, Maigetter RZ, Wampler DE, Miller WJ, Hilleman MR. Human hepatitis B vaccine from recombinant yeast. Nature 1984;307:178–180.

McCarty CE, Tekamp-Olson P, Rosenberg S, McAleer WJ, Maigetter RZ. Galactose-regulated expression of hepatitis B surface antigen by a recombinant yeast. Biotechnol Lett 1989;11:301–306.

Middelhoven WJ. History, habitat, variability, nomenclature and phylogenetic position of *Hansenula polymorpha*. In: Gellissen G, editor. *Hansenula polymorpha—Biology and Applications*. Weinheim: Wiley-VCH; 2002. p 1–7.

Milich DR, McLachlan A, Chisari FV, Kent BH, Thornton GB. Immune response to the preS1 region of the hepatitis B surface antigen: a preS1-specific T cell response can bypass non-responsiveness to the preS2 and S regions of HBsAg. J Immunol 1986;137:315–322.

Miyanohara A, Toh-E A, Nozaki C, Hamada F, Ohtomo N, Matsubara K. Expression of hepatitis B surface antigen gene in yeast. Proc Natl Acad Sci U S A 1983;80:1–5.

Neurath AR, Seto B, Strick N. Antibodies to synthetic peptides from the preS1 region of the hepatitis B virus envelope protein are virus-neutralizing and protective. Vaccine 1989;7:234–236.

Petre J, Rutgers T, Hauser P. Properties of a recombinant yeast-derived hepatitis B surface antigen containing S, preS2 and preS1 antigenic domains. Arch Virol 1992;4:137–141.

Petre J, Van Wijnendaele F, De Neys B, Conrath K, Opstal V, Hauser P, Rutgers T, Cabezon T, Capiau C, Harford N, De Wilde M, Stephenne J, Carr S, Hemling H, Swadesh J. Development of a hepatitis B vaccine from transformed yeast cells. Postgrad Med J 1987;63:73–81.

Rattray JB, Hambleton JE. The lipid components of *Candida boidinii* and *Hansenula polymorpha* grown on methanol. Can J Microbiol 1980;26:190–195.

Raz E, Koren R, Bass D. Safety and immunogenicity of a new mammalian cell-derived recombinant hepatitis B vaccine containing preS1 and preS2 antigens in adults. Isr Med Assoc J 2001;3:328–332.

Rodriguez M, Rubiera R, Penichet M, Montesinos R, Cremata J, Falcón V, Sanchez G, Bringas R, Coddovés C, Valdés M. High level expression of the *B. microplus* Bm86 antigen in the yeast *P. pastoris* forming highly immunogenic particles for cattle. J Biotechnol 1994;33:135–146.

Schaefer S, Piontek M, Ahn SJ, Papendieck A, Janowicz ZA, Timmermans I, Gellissen G. Recombinant hepatitis B vaccines—disease characterization and vaccine production. In: Gellissen G, editor. *Hansenula polymorpha—Biology and Applications.* Weinheim: Wiley-VCH; 2002. p 175–210.

Schulman CA, Ellis RW, Maigetter RZ. Production of hepatitis B surface antigen (preS2 + S) by high-cell density cultivations of a recombinant yeast. J Biotechnol 1991;21:109–126.

Sninsky JJ, Siddiqui A, Robinson WS, Cohen SN. Cloning and endonuclease mapping of the hepatitis B viral genome. Nature 1979;279:346–348.

Srienc F, Campbell JL, Bailey JE. Analysis of unstable recombinant *Saccharomyces cerevisiae* population growth in selective medium. Biotechnol Bioeng 1986;28:996–1006.

Stanley M, Lowy DR, Frazer I. Prophylactic HPV vaccines: underlying mechanisms. Vaccine 2006;24:S3/106–S3/113.

Stephenne J. Development and production aspects of a recombinant yeast-derived hepatitis B vaccine. Vaccine 1990;8:S69–S73.

Tong NK, Beran J, Kee SA, Mifuel JL, Sànchez C, Bayas JM, Vilella A, de Juanes JR, Arrazola P, Calbo-Torrecillas F, de Novales EL, Hamtiaux V, Lievens M, Stoffel M. Immunogenicity and safety of an adjuvanted hepatitis B vaccine in pre-hemodialysis and hemodialysis patients. Kidney Int 2005;68:2298–2303.

Trottier H, Franco EL. The epidemiology of genital human papillomavirus infection. Vaccine 2006;24:S3/1–S3/15.

Valenzuela P, Coit D, Kuo CH. Synthesis and assembly in yeast of hepatitis B surface antigen particles containing the polyalbumin receptor. Nat Biotechnol 1985;3:317–320.

Valenzuela P, Medina A, Rutter WJ, Ammerer G, Hall BD. Synthesis and assembly of hepatitis B virus surface antigen particles in yeast. Nature 1982;298:347–350.

Vandepapelière P, Rehermann B, Koutsoukos M, Moris P, Garcon N, Wettendorff M, Leroux-Roels G. Potent enhancement of cellular and humoral immune responses against recombinant hepatitis B antigens using AS02A adjuvant in healthy adults. Vaccine 2005;23:2591–2601.

Vlasuk GP, Waxman L, Davis LJ, Dixon RAF, Schzultz LD, Hofmann KJ, Tung JS, Schulman CA, Ellis RW, Bencen GH, Duong LT, Polokoff MA. Purification and characterization of human immunodeficiency virus core precursor (p55) expressed in *Saccharomyces cerevisiae.* J Biol Chem 1989;264:12106–12112.

Wampler DE, Lehman ED, Boger J, McAleer WJ, Scolnick EM. Multiple chemical forms of hepatitis B surface antigen produced in yeast. Proc Natl Acad Sci U S A 1985;82:6830–6834.

WHO Expert Committee on Biological Standardization. Requirements for hepatitis B vaccines made by recombinant DNA techniques. Technical Report Series 786, Annex 2; 1989; Geneva: World Health Organisation. p 38–71.

Yurimoto H, Sakai Y, Kato N. Methanol metabolism. In: Gellissen G, editor. *Hansenula polymorpha–Biology and Applications.* Weinheim: Wiley-VCH; 2002. p 61–75.

Zajac BA, West DJ, McAleer WJ, Scolnick EM. Overview of clinical studies with hepatitis B vaccine made by recombinant DNA. J Infect 1986;13(Suppl A):39–45.

Zepp F, Knuf M, Heininger U, Jahn K, Collard A, Habermehl P, Schuerman L, Sänger R. Safety, reactogenicity and immunogenicity of a combined hexavalent tetanus, diphtheria, acellular pertussis, hepatitis B, inactivated poliovirus vaccine and *Haemophilus influenzae* type B conjugate vaccine, for primary immunization of infants. Vaccine 2004;22: 2226–2233.

Zuckerman JN, Zuckerman AJ, Symington I, Du W, Williams A, Dickson B, Young MD; UK Hepacare Study Group. Evaluation of a new hepatitis B triple-antigen vaccine in inadequate responders to current vaccines. Hepatology 2001;34:798–802.

4

NOVEL EXPRESSION SYSTEMS FOR VACCINE PRODUCTION

SHAILAJA RABINDRAN

US Department of Agriculture Animal and Plant Health Inspection Service, Riverdale, MD, USA

VIDADI YUSIBOV

Fraunhofer USA Center for Molecular Biotechnology, Newark, DE, USA

4.1 INTRODUCTION

In 1796, when Edward Jenner demonstrated protection of individuals against smallpox after inoculation with cowpox virus, he established vaccines as an effective tool to combat infectious diseases. Since then, there has been significant progress in vaccine development, evolving from full pathogen-based, killed or live-attenuated, vaccines to subunit vaccines. Although 25–30 vaccines are now licensed for use in humans, developing a vaccine against every new pathogen continues to be a paramount challenge, and the global need for vaccines continues to grow. With advances in genomics and proteomics, there has been an explosion in new knowledge that has enabled better understanding of the molecular pathways underlying pathogenesis, the host immune system, and host–pathogen interactions. This new knowledge, coupled with the development of new and highly efficient production technologies, has created opportunities for the design and manufacture of new subunit vaccines and has ushered in a renaissance in the field of vaccinology.

Vaccine Development and Manufacturing, First Edition.
Edited by Emily P. Wen, Ronald Ellis, and Narahari S. Pujar.

4.2 SUBUNIT VACCINES

Although a majority of currently licensed vaccines is based on killed or live-attenuated pathogens, subunit vaccines that rely on specific antigens or toxins that induce protective immunity are becoming preferred alternatives. This is because recombinant subunit vaccines are safe and effective, and their production can be easily scaled-up.

Initially, subunit vaccines were based on toxins purified from culture supernatants of host organisms, such as tetanus and diphtheria toxins. With better understanding of the molecular basis of pathogenesis and with the availability of new methodologies, conjugate vaccines then emerged as a new class of subunit vaccines, in which protective immunity is generated by a polysaccharide molecule coupled to a protein carrier. Vaccines against *Haemophilus influenza* type B or *Neisseria meningitidis* are good examples of subunit conjugate vaccines. More recently, vaccines based on recombinant antigens produced in yeast or insect cell expression systems (Lowy and Schiller, 2006) have been approved for human use. The increase in the use of genomics-based approaches to subunit vaccine development has facilitated the identification of several new candidates. This, in its turn, requires expression systems that can accommodate rapid production of a broad variety of targets that are correctly folded, are safe, and that confer pathogen-specific immunity. For this reason, several new expression systems are being examined for subunit vaccine production.

4.3 EXPRESSION SYSTEMS

Over the last four to five decades, several systems for the expression of target proteins have been developed (Rogan and Babiuk, 2005), and new ones continue to emerge (Franklin and Mayfield, 2004; Gasdaska et al., 2003; Houdebine, 2000). Bacterial, yeast, mammalian, and insect cell cultures have been extensively used for producing target proteins, and both regulatory and manufacturing infrastructures for these systems are well established. Bacterial expression systems are excellent candidates for production. However, limited post-translational modification of proteins, the presence of endotoxins, and problems associated with protein solubility remain a concern. Thus, alternative expression systems that have the capacity to deliver soluble, safe, and appropriately post-translationally modified and correctly folded proteins are being sought after. A number of products made using these expression systems have been approved for human use, including, most recently, vaccines against *Human papillomavirus* (HPV; Gardasil produced in yeast by Merck & Company, Inc., and Cervarix produced in insect cells by GlaxoSmithKline) and *Hepatitis B virus* (Engerix-B by GlaxoSmithKline and Recombivax HB by Merck & Co. Inc., both produced in yeast). The emergence of new targets and the growing global demand for vaccines require continued improvement of current expression and production systems and discovery and development of new high capacity, high performance expression systems. Furthermore, during the past decade, more than 10 new pathogens that pose public health threats have emerged, an alarming trend, demanding technologies with rapid engineering and production capacity. In this chapter, several new systems are reviewed, with major focus on plants, which are being developed in an attempt to address several of the aforementioned concerns.

4.4 NOVEL EXPRESSION SYSTEMS

4.4.1 Transgenic Animals

Transgenic animals, such as rabbits, sheep, goats, pigs, and cows, have been studied as alternative systems for protein production, particularly for expressing targets that require complex post-translational modifications. Most targets produced in transgenic animals are complex enzymes, such as blood factors, antibodies, wound healing enzymes, and hormones (Houdebine, 2000), although they are also being used to produce vaccines. Two rotavirus antigens, VP2 and VP6, produced in the milk of transgenic rabbits were shown to be immunogenic, and they significantly reduced viral antigen shedding in a mouse model when delivered orally (Soler et al. 2005). At the industrial scale level, blood, urine, milk, and egg whites are among the sources of materials from transgenic animals for recombinant proteins. However, several issues related to the use of transgenic animals still remain to be addressed, which include efficiency of generating transgenic animals, speed of production for commercial purposes, and safety because of the potential to transmit infectious diseases (Larrick and Thomas, 2001).

4.4.2 Mushrooms

A recent report described a button variety of the edible mushroom, *Agaricus bisporus*, as a means for producing recombinant proteins on a large scale. The technology is based on genetic transformation of fruiting body explants, particularly the gills, to introduce the target gene. This new approach of introducing target genes via fruiting body explant transformation has overcome the inefficacy of fungal spore or vegetative mycelium-based introduction of target genes (Chen et al., 2000; Romaine and Schlagnhaufer, 2006). Using this new approach, transgenic mushrooms can be engineered to produce recombinant proteins at a large scale without further selection of transgenic lines. The technology has some definite advantages, including the ability for rapid expansion to produce bulk quantities, low cost infrastructure, contained facilities, and established practices of food grade mushroom production. However, analogous to all new technologies, further development is needed to demonstrate its feasibility for manufacturing of targets to be used in humans.

4.4.3 Algae

Chlamydomonas reinhardtii is a well-studied representative of green algae that has been a model organism for several studies, including light-induced gene expression (Franklin and Mayfield, 2004; Boynton et al., 1988). Features that make this alga attractive as a production platform include the ease of genetic manipulation to introduce the gene of interest into the nuclear, chloroplast, or mitochondrial genome, post-translational modification machinery, and simplicity of large-scale growth in a contained and cost-effective manner (Siripornadulsil et al., 2007). Target expression levels and issues related to gene silencing, however, need to be addressed before the system can be fully used for commercial manufacturing.

4.4.4 Lemna

The aquatic plant *Lemna* is another production system that is being examined for large-scale manufacturing of recombinant proteins. Key features of this novel expression system are that the growth requirement of the transgenic *Lemna* is simple, the duckweed proliferates rapidly with a biomass doubling time of 36 h, protein is secreted into the medium, thus simplifying the purification process, and the plants are grown in enclosed environments, thus permitting contained manufacturing (Gasdaska et al., 2003).

4.4.5 Plants

In the 1990s, plants emerged as an alternative platform for foreign protein production, with growing potential for commercial manufacturing. Plants offer several advantages as production systems, including possession of eukaryotic post-translational modification machinery, ability for simple low-cost scale-up for manufacturing, and safety, as plants do not harbor mammalian pathogens and plant pathogens do not infect humans. There are two main strategies by which plants can be used for producing recombinant proteins, which include the transgenic route in which the target gene is incorporated into the plant nuclear genome or chloroplast genome and the transient route that uses genetically engineered plant viruses to produce the recombinant protein on infection of the plant.

4.5 PRODUCTION OF RECOMBINANT PROTEINS IN PLANTS

Historically, recombinant proteins in plants were produced by the introduction of the target gene into the nuclear genome (Franken et al., 1997; Daniell et al., 2001). More recently, chloroplasts are being engineered for candidate vaccine production (Daniell, 2006; Koya et al., 2005; Molina et al., 2005; Tregoning et al., 2004). Most target proteins expressed in plants are vaccine antigens, including enterotoxigenic *Escherichia coli* Lt-B antigen (Haq et al., 1995), *Bacillus anthracis* protective antigen (Aziz et al., 2002), *Norwalk virus* capsid protein (Huang et al., 2005), and *Hepatitis B virus* surface antigen (Richter et al., 2000; Sunil Kumar et al., 2003). These plant-produced vaccine antigens generate pathogen-specific protective immune responses when administered into animals (Carrillo et al., 1998; Khandelwal et al., 2004; Tuboly et al., 2000). The transgenic approach is used for producing proteins in growing plants and plant cell cultures via conventional fermentation (Boehm, 2007;

Floss et al., 2007; Schillberg et al., 2005). A vaccine against Newcastle Disease virus (Dow AgroSciences LLC), produced using the transgenic plant cell culture approach, has recently been issued a license for commercial use to protect chickens against disease caused by this virus. This is the first plant-made product that has been licensed by the U.S. Department of Agriculture Animal and Plant Health Inspection Service.

Besides transgenic plants, plant RNA viruses are being used as vectors for foreign protein expression (Canizares et al., 2005; Grill et al., 2006; Pogue et al., 2002; Yusibov et al., 2006; Yusibov et al., 2013). The availability of infectious cDNA clones, small genome size, ease of genetic manipulations, and the short time in which a target protein can be expressed make this strategy particularly attractive. In addition, there is no need to genetically alter host plants. The expression is transient, with the target gene inserted into the viral genome so that on infection of the host plant, the transgene is amplified and the recombinant protein is produced. Both replication of the viral vector and expression of the target gene are limited to the cell cytoplasm. To date, several plant RNA viruses have been developed into expression vectors, including *Tobacco mosaic virus* (TMV), *Potato virus* X (PVX), *Alfalfa mosaic virus* (*AlMV*), and *Cowpea mosaic virus* (CPMV) (Pogue et al., 2002; Yusibov and Rabindran, 2004; Yusibov et al., 2013). There are different approaches for the expression of foreign sequences using plant viruses. The most commonly used approaches for producing soluble protein antigens are the following: (i) replacing nonessential viral genes such as coat protein (CP) with target sequences, or (ii) inserting target sequences into the viral genome as an additional gene whose expression is driven by a second CP subgenomic promoter. Several reviews are available on the use of this technology (Gleba et al., 2007; Scholthof et al., 1996; Yusibov and Rabindran, 2004; Yusibov et al., 1999). A number of candidate antigens have been produced using this plant virus-based approach, several of these have been shown to induce protective immunity and confer protection when challenged in animal models (see Table 4.1 and Yusibov et al., 2013), and some have undergone clinical development (Yusibov et al., 2011)).

Another approach that is most frequently used with plant viruses is based on fusing known target peptide epitopes to the viral CP to obtain virus-like particles (VLPs) that mimic native viruses and present the epitopes on their surfaces, but are devoid of infectious genetic material. These VLPs can then be used as immunogens. Several plant viral CPs have been used to produce and deliver antigenic determinants from a variety of viral and bacterial pathogens as VLPs, and these particles have conferred protective immunity against the target pathogen (Canizares et al., 2005; Grill et al., 2006; Pogue et al., 2002; Kushnir et al., 2012). The peptides range in size from a few amino acids up to >150 amino acids. Due to particulate structure and multivalent epitope organization, as well as the presence of residual host cell components, VLPs elicit stronger protective immune responses compared to soluble recombinant antigens (Chackerian 2007; Deml et al., 2005; Grgacic and Anderson, 2006). Using *Alfalfa mosaic virus* (AlMV), we have shown that recombinant AlMV particles presenting a 21-mer peptide from the *Respiratory syncytial virus* (RSV) G protein induced significant pathogen-specific immune responses *in vitro* using human dendritic cells and *in vivo* in nonhuman primates (Yusibov et al., 2005). The results showed that human dendritic cells armed with AlMV-RSVG

TABLE 4.1 Vaccine Antigens Produced Using Plant Virus-Based Expression Systems that Confer Protective Immunity

Production system	Antigen	Reference
Tobacco mosaic virus Soluble antigen vaccines	• *Foot and mouth disease virus* VP1 • *Bovine herpes virus* gD • *Cottontail rabbit papillomavirus* L1 • *Yersinia pestis* F1 and V, F1-V fusion • *Dengue virus* D2EIII • *Smallpox virus* • *Human papillomavirus* E7 • *Bacillus anthracis* PA domain 4 • *Bacillus anthracis* PA83 • A/California/04/09 (H1N1) *influenza virus* HA • A/Indonesia/05/05 (H5N1) *influenza virus* HA • *Plasmodium falciparum* Pfs25 • *Plasmodium falciparum* Pfs230	• Wigdorovitz et al., 1999 • Pérez Filgueira et al., 2003 • Kohl et al., 2006 • Santi et al., 2006; Mett et al., 2007 • Saejung et al., 2007 • Golovkin et al., 2007 • Massa et al., 2007 • Chichester et al., 2007 • Chichester et al., 2013 • Shoji et al., 2011 • Shoji et al., 2011 • Farrance et al., 2011a; Jones et al., In Press • Farrance et al., 2011b
Tobacco mosaic virus Coat protein–peptide fusions	• *Murine hepatitis virus* 5B19 • *Hepatitis C Virus* HVR1 • *Pseudomonas aeruginosa* F peptides • *Rabies virus* G peptide fused to *Alfalfa mosaic virus* CP • *Foot and mouth disease virus* VP1 • *Poliovirus* PVP • *Cottontail rabbit papillomavirus* L2 • *Rabbit oral papillomavirus* L2	• Koo et al., 1999 • Nemchinov et al., 2000 • Gilleland et al., 2000; Staczek et al., 2000 • Yusibov et al., 2002 • Wu et al., 2003 • Fujiyama et al., 2006 • Palmer et al., 2006 • Palmer et al., 2006
PVX	• *Toxoplasma gondii* SAG1	• Clemente et al., 2005
Alfalfa mosaic virus Coat protein–peptide fusions	• *Respiratory syncytial virus* G peptide • *Plasmodium falciparum* Pfs25	• Belanger et al., 2000 • Jones et al., 2013
Bamboo mosaic virus	• FMDV VP1 peptides	• Yang et al., 2007

TABLE 4.1 (*Continued*)

Production system	Antigen	Reference
Cowpea mosaic virus Coat protein–peptide fusions	• *Mink enteritis virus* VP2 • *Pseudomonas aeruginosa* F peptides • *Canine parvovirus* VP2 peptide • *Staphylococcus aureus* fibronectin-binding protein D2 domain	• Dalsgaard et al., 1997 • Gilleland et al., 2000; Brennan et al., 1999 • Langeveld et al., 2001 • Rennermalm et al., 2001

generated vigorous CD4+ and CD8+ T cell responses, and nonhuman primates that received these particles responded by mounting strong cellular and humoral immune responses. In a recent study, VLPs produced in *Nicotiana benthamiana* plants by genetic fusion of Pfs25, a sexual stage antigen of *Plasmodium falciparum*, to AlMV CP, have been shown to induce antibodies with persistent transmission blocking activity against the *Plasmodium* parasite in immunized mice (Jones et al., 2013).

Both the transgenic and viral vector-based approaches for producing target proteins in plants have some shortcomings. The transgenic approach suffers from long lead times, low levels of target expression, gene silencing, and nonuniform expression. Plant viral vectors, however, provide high levels of target protein in a time-efficient manner, although efficient target protein expression is dictated by the capability of the particular vector to spread throughout the plant. This requirement for spread throughout the plant, in its turn, has been shown to result in loss of expression of the foreign gene owing to the genetic instability of the viral vector, thus limiting the use of this technology for manufacturing purposes.

4.6 LAUNCH VECTOR SYSTEM

To overcome the shortcomings of the transgenic and plant virus-based approaches, we and other groups have taken advantage of the positive aspects of both systems by incorporating the plant viral vector genome into an agrobacterial binary plasmid (Gleba et al., 2005, Musiychuk et al., 2007). One of the plant viruses that we have engineered is TMV. In this "launch vector" system (Fig. 4.1), the target gene is engineered so that it replaces the CP coding sequence in the TMV genome, and *Agrobacterium* is used to introduce millions of copies of the launch vector into plants by vacuum infiltration. Primary transcripts, which contain the recombinant viral genome, are then produced and transported into the cytoplasm. Subsequently, viral RNA sequences replicate to very high copy numbers, and high-level target protein accumulation occurs in a matter of days. Levels of expression from hundred milligrams to gram quantities of target protein per kilogram of fresh plant tissue can be achieved. The vector design circumvents instability issues related to the presence

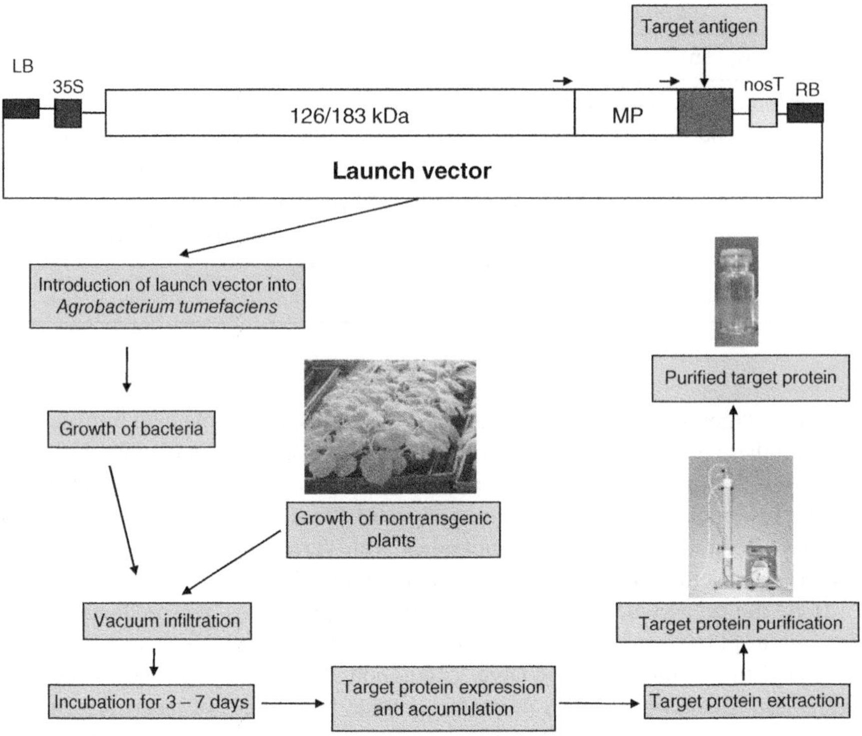

Figure 4.1 Schematic diagram of a *Tobacco mosaic virus*-based launch vector system for the production of vaccine antigens in nontransgenic plants. LB and RB refer to left and right borders, respectively, of the T-DNA in the agrobacterial binary vector; this T-DNA is transferred into the nuclei of the plant cells following agroinfiltration; 35S: 35S promoter from *Cauliflower mosaic virus* (a plant DNA virus) that drives transcription of the transgene; nosT: nos transcriptional terminator from Agrobacterium nopaline synthase gene; 126/183 kDa: replicase proteins of *Tobacco mosaic virus* required for replication of the virus; MP: movement protein required for cell-to-cell movement. Arrows indicate positions of subgenomic mRNA promoters. The target antigen replaces the coat protein coding sequence.

of CP and phloem-mediated movement and also provides additional environmental safety because the system does not produce infectious virus particles. Using this system, we have produced a wide variety of target antigens from several pathogens, including *Bacillus anthracis* (Chichester et al., 2013), *Yersinia pestis* (Chichester et al., 2009), *Influenza virus* (Shoji et al., 2011), *P. falciparum* (Farrance et al., 2011a, b; Jones et al., 2013), and HPV (Massa et al., 2007).

We have used the launch vector system, to produce Domain 4 of protective antigen (PA) from *B. anthracis* as a fusion with modified lichenase carrier (LicKM; Musiychuk et al., 2007), a thermostable protein derived from *Clostridium thermocellum* in *Nicotiana benthamiana* plants. When combined with purified plant-produced Domain 1 of lethal factor (LF), which was similarly expressed as a LicKM fusion protein in plants, and evaluated in mice, all animals developed high antibody titers that neutralized the effects of lethal toxin in an *in vitro* assay (Chichester et al., 2007). Subsequently, we produced in plants a full-length non-fusion version of PA (pp-PA83), which, in the presence of Alhydrogel adjuvant, elicited high toxin neutralizing antibody titers in mice and rabbits and conferred complete protection to rabbits against a lethal aerosolized *B. anthracis* challenge (Chichester et al., 2013). In yet another study, when purified E7 oncoprotein from HPV, expressed in plants using the launch vector system (as a fusion with LicKM), was evaluated in mice as a potential therapeutic vaccine candidate, target-specific IgG and cytotoxic T cell responses were induced, and mice were protected when challenged with tumor cells that expressed E7 (Massa et al., 2007). Furthermore, when animals previously challenged with E7-expressing tumor cells were immunized with the plant-produced vaccine candidates, all animals remained tumor-free for the duration of the 10-week study, whereas only 40% of animals immunized with *E. coli* produced E7 were protected from tumor development. Animals immunized with the thermostable carrier protein LicKM alone, developed tumors in 4 weeks. Purified F1 and LcrV of *Y. pestis* produced in plants, again as fusions to LicKM, when administered to Cynomolgus macaques induced target-specific serum IgG and IgA and conferred complete protection to the animals against lethal challenge with *Y. pestis* (Mett et al., 2007). These results demonstrate that plant-produced vaccines are effective in inducing protective responses not only in animals such as mice, but also in nonhuman primate models. More recently, the launch vector system has successfully been used to produce several other subunit vaccine candidates, such as non-fused HA antigens from A/California/04/09 (H1N1) and A/Indonesia/05/05 (H5N1) strains of influenza A virus (Shoji et al., 2011); a portion of the Pfs230 surface molecule of *P. falciparum* (a transmission blocking vaccine target) (Farrance et al., 2011b); a non-glycosylated Pfs25-LicKM fusion molecule (Farrance et al., 2011a; Jones et al., In Press); Pfs25-CP VLPs (Jones et al. 2013); and full-length non-fused PA from *B. anthracis* (Chichester et al., 2013). The plant-produced H1 and H5 HA products have been tested in clinical trials (Chichester et al., 2012; Cummings et al., 2014), and Pfs25-CP VLP is currently being evaluated in humans as a transmission blocking vaccine candidate (ClinicalTrials.gov Identifier NCT02013687).

The launch vector system provides high levels of expression and is highly amenable to rapid large-scale production of a wide range of recombinant proteins and VLPs. Thus, it is a very viable platform for the rapid manufacture of recombinant proteins for commercial purposes. A further advantage of the launch vector technology is that it lends itself to the creation of production modules with predetermined capacity, and by simply adding more modules, manufacturing capacity can be rapidly increased.

4.7 CONCLUSIONS

Vaccines are vital to public health. An effective vaccine should be safe, easy to administer, stable, and inexpensive, and provide protective immunity, which is sustained for long periods with few side effects. There are several diseases for which vaccines are not available, or there are limitations in current manufacturing technologies. As the industry moves forward, the collaborative efforts of researchers, immunologists, chemical engineers, and protein chemists are vital for the successful development of vaccines targeting a wide range of diseases and reaching the global population. Several novel expressions systems are being examined for the production of vaccine antigens, including transgenic animals, mushrooms, duckweed, algae, and plants. One promising plant-based technology that we have developed, the launch vector-based transient protein expression, combines the use of highly expressing plant virus-based systems and efficient delivery of target genes by *Agrobacterium*. This system shows great promise for the rapid, large-scale manufacture of recombinant proteins for subunit vaccine development. We have demonstrated this system's capability to be scaled up and produce vaccine antigens in plants under current Good Manufacturing Practices guidelines, and several vaccine candidates produced using this system have reached clinical development.

REFERENCES

Aziz MA, Singh S, Anand Kumar P, Bhatnagar R. Expression of protective antigen in transgenic plants: a step towards edible vaccine against anthrax. Biochem Biophys Res Commun 2002;299:345–351.

Belanger H, Fleysh N, Cox S, Bartman G, Deka D, Trudel M, Koprowski H, Yusibov V. Human respiratory syncytial virus vaccine antigen produced in plants. Faseb J 2000;14: 2323–2328.

Boehm R. Bioproduction of therapeutic proteins in the 21st century and the role of plants and plant cells as production platforms. Ann N Y Acad Sci 2007;1102:121–134.

Boynton JE, Gillham NW, Harris EH, Hosler JP, Johnson AM, Jones AR, Randolph-Anderson BL, Robertson D, Klein TM, Shark KB. Chloroplast transformation in Chlamydomonas with high velocity microprojectiles. Science 1988;240:1534–1538.

Brennan FR, Jones TD, Gilleland LB, Bellaby T, Xu F, North PC, Thompson A, Staczek J, Lin T, Johnson JE, Hamilton WD, Gilleland HE Jr. *Pseudomonas aeruginosa* outer-membrane protein F epitopes are highly immunogenic in mice when expressed on a plant virus. Microbiology 1999;145:211–220.

Canizares MC, Lomonossoff GP, Nicholson L. Use of viral vectors for vaccine production in plants. Immunol Cell Biol 2005;83:263–270.

Carrillo C, Wigdorovitz A, Oliveros JC, Zamorano PI, Sadir AM, Gomez N, Salinas J, Escribano JM, Borca MV. Protective immune response to foot-and-mouth disease virus with VP1 expressed in transgenic plants. J Virol 1998;72:1688–1690.

Chackerian B. Virus-like particles: flexible platforms for vaccine development. Expert Rev Vaccines 2007;6:381–390.

Chen X, Stone M, Schlagnhaufer C, Romaine CP. A fruiting body tissue method for efficient Agrobacterium-mediated transformation of *Agaricus bisporus*. Appl Environ Microbiol 2000;66:4510–4513.

Chichester JA, Musiychuk K, de la Rosa P, Horsey A, Stevenson N, Ugulava N, Rabindran S, Palmer GA, Mett V, Yusibov V. Immunogenicity of a subunit vaccine against *Bacillus anthracis*. Vaccine 2007;25:3111–3114.

Chichester JA, Musiychuk K, Farrance CE, Mett V, Lyons J, Mett V, Yusibov V. A single component two-valent LcrV-F1 vaccine protects non-human primates against pneumonic plague. Vaccine 2009;27:3471–3474.

Chichester JA, Jones RM, Green BJ, Stow M, Miao F, Moonsammy G, Streatfield SJ, Yusibov V. Safety and immunogenicity of a plant-produced recombinant hemagglutinin-based influenza vaccine (HAI-05) derived from A/Indonesia/05/2005 (H5N1) influenza virus: a phase 1 randomized, double-blind, placebo-controlled, dose-escalation study in healthy adults. Viruses 2012;4:3227–3244.

Chichester JA, Manceva SD, Rhee A, Coffin MV, Musiychuk K, Mett V, Shamloul M, Norikane J, Streatfield SJ, Yusibov V. A plant-produced protective antigen vaccine confers protection in rabbits against a lethal aerosolized challenge with Bacillus anthracis Ames spores. Hum Vaccin Immunother 2013;9(3). [Epub ahead of print].

Clemente M, Curilovic R, Sassone A, Zelada A, Angel SO, Mentaberry AN. Production of the main surface antigen of *Toxoplasma gondii* in tobacco leaves and analysis of its antigenicity and immunogenicity. Mol Biotechnol 2005;30:41–50.

Cummings JF, Guerrero ML, Moon JE, Waterman P, Nielsen RK, Jefferson S, Gross FL, Hancock K, Katz JM, Yusibov V. Fraunhofer USA Center for Molecular Biotechnology Study Group. Safety and immunogenicity of a plant-produced recombinant monomer hemagglutinin-based influenza vaccine derived from influenza A (H1N1)pdm09 virus: A Phase 1 dose-escalation study in healthy adults. Vaccine 2014;32:2251–2259.

Dalsgaard K, Uttenthal A, Jones TD, Xu F, Merryweather A, Hamilton WD, Langeveld JP, Boshuizen RS, Kamstrup S, Lomonossoff GP, Porta C, Vela C, Casal JI, Meloen RH, Rodgers PB. Plant-derived vaccine protects target animals against a viral disease. Nat Biotechnol 1997;15:248–252.

Daniell H. Production of biopharmaceuticals and vaccines in plants via the chloroplast genome. Biotechnol J 2006;1:1071–1079.

Daniell H, Streatfield SJ, Wycoff K. Medical molecular farming: production of antibodies, biopharmaceuticals and edible vaccines in plants. Trends Plant Sci 2001;6:219–226.

Deml L, Speth C, Dierich MP, Wolf H, Wagner R. Recombinant HIV-1 Pr55gag virus-like particles: potent stimulators of innate and acquired immune responses. Mol Immunol 2005;42:259–277.

Farrance CE, Chichester JA, Musiychuk K, Shamloul M, Rhee A, Manceva SD, Jones RM, Mamedov T, Sharma S, Mett V, Streatfield SJ, Roeffen W, van de Vegte-Bolmer M, Sauerwein RW, Wu Y, Muratova O, Miller L, Duffy P, Sinden R, Yusibov V. Antibodies to plant-produced Plasmodium falciparum sexual stage protein Pfs25 exhibit transmission blocking activity. Hum Vaccin 2011a;7(Suppl):191–198.

Farrance CE, Rhee A, Jones RM, Musiychuk K, Shamloul M, Sharma S, Mett V, Chichester JA, Streatfield SJ, Roeffen W, van de Vegte-Bolmer M, Sauerwein RW, Tsuboi T, Muratova OV, Wu Y, Yusibov V. A Plant-Produced Pfs230 Vaccine Candidate Blocks Transmission of Plasmodium falciparum. Clin Vaccine Immunol 2011b;18:1351–1357.

Floss DM, Falkenburg D, Conrad U. Production of vaccines and therapeutic antibodies for veterinary applications in transgenic plants: an overview. Transgenic Res 2007;16:315–332.

Franken E, Teuschel U, Hain R. Recombinant proteins from transgenic plants. Curr Opin Biotechnol 1997;8:411–416.

Franklin SE, Mayfield SP. Prospects for molecular farming in the green alga Chlamydomonas. Curr Opin Plant Biol 2004;7:159–165.

Fujiyama K, Saejung W, Yanagihara I, Nakado J, Misaki R, Honda T, Watanabe Y, Seki T. In Planta production of immunogenic poliovirus peptide using tobacco mosaic virus-based vector system. J Biosci Bioeng 2006;101:398–402.

Gasdaska JR, Spencer D, Dickey L. Advantages of therapeutic protein production in the aquatic plant lemna. BioProcessing J 2003;49–56.

Gilleland HE, Gilleland LB, Staczek J, Harty RN, Garcia-Sastre A, Palese P, Brennan FR, Hamilton WD, Bendahmane M, Beachy RN. Chimeric animal and plant viruses expressing epitopes of outer membrane protein F as a combined vaccine against *Pseudomonas aeruginosa* lung infection. FEMS Immunol Med Microbiol 2000;27:291–297.

Gleba Y, Klimyuk V, Marillonnet S. Magnifection—a new platform for expressing recombinant vaccines in plants. Vaccine 2005;23:2042–2048.

Gleba Y, Klimyuk V, Marillonnet S. Viral vectors for the expression of proteins in plants. Curr Opin Biotechnol 2007;1:134–141.

Golovkin M, Spitsin S, Andrianov V, Smirnov Y, Xiao Y, Pogrebnyak N, Markley K, Brodzik R, Gleba Y, Isaacs SN, Koprowski H. Smallpox subunit vaccine produced in planta confers protection in mice. Proc Natl Acad Sci U S A 2007;104:6864–6869.

Grgacic EV, Anderson DA. Virus-like particles: passport to immune recognition. Methods 2006;40:60–65.

Grill LK, Palmer KE, Pogue GP. Use of plant viruses for production of plant-derived vaccines. Crit Rev Plant Sci 2006;24:309–323.

Haq TA, Mason HS, Clements JD, Arntzen CJ. Oral immunization with a recombinant bacterial antigen produced in transgenic plants. Science 1995;268:714–716.

Houdebine LM. Transgenic animal bioreactors. Transgenic Res 2000;9:305–320.

Huang Z, Elkin G, Maloney BJ, Beuhner N, Arntzen CJ, Thanavala Y, Mason HS. Virus-like particle expression and assembly in plants: Hepatitis B and Norwalk viruses. Vaccine 2005;23:1851–1858.

Jones RM, Chichester JA, Manceva S, Gibbs SK, Musiychuk K, Shamloul M, Norikane J, Streatfield SJ, van de Vegte-Bolmer M, Roeffen W, Sauerwein RW, Yusibov V. A novel plant-produced Pfs25 fusion subunit vaccine induces long-lasting transmission blocking antibody responses. Hum Vaccin Immunother. In Press.

Jones RM, Chichester JA, Mett V, Jaje J, Tottey S, Manceva S, Casta LJ, Gibbs SK, Musiychuk K, Shamloul M, Norikane J, Mett V, Streatfield SJ, van de Vegte-Bolmer M, Roeffen W, Sauerwein RW, Yusibov V. A Plant-produced Pfs25 VLP Malaria Vaccine Candidate Induces Persistent Transmission Blocking Antibodies against Plasmodium falciparum in Immunized Mice. PLoS One 2013;8:e79538.

Khandelwal A, Renukaradhya GJ, Rajasekhar M, Sita GL, Shaila MS. Systemic and oral immunogenicity of hemagglutinin protein of rinderpest virus expressed by transgenic peanut plants in a mouse model. Virology 2004;323:284–291.

Kohl T, Hitzeroth II, Stewart D, Varsani A, Govan VA, Christensen ND, Williamson AL, Rybicki EP. Plant-produced cottontail rabbit papillomavirus L1 protein protects against tumor challenge: a proof-of-concept study. Clin Vaccine Immunol 2006;13: 845–853.

Koo M, Bendahmane M, Lettieri GA, Paoletti AD, Lane TE, Fitchen JH, Buchmeier MJ, Beachy RN. Protective immunity against murine hepatitis virus (MHV) induced by intranasal or subcutaneous administration of hybrids of tobacco mosaic virus that carries an MHV epitope. Proc Natl Acad Sci USA 1999;96:7774–7779.

Koya V, Moayeri M, Leppla SH, Daniell H. Plant-based vaccine: mice immunized with chloroplast-derived anthrax protective antigen survive anthrax lethal toxin challenge. Infect Immun 2005;73:8266–8274.

Kushnir N, Streatfield SJ, Yusibov V. Virus-like particles as a highly efficient vaccine platform: diversity of targets and production systems and advances in clinical development. Vaccine 2012;31:58–83.

Langeveld JP, Brennan FR, Martínez-Torrecuadrada JL, Jones TD, Boshuizen RS, Vela C, Casal JI, Kamstrup S, Dalsgaard K, Meloen RH, Bendig MM, Hamilton WD. Inactivated recombinant plant virus protects dogs from a lethal challenge with canine parvovirus. Vaccine 2001;19:3661–3670.

Larrick JW, Thomas DW. Producing proteins in transgenic plants and animals. Curr Opin Biotech 2001;12:411–418.

Lowy DR, Schiller JT. Prophylactic human papillomavirus vaccines. J Clin Invest 2006;116: 1167–1173.

Massa S, Franconi R, Brandi R, Muller A, Mett V, Yusibov V, Venuti A. Anti-cancer activity of plant-produced HPV16 E7 vaccine. Vaccine 2007;25:3018–3021.

Mett V, Lyons J, Musiychuk K, Chichester JA, Brasil T, Couch R, Sherwood R, Palmer GA, Streatfield SJ, Yusibov V. A plant-produced plague vaccine candidate confers protection to monkeys. Vaccine 2007;25:3014–3017.

Molina A, Veramendi J, Hervas-Stubbs S. Induction of neutralizing antibodies by a tobacco chloroplast-derived vaccine based on a B cell epitope from canine parvovirus. Virology 2005;342:266–275.

Musiychuk K, Stevenson N, Bi H, Farrance CE, Orozovic G, Brodelius M, Brodelius P, Horsey A, Ugulava N, Shamloul AM, Mett V, Rabindran S, Streatfield SJ, Yusibov V. A launch vector for the production of vaccine antigens in plants. Influenza Other Resp Viruses 2007;1:19–25.

Nemchinov LG, Liang TJ, Rifaat MM, Mazyad HM, Hadidi A, Keith JM. Development of a plant-derived subunit vaccine candidate against hepatitis C virus. Arch Virol 2000;145:2557–2573.

Palmer KE, Benko A, Doucette SA, Cameron TI, Foster T, Hanley KM, McCormick AA, McCulloch M, Pogue GP, Smith ML, Christensen ND. Protection of rabbits against cutaneous papillomavirus infection using recombinant tobacco mosaic virus containing L2 capsid epitopes. Vaccine 2006;24:5516–5525.

Pérez Filgueira DM, Zamorano PI, Domínguez MG, Taboga O, Del Médico Zajac MP, Puntel M, Romera SA, Morris TJ, Borca MV, Sadir AM. Bovine herpes virus gD protein produced in plants using a recombinant tobacco mosaic virus (TMV) vector possesses authentic antigenicity. Vaccine 2003;21:4201–4209.

Pogue GP, Lindbo JA, Garger SJ, Fitzmaurice WP. Making an ally from an enemy: plant virology and the new agriculture. Annu Rev Phytopathol 2002;40:45–74.

Rennermalm A, Li YH, Bohaufs L, Jarstrand C, Brauner A, Brennan FR, Flock JI. Antibodies against a truncated *Staphylococcus aureus* fibronectin-binding protein protect against dissemination of infection in the rat. Vaccine 2001;19:3376–3383.

Richter LJ, Thanavala Y, Arntzen CJ, Mason HS. Production of Hepatitis B surface antigen in transgenic plants for oral immunization. Nat Biotechnol 2000;1:1167–1171.

Rogan D, Babiuk LA. Novel vaccines from biotechnology. Rev Sci Tech 2005;24: 159–174.

Romaine CP, Schlagnhaufer C. Mushroom (*Agaricus bisporus*). Methods Mol Biol 2006;344: 453–463.

Saejung W, Fujiyama K, Takasaki T, Ito M, Hori K, Malasit P, Watanabe Y, Kurane I, Seki T. Production of dengue 2 envelope domain III in plant using TMV-based vector system. Vaccine 2007;25:6646–6654.

Santi L, Giritch A, Roy CJ, Marillonnet S, Klimyuk V, Gleba Y, Webb R, Arntzen CJ, Mason HS. Protection conferred by recombinant *Yersinia pestis* antigens produced by a rapid and highly scalable plant expression system. Proc Natl Acad Sci USA 2006;103: 861–866.

Schillberg S, Twyman RM, Fischer R. Opportunities for recombinant antigen and antibody expression in transgenic plants—technology assessment. Vaccine 2005;23:1764–1769.

Scholthof HB, Scholthof KB, Jackson AO. Plant virus gene vectors for transient expression of foreign proteins in plants. Annu Rev Phytopathol 1996;34:299–323.

Shoji Y, Chichester JA, Jones M, Manceva SD, Damon E, Mett V, Musiychuk K, Bi H, Farrance C, Shamloul M, Kushnir N, Sharma S, Yusibov V. Plant-based rapid production of recombinant subunit hemagglutinin vaccines targeting H1N1 and H5N1 influenza. Hum Vaccin 2011;7(Suppl):41–50.

Siripornadulsil S, Dabrowski K, Sayre R. Microalgal vaccines. Adv Exp Med Biol 2007;616:, 122–128.

Soler E, Le Saux A, Guinut F, Passet B, Cohen R, Merle C, Charpilienne A, Fourgeux C, Sorel V, Piriou A, Schwartz-Cornil I, Cohen J, Houdebine LM. Production of two vaccinating recombinant rotavirus proteins in the milk of transgenic rabbits. Transgenic Res 2005;14:833–844.

Staczek J, Bendahmane M, Gilleland LB, Beachy RN, Gilleland HE Jr. Immunization with a chimeric tobacco mosaic virus containing an epitope of outer membrane protein F of *Pseudomonas aeruginosa* provides protection against challenge with *P. aeruginosa*. Vaccine 2000;18:2266–2274.

Sunil Kumar GB, Ganapathi TR, Revathi CJ, Prasad KS, Bapat VA. Expression of hepatitis B surface antigen in tobacco cell suspension cultures. Protein Expr Purif 2003;32: 10–17.

Tregoning J, Maliga P, Dougan G, Nixon PJ. New advances in the production of edible plant vaccines: chloroplast expression of a tetanus vaccine antigen, TetC. Phytochemistry 2004;65:989–994.

Tuboly T, Yu W, Bailey A, Degrandis S, Du S, Erickson L, Nagy E. Immunogenicity of porcine transmissible gastroenteritis virus spike protein expressed in plants. Vaccine 2000;18: 2023–2028.

Wigdorovitz A, Carrillo C, Dus Santos MJ, Trono K, Peralta A, Gomez MC, Rios RD, Franzone PM, Sadir AM, Escribano JM, Borca MV. Induction of a protective antibody response to foot and mouth disease virus in mice following oral or parenteral immunization with alfalfa transgenic plants expressing the viral structural protein VP1. Virology 1999;255:347–353.

Wu L, Jiang L, Zhou Z, Fan J, Zhang Q, Zhu H, Han Q, Xu Z. Expression of foot-and-mouth disease virus epitopes in tobacco by a tobacco mosaic virus-based vector. Vaccine 2003;21:4390–4398.

Yang CD, Liao JT, Lai CY, Jong MH, Liang CM, Lin YL, Lin NS, Hsu YH, Liang SM. Induction of protective immunity in swine by recombinant bamboo mosaic virus expressing foot-and-mouth disease virus epitopes. BMC Biotechnol 2007;7:62–72.

Yusibov V, Hooper DC, Spitsin SV, Fleysh N, Kean RB, Mikheeva T, Deka D, Karasev A, Cox S, Randall J, Koprowski H. Expression in plants and immunogenicity of plant virus-based experimental rabies vaccine. Vaccine 2002;20:3155–3164.

Yusibov V, Mett V, Mett V, Davidson C, Musiychuk K, Gilliam S, Farese A, Macvittie T Mann D. Peptide-based candidate vaccine against respiratory syncytial virus. Vaccine 2005;23:2261–2265.

Yusibov, V, Rabindran, S, Plant viral expression vectors: History and Developments. In: Fischer, R, Schillberg, S. *Molecular Farming*. Weinheim: Wiley-VCH Verlag GmbH and Co. KgaA 2004; 77–90.

Yusibov V, Rabindran S, Commandeur U, Twyman RM, Fischer R. The potential of plant virus vectors for vaccine production. Drugs R&D 2006;7:203–217.

Yusibov V, Shivprasad S, Turpen TH, Dawson W, Koprowski H. Plant viral vectors based on tobamoviruses. Curr Top Microbiol Immunol 1999;240:81–94.

Yusibov V, Streatfield SJ, Kushnir N. Clinical development of plant-produced recombinant pharmaceuticals: Vaccines, antibodies and beyond. Hum Vaccin 2011;7:313–321.

Yusibov V, Streatfield SJ, Kushnir N, Roy G, Padmanaban A. Hybrid viral vectors for vaccine and antibody production in plants. Curr Pharm Des 2013;19:5574–5586.

5

VIRAL VACCINES PURIFICATION

BERND KALBFUSS-ZIMMERMANN

Novartis Pharma AG, Basel, Switzerland

UDO REICHL

Max Planck Institute for Dynamics of Complex Technical Systems, Bioprocess Engineering, Magdeburg, Germany; Otto-von-Guericke University, Magdeburg, Germany

5.1 INTRODUCTION

Immunoprophylaxis by vaccination provides an effective means for the protection of human beings and animals against a number of severe and often fatal diseases. Of these, a significant proportion is caused by viral pathogens (Table 5.1). Fortunately, a multitude of viral vaccines have become available over the last decades—many of them being used in routine vaccination today (see e.g., vaccines against poliovirus, hepatitis A, mumps, measles, and rubella virus in childhood vaccination; Baker and Katz, 2004). The downstream processing of corresponding viruses (or viral components) poses a challenging task, which involves the purification of high amounts of virus particles or viral antigens in a combination of validated purification procedures. These must be shown to meet quality, safety, and efficacy standards that apply to the production of vaccines or biologicals in general (Gregersen, 1994; Josefsberg and Buckland, 2012). In particular, requirements on potency, final levels of impurities, and contaminants such as endotoxins—as specified by regulatory bodies—have to be matched at the end of a process. Moreover, all unit operations should be performed under sanitary (preferably sterile) conditions to guaranty absence of adventitious agents such as fungi, bacteria, mycoplasmas, and viruses. Owing to the nature of viral replication, large variations in virus yield and consequently in the composition

Vaccine Development and Manufacturing, First Edition.
Edited by Emily P. Wen, Ronald Ellis, and Narahari S. Pujar.

TABLE 5.1 Overview of Vaccine-Relevant Viruses

Virus *(Family/Genus)*	Disease	Group	Env.	CH	Size/nm	MW/MDa	Density/ g/cm^3	Morphology	Surface Antigens
Flaviviruses *(Flaviviridae/ Flavivirus)*	Japanese/ tick-borne encephalitis, yel- low/dengue fever	IV	Yes	Yes	40–60	N.a.	1.19–1.23	Spherical	E
Hepatitis A virus *(Picornaviridae/ Hepatovirus)*	Hepatitis A	IV	No	No	30	5	1.32–1.34 empty: 1.20–1.29	Icosahedral	VP1, VP2, VP3
Hepatitis B virus *(Hepadnaviridae/ Orthohepadnavirus)*	Hepatitis B	VII	Yes	Yes	DS: 42–47, S: 20F: 20 (diameter) × variable length	N.a.	N.a.	Spherical, filamentous	HbsAg
Hepatitis C virus *(Flaviviridae/ Hepaciviruses)*	Hepatitis C	IV	Yes	Yes	30–60	N.a.	LD: 1.06–1 .13HD: 1.17–1.25	Spherical	E1, E2
Influenza viruses *(Orthomyxoviridae/ Influenzavirus A, B, and C)*	Flu	V	Yes	Yes	80–120	N.a.	N.a.	Pleomorphic, spherical	A/B: HA, NA C: HEF

Measles virus *(Paramyxoviridae/ Morbillivirus)*	Measles	V	yes	yes	100–300	N.a.	N.a.	Pleomorphic	H, F
Mumps virus *(Paramyxoviridae/ Rubulavirus)*	Mumps	V	Yes	Yes	100–600	N.a.	N.a.	Pleomorphic (irregular, filamentous)	HN, F
Papillomavirus *(Papillomaviridae /Alpha-, Gamma-, Mupapillomaviruses and unclassified)*	Cancer	I	No	N.a.	52–55	N.a.	1.34	Icosahedral	L1, L2
Poliovirus *(Picornaviridae/ Enterovirus)*	Poliomyelitis	IV	No	N.a.	30	157–160[a]	N.a.	Spherical	VP1, VP2, VP3
Rabies virus *(Rhabdoviridae/ Lyssavirus)*	Rabies	V	Yes	Yes	100 – 430 × 45–100	300–1000	1.19–1.20	Bullet shaped	G
Rotaviruses *(Reoviridae/ Rotavirus)*	Vomiting, diarrhea	III	No	Yes	DL: 70 TL: 100	N.a.	DL: 1.38 TL: 1.36	Spherical	TL: VP4, VP7 DL: VP6

(*continued*)

TABLE 5.1 (*Continued*)

Virus (*Family/Genus*)	Disease	Group	Env.	CH	Size/nm	MW/MDa	Density/ g/cm^3	Morphology	Surface Antigens
Rubella virus (*Togaviridae/ Rubivirus*)	Rubella	IV	Yes	Yes	60–70	N.a.	1.17–1.19	Spherical	E1, E2
Vaccinia virus (*Poxviridae/ Orthopoxvirus*)	Cow pox	I	Yes	Yes	350 × 270	3000	N.a.	Brick-shaped	A33R, A34R, A36R, A56R, B5R
Varicella-Zoster virus(*Herpesviridae/ Varicellovirus*)	Chickenpox	I	Yes	Yes	180–200	N.a.	1.27	Pleomorphic to spherical	N.a.

Note: list of vaccine-relevant viruses was compiled from the Biologicals/Vaccine section of the WHO web page (http://www.who.int/biologicals/areas/vaccines/en/index.html). Data on viruses was taken from (Knipe and Howley, 2001). Virus classification according to NCBI taxonomy browser (http://www.ncbi.nlm.nih.gov). Env.: enveloped, CH: carbohydrates (glycosylated proteins), DS: double-shelled, S: spherical, F: filamentous, LD: low density, HD: high density, DL: double-layered, TL: triple-layered. Grouping according to Baltimore classification: I—double-stranded DNA, II—single-stranded DNA, III—double-stranded RNA, IV—single-stranded RNA(+), V—single-stranded RNA(−), VI—reverse transcribing RNA, VII—reverse transcribing DNA.

of cultivation broths have to be dealt with. Besides, improvements and changes in upstream processing—particularly, the trend toward higher cell concentrations and higher titers—regularly demand for modification and improvement of the existing purification processes. Noteworthy, the task is often complicated by the fact that precision of assays for the quantitation of virus particles (or viral antigens) is often limited, and analytical methods for an extensive characterization of the final product are not always available. Finally, all unit operations have to be robust, scalable, and allow for the production of vaccines in a cost-effective manner (Kemp, 2007; Wolff and Reichl, 2011).

Generally, viral vaccines are categorized into live and dead vaccines. While the first group comprises all vaccines containing avirulent or attenuated viruses, vaccines of the second group contain only virions that have been inactivated by physical or chemical means or components of the latter. Dead vaccines can be further divided into whole-virion, split virion, and subvirion vaccines corresponding to inactivated, intact virions purified from viral culture, chemically or physically disrupted virions, or specific viral antigens. Of these, the latter is either extracted from naturally occurring viruses or, nowadays, produced by recombinant DNA technology.

While live vaccines are usually given orally or nasally mimicking the natural route of infection, inactivated or dead vaccines are applied either subcutaneously or intramuscularly. Typically, lower doses of virus are required for live vaccination, as the virus is able to replicate to some extent. Another consequence of oral or nasal application is that live vaccines need to be purified only to a limited extent because the mucosa poses an effective barrier against residues from viral culture. Dead vaccines, in contrast, need to be highly purified, particularly to avoid anaphylactic reaction, inflammation, and intrusion of host cell DNA, which can code for harmful oncogenes.

In this chapter, discussion is limited to the purification of viral pathogens for use in inactivated whole-virion vaccines. Since in the majority of cases, veterinary vaccines are only partially purified, the scope was further restricted to human vaccines. However, examples of other viruses have been included wherever this seemed appropriate and instructive. Moreover, purification of influenza virus serves as the predominant example throughout this chapter—primarily because a considerable number of publications on the purification of influenza virus have accumulated over the last decades, but also because influenza virus has recently moved into the focus of public interest and contemporary research because of the pandemic threat in form of avian influenza A/(H5N1) and swine influenza A/(H1N1) (Barrett et al., 2010; Collin and de Radiguès, 2009; Genzel and Reichl, 2009; Howard et al., 2008; Iskander and Broder, 2008).

Evidently, when dealing with whole-virion vaccines, the question of relevance from a today's perspective emerges. On the one hand, various live vaccines have been developed to date that are highly efficacious (Bandell et al., 2011; Gasparini et al., 2011), convenient to apply, and do not require the development of sophisticated purification processes. Moreover, at least in the case of influenza virus, they have been shown to provide long-lasting and broad protection (Belshe et al., 2004), particularly in children and young adults (Belshe et al., 2007). Furthermore, influenza live vaccines appear to be more efficacious in naive individuals (Cinatl et al., 2007) than dead vaccines. However, despite these advantages, it has to be considered that attenuated strains suitable for live vaccine production are not always available from the beginning but need to be generated first—a procedure that is often time-consuming and not guaranteed to succeed. In addition, attenuated strains are at least hypothetically linked to the risk of genetic reversal or insufficient attenuation. The occurrence of vaccine-associated paralysis in childhood vaccination at a rate of only one per 2.4 million doses, for instance, led to the replacement of the highly efficacious oral poliovirus vaccine by its killed vaccine counterpart in the United States (Song and Katial, 2004). In the case of influenza virus, it was further shown that live and dead vaccines stimulate different compartments of the immune system and may be combined to achieve better protection (Cox et al., 2004). On the other hand, highly developed subvirion vaccines have become available that provide similar protection compared to whole-virion vaccines but appear to suffer less from adverse reactions (Fukuda et al., 2004). Concerning subvirion vaccines, however, the latter has been observed to be less efficacious if applied without appropriate adjuvant (Cinatl et al., 2007; Geeraedts et al. 2008), requiring higher doses of antigen. Moreover, subvirion vaccines—if not produced by recombinant DNA technology—are usually prepared from natural virions, thus crossing the stage of at least partially purified virions. Another point that stresses the persisting relevance of inactivated whole-virion vaccines is that a number of such vaccines can be found in the current lists of candidates against pandemic influenza virus (Cinatl et al., 2007; Keitel and Atmar, 2007; Wood and Robertson, 2004).

However, the methodology discussed in this chapter is by no means restricted to the purification of vaccine-relevant natural virions. It should be rather considered universal for the purification of not only virions, but also virus-like particles (VLPs). Virus-like particles are self-assembling, nonreplicating particles similar in size to natural virions, which result after expression of certain proteins in bacterial, insect, or mammalian cell culture (Chackerian, 2007; Ramqvist et al., 2007). Before their use as vaccines or gene therapy vectors, VLPs have to be stripped from impurities similarly to natural virions. Last but not least, the closely related task of purifying virions as gene therapy vectors should be pointed out. Despite the different viruses being targeted, the methods applied (Braas et al., 1996; Morenweiser, 2005; Segura et al., 2006) are very similar and can often be transferred between the fields.

In the following section, common approaches in the purification of whole virions are discussed. Firstly, a general overview is given in Section 5.2, introducing the concept of process tasks. Subsequently, detailed summaries of applicable methods for harvesting, inactivation, purification, and concentration of virions on the basis of published records are given. Although the main aim is to provide a comprehensive overview of available literature on the subject, it was attempted to present more than a mere listing of examples. Wherever possible, underlying engineering principles are highlighted, and reference is made to related literature from other fields. Ideally, methods addressed would have also been ranked in terms of hard figures such as yield, purity, productivity, and economical factors. It was found, however, that publications often do not provide sufficient detail. Besides, every result has to be judged in its particular context, such as the source of feed material and the virus purified, which further hampers a side-by-side comparison of different studies. Consequently, a neutral presentation was chosen, leaving final judgment to the expertise of readers. However, general features and advantages or disadvantages were discussed, wherever this seemed appropriate.

5.2 PROCESS TASKS

The particular choice of unit operations and the consecutive order used to design a purification process largely depend on the type of virus to be purified and the source of the crude starting material (fertilized eggs vs. cell culture). As an example, two downstream processes, one for the purification of influenza virus cultivated in fertilized eggs and one for hepatitis A virus from mammalian cell culture are shown in Figure 5.1. While the first process mainly relies on precipitation and density gradient centrifugation as the main purification steps, nuclease treatment, extraction, and chromatography are used in the second process. On a functional level, however, a number of tasks can be named that are more or less generic for all downstream processes—independent of the virus type or strain and upstream conditions.

To begin with, cell debris (or solid matter) needs to be separated after propagation of the virus. If virus replication does not involve a lytic cycle or the release of virions is incomplete, a disruption of host cells may be required in addition. Next, virions have to be concentrated, purified, and inactivated, whereby the actual order of unit operations depends on the overall strategy pursued. Finally, the vaccine is blended from purified virus bulk, adjuvanted, and filled (not covered in this review). Generally, all unit operations should be performed under sterile conditions whenever this is possible.

Analogous to the production of other biologicals, separation of cell debris is commonly achieved by centrifugation or depth filtration—optionally followed by normal flow microfiltration with membrane filters. Tangential-flow microfiltration is another technique that has been used for this purpose. Lysis of host cells may be accomplished chemically, for example, by the addition of detergents, mechanically by exerting shear forces on the cells, or a combination of both in the form of freeze-thawing. For the purification of virions, a vast number of possibilities exist. Traditional processes often incorporate the selective precipitation of virions or impurities. Density gradient centrifugation is another technique among the first to be described in literature. More recently, tangential-flow ultrafiltration (TFUF) has evolved as a universal tool for the concentration of virions that can simultaneously be used for the conditioning of concentrates and separation of low molecular weight impurities. Similarly, size-exclusion chromatography (SEC) has been routinely used for the separation of small impurities and buffer exchange. Adsorptive chromatography, that is, mainly ion-exchange chromatography (IEC) and affinity chromatography (AC), which used to suffer from low capacity in the past, is gaining more and more importance. New materials such as adsorptive membranes, monolithic supports, and nonporous media have opened new

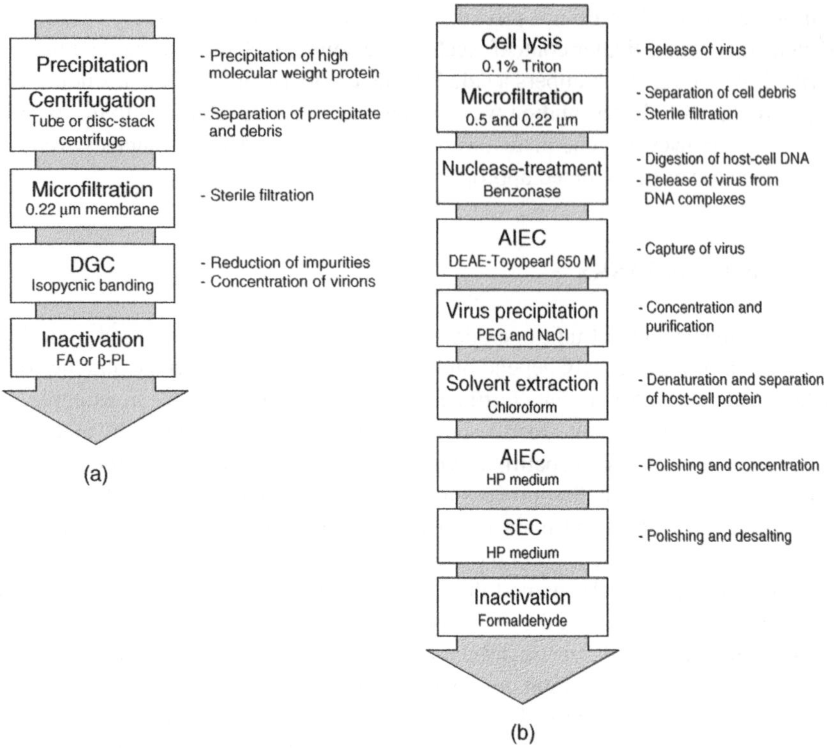

Figure 5.1 Traditional downstream process for the purification of egg-derived influenza virus based on continuous-flow density gradient centrifugation (DGC) (a) Purified virus is inactivated by formaldehyde (FA) or β-propiolactone (β-PL); process scheme assembled according to Gruschkau et al. (1973), Hilfenhaus et al. (1976a), and Bardiya and Bae (2005). Modern process for the purification of hepatitis A virus derived from mammalian cell culture involving anion-exchange (AIEC) and size-exclusion (SEC) chromatography (b) Process scheme assembled according to Hagen et al. (1996a, 1996b, 1997, 2000).

possibilities, making chromatography an attractive choice for the purification of virus particles in particular because of its high resolving power. Inactivation of infectious virions can take place either toward the end of a process or directly after clarification. In the latter case, handling of infectious material is reduced to a minimum, facilitating handling of intermediates in downstream processing. Inactivation conditions for crude starting materials, however, are less defined because of variations in the composition of viral harvests. Common ways of inactivation are by chemical agents such as formaldehyde (FA), β-propiolactone, or aziridines. Moreover, UV irradiation has been proposed as a gentle method reducing incubation time and leaving no residues.

For optimal process design and operation, current Good Manufacturing Practice (cGMP), guidelines of the International Standardization Organization (ISO) and International Conference on Harmonization (ICH), basic guides of the International

Society of Pharmaceutical Engineers (ISPE), and legal aspects have to be taken into account. Of particular importance are the respective documents of the World Health Organization (WHO) and regional pharmacopoeias published by regulatory bodies, which give detailed recommendations for manufacturing, production control, and final lot testing. Usually, as part of these documents, assays for the quantitation of antigen are described, and recommendations for the amount of antigen per dose are given. In addition, limits for the content of certain impurities are specified. Very often, these include limits on the specific content of host cell or total protein, host cell DNA, and endotoxins. Sometimes, additional limits for certain markers (e.g., bovine serum albumin for serum content), the residual content of inactivating agent (e.g., FA), or antibiotics are specified. As an example, release criteria for cell culture and egg-derived inactivated whole-virion influenza vaccines as stated by the WHO and European Pharmacopoeia have been summarized in Table 5.2.

In the following sections, a summary of common unit operations is given that have been reported useful with respect to the purification of whole virus particles. In addition, reference to new techniques or related areas is made wherever this seems appropriate, highlighting potentially new applications in the field. According to the concept of process functions, unit operations were categorized into the sections harvest, inactivation and purification, and concentration—the latter not being clearly separable for most unit operations. It should be mentioned here that the extent of chapters does not necessarily reflect the importance of particular unit operations but

TABLE 5.2 Specifications for Inactivated Whole-Virion Influenza Vaccines

Characteristic	WHO[a]	EP (egg-derived)[b]	EP (cell culture)[c]
HA antigen	>15 μg per strain	15 μg per strain[d]	15 μg per strain[d]
DNA	<10 ng[e]		<10 ng
Protein	<100 μg per strain <300 ug per dose	<6 × HA antigen content <100 μg per strain	<6 × HA antigen content <100 μg per strain
Endotoxins	To be tested	<100 IU	<25 IU
Sterility	To be tested	To be tested	To be tested
Formaldehyde	<0.1%[f]	<0.2 g/l[f]	<0.2 g/l
β-Propiolactone	<0.1%[f]	<0.1%[f]	
Ovalbumin	<5 μg	<1 μg	
BSA (from serum)			<50 ng
Residual infectivity	To be tested in fertilized eggs or cell culture, respectively	Amplification test in fertilized eggs over two passages	Amplification test in cell culture over two passages

[a](WHO Technical Report Series, 2005).
[b](European Pharmacopoeia Commission, 2012a).
[c](European Pharmacopoeia Commission, 2012b).
[d]Unless clinical evidence supports the use of a different amount.
[e]For virus grown in cell culture.
[f]At any time during inactivation.

rather corresponds to the amount of literature available. In fact, despite the long history of viral vaccines, information in some areas remains rather limited. Therefore, wherever possible, cross-links to the general theory were drawn, and reference to related work from other field (such as the purification of proteins from mammalian cell culture or studies with colloidal model systems) is made.

5.2.1 Harvest

5.2.1.1 Lysis of Host Cells Eventually, after infection, newly produced virions will be released from host cells as part of their natural infection cycle. Release occurs either by budding from the cell membrane (enveloped viruses) or by virus-induced lysis of host cells (naked viruses). If the virus to be purified is assembled intracellularly, it may sometimes be advantageous to lyse host cells on purpose in order to maximize virus yield. At the laboratory scale, this is often achieved by freeze-thawing of cells followed by centrifugation or filtration (Divizia et al., 1989; Guskey and Wolff, 1972; Hu et al. 2010; Peixoto et al., 2007; Peixoto et al., 2006). Obviously, this procedure is fairly energy intensive and not suitable for large-scale manufacturing. Alternatively, detergents may be added to viral cultures in order to permeabilize host cell membranes (Hagen et al., 1996a; Hagen et al., 1996b; Peixoto et al., 2007). Although detergent lysis can be performed at arbitrary scale, the disadvantage is that detergent needs to be removed again and may have an impact on subsequent unit operations. In principle, mechanical disintegration such as milling or high pressure homogenization could be applied as well. Mechanical disintegration is often used in the purification of cytosolic products from bacterial or yeast culture. In contrast to microorganisms, much lower energy input would be required for the lysis of mammalian cells. Possibly, shearing at the inlet of continuous centrifuges would already be sufficient for the complete release of virions. However, independently of the method used, it has to be considered that lysis of host cells leads to an extra burden of impurities. Gains in virus yield therefore have to be traded off against the extra effort required to achieve the desired level of product purity.

5.2.1.2 Normal Flow Filtration Normal flow filtration probably represents the simplest unit operation for the separation of cell debris. It has been frequently described for the harvest of virus-containing supernatant subsequent to virus propagation (Brands et al., 1999; Hagen et al., 2000; Kalbfuss et al., 2007a; Montagnon and Fanget, 1985; Peixoto et al., 2007; Wiktor et al., 1987). In some cases, direct application of membrane filters has been reported (Hagen et al., 2000; Montagnon and Fanget, 1985; Wiktor et al., 1987), as well as the application of depth filtration alone (Peixoto et al., 2007). In order to enhance the capacity of filters, it is usually advisable to combine depth or prefiltration with a fibrous media and membrane microfiltration (e.g., Kalbfuss et al., 2007a). This is particularly true for feed streams of high solid content (e.g., microcarrier or high celldensity cultivations). Alternatively, normal flow filtration can be combined with centrifugation (Hong et al., 2001). In this combination, centrifugation takes the part of the depth filter, while separation of fines is achieved using a microfilter. Although normal flow filtration appears to be preferred for the harvest of biologicals because of its low investment costs and simplicity, the use of tangential-flow microfiltration has been described as well (Berthold and Kempken, 1994; Guo et al. 2009; Maiorella et al., 1991; Saxena et al., 2009; van Reis et al., 1991). In general, tangential-flow microfiltration provides better fouling control and filter capacity than its normal flow counterpart but at the cost of increased process complexity and higher cost of investment.

Depth filters used in bioprocessing are typically composed of a fibrous support (cellulose or polypropylene) and a filter aid (diatomaceous earth, perlite, or activated carbon), which is structured into sheets by a binder polymer. Several of these filter sheets are then stacked into special filter housings (van Reis and Zydney, 2007). Filtration occurs by gravitational settling, direct interception of particles, inertial impaction, diffusional interception, and electrostatic deposition (Davis and Grant, 1992). Importantly, separation is not exclusively controlled by size, but the adsorptive properties of filter aids are equally important (Yigzaw et al., 2006). Polymer microfiltration membranes are commonly cast from regenerated cellulose, polysulfone, polyethersulfone, polyvinylidene fluoride, or polycarbonate (Zeman and Zydney, 1996). Available membrane cutoffs range from about 0.1 to several micrometers. The corresponding modules are composed of one or several layers of a pleated membrane on top of a fibrous support. Pleated layers are wrapped around a tubular core giving rise to the dome-shaped appearance of current filter modules (van Reis and Zydney, 2007). A compendium on the properties, design, and manufacture of filter media composed by Purchas and Sutherland (2002) is recommended for further reading.

Cutoffs of membrane filters used for the harvest of viruses typically range from 0.2 to 0.5 μm depending on the size of the virus and fouling characteristics. If membrane filters with 0.2 μm cutoff or lower are used, filtration further serves as a sterile barrier adding safety to the process. At low solid content and pores smaller than the size of solids, filtration is exclusively controlled by the pore-size distribution of the membrane (surface filtration; Davis and Grant, 1992). But the cutoff of membranes may be altered during filtration by pore constriction (Trilisky and Lenhoff, 2009) and pore blockage. In addition, eventually, a cake will form further impacting sieving characteristics. Consequently, depending on the size of virus particles and the nature and concentration of solids, loss of virus may be observed even in the case of sufficiently large pores. Sometimes, a fibrous prefilter made from glass or polypropylene is used to prolong the lifetime of membrane filters. These prefilters are either integrated into the same module (as an additional layer) or packaged as a separate module for operation in line.

Today, both—normal flow depth and membrane filters—are almost exclusively designed as disposable devices, totally avoiding the need for filter cleaning and cleaning validation. Tangential-flow microfilters, in contrast, may be too expensive for single-use operation. In addition, a filtration rig is required for operation, increasing the costs of investment. However, tangential-flow microfiltration provides better fouling control and can be used directly for the clarification of feed streams with high solid content. This may further allow for the selection of membrane cutoffs closer to the dimensions of the product. Which technique is more adequate cannot be predicted per se but depends on individual process requirements or is a matter of process design approach. For a final decision, thorough experimental characterization and experience with similar processes are usually required.

Both normal flow and tangential-flow filtration can be directly conducted out of bioreactors or harvest vessels. In the case of normal flow filtration, this is achieved either by pressurizing the vessel or by using a pump. Various strategies exist for controlling the driving force, of which, filtration at a constant pressure drop or constant flux is the most convenient. Since, however, operation of filters at low flux has been demonstrated to result in a significant gain in capacity (Singhvi et al., 1996), operation at constant flux should be preferred. Alternatively, the pressure drop may be successively increased starting at a very low pressure drop first. Despite the frequent use of normal flow filtration, hardly any data on the clarification of virus-containing cell culture supernatant or related feed streams have been reported in literature. Accordingly, only a general guideline for the development of normal flow filtration operations can be provided.

An obvious approach for the characterization of flux decay and filter capacity is scale-down experiments with real samples. In such experiments, the samples are pumped through a scale-down variant of the filter to be used—either at a constant flux or driven by a constant pressure drop. Pressure drop or filtrate flux is then recorded over time (Fig. 5.2a). Afterward, the capacity of filters is defined by a critical mark (either maximum pressure drop or a certain fraction of the initial flux). The disadvantage of such an approach is the relatively large amount of sample volume required. This is particularly true because experiments should be repeated multiple times with different lots of the filter material and the sample. In order to cut down on the volume of samples, it is desirable to terminate filtration at an early stage and extrapolate the data using an appropriate filtration model. Evidently, such extrapolation is only valid if the filtration model applied includes all the relevant mechanisms and if parameters can be identified accurately at the initial period of filtration. In addition, there will be no indication whether the capacity of filters can truly be exploited or a significant loss of product will occur much earlier because of altered sieving characteristics of filters as a consequence of pore constriction and cake formation.

Several laws for the description of filtration at constant pressure drop have been summarized by Hermia (1982). Independent of the dominating mechanism, these models can be summarized by the relation,

$$\frac{d^2t}{dV^2} = k\left(\frac{dt}{dV}\right)^n \tag{5.1}$$

with dt/dV and d^2t/dV^2 denoting the reciprocals of the first and second derivative of filtrate volume with respect to the time t. If a single mechanism is dominant, n takes discrete values between 0 and 2 indicating either cake filtration ($n = 0$), intermediate blocking ($n = 1$), pore constriction ($n = 3/2$), or complete pore blocking ($n = 2$). More likely, however, distinct phases of filtration are to be expected over time (Fig. 5.2b). A drawback of this approach is that derivatives of experimental data need to be calculated, which are very sensitive to noise. The problem can be overcome

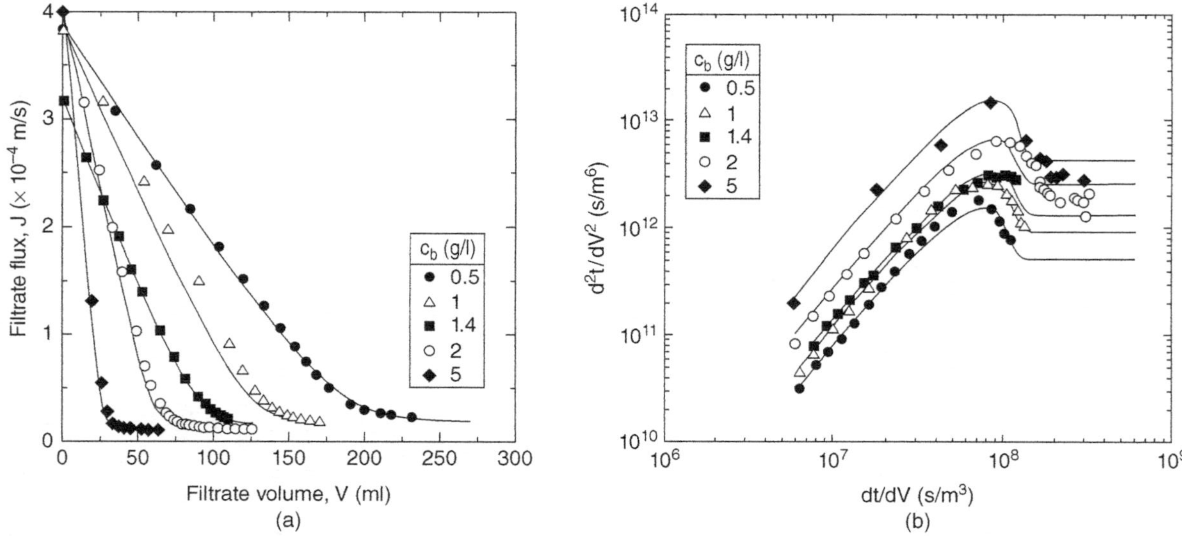

Figure 5.2 Flux decline (a) and flux decline analysis (b) for BSA filtration at different bulk protein concentrations. Solid curves represent model calculations using a combined pore blockage and cake filtration model. Reproduced with permission from Elsevier, Journal of Colloid and Interface Science, 2000.

at least partially by advanced numerical methods such as smoothing splines (Craven and Wahba, 1979; Reinsch, 1967) or Tikhonov regularization (Lubansky et al., 2006).

For the special case of $n = 3/2$ (pore constriction), filter capacity can be determined by the V_{max} method (Badmington et al., 1995; Zydney and Ho, 2002). Firstly, the sample is filtered at a constant pressure drop until flow rate has reduced to 90% or 80% of its initial value. Secondly, the linearized form of the pore constriction model,

$$\frac{t}{V} = \frac{1}{Q_0} + \left(\frac{1}{V_{max}}\right) t \tag{5.2}$$

is fitted to the data by linear regression. In this equation, V denotes the filtrate volume as a function of time t. The initial flow rate Q_0 and maximum filtrate volume V_{max} are determined as the result of regression analysis. In the following, relative flow rate Q/Q_0 as a function of time can be extrapolated according to,

$$\frac{Q}{Q_0} = \left(1 + \frac{Q_0 t}{V_{max}}\right)^{-2} \tag{5.3}$$

In most practical applications, filter capacity V_{cap} is defined as the filtrate volume after which the current flow rate has dropped to values between 10% and 20% of the initial value. It can be obtained from the equation,

$$V_{cap} = V_{max}\left(1 - \sqrt{\frac{Q_{min}}{Q_0}}\right) \tag{5.4}$$

Although accurate prediction of filter capacity by the V_{max} method has been achieved for the filtration of calf serum, dilute milk solution, and tap water (Badmington et al., 1995), often a combination of pore constriction and cake formation occurs. This is particularly true if the content of depositing solid in the feed is significant. For such cases, a combined pore blockage and cake filtration model has been developed by Ho and Zydney (Ho and Zydney, 2000; Palacio et al., 2002). This model has further been extended to the description of filtration at constant flux (Ho and Zydney, 2002). Prediction of filter capacity based on the combined model proved superior to that by the V_{max} method for the filtration of protein solutions (Zydney and Ho, 2002). In order to obtain accurate prediction, however, exact solutions of the model had to be calculated, which required numerical integration in addition to nonlinear regression analysis for the identification of parameters.

5.2.1.3 Continuous Centrifugation Centrifugation in disc-stack or tubular bowl centrifuges is probably the most common method for the clarification of culture broth at large scales. In comparison to dead-end filtration, the cost of investment is fairly high and sanitization, as well as cleaning is often considered critical. However, significant savings in operating costs may be the benefit when centrifugation is used. Moreover, centrifugation can be operated as a continuous operation at a constant flow rate in contrast to the limited capacity of dead-end filters. In addition, the risk of early filter blockage is eliminated. However, centrifugal clarification may be insufficient for the protection of chromatography operations and may require additional clarification by microfiltration (Berthold and Kempken, 1994; Kempken et al., 1995).

In contrast to filtration, separation in centrifuges is governed by the sedimentation velocity of particles (and not size or adsorptive properties). According to sigma theory, the cutoff sedimentation velocity is equivalent to $u_s = Q/2\Sigma$, where Q is the volumetric flow rate and Σ the equivalent area of a settling tank. The ratio Q/Σ corresponds to the load of the centrifuge (Ambler, 1959). Note that for noncontinuous centrifuges, the flow rate is replaced by the ratio of batch volume and centrifugation time V/t. By definition, in ideal systems, half of the particle population having cutoff sedimentation velocity will be recovered after centrifugation. Various expressions have been derived for the calculation of Σ, including laboratory, bowl, and disc-stack centrifuges (Ambler, 1959). Concerning scale-up, the only criterion to be fulfilled (at least in theory) is an equivalent load of centrifuges $Q_1/\Sigma_1 = Q_2/\Sigma_2$. In reality, however, correction factors μ_i have to be introduced such that $Q_1/\mu_1\Sigma_1 = Q_2/\mu_2\Sigma_2$, with values ranging from 0.4 to 1 (Maybury et al., 2000). The correction factor of laboratory centrifuges is typically assumed as unity.

Practically, the distribution of the settling velocity is almost never available. It is therefore necessary to characterize the clarification efficiency as a function of the centrifugal load. In these experiments, the clarification efficiency is followed by measures for the content of solid in feed and supernatant. Often, turbidity is measured for this purpose. A possible definition of clarification efficiency could be $1 - c_{super}/c_{feed}$, with c_{super} and c_{feed} denoting concentrations in the supernatant and feed, respectively. Finally, the critical clarification efficiency has to be defined, which is considered acceptable for the process. The corresponding load is then used for the definition of appropriate operating conditions and scale-up.

Clarification efficiency can be characterized either directly on the system of interest (typically a bowl or disc-stack centrifuge) or by using scale-down models. Although the first approach is less likely to fail, it is also very expensive, requiring large volumes of feed material and a production-scale centrifuge at the stage of process development. Maybury et al. (1998) reported on how to minimize the hold-up volume and separation area of a disc-stack centrifuge without affecting separation behavior. Even simpler, initial studies can be conducted in laboratory centrifuges, which require only a minimum amount of feed (Maybury et al., 2000). As long as the time for acceleration and deceleration remains negligible, the equivalent settling tank area of a laboratory centrifuge can be be calculated.

$$\Sigma_{lab} = \frac{V\omega^2}{2g \cdot \ln\left(\frac{2r_2}{r_2+r_1}\right)} \tag{5.5}$$

with r_1 and r_2 denoting the inner and outer radii of the liquid volume V and angular velocity ω, respectively (Ambler, 1959). For very short centrifugation times, the acceleration and deceleration phases have to be considered, and the approach described by Maybury et al. (2000) is more appropriate.

Although successful scale-up from laboratory to continuous centrifuges has been demonstrated for rigid particles (Boychyn et al., 2000; Maybury et al., 2000), shear stress at the inlet of continuous centrifuges regularly affects the size distribution of shear-sensitive matter (such as biomass), leading to a reduction in the clarification efficiency (Boychyn et al., 2000; Hutchinson et al., 2006; Maybury et al., 2000). It was estimated by computational fluid dynamics that the maximum energy dissipation of a multichamber bowl centrifuge occurs at the inlet, with rates being as high as $6 \cdot 10^5$ W/kg (fully flooded inlet; Boychyn et al., 2001). However, lysis of mammalian cells already occurs at much lower energy dissipation rates (Hutchinson et al., 2006). Similar studies on a tubular bowl centrifuge predicted shear rates up to 25,000/s near the inlet (close to the deflector plate; Jain et al., 2005). Again, disintegration of mammalian cells has been observed during cross-flow filtration for shear rates exceeding 3000/s (Maiorella et al., 1991). A simple yet effective approach to simulate these conditions is by pretreating samples in a shear device, mimicking the high energy dissipation rates at centrifuge inlets (Boychyn et al., 2001). By doing so, fairly accurate prediction of centrifugal performance has been achieved for yeast protein, plasma precipitate (Boychyn et al., 2004), and mammalian cells (Hutchinson et al., 2006).

Despite the value of sigma theory, no published data on the clarification of virus-containing cell culture supernatant or virus-containing allantoic fluid appear to exist. Therefore, only an example for the clarification of influenza virus-containing cell culture supernatant (unpublished data) can be provided (Fig. 5.3). Independently of the cultivation system (roller bottles, wave bag, and stirred tank), about 98% clarification appeared to be feasible after centrifugation at $V/\Sigma t = 2 \times 10^{-8}$ m/s

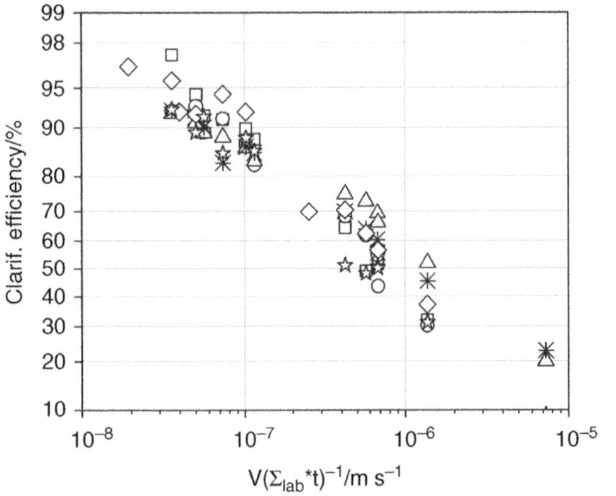

Figure 5.3 Clarification of influenza virus-containing cell culture supernatant by centrifugation (unpublished data). Supernatant from various MDCK cell cultures (roller bottles, wave bag, and stirred tank) infected with influenza virus A/PR/8/34 (H1N1) was clarified 3 days after infection using a laboratory centrifuge. Clarification efficiency was determined by the measurement of light extinction at 700 nm.

(extrapolated from the data). Scalability between different types of laboratory centrifuges was confirmed, but investigations of the impact of shear stress on settling behavior are still required. A similar correlation was found by Hutchinson et al. (circa 98.5% clarification at $V/\Sigma t = 2 \times 10^{-8}$ m/s; Hutchinson et al., 2006). In their work, a mammalian cell suspension (myeloma cell line producing antibody) at the late culture phase (<10% viability) was used for experiments. A slightly different definition of the clarification efficiency was employed, however. Pretreatment of the suspension in a shear device (simulating shear at the inlet of continuous centrifuges) led to up to fivefold increase in the remaining solid content depending on the maximum energy dissipation rate. A somewhat lower ratio may be expected for cells after virus infection, owing to cell lysis during the infection phase, but the factor of five can be used for estimation of the worst-case scenario.

5.2.2 Inactivation

Inactivation of infectious virus is a key process in the manufacture of inactivated whole-virion vaccines for human and veterinary use. While for subunit vaccines inactivation usually occurs as part of the dismantling process, dedicated unit operations have to be integrated into the process for inactivated whole-virion vaccines. Inactivation has to be safe, complete, and irreversible, but the potency of the vaccine should not be affected. Although a large number of inactivation methods exist (see e.g., Benedictis et al., 2007), the latter requirement dramatically reduces the number of viable options.

Traditionally, vaccines have been inactivated by FA and still appear to be (Armstrong et al., 1993; Kistner et al., 1998; Lauffer and Wheatley, 1949; Timm et al., 1956). A finding that is surprising in the context of several outbreaks of disease after vaccination with FA-inactivated poliovirus in the 1930s and 1955 and FMD virus in the 1970s and 1980s, which seemed to be related to the incomplete inactivation of virions (King et al., 1981). Of these, the Cutter incident, which occurred in the United States in 1955, was propably the most severe. During a 10-day period in April, approximately 400,000 persons—primarily grade-school children—had been inoculated with Cutter vaccine (FA-inactivated poliovirus). In the following 2 months, an extraordinarily high rate of poliomyelitis incidents were recorded, which were later related to two lots of Cutter vaccine containing residual virulent virus. Of the children who had received Cutter vaccine, abortive poliomyelitis developed in about 40,000 individuals; 51 were permanently paralyzed, and five died. Moreover, more than 100 cases of poliomyelitis were detected in family and community contacts (Nathanson et al., 1995; Offit, 2005). Fault of the inactivation procedure was generally ascribed to the presence of virus aggregates, which restricted access of FA to virions (Melnick, 1991). It was further demonstrated that not only physicochemical conditions such as temperature and pH value, but also the microenvironment and heterogenity of virions do play a role in the inactivation process (Salk et al., 1960). Neither should the consumption of FA by unspecific side reactions be neglected, as has been discussed for β-propiolactone (see the following section). Somewhat later, additional concerns about the safety of FA inactivation because of only reversible modification of viral genomes emerged (Beck and Strohmaier, 1987; Budowsky, 1991; King et al., 1981). In a search for alternatives, new reagents were suggested, which were considered safer and believed to target nucleic acids (i.e., viral genomes) more specifically. Of these, inactivation by aziridines and β-propiolactone (β-PL) is discussed in this chapter. Other methods such as inactivation by UV irradiation (Budowsky et al., 1981; Cutler et al., 2011; Loewinger and Katz, 2002; Simonet and Gantzer, 2006; Wang et al., 1995), pasteurization (Arita and Matumoto, 1968; Darnell et al., 2004; Lauffer and Carnelly, 1945; Rueda et al., 2000), or high pressure inactivation (Freitas et al., 2003; Grove et al., 2006) have not been considered for large-scale application because their role in the manufacture of viral vaccines remains unclear.

The degree of inactivation is commonly described by survival curves of type $S(t) = lg(X_0/X(t))$, where X denotes either the concentration or the total amount of infectious virions. The shape of survival curves very much depends on the virus to be inactivated (very often the type of genome) and, obviously, the method of inactivation (Budowsky, 1991). In the simplest case, an exponential decay (first order process) can be observed. The probability of finding a single infectious virion per dose is equal to $X(t)$ (denoting the total amount of virions) in the limit of $X(t) \rightarrow 0$ (Storhas, 1994). Typically, inactivation of 15–20 orders of magnitude will be required for the probability of an infectious virus being present in any annual production of the vaccine not exceeding 10^{-1} to 10^{-2} (Budowsky, 1991). Experimentally, however, reduction can only be controlled by 10 orders of magnitude at most. Safety of inactivation methods must hence be inferred from proper description of inactivation kinetics, requiring a profound understanding of mechanisms. In addition, in-process safety testing of inactivation for every lot by inoccuity tests is usually required (European Pharmacopoeia Commission, 2012a; European Pharmacopoeia Commission, 2012b; WHO Technical Report Series, 2005). However, such innocuity testing can only provide an additional level of safety. Especially, a low level of residual infectivity after inactivation is not necessarily detected because of limited sampling volumes. Finally, the risk of virus particles escaping the inactivation process has to be minimized. In particular, dead ends in inactivation vessels (e.g., dip tubes, sampling ports, and valves) have to be avoided. After addition of the inactivant, the virus-inactivant mixture should be transferred into a second vessel for completion of the inactivation process, whereas inactivation conditions (pH value and °C) need to be tightly controlled to guaranty innocuity of inactivated vaccines.

Chemical inactivation of virions by numerous agents has been reported in the past, including the use of FA, aziridines, and β-PL (Table 5.3). In particular, aziridines (mostly in the form of "binary ethyleneimine"; BEI) and β-PL have been frequently used as specific agents for the modification of viral genomes. Both aziridines and lactones are highly strained molecules that react with nucleophilic compounds by ring-opening (Bartlett and Small, 1950; Vollhardt and Schore, 1999a; Vollhardt and Schore, 1999b). While β-PL is available as a pure liquid that can be stably stored at −20°C, ethyleneimine in the form of BEI is usually synthesized from 2-bromo-ethylamine under alkaline conditions (Bahnemann, 1990). Both reagents are extremely toxic (Bahnemann, 1990; Brusick, 1977) and need to be handled with special precaution. They are hydrolyzed in (acidic) aqueous solution (Bartlett and

TABLE 5.3 Studies on Virus Inactivation

Virus	Reagent	Reference
Hepatitis A virus	FA	Armstrong et al. (1993)
HIV-1	β-PL, BEI	Race et al. (1995)
Influenza virus	FA	Lauffer and Wheatley (1949)
	β-PL	Budowsky et al. (1991) Budowsky et al. (1993)
	BEI	King (1991)
Rabies virus	BEI	Larghi and Nebel (1980)
Poliovirus	FA	Timm et al. (1956) Lycke (1958)
	BEI, AEI	Brown (2002)
Vaccinia virus (recombinant)	BEI	Hulskotte et al. (1997)

FA: formaldehyde, β-PL: β-propiolactone, BEI: binary ethyleneimine, AEI: N-acetyl-ethyleneimine.

Small, 1950; Vollhardt and Schore, 1999a; Vollhardt and Schore, 1999b). Thiosulfate may be equally used not only for neutralization (Bahnemann, 1990), but also for titration of β-PL and ethyleneimine in analytical assays for the determination of residual concentration (Bartlett and Small, 1950; Budowsky et al., 1991). In addition, colorimetric quantitation by reaction with 4-(p-nitrobenzyl)pyridine has been described for aziridines (Epstein et al., 1955; Tsvetkova and Nepomnyaschaya, 2001).

β-PL has been demonstrated to alkylate nucleic acids (RNA and DNA) both *in vitro* (Chen et al., 1981; Morgeaux et al., 1993; Roberts and Warwick, 1963) and *in vivo* (Boutwell et al., 1969; Morgeaux et al., 1993). At elevated concentrations, it has been shown to induce nicks into DNA and lead to cross-linking between DNA and proteins, as well as between DNA-strands in the double helix (Perrin and Morgeaux, 1995). In addition, β-PL is able to react with amino acids (cysteine and probably also methionine) (Dickens and Jones, 1961) and proteins (Boutwell et al., 1969). In a more recent study, β-PL treatment of two H1N1 influenza A strains indicated that the first step of virus membrane fusion was inhibited and therefore virus entry into host cells impaired (Desbat and Lancelot, 2011). Furthermore, the application of β-PL for inactivation of influenza virus, for example, resulted in a partial inactivation of hemagglutination activity (King, 1991) and a chemical modification of the hemagglutinine (Desbat and Lancelot, 2011).

The use of aziridines, mostly in the form of BEI, was first reviewed by Bahnemann, 1990. Analogous to β-PL, the supposed mechanism of inactivation is by alkylation of nucleic acids (Brown, 2002). It was claimed that BEI shows higher specificity for nucleic acids than β-PL. *In vitro* experiments with various test proteins, however, demonstrated that aziridines may react with proteins as well (Käsermann et al., 2001; Tsvetkova and Nepomnyaschaya, 2001). Interestingly, not only selectivity but also the rate of inactivation very much depended on the type of aziridine used (monomer to tetramer; Tsvetkova and Nepomnyaschaya, 2001). In contrast to β-PL, no reduction in hemagglutination activity was detected on inactivation of Newcastle disease virus and avian influenza virus at doses until 10 mM (King, 1991). A fact, which may, however, be related to the lower maximum concentration applied.

Despite the fact that inactivation kinetics of the experimentally controllable region often appears of the first order, deviation from first order kinetics is to be expected whenever the inactivating agent is consumed in the process (Budowsky et al., 1991). Since conditions for safe inactivation have to be inferred from proper description of inactivation kinetics, consumption of the inactivating agent should not be ignored. Still, the inactivation of many viruses with BEI has been described as a first order process (Bahnemann, 1990). Data for Semliki forest virus and mouse minute virus inactivated with BEI and trimeric ethyleneimine, however, clearly indicate that the consumption of aziridines cannot be neglected (Käsermann et al., 2001).

An excellent example for adequate description of inactivation kinetics is given by Budowsky et al., who characterized the inactivation of bacterial phage MS2 (Budowsky et al., and Zalesskaya 1991) and egg-derived influenza virus (three strains) by β-PL (Budowsky et al., 1991; Budowsky et al., 1993). The inactivation of infectious virions was found to follow second order kinetics, whereas β-PL was consumed in a first order reaction. No lag time in the reduction of viral infectivity could be detected in either case, indicating complete inactivation of virions after the first lesion (Budowsky, 1991). However, a heterogeneous population was observed for influenza virus A/WSN/33 (H1N1) such that analysis had to be restricted to the haploid form of virions (containing a single genome copy per virion only; Budowsky et al., 1993). Inactivation kinetics could be appropriately described by the equation,

$$S(t, c_0) = 0.434 \cdot c_0 \frac{k_2}{k_1}(1 - e^{-k_1 t}) \tag{5.6}$$

with the initial concentration of β-PL c_0, incubation time t, and rate constants k_1 for the first order decay of β-PL and k_2 for the second order inactivation of infectious virions. In addition, in the case of phage MS2, the Arrhenius law was applied to describe temperature dependency of rate constants (Budowsky et al., 1991).

Parameters for the different strains of influenza virus and rate constants for reaction of β-PL with water and thiosulfate are summarized in Table 5.4. The degree of inactivation of influenza virus as a function of initial concentration of β-PL and incubation time (assuming the most unfavorable parameters $k_1 = 8 \cdot 10^{-3}$/min and $k_2 = 50$ l/mol/h) is illustrated in Fig. 5.4. As can be seen, the maximum degree of inactivation $S(t, c_0) = 0.434 \cdot c_0 \frac{k_2}{k_1}$ for $t \to \infty$ is reached after about 8 h, independently of the initial concentration used.

5.2.3 Purification and Concentration

5.2.3.1 Density Gradient Centrifugation It was in the early 1960s when Anderson reported on the development of the first continuous-flow zonal ultracentrifuge (Anderson, 1962) having preparative separations of particles mixtures in mind.

TABLE 5.4 Rate Constants for the Inactivation of Influenza Virus with *β*-Propiolactone

Virus or Reactant	Medium	pH Value	Temp. /°C	$k_1/10^{-3}$ /min	k_2/l/ mol/min	Reference
B/Leningrad/ 489/80	Allantoic fluid[a]	7.2–7.3	20	6.9	50	Budowsky et al. (1991)
	Purified virus[b]	7.2–7.4	20	5.1	80	
A/Leningrad/ 385 (H3N2)	Allantoic fluid[a]	7.2–7.3	20	8.0	50	
	Purified virus[b]	7.2–7.4	20	5.1	120	
A/WSN/33 (H1N1)	Allantoic fluid[a]		20	2.3	110	Budowksky et al. (1993)
Water (acidic solution)	Purified virus[b]		20	1.3	250	
	0.01–0.05 M perchloric acid	1.3–2.0	25	3.35[c]		Bartlett and Small (1950)
Sodium thiosulfate		N.A.	25		11.2[d]	

[a]0.2 M phosphate buffer added.
[b]In 0.15 M NaCl + 0.2 M phosphate buffer.
[c]First-order reaction.
[d]Second-order reaction.

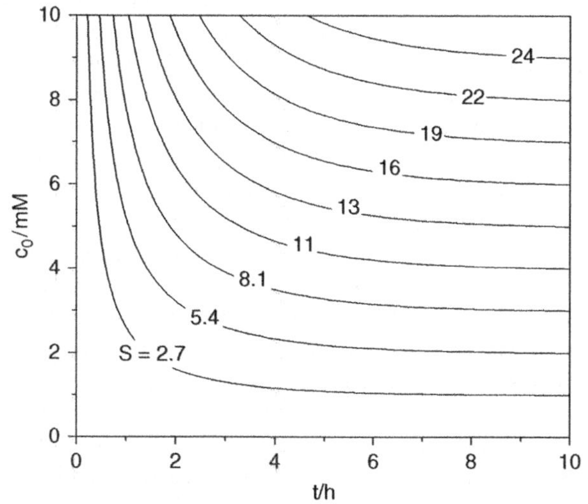

Figure 5.4 Inactivation of influenza virus with *β*-propiolactone. The degree of inactivation S (contour lines) is given as a function of the initial concentration of *β*-propiolactone c_0 and incubation time. Most unfavorable parameters from literature have been assumed for calculation ($k_1 = 8 \cdot 10^{-3}$/min and $k_2 = 50$ l/mol/h) (Budowsky et al., 1991).

Until then, zonal ultracentrifugation had been exclusively an analytical or semipreparative method. First applications comprised the separation of cellular components (Anderson and Burger, 1962) and purification of bacterial phage T3 (Anderson, 1963). Soon, continuous-flow zonal ultracentrifugation developed into a powerful method for the purification of influenza virions propagated in the allantois of embryonated chicken eggs (Reimer et al., 1966a; Reimer et al., 1966b; Reimer et al., 1967; Fig. 5.6). Consequently, the development of centrifuges and rotors was continued until it yielded the first centrifuge (K-II type) primarily intended for the preparation of viral vaccines at large scale (Anderson et al., 1969; Perardi et al., 1969). Suitability was again demonstrated in the example of influenza virus (Gerin and Anderson, 1969). In contrast to first designs, the K-II rotor was operated by the principle of reorienting gradients and allowed for the continuous loading of sample. Previously, concentration of samples before zonal centrifugation, for example, by precipitation (Reimer et al., 1966b), batch adsorption (Reimer et al., 1967), or pelleting in an ultracentrifuge (Reimer et al., 1966a) was necessary for economic operation. However, concentration before density centrifugation may still be required for small viruses that sediment slowly in the centrifugal field (Hilfenhaus et al., 1976c).

A growing number of applications evolved accompanied by a steady improvement of rotor designs (e.g., Round et al., 1981; McAleer et al., 1979). Continuous-flow zonal ultracentrifugation has been described for the preparation of traditional vaccines (Table 5.5), new vaccines (Hilfenhaus et al., 1976a; Hilfenhaus et al., 1976c; Pyke et al., 2004), viral vectors (Eglon et al., 2009), or simply for the purpose of research (Gerin et al., 1968; Grandgenett et al., 1973; Toplin and Sottong, 1972). In addition, a multitude of information on the purification of virions from laboratory-scale experiments with analytical ultracentrifuges exists (e.g., Dubois et al., 1991; McCombs and Rawls, 1968; Trudel and Payment, 1980; Sokolov et al., 1971). Even today, zonal ultracentrifugation appears to be a method of choice for the preparation of influenza vaccines (Andre and Champluvier, 2010; Bardiya and Bae, 2005; Kistner et al., 1998). A fact that may partially be ascribed to advances in the technology such as autoclavable rotors compatible with caustic agents (Aizawa and Tobita, 2006) and centrifugal forces up 120,000 g.

With respect to operation, two alternatives exist: centrifugation can be conducted either under equilibrium conditions (referred to as *isopycnic banding*) or instationary (referred to as *rate-zonal centrifugation*; Price, 1982). It should be noted, however, that only isopycnic banding is compatible with continuous loading of the sample. In this case, particles migrate to the point at which their density matches that of the density gradient. The density gradient in turn is formed by a gradient-forming solute (sucrose in most cases) either dynamically during centrifugation or before application of the sample. Noteworthy, particle density is not necessarily an intrinsic property of particle species but may be influenced by the surrounding medium. During rate-zonal centrifugation, the difference in migration velocity, which depends on the size and shape in addition to density, is used for the separation of particles of similar density. The migration velocity is generally characterized by the Svedberg coefficient s (Lebowitz et al., 2002; Price, 1982). It is defined as the radial migration velocity dr/dt

TABLE 5.5 Sucrose Gradient Purification of Viruses in Continuous-Flow Rate Zonal Centrifuges

Virus	Host	Rotor	Dens./g/cm^3	Sed./S	Yield/%	Conc.	Purif.	Ref.
Mumps virus	CE	RK-6	1.19	N.a.	61[a]	30	N.a.	Hilfenhaus et al. (1976a); Hilfenhaus et al. (1976b); Hilfenhaus et al. (1976c)
Influenza virus	CE	RK-3	1.19	N.a.	76[a]	N.a.	N.a.	
	PBKC	K-II	1.19	N.a.	N.a.	125[a]	16[b]	Gerin and Anderson (1969)
	CE	B-IV	1.19	722	N.a.	120	>10[c]	Reimer et al. (1966)
Japanese encephalitis virus	Mouse brain	K-III	1.20	N.a.	N.a.	N.a.	>20[b,d]	Okuda et al. (1975)
Rabies virus	WI-38 CEC	RK-3	1.16	N.a.	70[e]	100	N.a.	Hilfenhaus et al. (1976a); Hilfenhaus et al. (1976b); Hilfenhaus et al. (1976c)
	DEC	K-VI, B-IX	1.16[d]	N.a.	N.a.	870[e]	N.a.	Neurath et al. (1966)
Tick-borne encephalitis virus	CEC	RK-3	1.17	200	N.a.	N.a.	N.a.	Heinz et al. (1980)
Vaccinia virus	PRKC	RK-3, Ti-14	1.23	N.a.	65[f]	26	N.a.	Hilfenhaus et al. (1976a); Hilfenhaus et al. (1976b); Hilfenhaus et al. (1976c)

Dens.: density, Sed.: sedimentation coefficient, N.a.: not available, CE: embryonated chicken eggs, CEC: chicken embryo cell culture, DEC: duck embryo cell culture, PRKC: primary rabbit kidney cell culture, PBKC: primary bovine kidney cells.

[a]HA activity.

[b]Estimated from banding profile, e: protein-based.

[c]UV-based.

[d]PFU.

[e]LD50.

[f]ID50.

normalized by centrifugal acceleration $\omega^2 r$

$$s = \frac{1}{\omega^2 r}\frac{dr}{dt} \tag{5.7}$$

and is commonly specified in Svedberg units s, which correspond to 10^{-13} s. Reference values are usually provided for water at 20°C and need to be corrected for the influence of the medium. For the purpose of illustration, a Svedberg-density map of subcellular particles and certain viruses was included in Figure 5.5. More reference values can be found in the study by Mazzone, 1998.

In principle, sedimentation behavior can be predicted by solution of the Lamm equation for sector-shaped centrifuges (Lamm, 1929). Many systems are, however, too complex for the equation be solved analytically, requiring the use of advanced numerical methods (e.g., Sartory et al., 1976). An example for the purification of influenza virus by rate-zonal centrifugation was given by Reimer et al. (1966b). Most researchers, however, have made use of the continuous sample loading technique involving isopycnic banding (Hilfenhaus et al., 1976a; Hilfenhaus et al., 1976b; Hilfenhaus et al., 1976c; Okuda et al., 1975). In some cases, both techniques (rate-zonal centrifugation and isopycnic banding) have been combined either for preparative

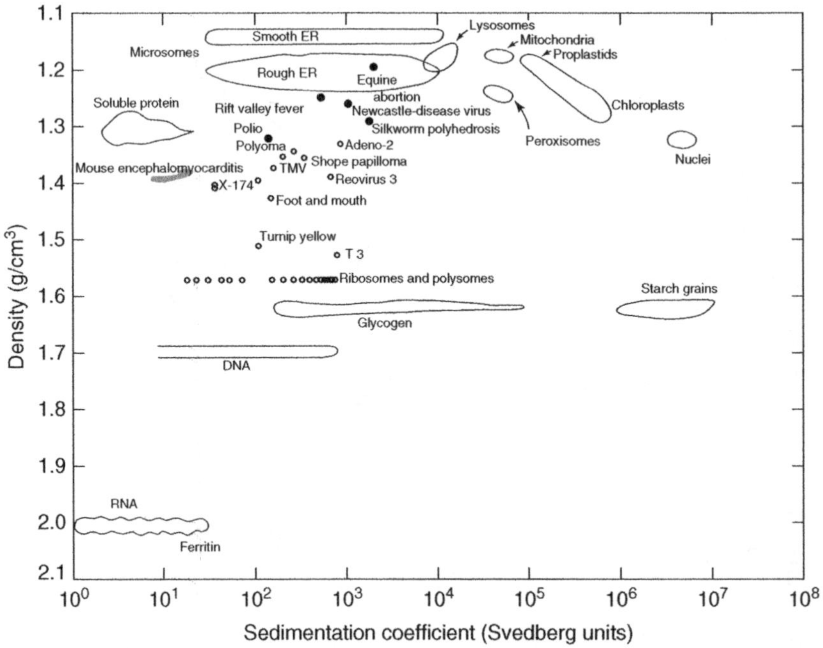

Figure 5.5 Svedberg-density map for subcellular particles and viruses. Note that actual values are dependent on the nature of the medium. Reproduced with permission from Academic Press, Centrifugation in Density Gradients, 1988.

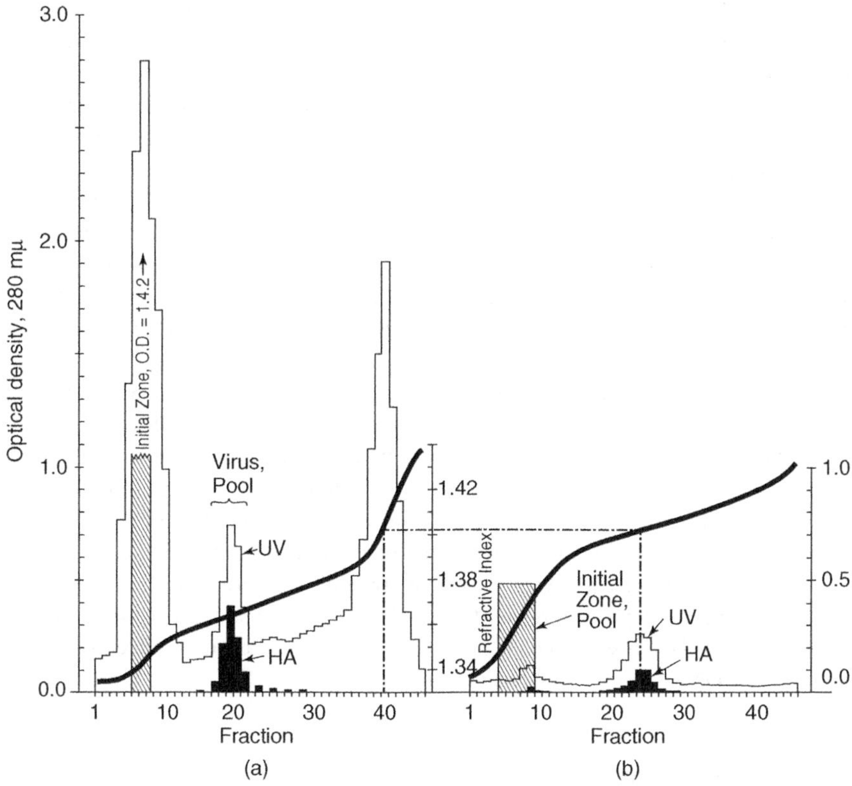

Figure 5.6 Rate-zonal centrifugation of influenza virus A/PR/8 (H1N1) propagated in embryonated chicken eggs (a) Virus harvested in allantoic fluid was concentrated about 10-fold by differential centrifugation before density gradient centrifugation. Equilibrium-zonal centrifugation of virus pool obtained after rate-zonal centrifugation (b). Reproduced with permission from AAAS, Journal of Virology, 1967.

(Reimer et al., 1966a; Reimer et al., 1967; also see Fig. 5.6) or for analytical purposes (Heinz et al., 1980).

5.2.3.2 ***Precipitation, Flocculation, and Batch Adsorption*** Among the first methods described for the purification and concentration of viruses are precipitation, flocculation, and batch adsorption. While precipitation refers to the process of recovering solutes as solids by changing their solubility (e.g., by salting out or addition of solvent), flocculation describes the formation of large colloidal clusters mediated by a flocculant. For simplicity, however, the term *precipitation* will be used in the following section for both phenomena—particularly because it is sometimes difficult to decide which term is more appropriate in the context of a certain technique. The term *batch adsorption* refers to the process of adsorbing solutes onto a dispersed particular adsorbent that can be easily recovered from suspension for consecutive elution of captured solutes.

Despite their old-fashioned appearance, the potential of precipitation and batch adsorption should not be underestimated. Both processes are relatively simple to operate (but not necessarily to develop), and a variety of procedures exists for the fractionation of biological compounds. Moreover, purification is typically accompanied by a concentration of the precipitated or adsorbed solute by one or two orders of magnitude. Accordingly, both operations are most efficient at early stages of a downstream process where volume reduction is the top priority. Adequate choice of precipitating agents or use of affinity ligands in batch adsorption further allows for highly selective capture of target compounds. In contrast to membrane operations or chromatography, precipitation and batch adsorption both scale with volume (and not area such as chromatography columns that are usually scaled by diameter) and are therefore almost unlimitedly scalable.

Precipitation can be either conducted in stirred tank reactors to which the precipitating agent is successively added or in tube reactors, which allow for continuous operation. Batch adsorption to fluidized beds can be realized in stirred tanks or hydraulic reactors. The separation of solids (precipitate or adsorbate) from the liquid phase is typically achieved by centrifugation or, in the case of rigid particles, with nutsche-type filters. If the solid is not to be recovered as in the case of precipitated DNA, disposable filter cartridges provide a convenient alternative. In the following section, some general procedures for the precipitation and batch adsorption of viruses are summarized (see also Table 5.6). Owing to the particular importance of eliminating host cell DNA, an additional section was dedicated to the selective precipitation of nucleic acids.

Precipitation of Virus Probably, most of the knowledge on the precipitation of biomolecules has been obtained from purification of proteins. For a comprehensive review on the subject see, for example, Bell et al. (1983). Similarly to proteins, viruses may be precipitated by the addition of salts such as ammonia sulfate or sodium phosphate at elevated concentrations—the effectiveness of salts thereby given by the Hofmeister series (Hofmeister, 1887). Even today, the mechanisms of precipitation are not fully understood, but it is assumed that precipitation occurs because of direct interaction of ions with macromolecules or water in the first hydration shell (Zhang and Cremer, 2006). A thermodynamic model including both the salting-in and salting-out effect has been formulated by Melander and Horvarth (Melander and Horvath, 1977). At low salt concentrations, solubility increases first because of a salting-in effect. At elevated salt concentrations, solubility decreases again. Beyond a certain concentration, an exponential dependency of the relative solubility S/S_0 on the salt concentrations exists, which can be formulated as,

$$\frac{\log S}{S_0} = \beta - Kc_s \qquad (5.8)$$

where, S_0 denotes the solubility in pure water and c_s the molar concentration of salt. The intercept β is a function of the precipitated colloid and independent of the salt concentration. K is called *the salting-out constant.* Analogous to β, it depends on the

TABLE 5.6 Some Examples for Purification of Viruses by Precipitation and Batch Adsorption

Agent/Adsorb.	Virus *(Source)*	Conditions	Resuspension/Elution	Ref.
Precipitation				
$(NH_4)_2SO_4$	Rubella virus *(cell culture supernatant)*	50% saturation, pH 7.4, 2 h at 4°C, 2000 g for 30 min	1:50 of initial volume in NTE buffer (0.15 M NaCl, 0.05 M Tris-Cl, 0.001 M EDTA), pH 7.4	Trudel and Payment (1980)
$(NH_4)_2SO_4$	Rubella virus *(cell culture supernatant)*	50 g solid per 100 ml supernatant, 25°C	1:10 of initial volume in NTE buffer (0.1 M NaCl, 0.01 M Tris. 0.001 M EDTA, pH 7.5)	Liebhaber and Gross (1972)
Methanol	Influenza virus *(allantoic fluid)*	20–30%, pH~7.0	0.3 M phosphate buffer, pH 7.0	Moyer et al. (1950)
Methanol	Mouse poliovirus *(partially purified)*	25–30%, −4 to 4°C for 1–4 h, centrifuged for 1 h	0.1 M phosphate buffer, pH 7	Brumfield et al. (1948)
Methanol	Mumps virus *(allantoic fluid)*	9–30%, −5 to −10°C for 2.5 h, centrifuged for 30 min	1:10 of initial volume in nutrient broth	Forster and Carson (1949)
Methanol/ethanol	Influenza virus *(allantoic fluid)*	15–30%, −5°C for 5 h, centrifuged for 3 h	50% of initial volume in 0.1 M phosphate buffer, pH 7.0	Cox (1946)

(continued)

TABLE 5.6 (*Continued*)

Agent/Adsorb.	Virus (*Source*)	Conditions	Resuspension/Elution	Ref.
PEG and NaCl	Hepatitis A virus (*partially purified*)	2.7–7% and 0.35–1 M, pH 7.5, 2–8°C for 1 h, 1000 g for 10 min	10–20% of initial volume in PBS (0.12 M NaCl, 6.2 mM sodium phosphate, 1 mM EDTA), pH 7.5	Hagen et al. (1996a); Hagen et al. (1996b)
PEG,6000 g/mol	Influenza virus (*allantoic fluid*)	1–8%, RT for 30 min, 1000 g for 30 min	Initial volume in 0.066 M phosphate buffer, pH 7.0	Polson (1974)
PEG, 6000 g/mol and NaCl	Rubella virus (*cell culture supernatant*)	10% and 0.5 M, pH 7.2, 2 h at 4° C, 2000 g for 30 min	1:50 of initial volume in NTE buffer (0.15 M NaCl, 0.05 M Tris-Cl, 0.001 M EDTA), pH 7.4	Trudel and Payment (1980)
PEG, 6000 g/mol and NaCl	Jap. enc, virus (*clarified cell culture supernatant*)	8% and 0.5 M, 8500 g for 15 min	1:20 of initial volume in STE buffer (0.1 M NaCl, 0.01 M Tris-Cl, 0.001 M EDTA), pH 7.6	Igarashi et al. (1973)
PEG, 8000 g/mol and NaCl	Bovine rotavirus (*clarified cell culture supernatant*)	8% and 0.4 M, 4°C overnight, 10 000 g for 30 min	1:100 in NTE buffer (10 mM Tris, 1 mM EDTA, 100 mM NaCl), pH 7.2	Fontes et al. (2005)
Zinc acetate	Rabies virus (*clarified cell culture supernatant*)	20 mM, pH 6.7–6.9, 4°C for 20 min, 1000 g for 20 min	1.25% of initial volume in saturated solution of Tris-EDTA, pH 7.8	Sokol et al. (1968)

Batch Adsorption				
Amberlite XE-67 Anion-Exchanger	Poliovirus(*human stool*)	200 g/l added to 10% fecal suspension, RT for 20 min, filtration	10% Na_2HPO_4	LoGrippo (1950)
$BaSO_4$	Influenza virus *(allantoic fluid)*	125 g/l, 0–37°C 10 min, settling at 4°C overnight	0.15–0.5 M sodium citrate, pH 7.2–8.2	Mizutani (1963)
$Ca_3(PO_4)_2$	Influenza virus *(conc. and purified)*	pH 8.1–8.7, centrifugation		Stanley (1945)
Disulfide-linked antibodies	Influenza virus *(allantoic fluid)*	5°C for 17 h, 2500 g for 15 min	5°C for 30 min, alkaline buffer (Glycine, NaCl, NaOH), pH 11.3–12.5	Sweet et al. (1974a)
Human erythrocytes	Influenza virus *(allantoic fluid)*	0.125–2%, 2°C for 30 min, centrifuged for 3 min	Dilution in sterile physiological saline at 37°C for 20 min	Sheffield et al. (1954)

PBS: phosphate-buffered saline, NTE: Sodium-Tris-EDTA.

precipitated colloid as well as on pH value, and its value decreases inversely with temperature.

In literature, examples for the salting-out of porcine parvovirus-like particles (Maranga et al., 2002), rubella virus (Liebhaber and Gross, 1972; Trudel and Payment, 1980), and influenza virus (Reimer et al., 1966b) by ammonia sulfate can be found. Another report on the precipitation of rabies virus with zinc acetate at rather low concentrations (<0.5 mol/l) is probably not because of a pure salting-out effect but involves the specific interaction of polyvalent zinc ions with virions. This speculation is supported by the fact that EDTA could be used to redissolve the virus.

A second possibility for the precipitation of macromolecules is by the addition of weakly polar solvents. The addition of solvents results in a decrease in dielectricity of the mixture and causes an increase in the strength of intramolecular and intermolecular electrostatic attraction forces (Bell et al., 1983; Green and Hughes, 1955). The latter favors nucleation and aggregation, and finally induces precipitation from the solution. Owing to their ability to shield charge, salts can be further used to tune the precipitation process. As demonstrated for BSA precipitated with ethanol at its isoelectric point (and confirmed for glycolic acid oxidase precipitated with acetone), relative solubility S/S_0 toward a reference state can be expressed by,

$$\frac{\log S}{S_0} = K\frac{\epsilon_{r,0}^2}{e_r^2} \tag{5.9}$$

with ϵ_r and $\epsilon_{r,0}$ denoting relative dielectric constants of the current solvent mixture and that of the reference state (Frigerio and Hettinger, 1962). The constant K primarily depends not only on the precipitated macromolecule, but also on ionic strength and temperature.

Precipitation of viruses by solvent addition has been described for influenza virus (Cox et al., 1946; Moyer et al., 1950), poliovirus (Brumfield et al., 1948), and mumps virus (Forster and Carson, 1949). A comparative study comprising the precipitation of all three viruses with methanol was conducted by Pollard et al. (1949). A principle disadvantage of the method is the risk of denaturation of proteins by the solvent, which has been studied in detail for catalase (Schubert and Finn, 1981). In the case of enveloped viruses, there is a further risk of damaging the lipid envelope with increasing nonpolarity of the solvent. However, successful extraction of host cell proteins with chloroform from solution containing nonenveloped hepatitis A virus has been reported (Hagen et al., 1997). Therefore, no general recommendation concerning the stability of viruses with respect to solvents can be made.

A third possibility for the precipitation of macromolecules is by the addition of nonionic polymers such as polyethylene glycol (PEG). In fact, such separation is rather based on a phase separation and is thus closely related to the method of aqueous two-phase extraction (see e.g., Albertsson, 1977; Kroner and Kular, 1978). Phase separation occurs because of the impenetrability of volumes occupied by the charged colloids and coiled polymers. If the surface distance between colloids becomes low (favored at high salt concentrations), the polymer is excluded from a certain fraction of the total volume, leading to an osmotic driving force. Under conditions where the

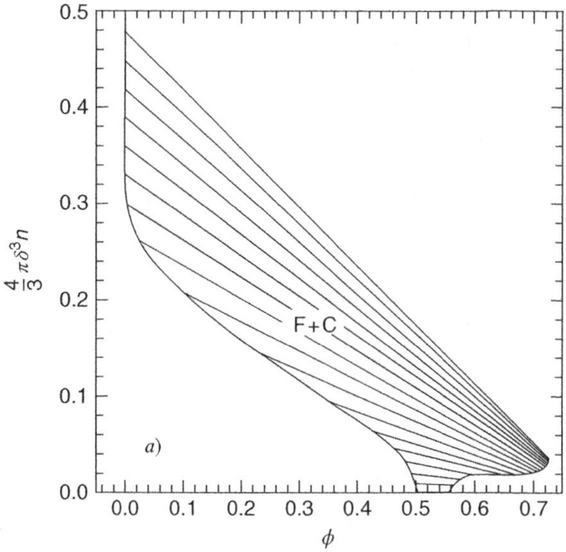

Figure 5.7 Phase diagram of a colloid–polymer mixture as a function of colloid volume fraction ϕ against dimensionless polymer concentration $4/3\pi\delta^3$n for δ/a = 0.1. Tie lines are shown in the two-phase region whose composition is fluid and crystalline (F + C). Reproduced with permission from EDP Sciences, EPL (Europhysics Letters), 1992, 20, http://epljournal.edpsciences.org/.

concentration of polymer is sufficiently high, separation into two phases occurs, of which, one is rich in polymer and one in the colloid (Fortini et al., 2005; Lekkerkerker et al., 1992). An example for a theoretically derived phase diagram is given in Figure 5.7. It was calculated for a diameter ratio of polymer to spherical colloid (δ/a) of 0.1.

With respect to virus purification, preparation of plant viruses (Leberman, 1966; Hebert, 1963) and bacteriophages (Yamamoto et al., 1970) by PEG precipitation appears to be the first application of the technique. Further examples include the precipitation of influenza virus (Heyward et al., 1977; Kanarek and Tribe, 1967; Polson, 1974, 1993), rotavirus (Fontes et al., 2005; Lewis and Metcalf, 1988), hepatitis A virus (Hagen et al., 1996a; Hagen et al., 1996b; Lewis and Metcalf, 1988), rubella virus (Trudel and Payment, 1980), and Japanese encephalitis virus (Igarashi et al., 1973). A comprehensive review covering many viruses and bacteriophages has been provided by Vajda (1978). In most cases, PEG with a molecular weight of 6000 or 8000 g/mol was used. PEG at lower molecular weight can still be used for the precipitation of virions but was found to be less efficient (Yamamoto et al., 1970). Concentrations of PEG required for quantitative precipitation range between about 4% and 10% (Table 5.6). In most cases, salt was added for better shielding of electric charge, favoring phase separation (Fortini et al., 2005; Leberman, 1966).

In addition to solubility, kinetics of precipitation, that is, nucleation and floc growth, are of importance. In particular, relaxation times toward a steady-state size distribution of flocs need to be determined for the design of operations. Moreover, it has to be kept in mind that only flocs sufficiently large and stable will be separable from the bulk liquid by centrifugation or filtration. Kinetics of flocculation is complex and difficult to state in mathematical form (Thomas et al., 1999). In general, the steady-state size distribution of flocs appears to be determined by energy dissipation rates in reactors and the resulting maximum shear stress exerted on flocs (Bell and Dunnill, 1982b). However, shearing in pumps (Hoare et al., 1982) and at the inlet of centrifuges should not be neglected (Maybury et al., 2000). Furthermore, the stability of flocs is subject to a process called *maturation* and was shown to be a function of the nondimensional Camp number $C_a = \overline{G}t$ (Camp and Stein, 1943). It is the product of root-mean-square shear rate $\overline{G}$ and incubation time t. In stirred vessels, the root-mean-square shear rate is given by,

$$\overline{G} = \left(\frac{\epsilon}{\nu}\right)^{1/2} \tag{5.10}$$

with ϵ denoting the volumetric power dissipation rate and ν the kinematic viscosity of the suspension. It was found in two studies (precipitation of soy protein and lysozyme) that maximum stability of flocs is reached for $C_a > 10^5$ (Bell and Dunnill, 1982a; Kim et al., 2001).

Precipitation of DNA Selective precipitation of DNA appears to be an attractive choice for the early depletion of host cell DNA, as it is simple to conduct and comparably inexpensive. It can be implemented either as an additional clearance step right after primary clarification or later in the process under more defined conditions. The principal prerequisite is the availability of a selective agent that allows for the quantitative precipitation of DNA while virions remain in the supernatant.

Precipitation of DNA has been achieved by salting-out (LiCl) (Wolf et al., 1977), addition of divalent ions (Ca^{2+}, Mg^{2+}) (de Frutos et al., 2001), alcohol (ethanol and isopropanol) (Eickbush and Moudrianakis, 1978; Moore and Dowhan, 2007), PEG (Lis, 1980; Volkening et al., 2009), detergents (CTAB, CPC, DB) (Goerke et al., 2005; Gustincich et al., 1991), protamine sulfate (Amosenko et al., 1991), poly-L-lysine (Shapiro et al., 1969), cobalthexamide (Pelta et al., 1996; Widom and Baldwin, 1980), or polyamines such as spermine or spermidine (Hoopes and McClure, 1981; Pelta et al., 1996; Raspaud et al., 1999) and polyethylenimine (PEI) (Cordes et al., 1990; Jendrisak, 1987; Kröber et al., 2010). Moreover, harsh methods such as the precipitation of genomic DNA by boiling and acidification or alkalinization play a role in the purification of plasmid DNA (Babu and Rajamanickam, 1998). Noteworthy, when interpreting the results of these studies, the specific type of DNA should be kept in mind because different behavior may be observable among different types of DNA. It needs to be distinguished between chromosomal DNA or nucleosomes, naked DNA, and supercoiled circular DNA (i.e., plasmid DNA). In the context of virus purification, only the precipitation of chromosomal DNA is of practical interest. Basically, by definition, such DNA incorporates structural proteins and may be decorated with other proteins in complex mixtures. Moreover, the size distribution of DNA fragments may play a role in the precipitation process.

Several examples for the selective precipitation of DNA have been reported in literature. Selective precipitation has been used in the purification of poliovirus (Amosenko et al., 1991) and Japanese encephalitis virus (protamine sulfate) (Hong et al., 2001; Srivastava et al., 2001), adenovirus (detergents) (Goerke et al., 2005), and in the general clarification of microbial lysates (spermine and PEI) (Choe and Middelberg, 2001; DeWalt et al., 2003; Salt et al., 1995). Another important application is the purification of plasmid DNA by selective precipitation of plasmids with isopropanol or ammonium sulfate (Freitas et al., 2006), poly(N,N'-dimethyldiallylammoium (Nicoletti and Condorelli, 1993), spermidine (Murphy et al., 1999), and PEG (Wahlund et al., 2004).

Crucial for the performance of DNA clearance operations is the selectivity of precipitating agents and operation under mild conditions that are compatible with the product. Methods such as salting-out or solvent addition are usually fairly unspecific and have been described for the precipitation of viruses as well. The same applies for the precipitation with PEG (see the previous section). Although acceptable selectivity may be achievable under appropriate conditions, method development can be rather tedious, and robustness of the operation may be insufficient. Other methods such as boiling or precipitation at extreme pH will most certainly damage the product and can usually be excluded a priori for the purification of virions. Protamine sulfate, however, may be fairly selective but is of biological origin and should therefore be avoided in production processes. Polyamines such as spermidine, spermine, and PEI, in contrast, are synthetic polymers that posses a high affinity toward DNA and are effective even at low concentrations (Pelta et al., 1996; Raspaud et al., 1999). However, when used as precipitating agents, some loss of protein and lipid is typically observed (Cordes et al., 1990; Hoopes and McClure, 1981; Salt et al., 1995). In the case of PEI, direct interaction with proteins has even been demonstrated by chromatography (Atkinson and Jack, 1973). PEI further involves the risk of *in vivo* toxicity because of its ability to agglutinate erythrocytes (Boeckle, 2004) and has to be removed (analogous to most other agents) in subsequent unit operations.

One of the main characteristics of DNA is the high negative charge density along its backbone. Respectively, it is to be assigned to the class of highly charged polyelectrolyte chains (de la Cruz et al., 1995)—a class whose members appear to behave similarly in the presence of monovalent and polyvalent counter-ions (Delsanti et al., 1994; Manning, 1978; Tang et al., 1996). In the presence of counter-ions, condensation of the latter along the polymer chain occurs. The term *condensation* refers to the accumulation of counter-ions within a small volume around the polymer chain, which is because of coulombic attraction forces between ions that are balanced by an entropic driving force. Yet, condensed counter-ions typically remain fully hydrated and delocalized, including rapid exchange of ions with the bulk liquid.

Condensation of counter-ions leads to partial neutralization of polymer charge, which can be predicted by the theory of Manning (1978). The degree of charge neutralization at low salt concentration solely depends on the valence of counter-ions and was predicted to be 76% for monovalent, 88% for divalent, and 92% for trivalent ions in water. Beyond a certain degree of charge neutralization, compaction of the polymer chain occurs because of shielding of intramolecular repulsive forces.

Counter-ions capable of inducing DNA compaction are respectively referred to as *compacting agents*. A threshold value of about 90% charge neutralization was determined experimentally for the compaction of T7 DNA by spermine in the presence of Na^+ or Mg^{2+} and Mg^{2+} or putrescine in 50% methanol (Wilson and Bloomfield, 1979). At elevated concentrations of DNA and compacting agent, a second effect called *ion-bridging* leads to aggregation of DNA chains and finally precipitation. Depending on the concentration of monovalent salt, hexagonally packed or loose bundles formed by DNA and compacting agent have been detected (DeRouchey, 2005). Under certain circumstances, more complex structures such as toroids can be observed (Arscott et al., 1990). If, however, the concentration of compacting agent exceeds a certain critical concentration, reversal of charge occurs, restabilizing the polymer in solution (Delsanti et al., 1994; Pelta et al., 1996; Raspaud et al., 1998).

The phenomena of intramolecular compaction and intermolecular aggregation were shown to occur on different time scales by light scattering studies (Porschke, 1984). While compaction because of ion condensation occurred within a few milliseconds, kinetics of aggregation because of ion-bridging was slower, requiring several seconds until steady state. Aggregation further showed a clear dependency on the concentration of compaction agent and DNA. The critical concentration of compacting agent $c_{precip.}$ beyond which aggregation in the presence of monovalent salt at concentration c_s occurs was found to be a linear function of DNA equivalent concentration c_{DNA} as long as $c_{\mathrm{DNA}} \ll c_s$ (Burak et al., 2003):

$$c_{\mathrm{precip.}} = \alpha \cdot c_{\mathrm{DNA}} + \beta \tag{5.11}$$

The DNA equivalent concentration is defined as the concentration of charged phosphate groups in the DNA backbone. Slope α denotes the stoichiometric ratio of DNA and compacting agent. Offset β is the bulk concentration of compacting agent, which is a function of monovalent salt concentration. The critical concentration of the compacting agent $c_{\mathrm{redissol.}}$ beyond which DNA is stabilized in solution was found to be constant independent of DNA and monovalent salt concentration (Pelta et al., 1996; Raspaud et al., 1998). For the precipitation of a 150 base pairs, DNA fragment with spermine a stoichiometric ratio of $\alpha = 0.2$ and a critical concentration for stabilization of 105 mM has been determined (Raspaud et al., 1998). The corresponding phase diagram showing spinodal lines for the precipitation and stabilization of DNA is shown in Figure 5.8.

The residual content of DNA after precipitation primarily depends on phase separation, which is characterized by tie lines in phase diagrams (not shown). Moreover, the size of aggregates and the method of solid separation are equally important. Concerning this aspect, similar principles as for the precipitation of proteins should apply. Another point to consider is the complex nature of most virus-containing solutions. So far, all detailed studies on the compaction of DNA have been conducted under defined conditions. Deviation from ideal behavior in real world applications has to be expected. Particularly, the coprecipitation of DNA and virus needs to be avoided under all circumstances. Thorough experimental design studies or at least process

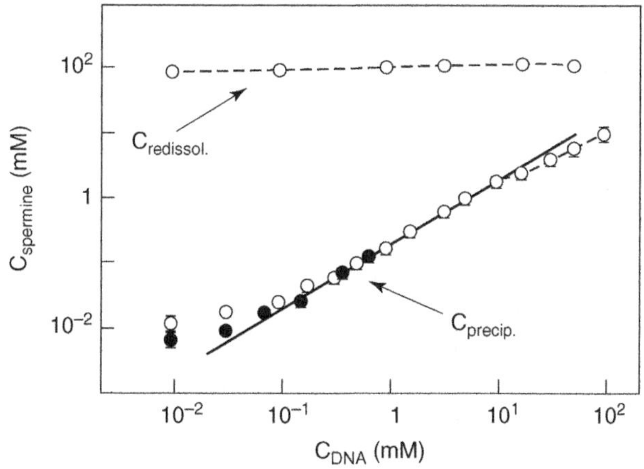

Figure 5.8 Spermine concentrations $c_{precip.}$ and $c_{redissol.}$ versus DNA concentration. A constant ratio of $c_{precip.}/cDNA = 0.20 \pm 0.02$ was determined over a wide range of spermine and DNA concentrations. The critical concentration of redissolution was independent of the DNA concentration. Both lines confine the two phase region where aggregation occurs. Reproduced with permission from Elsevier, Biophysical Journal, 1998.

validation will therefore be required with pH, ionic strength, and concentration of compacting agent being the most important parameters.

Batch Adsorption An alternative to the precipitation of virions from solution is adsorption to the surface of suitable adsorbents, which are finely dispersed throughout the bulk liquid. In a second step, the adsorbent is recollected and virions are eluted under appropriate conditions. In principle, batch adsorption can be regarded as an inefficient chromatography step using a column with only one plate. Adsorption isotherms characterizing the virus–adsorbent interaction therefore have to be very steep for quantitative adsorption of virions. Moreover, adsorbents have to be fairly selective not only for the efficient separation of virions from impurities, but also to prevent impurities from consuming a large share of the capacity.

An early application of the batch adsorption principle is the capture of influenza virus with insoluble calcium (Salk, 1945; Stanley, 1945) and barium salts (Klembala and Szekacs, 1965; Mizutani, 1963). While soluble Ca^{2+} was precipitated from solution by the addition of phosphate in the first case, insoluble $BaSO_4$ directly added to the virus-containing solution was used in the second case. Another example is the use of ion-exchange resins as demonstrated for poliomyelitis and Theiler virus (LoGrippo, 1950). However, batch adsorption with ion-exchangers is not restricted to the capture of virions. Nucleic acids, because of their high charge density, can also be depleted efficiently by the addition of anion-ion exchange resins even at fairly high salt concentrations (Ferreira et al., 2000). One possible application would be the immediate addition of anion-exchangers during virus propagation. In fact, this is already done unintentionally in microcarrier cultures with Cytodex-1 carriers, which are nothing but DEAE anion-exchange resins (GE Healthcare, 2007). As a consequence, microcarrier cultivations frequently result in lower content of cellular DNA after virus infection (approximately 5-fold to 10-fold lower with $2 \cdot 10^6$ cells/ml[1] and 2 g/l of Cytodex-1) than roller bottle cultivations (unpublished data).

In order to achieve extraordinary selectivity, the use of affinity ligands in the form of cross-linked antibodies has been made (Gallop et al., 1966; Stephen et al., 1966). Successful application has been demonstrated for a number of plant viruses (Galvez, 1966; Ladipo and Zoeten, 1971) and influenza virus (Sweet et al., 1974a; Sweet et al., 1974b). Another example is the purification of influenza virus by repeated adsorption to and elution from erythrocytes, which is based on the selective binding of viral hemagglutinin to sugar moieties on the surface of cells (Sheffield et al., 1954). It is representative for all strategies exploiting viral receptor activities, which are present in most enveloped viruses.

In general, the separation of solid adsorbate is similar to the recovery of precipitated matter. If the matrix of sorbents is sufficiently rigid, chromatography-like elution from packed beds should be preferred in order to allow for simplified washing and selective elution (see e.g., Pepper, 1967). Such packed beds may be obtained by sedimentation, nutsche-type filtration, or hydrodynamic compaction after adsorption in a slim fluidized bed reactor. Another interesting and comparatively new technique is the use of magnetic beads, which are easily separable in magnetic fields and have proven valuable in a number of applications (Franzreb et al., 2006; Horak et al., 2007).

5.2.3.3 ***Tangential-Flow Ultrafiltration*** TFUF can nowadays probably be considered the default method for concentrating virions (Kalbfuss et al., 2007a; Kim et al., 1999; Paul et al., 1993; Peixoto et al., 2007; Srivastava et al., 2001). By the use of diafiltration (DF), which often follows the concentration step, its function can be further extended to purification and conditioning (Cruz et al., 2000; Czermak et al., 2008; Grzenia et al., 2008; Guo et al., 2009; Hensgen et al., 2010; Maranga et al., 2002; Valeri et al., 1977). However, despite its frequent use, filtration conditions and performance are often poorly described or characterized in literature. In many instances, the use of TFUF is only briefly mentioned without providing enough details that would be required for successful reproduction or evaluation of performance (e.g., Frazatti-Gallina et al., 2004; Hong et al., 2001; Kistner et al., 1998; Montagnon et al., 1984).

Since viral harvests are typically dilute (concentrations in the range of a few micrograms per milliliters only), TFUF is often used as a first step to enrich the product (Frazatti-Gallina et al., 2004; Hong et al., 2001; Kalbfuss et al., 2007a; Kim et al., 1999; Montagnon et al., 1984; Peixoto et al., 2007; Srivastava et al., 2001). Volume reduction in the range of 20-fold to 50-fold can usually be achieved while more than 80% of the product is recovered (Hong et al., 2001; Kalbfuss et al., 2007a; Peixoto et al., 2007; Trudel et al., 1983). If higher volume reduction is required, TFUF operations can be cascaded using filtration rigs of different scale (Trudel et al., 1983). Alternatively, devices optimized with respect to hold-up volume can be used (Schu and Mitra, 2001). Diafiltration may be employed to wash out small impurities and condition concentrates for subsequent unit operations (such as chromatography).

If conducted at a constant volume (assuming an ideal system), the residual content of fully permeable impurities may be estimated according to the equation,

$$c(V_{\text{dia}}) = c_0 \cdot e^{-V_{\text{dia}}/V_t} \qquad (5.12)$$

with V_{dia}/V_t denoting the number of buffer exchanges. Since most virions are comparatively large (Table 5.1), small molecules and proteins are easily withdrawn, whereas large genomic DNA fragments are rejected by the membrane (Fig. 5.9).

The choice of membrane cutoff obviously depends on the dimensions of the product. It should be maximized at early process stages for a maximum reduction of impurities. However, a membrane with large pores close to the dimensions of the product may be more prone to fouling (Bacchin et al., 2006; Wu et al., 1999). The material of the membrane should be chosen such that unspecific adsorption is minimized, which is particularly important during DF. Unspecific adsorption has been addressed in the context of concentrating viruses from ground and waste water (Divizia et al., 1989; Jansons and Bucens, 1986; Winona et al., 2001). In all cases high, recoveries were only achieved by the addition of blocking agents such as beef extract stressing not only the importance of the membrane material, but also composition of the DF buffer. In another report dealing with DF of hepatitis B surface antigen, pretreatment of the membrane with 0.1% Tween 20 solution was required (Schu and Mitra, 2001). Besides chemical and physical stability (with respect to cleaning-in-place, steaming-in-place, storage, etc.) and cost also play a role in the membrane selection process. The choice of module design (hollow-fibers, flat-sheet, or spiral-wound

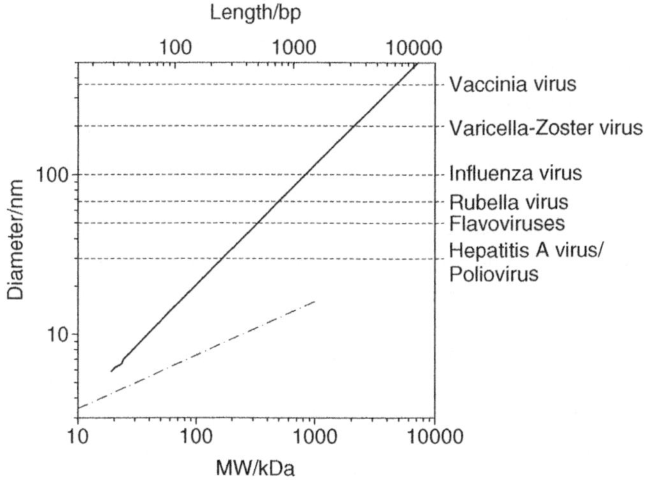

Figure 5.9 Characteristic size of DNA (–), protein (---) and various viruses. The size of DNA (chromatographic diameter at I = 200 mM, pH 6.85) was calculated from the size–length correlation reported by Potschka (1991). Hydrodynamic diameters of proteins were derived from experimentally determined diffusion coefficients (Li et al., 1998). Concerning viruses, the largest dimension is reported (see Table 5.1).

membranes), in contrast, may be rather a question of philosophy or availability. While hollow-fiber modules are probably best characterized (Belfort et al., 1994), flat-sheet and spiral-wound membrane modules may yield higher productivity and better control of fouling (Schwinge et al., 2004). When choosing the latter designs, one should consider that filtration behavior is a lot more difficult to predict because it does not only depend on membrane characteristics and geometry, but also on the type of spacers used, their orientation, and the flow distribution in channels.

It remains the task of the process engineer to find appropriate operating conditions (i.e., wall shear rate or Reynolds number on the retentate side; transmembrane pressure or flux on the permeate side) and configurations of filtration modules (serial, parallel, or tapered array (Schwinge et al., 2004)). A first estimate for the maximum productivity of hollow-fiber modules can be obtained by the limiting flux concept. The limiting flux is reached when flux becomes independent of driving force (Fig. 5.10a). In the case of submicron-sized particles such as virions, Brownian diffusion is the dominant driving force for back migration from the membrane (Belfort et al., 1994; Davis, 1992). Hence, the similarity solution by Tretin and Doshi (Trettin and Doshi, 1980) can be used for estimation of the limiting flux:

$$J = 1.31\left(\frac{\dot{\gamma}_0 D^2 \phi_w}{\phi_b L}\right)^{1/2} \tag{5.13}$$

It depends on the length of fibers L, the wall shear rate $\dot{\gamma}_0$, diffusivity D of particles, and their volume fractions in the bulk liquid (φ_b) and at the membrane (φ_w). Alternatively, film theory can be used to predict the limiting flux (Porter, 1972).

Since the limiting flux concept exclusively considers hydrodynamic mechanisms, it is, however, only partially applicable to the filtration of viruses. In the submicron range, surface interactions usually play a role such that the achievable productivity may differ significantly (Bacchin et al., 2006). For such systems, it has been observed that fouling often occurs if a certain flux is exceeded but remains negligible otherwise (Wu et al., 1999). This led to the development of the critical flux concept, defining a critical flux beyond which irreversible fouling occurs (Field et al., 1995; Bacchin et al., 2006) and that is distinct from the limiting flux (Fig. 5.10a). In contrast to the limiting flux, it is a local concept characterized by a local critical Peclet number (Bacchin et al., 2002). It has been further distinguished between the strong and weak form of the concept in the absence or presence of flux-independent fouling (Bacchin et al., 2006; Field et al., 1995).

Although fouling should be in general avoided or at least minimized, this is particularly important for the concentration of virions. Owing to the very low content of biomass in viral feed streams, flux-dependent fouling as caused by excessive transmembrane pressure or forced flux very often coincides with a loss of product (Kalbfuss et al., 2007a; Paul et al., 1993; Peixoto et al., 2007). In addition, deposits on the membrane can alter rejection behavior (sieving effect of a gel layer or by pore constriction/blocking) such that impurities are no longer separable from the product. Presently, different approaches exist for the inclusion of surface interactions into filtration models (Bacchin et al., 2002; Baruah et al., 2005; Harmant and Aimar, 1998;

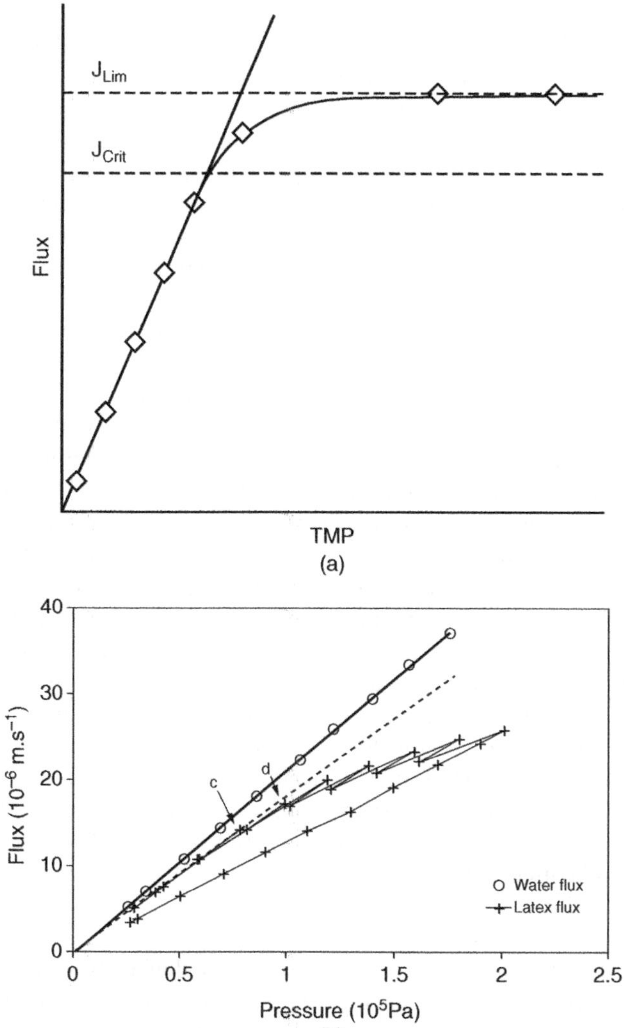

Figure 5.10 Critical and limiting flux in tangential-flow filtration (a) The critical flux $J_{critical}$ denotes the flux below which there is no increase in transmembrane pressure (Δ) P with time or particle deposition on the membrane, whereas the limiting flux $J_{limiting}$ is the value for which flux becomes independent of the driving force. Reproduced from Schwinge et al. (2004) with kind permission of Elsevier. Determination of the critical flux by flux cycling (b) Relationship between transmembrane pressure and flux for the filtration of water (o) and PVC latex (+) at $7.1 \cdot 10-4\,g\,l^{-1}$ without salt. The dotted line corresponds to the permeability measured on the first points of the filtration of latex. Points c and d correspond to the range of critical flux. Reproduced from Espinasse et al. (2002). Reproduced with permission from Elsevier, Desalination, 2002.

Rabiller-Baudry et al., 2000). The history of development has been summarized by Bacchin et al. (2006). However, all of them are fairly complex and difficult to apply because the required information on particle characteristics (size distribution, zeta or surface potential, electrophoretic mobility, etc.) is often not available. Properties such as the surface potential further depend on the environment (pH, ionic strength, and temperature; Lucas et al., 1998), and, in addition, specific adsorption of ions to the surface of colloids may play a role (Rabiller-Baudry and Chaufer, 2003). Finally, none of these models is able to deal with the highly complex mixtures of particles that are typically found at the early stages of purification processes. Experimental determination of filtration behavior (flux-pressure dependency, flux decline, concentration dependence, and hysteresis behavior) therefore remains essential.

A safe but not necessarily the best strategy could be to operate filtration always just below the critical flux of the system, thereby totally avoiding fouling. Determination of the critical flux by several methods has been reported in the past, leading to different definitions of the latter (Schwinge et al., 2004). Critical flux can be determined by monitoring either the transmembrane pressure increase for a constant flux or flux decline at a constant pressure (Espinasse et al., 2002; Kwon et al., 2000) by mass balancing of particles (Kwon et al., 2000) or by direct observation of particle deposition on the membrane (Chen et al., 2004; Li et al., 1998a; Li et al., 1998b). An example for the determination of critical flux based on the detection of flux decline is given in Figure 5.10b. Interestingly, values for the critical flux determined by different methods do not necessarily coincide. Deposition on the membrane seems to appear earlier than can be detected by a rise in transmembrane pressure or flux decline (Kwon et al., 2000). Since, however, for the production of vaccines recovery of virions is most important, the method of mass balancing seems to be most appropriate. Once filtration has been characterized experimentally, relevant filtration mechanisms may be identified by fitting existing models to experimental data. The so-gained knowledge can then be used to maximize performance or at least to find safe and robust operating conditions.

5.2.3.4 Chromatography Chromatography is undoubtedly one of the most powerful unit operations in the downstream processing of biologicals. Owing to the repeated exchange of solutes between the stationary and mobile phase, separation can be achieved even under conditions, where the selectivity of a chromatography medium remains rather low. Using gradient chromatography, it is further possible to concentrate a product—an important feature if chromatography is to be used at the early stages of a downstream process. Since chromatography usually constitutes the backbone in protein purification these days (Curling, 2007), an abundance of chromatography media (built from different matrices and ligands) has become available. However, materials for the chromatographic purification of viruses (or bioparticles in general) need to be carefully chosen. Most biochromatography media have been designed for the purification of macromolecules in the order of a few nanometers only. The majority of their pores is not accessible for virions. But even if pores were designed to be sufficiently large, mass transfer would be limiting because of the low diffusivity of large colloids. Moreover, broadening of peaks and low resolution would be obtained at flow velocities that are usually required for economic operation. A common solution to this problem is the use of media with large through pores such as stacks of adsorptive membranes and monolithic columns (Podgornik et al., 2010), which permit convective flow through the porous space. Alternatively, packing of small nonporous particles can be used, but chromatography equipment capable of dealing with the resulting high backpressures has to be employed.

Neglecting dispersion, chromatographic processes can be described by the following system of partial differential equations (de Bokx et al., 1992):

$$\left(\frac{\partial}{\partial t^*} + \frac{\partial}{\partial z^*} c_i\right) + \phi \frac{\partial q_i}{\partial t^*} = 0 \tag{5.14}$$

where, variables c_i and q_i denote bulk concentrations in the mobile and average concentrations in the stationary phase. Index i refers to the different solute species involved. The phase ratio ϕ is defined as $\phi = (1 - \epsilon)/\epsilon$, where ϵ denotes the void fraction of the packing (or volume fraction of mesopores). Nondimensional variables t^* and z^* are defined as $t^* = t \cdot u/L$ and $z^* = z/L$, with time after injection t, linear flow rate u, and column length L, respectively. In addition, owing to the low diffusivity of virions, description of mass transfer is typically required. Depending on the type of matrix (packed-bed, stacked membrane, or monolith), appropriate descriptions for surface transport and pore diffusion remain to be integrated (Carta et al., 2005; Deen, 1987). If the efficiency of columns (or the chromatography system in general) is low, axial dispersion needs to be accounted for, for example, by considering eddy diffusion (Chung and Wen, 1968) or (cascades of) continuous stirred tank reactors (Boi et al., 2007). Moreover, adequate adsorption isotherms are required to describe virion-ligand as well as impurity–ligand interactions (Mollerup, 2007; Shukla and Yigzaw, 2007). Since maximum exploitation of the capacity of media is usually desired, competitive interactions and nonlinearity (i.e., saturation effects) have to be dealt with. An exception is SEC, where solute interactions are often negligible. Once an appropriate model and corresponding parameters have been identified, productivity and resolution can be optimized in silico. However, if the number of solutes is large (e.g., in capture and intermediate purification steps), parameterization is often infeasible because of a lack of information. In these cases, either simplification of the model is required or one still has to rely on fully empirical optimization.

In the following sections, purification of whole virions using SEC, IEC, and AC is discussed in detail, including some examples of application. In addition, some examples for bead-based purification of viruses from literature are summarized in Table 5.7. Noteworthy, the fact that other kinds of chromatography are not addressed in detail does not pose any judgment of their value. It rather reflects the frequency of their occurrence in literature and the amount of information available.

Size-Exclusion Chromatography SEC is a universal method for the separation of solutes by size. It dates back to the late 1950s when Porath and Flodin (1959) reported on the first chromatography media made from cross-linked dextran, leading to a diversity of chromatography media and applications in the following.

TABLE 5.7 Some Examples for the Purification of Viruses by Chromatography

Virus *(Source)*	Medium *(Manufacturer)*	Conditions	Ref.
Size-exclusion chromatography			
Influenza virus *(chicken eggs)*	Sepharose 2B *(GE Healthcare, Sweden)*	**I:** clarified and concentrated, up to 13% CV; **E:** 0.1 M PBS, pH 7.2, 1.9–2.5 cm/h	Valeri et al. (1981)
	Sepharose 6B *(GE Healthcare, Sweden)*	**I:** concentrated and inactivated, 3–13% CV; **E:** PBS (3.12 g NaH_2PO_4, 11.4 g Na_2HPO_4, 8 g NaCl), 3.6 cm h^{-1}	Tomita and Asahara (1971)
	700 Å Controlled Pore Glass *(Electro-Nucleonics, United States)*	**I:** clarified and concentrated, 5% CV; **E:** TNE-PEG (0.15 M NaCl, 20 mM EDTA, 0.1% PEG-20000, 10 mM Tris-Cl, pH 7.8), 95 cm h^{-1}	Heyward et al. (1977)
Influenza virus *(cell culture)*	Sepharose CL-2B *(GE Healthcare, Sweden)*	**I:** clarified, inactivated and concentrated, 5% CV; **E:** PBS (circa 0.15 M NaCl, 10 mM phosphate, pH 7.3), 30 cm/h	Nayak et al. (2005)
	Sepharose 4-FF *(GE Healthcare, Sweden)*	**I:** clarified, inactivated and concentrated, 7–28% CV; **E:** PBS (0.65 M NaCl, 20 mM phospate, pH 7.3), 60 cm/h	Kalbfuss et al. (2007a); Kalbfuss et al. (2007b); Kalbfuss et al. (2007c)
Rubella virus *(cell culture)*	Sepharose 2B *(GE Healthcare, Sweden)*	**I:** clarified and concentrated, 0.5% CV; **E:** TNE (0.15 M NaCl, 1 mM EDTA, 50 mM Tris-Cl, pH 7.4), 2 cm/h	Trudel et al. (1981)

Tick-borne encephalitis virus *(mouse brain)*	Sephacryl S-300 *(GE Healthcare, Sweden)*	**I:** clarified and concentrated, 7.5% CV, **E:** PBS (0.13 M NaCl, 20 mM phosphate, pH 8.0), 19 cm/h	Crooks et al. (1990)
Rotavirus-like particles *(cell culture)*	Sephacryl S-1000 *(GE Healthcare, Sweden)*	**I:** clarified and concentrated, 5% CV; **E:** D-PBS, 22 cm/h	Peixoto et al. (2007)
Ion-exchange chromatography			
Influenza A virus *(chicken eggs)*	Amberlite XE-64 *(Rohm and Haas, Philadelphia)*	**Eq:** distilled water; **A:** clarified, ca. 7.5 cv/h ; **D:** 10% sodium chloride	Muller and Rose (1952)
Influenza A virus *(cell culture)*	Sartobind Q and D *(Sartorius, Göttingen)*	**Eq:** 50 mM NaCl, 20 mM HEPES, pH 7.3; **A:** clarified and inactivated, loaded until 10% breakthrough; **D:** step and linear gradient to 1.5 M NaCl, 20 mM HEPES, pH 7.3	Kalbfuss et al. (2007a); Kalbfuss et al. (2007b); Kalbfuss et al. (2007c)
Rotavirus-like particles *(cell culture)*	Sartobind D *(Sartorius, Göttingen)*	**Eq:** low-salt buffer (50 mM NaCl + 20 mM HEPES, pH 7.3); A: concentrated and diafiltered against low-salt buffer; D: linear gradient to 1.5 M NaCl	Vicente et al. (2008)
Hepatitis A Virus *(cell culture)*	DEAE-Toyopearl 650 M *(TosoHaas, Philadelphia)*	**Eq:** 90 mM NaCl, 4.7 mM phosphate, pH 6.5–7; **A:** clarified and nuclease-treated lysate; **D:** 0.35 M NaCl, 1 mM EDTA. 120 mM phosphate buffer, pH 7.5	Hagen et al. (1996a); Hagen et al. (1996b)

(continued)

TABLE 5.7 (*Continued*)

Virus *(Source)*	Medium *(Manufacturer)*	Conditions	Ref.
Affinity chromatography			
Hepatitis A virus *(human feces)*	Antiserum on Sepharose 4B *(GE Healthcare, Sweden)*	Eq**:** PBS; A**:** 10% extract in PBS; D**:** 4 M sodium iodide, 4 M thiocyanate or 5 M sodium perchlorate	Elkana et al. (1979)
Hepatitis B and C virus *(human plasma)*	HiTrap heparin *(GE Healthcare, Sweden)*	Eq**:** TN buffer (0.15 M NaCl, 20 mM Tris-Cl, pH 7.4); A**:** diluted in E buffer or plasma, circulated at RT for 1 h; D**:** TN buffer (0.4 M NaCl, 20 mM Tris-Cl, pH 7.4)	Zahn and Allain (2005)
Influenza A virus *(cell culture)*	EE and EC lectin on polymer matrix *(GE Healthcare, Sweden)*	Eq**:** CEWB (0.15 M NaCl, 50 mM Tris-Cl, 1 mM $MnCl_2$, 1 mM $CaCl_2$, 1 mM $MgCl_2$), pH 7.4; A**:** clarified and concentrated by tangential-flow filtration, 0.2–0.5 CV/min or recycled ON at 4°C; D**:** 0.5 M lactose in CWEB followed by 0.5 M lactose and 2 M NaCl in CWEB, stop-flow elution at 4°C	Opitz et al. (2007a); Opitz et al. (2007b)

Influenza A virus *(chicken eggs)*	Disulfide-linked antibodies mixed with Sephadex G-15 *(GE Healthcare, Sweden)*	Eq: PBS (pH 7.0); A: RT; D: glycine-Na (pH 11.3–12.5)	Sweet et al. (1974a)
Measles virus *(cell culture)*	Antiserum on glass beads	A: clarified cellular extract, recycled ON at 4°C ; D: 0.1 M glycine-Cl (pH 2.3), 4°C	Njayou and Quash (1991)
Rubella virus *(cell culture)*	Monoclonal antibody on Sepharose 4B *(GE Healthcare, Sweden)*	Eq: TNE buffer (10 mM Tris-Cl, 0.15 M NaCl, 1 mM EDTA, pH 7.8); A: clarified and concentrated by PEG precipitation, 2 h at 4°C; D: 5% Diethanolamine + 0.15 M NaCl (pH 11.5)	Chong and Gillam (1985)
Poliovirus *(cell culture)*	Antiserum on Sepharose 4B *(GE Healthcare, Sweden)*	Eq: PBS + 1% serum; D: 3 M potassium thiocyanate	Brown et al. (1979)
Tick-borne encephalitis virus*(cell culture)*	Monoclonal antibody on CNBr-Sepharose *(GE Healthcare, Sweden)*	Eq: PBS; A: clarified and concentrated by centrifugation, resuspended in borate buffer, pH 9.0; D: glycine buffer (pH 2.4 or 3.4)	Gresikova et al. (1984)
Vaccinia virus *(cell culture)*	Disulfide-linked antibodies mixed with Sephadex G-200 *(GE Healthcare, Sweden)*	Eq: PBS (pH 7.0); A: extracted by grinding and clarified; recycled; D: glycine-Cl (pH 2.2)	Birkbeck and Stephen (1970)

(continued)

TABLE 5.7 ***(Continued)***

Virus *(Source)*	Medium *(Manufacturer)*	Conditions	Ref.
Adsorption chromatography			
Influenza virus *(chicken eggs)*	Aluminum phosphate mixed with silica	**Eq:** 0.125 M phosphate buffer (pH ~6); **A:** allantoic fluid pre-conditioned to appropriate buffer, ca. 10 CV; **D:** 0.25 M phosphate buffer (pH ~7)	Miller and Schlesinger (1955)
	Calcium phosphate	**Eq:** 0.15 M phosphate buffer (pH 7.5); **A:** allantoic fluid adjusted to 0.15 M phosphate buffer (pH 7.5), 20 CV; **D:** 0.9 M phosphate buffer, pH 7.5	Pepper (1967)
Poliovirus *(cell culture)*	Calcium phosphate	**A:** 1 CV of virus suspension, D: 0.05–0.5 M phosphate buffer, pH 7.0	Ozaki et al. (1965)

I: injection, E: elution, Eq: equilibration, A: adsorption, D: desorption, CV: column volume, ON: over night, RT: room temperature, TNE: Tris-NaCl-EDTA, TN: Tris-NaCl, PBS: phosphate-buffered saline, PEG: polyethyleneglycol, CEWB: cleaning, equilibration and washing buffer.

While first media were cast from cross-linked dextran, a variety of chemistries are in use today including matrices from silica, agarose, polyacrylamide, polyacrylates, and their copolymers (Eriksson, 2002; Mori and Barth, 1999). Historically, media made from controlled pore glass also played a role because they can be cast with narrow pore size distributions (Haller, 1965a, Haller, 1965b). The surface of controlled pore glass, however, is barely inert and therefore not truly suited for SEC without surface modification (Mizutani, 1985; Schnabel and Langer, 1991). Nowadays, SEC (also known as *gel filtration*) is a well-established technique having its place in analytical and preparative applications (Eriksson, 2002; Janca, 1983; Mori and Barth, 1999). Concerning the purification of viruses, SEC is probably the most widely used type of chromatography. Published records include the chromatography of influenza virus (Abraham et al., 1984; Heyward et al., 1977; Kalbfuss et al., 2007c; Nayak et al., 2005), rubella virus (Trudel et al., 1981), tick-borne encephalitis virus (Crooks et al., 1990), rotavirus-like particles (Peixoto et al., 2007), coronavirus (Loa et al., 2002; Nagano et al., 1989), baculovirus (Transfiguracion et al., 2007), bacteriophages (Gschwender et al., 1969), and retroviral vectors (Segura et al., 2005; Transfiguracion et al., 2003). SEC has been further mentioned in the context of industrial vaccine manufacturing (Hagen et al., 2000; Montagnon and Fanget, 1985; Wiktor et al., 1987).

Preparative SEC is typically operated in group separation mode aiming at the separation of smaller colloids such as proteins from virions. Simultaneously, the product fraction can be conditioned for subsequent unit operations or desalted after IEC and AC (see e.g., Kalbfuss et al., 2007c; Segura et al., 2005). Noteworthy, it was Porath and Flodin (1959) who introduced the term *group separation* within the context of preparative SEC. In this mode, the chromatography medium is chosen such that virions are totally excluded from the stationary phase. Owing to the absence of mass transfer, virions and other excluded solutes elute in a narrow peak almost independent of flow rate (Fig. 5.11a), thus providing high resolution and low dilution of the product. Chromatography media with pores sufficiently large for virus entry may in fact exist—theoretically allowing for the separation of larger impurities as well. However, operation would be restricted to very low flow rates in order to avoid excessive band broadening because of the low diffusivity of virions (Fig. 5.11b).

SEC is operated strictly isocratically and hence a diluting chromatography operation. The concentration of the sample as in gradient chromatography is not possible because of the separation principle (nonadsorptive, molecular sieving effect). But dilution can be minimized by reducing axial dispersion (i.e., maximizing column efficiency) and choosing a sufficiently large injection volume. On the other hand, SEC does not suffer from a limited capacity for virus particles that is typical for most chromatography media. Accordingly, the columns may be loaded with highly concentrated feed streams. In general, productivity and dilution have to be balanced with resolution and hence the degree of purification by selecting an appropriate injection volume, flow rate, and column length. Although operation under analytical conditions (low injection volume, low flow rate, and long column) will result in the highest purity, it is typically economically unfeasible. But even after careful optimization

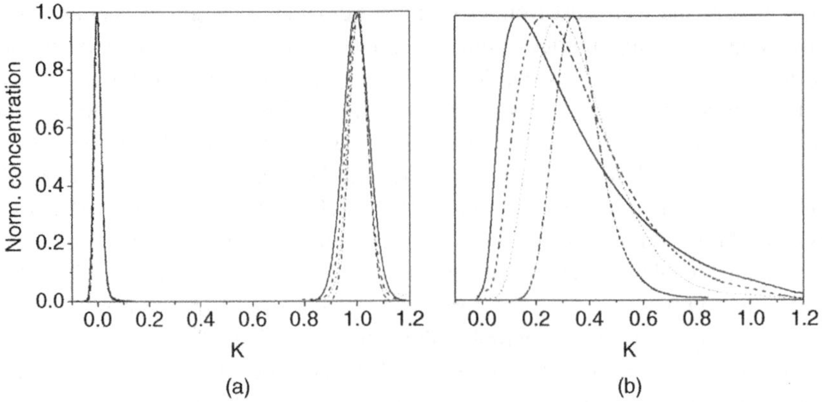

Figure 5.11 Band broadening in size-exclusion chromatography. 100 nm BSA-coated polystyrene beads (a, left), acetone (a, right), and a 201-kDa polymethacrylic acid marker (b) were injected onto a 30-cm column packed with Sepharose 4 FF. Markers were eluted at linear flow rates of 120 (—), 60 (---), 30 (···), and 7.5 (-··) cm/h. The injection volume was less than 0.1% of the column volume. Chromatograms were normalized to the maximum concentration.

of operating conditions, SEC may still pose a bottleneck in large-scale manufacturing of viral vaccines. In such cases, simulated moving-bed (SMB)-SEC could be an alternative (Hashimoto et al., 1988; Paredes et al., 2005; Xie et al., 2002). SMB-SEC has been demonstrated to provide higher productivity and/or purity compared to the batch process (Xie et al., 2002). Its design and realization are further comparatively straightforward (Zhong and Guiochon, 1996; Zhong and Guiochon, 1998). The principle as such, however, has been patented and likely requires the payment of royalties (Merck Patent GmbH, 2000).

A general concern in SEC is the high surface to volume ratio combined with the typically low concentrations of biomass in feed streams. Similarly to TFUF, unspecific adsorption of virions to the stationary phase may occur, leading to recoveries far below 100% (Nayak et al., 2005; Peixoto et al., 2007; Segura et al., 2005). Selection of an appropriate medium–eluent combination is therefore crucial. In some instances, additional supplementation of eluents may help to overcome surface interactions (Ejima et al., 2005).

SEC at moderate concentrations belongs to the realm of linear chromatography. Moderate means that particle–particle interactions are still negligible with respect to mass transfer. Historically, the propagation of band profiles has been described using plate models (Giddings and Mallik, 1966; Yamamoto et al., 1990) and continuum approaches (Li et al., 1998a; Li et al., 1998b; Zelic and Nesek, 2006). A more recent and distinct view is given by the stochastic theory of SEC, which builds on the stochastic processes of single solutes (pore ingress and egress; Dondi et al., 2002). In the simplest case, attention is paid only to the location of peaks (i.e., mean elution volume or retention time) after short injections (<1% column volume), which can be predicted from the distribution coefficient K_{SEC} between phases (Eriksson, 2002; Mori and Barth, 1999):

$$K_{SEC} = \frac{c_p}{c_b} = \frac{(V_e - V_0)}{(V_l - V_0)} \tag{5.15}$$

The distribution coefficient is defined as the ratio of concentrations in the stationary (c_p) and mobile phase (c_b). It is related to the mean elution volume V_e of a solute and can be calculated once the column void volume V_0 and total liquid volume V_l have been determined. In general, the use of K_{SEC} is preferable over V_e because it is independent of column dimensions and can be directly used to compare the selectivity of chromatography media. For convenience, a similar definition of an apparent distribution coefficient K_{av} exists, which is based on the volume of the column and not on the total liquid volume. It is sometimes used in cases where a total inclusion marker for the determination of V_l is not available or the volume fraction of the solid is negligible. Importantly, values of K_{SEC} in true SEC are always in the range from 0 (total exclusion) to 1 (total inclusion). Solutes therefore have to elute within one liquid volume of the column. Values of $K_{SEC} > 1$ indicate nonspecific interaction with the stationary phase. For colloids significantly larger than the largest pores, the stationary phase is practically nonporous, and SEC passes over to the principle of hydrodynamic chromatography (Stegeman et al., 1993a; Stegeman et al., 1993b).

The choice of chromatography media mainly depends on the size and geometry of the virus to be purified (Table 5.1). The selection of a proper medium will normally be based on experiments with the true sample. However, if calibration data are available (ideally provided through the suppliers), the theory of universal calibration (Rudin and Hoegy, 1972) can be used for a rational preselection. Calibration data usually exist as a table of elution volumes for a number of homogeneous markers (same type of polymer) linking molecular weight and distribution coefficients or elution volumes. If the logarithm of molecular weight is plotted over K_{SEC}, a sigmoid curve is typically obtained with poles at $K_{SEC} = 0$ and 1 (Dawkins, 1984). Results for different types of markers are, however, not comparable. Universal calibration provides a general framework to convert the molecular weight of linear flexible polymers into their equivalent hydrodynamic volume (Rudin and Hoegy, 1972). The limiting viscosity number (η) (also known as *intrinsic viscosity*) of such polymers is related to their molecular weight M by the Mark-Houwink-Sakurada equation (Brandrup et al., 1999).

$$[\eta] = KM^{\alpha} \tag{5.16}$$

The coefficients K and α depend on the polymer, solvent, and temperature and are subject to experimental determination. However, data for many combinations are available in literature (see e.g., Brandrup et al., 1999 for a comprehensive compilation). Of these, polyethylene oxide, dextran, and pullulan are probably the most common markers for calibration in aqueous solution (Kato et al., 1983). Using the

Einstein viscosity relation for dilute solutions of rigid spheres, the limiting viscosity number can be converted into the hydrodynamic volume V_m of the polymer (Rudin and Hoegy, 1972) (N_A denotes Avogadro's number).

$$V_m = [\eta]\frac{M}{2.5N_A} \quad (5.17)$$

From this volume, the diameter of the volume-equivalent sphere is readily calculated and therewith a characteristic measure of size derived. Apart from a priori estimation of distribution coefficients, calibration data may further be used to estimate the separability of certain impurities by SEC (Fig. 5.9). The fragment length distribution of residual host cell DNA, for instance, can be determined by agarose gel electrophoresis (Kalbfuss et al., 2007c) and then converted into a distribution of hydrodynamic diameter using the length-size correlation reported by Potschka (1991). Alternatively, the size of molecules for which a diffusion coefficient has been determined may be estimated by application of the Einstein-Stokes equation (Li et al., 1998a; Li et al., 1998b). It should be kept in mind, however, that such calculations only provide a rough orientation and always have to be validated experimentally.

The description of peak broadening and finally the prediction of elution profiles is a much more delicate matter. On the one hand, peak broadening is affected by axial dispersion and mass transfer. On the other hand, effects related to volume overloading have to be considered. As seen in Fig. 5.11, peak broadening as a function of flow rate is closely related to the distribution coefficient. While the shape of peaks of totally excluded solutes is solely affected by axial dispersion (which is almost independent of flow rate), other solutes suffer from significant broadening of peaks because of limitations in mass transfer. In particular, solutes close to the exclusion limit are strongly affected, and a shift of modal values toward earlier elution volumes can be observed together with an increase in peak asymmetry.

An adequate mathematical description for the prediction of elution profiles in SEC has been given in the form of a general rate model (Li et al., 1998a; Li et al., 1998b; Zelic and, 2006). It accounts for the phenomena of convective transport, molecular sieving, axial dispersion, film diffusion, and pore diffusion. It is further capable of dealing with alterations in column length and arbitrary injection profiles. Once reliable prediction of elution profiles has been achieved, benchmarks of the unit operation such as yield, purity, dilution, and productivity as a function of operating conditions and fractionation can be calculated from simulations. However, although this model has been validated experimentally for a number of proteins, it is less suited for application to separation problems involving complex mixtures. Apart from the numerical difficulties associated with solving systems of coupled partial differential equations, such models require a detailed knowledge on the composition of feed streams, including solute characteristics such as distribution and diffusion coefficients of all compounds involved. Appropriate inverse methods starting from a limited set of experimental data with real sample are not available until date. Owing to these limitations, the determination of elution profiles, purity, dilution, and productivity as a function of operating conditions and column length mainly remains an experimental task (see e.g., Kalbfuss et al., 2007c; Kalbfuss-Zimmermann et al., 2008).

The isolated effect of volume overloading, in contrast to flow rate and column length, can be readily predicted by application of the superposition principle. Mathematically, the elution profile of an overloaded preparative run $c(t)$ can be predicted from the ideal profile after injection of an infinitely short pulse $c_\delta(t)$ by solving the convolution integral (Kalbfuss-Zimmermann et al., 2008; Zoran, 2003),

$$c(t) = \int_0^{+\infty} c_{\text{inj}}(\tau) \cdot c_\partial(t - \tau) d\tau \tag{5.18}$$

The shape of the injection pulse is provided by $c_{\text{inj}}(t)$ and is usually (but not necessarily) rectangular. The main difficulty is the determination of $c_\delta(t)$, which has to be approximated either from a finite but short injection or by deconvolution of experimental data.

Ion-Exchange Chromatography The principle of IEC is based on electrostatic (coulombic) interactions between charged solutes and immobilized charge on the stationary phase. Common ligands in anion-exchange chromatography (AIEC) include quaternary ammonia and diethylaminoethyl and those in cation-exchange chromatography (CIEC) are sulphonyl and carboxyl. Functional groups may either be directly coupled to the stationary phase or via spacers (also called *tentacles*), allowing for more flexibility in the binding of macromolecules. Under appropriate conditions (ionic strength and pH), solutes adsorb to the oppositely charged stationary phase and are separated from other compounds on the basis of differential retention. For macromolecules with multiple interaction sites, often a very strong bond with affinity-like character can be observed. In this case, it is more favorable to operate in gradient mode. Firstly, product and a share of impurities are adsorbed to the column under conditions that maximize not only selectivity but also dynamic capacity—a process referred to as *frontal chromatography*. Secondly, desorption of the product is achieved either by displacement with an increasing concentration of salt or by gradual changes in pH reducing and eventually reversing the charge of adsorbed solutes. Comprehensive overviews on the subject have been provided by Yamamoto et al. (1988) and Choudhary and Horvath (1996).

Virions are polyelectrolytes such that IEC is almost always applicable, presuming the proper choice of ion-exchanger and supporting matrix. Chromatographic purification by IEC has been described for a variety of viruses. Examples using packed-bed chromatography comprise the purification of influenza virus (Muller and Rose, 1952), hepatitis A virus (Hagen et al., 1996a; Hagen et al., 1996b), adenovirus (Brument et al., 2002; Green et al., 2002; Kaludov et al., 2002; Konz et al., 2005;), adeno-associated virus (O'Riordan et al., 2000; Smith et al., 2003), and retroviral vectors (Rodrigues et al., 2006). Ion-exchange membrane chromatography has been described for influenza virus (Goyal et al., 1980; Kalbfuss et al., 2007b), rotavirus-like and VLP-based particles (Vicente et al., 2008; Vicente et al., 2011a), alphaherpesviruses (Karger et al., 1998), baculovirus (Vicente et al., 2010a; Vicente et al., 2011b; Wu et al., 2007), densonucleosis virus (Specht et al., 2004), and bacteriophage PRD1 (Walin et al., 1994). Regarding monoliths, examples for tomato mosaic virus (Kramberger et al., 2007), rubella virus (Forcic et al., 2011), and bacteriophage T4 (Smrekar et al., 2007) can be found. Besides, a patent describing AIEC of influenza virus with different media including adsorptive membranes and monoliths has been granted (Peterka et al., 2008).

The choice of ion-exchanger mostly depends on the net charge of virions. If the pH value is above the isoelectric point, virions are negatively charged and anion-exchangers are most appropriate. Otherwise, cation-exchangers should be used. Although net charge can be influenced via pH value (e.g., Specht et al., 2004), the stability of viruses often limits the pH working range. In the case of influenza virus, a pH value below 5 induces conformational changes in the hemagglutinin protein (Lamb and Krug, 2001), culminating in a loss of infectivity (Scholtissek, 1985) and viral aggregation (Campbell et al., 2004). Similarly, a loss of HA activity has already been observed not only under mildly acidic conditions but also at alkaline pH value (Kalbfuss et al., 2007c). The acceptable pH working range therefore always needs to be determined experimentally ahead of developing IEC operations.

The isoelectric point of virions can be determined by isoelectric focusing or isoelectric titration (i.e., measurement of zeta potential or electrophoretic mobility as a function of the pH value). The latter provides additional information on the quantity of charge in addition to sign. From the electrophoretic methods available, at least agarose gels or free-flow electrophoresis need to be used because of the size of virions. The isoelectric point of influenza virus A2/Singapore/57, for example, has been determined as 5.0 (Zhilinskaya et al., 1972), that of poliovirus (Mahoney strain) as 8.2 (Floyd and Sharp, 1978) by isoelectric focusing, that of influenza virus A/PR/8/34 (H1N1) as 5.3 (Miller et al., 1944), and that of measles virus as 7.0 (Herzer et al., 2003) by isoelectric titration. Theoretical calculations of isoelectric points, in contrast, are highly unreliable because the precise composition of virions is often not known, neither is the fraction of proteins that is exposed on the viral surface. Moreover, post-translational modifications such as glycosylation can severely alter the charge of virions. A peculiarity of macromolecules and virions is that even if the net charge has been determined, patches of the opposite charge may still exist. Respectively, purification of influenza virus A/PR/8/34 (H1N1) at neutral pH value has been reported not only by AIEC (Kalbfuss et al., 2007b), but also by CIEC (Muller and Rose, 1952). Suitability of ion-exchangers therefore always remains to be confirmed experimentally.

Two applications of IEC are usually considered: in the first one, virus is to be gross-purified and concentrated early in the process (referred to as *capture*, e.g., Hagen et al., 1996a; Hagen et al., 1996b; Kalbfuss et al., 2007b). In some of these cases, buffer exchange may be required in advance (e.g., Rodrigues et al., 2007). During capture, the focus is set on productivity because large volumes of feed material have to be processed. In addition, conditions on adsorption need to be carefully optimized in order to maximize selectivity. Otherwise, a large share of the dynamic capacity may be consumed by impurities. Direct capture of influenza virus from cell culture by membrane AIEC, for example, resulted in about fivefold concentration of the virus and 70% recovery (Kalbfuss et al., 2007b). At the same time, total protein was reduced to 23%. The content of host cell DNA, in contrast, remained unchanged.

Owing to the low bed height of the adsorbent, chromatography could be operated at the high flow rate of 10 column volumes per hour, thus providing the productivity required at this process stage. Alternatively, virus is separated from minor yet critical amounts of particular impurities at an intermediate or late stage of the purification process (referred to as *intermediate purification* or *polishing*, e.g., Hagen et al., 2000; Konz et al., 2005). In this case, it is mainly resolution (i.e., high selectivity and column efficiency) that is the crucial feature.

A third possibility is the operation of AIEC in flow-through mode particularly for the depletion of nucleic acids and proteins (Iyer et al., 2011; Knudsen et al., 2001; Sakata et al., 2005). This option should be considered whenever appropriate ion-exchangers for the adsorption of virus do not exist or adsorptive purification is too inefficient because of low recovery or capacity. Noteworthy, it is not necessarily electrostatic interaction alone but a combination of electrostatic and hydrophobic interactions that is involved in the binding of nucleic acids (Charlton et al., 1999). An example of virus purification by AIEC in flow-through mode has been given by Kalbfuss et al. (2007c). In order to prevent viral adsorption, preconditioning to 0.65 M NaCl in a previous step was required. Resulting reduction in DNA was about 60-fold, while more than 80% of the product could be recovered.

If IEC is to be described mathematically, appropriate choice of adsorption isotherms is crucial. In this context, the steric mass action (SMA) formalism (Brooks and Cramer, 1992) is briefly introduced—an extension of the steric displacement model (Drager and Regnier, 1986), which additionally considers steric effects of large solutes and can be easily extended to the multicomponent case (Gallant et al., 1995). The SMA formalism is built on the stoichiometric exchange of solute and salt on the ion-exchange resin according to the equation,

$$C_a + \nu_a \overline{Q}_s \Longleftrightarrow Q_a + \nu_a C_s \qquad (5.19)$$

C_a and C_s hereby denote solute and salt in the mobile phase, while Q_a and Q_s refer to their adsorbed counterparts. $\overline{Q}_s$ refers explicitly to the fraction of exchangeable salt (in contrast to shielded salt). The stoichiometric coefficient is given by ν_a. Corresponding concentrations of solute and salt will be referred to by small letters c and q in the following sections. The corresponding equilibrium constant K_a for the ion-exchange process is defined as,

$$K_a = \left(\frac{q_a}{c_a}\right)\left(\frac{c_s}{\overline{q}_s}\right)^{\nu_a} \qquad (5.20)$$

Adsorbed solute further shields a fraction of charge according to $\hat{q}_s = \sigma_a q_a$, which is characterized by the steric factor σ_a. Electroneutrality on the stationary phase requires that $\Lambda = \overline{q}_s + (\nu_a + \sigma_a) q_a$, with Λ being the ion capacity of the stationary phase. By substitution and rearrangement the implicit isotherm, the equation

$$c_a = \left(\frac{q_a}{K_a}\right)\left(\frac{c_s}{\Lambda - (\nu_a + \sigma_a)\, q_a}\right)^{\nu_a} \qquad (5.21)$$

can be derived. In the limiting case of $c_a \rightarrow 0$ and $q_a \approx 0$ (diluted conditions), a linear isotherm is approached with reciprocal dependence on the salt concentration (Brooks and Cramer, 1992).

The application of the SMA formalism to IEC of rotavirus-like particles has been reported only recently by Vicente et al. (2008). Equilibrium constants and stoichiometric factors were determined in linear gradient elution experiments with purified VLPs. Steric factors were, however, neglected. Instead, saturation and competitive binding of impurities were simulated by reducing the ion capacity of the stationary phase. Still, a fairly good match between the prediction of a preparative run and experimental data were achieved (Fig. 5.12).

Affinity Chromatography The principle requirement for AC or affinity methods in general is the availability of a highly selective ligand. Affinity bonds further need to be reversible, and ligands should be sufficiently robust to allow for multiple injection–elution cycles and with respect to regeneration and sanitization. Most often, natural interactions between molecules are being exploited. Common examples include antibody–antigen, lectin–sugar, receptor–ligand, and enzyme–inhibitor complexes. If no suitable ligands are available, the product may be genetically tagged (e.g., his or GST-tag) and purified using specifically designed chromatography media (Labrou and Clonis, 1994; Turkova, 2002).

AC belongs to the finest methods available in downstream processing. It is highly selective and capable of achieving purification efficacy that is unmatched by other unit operations. AC is therefore often used as the first step in purification processes

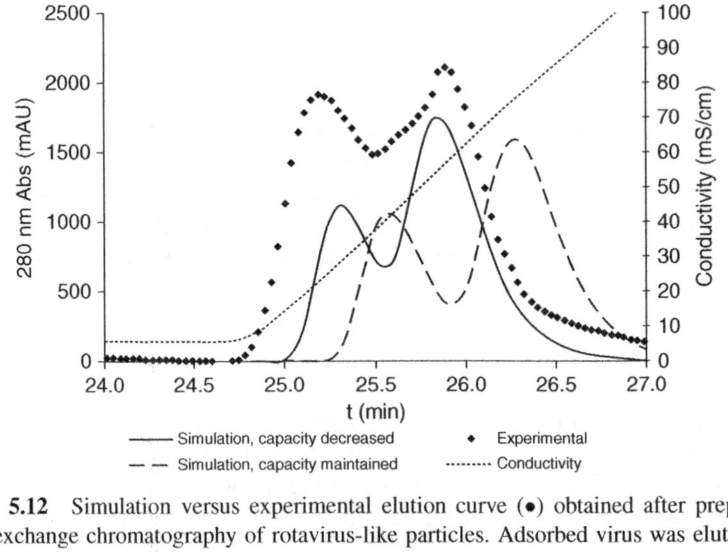

Figure 5.12 Simulation versus experimental elution curve (•) obtained after preparative anion-exchange chromatography of rotavirus-like particles. Adsorbed virus was eluted by a linear salt gradient (···). Simulations were performed using either the true (---) or an artificially reduced ion capacity (—). Reproduced with permission from Elsevier, Journal of Membrane Science, 2008.

(termed *capture*) or for single step purification. It can be applied directly either after solid separation or after a first concentrating step (e.g., TFUF) if the concentration of product should be insufficient. If chromatography is realized with an expanded bed (Sonnenfeld and Thömmes, 2007), solid separation can even be skipped and crude viral harvests may be directly applied to the column. Moreover, AC is the only type of chromatography for which column efficiency is usually considered negligible. Sometimes, selective separation can even be achieved in batch adsorption mode (see previous section). Longer columns providing higher efficiency, may, however, be beneficial in order to increase capacity (but not necessarily productivity; Fahrner et al., 1999).

Although AC provides a number of advantages and is often considered ideal, certain disadvantages have to be kept in mind. Affinity ligands are often very expensive, difficult to produce, or require genetic modification of the product. Possibly, the desired affinity medium is not even available commercially or only in insufficient quantities. Moreover, biological ligands such as antibodies or lectins are significantly less stable than small synthetic functional groups, resulting in a limited lifetime of columns. Harsh conditions on cleaning and sanitization have to be avoided in these cases. If ligands are of natural origin, additionally, innocuousness needs to be confirmed because leaching of columns can usually not be avoided.

An obvious approach for the generation of AC media is by coupling specific antibodies to a porous support. Hereby, antibodies are used either in the form of polyclonal sera or preferentially monoclonal antibodies. Indeed, this approach has been frequently pursued. Affinity media already described in the section on batch adsorption for the purification of plant viruses (Galvez, 1966; Ladipo and Zoeten, 1971), influenza (Sweet et al., 1974a; Sweet et al., 1974b), and vaccinia virus (Birkbeck and Stephen, 1970) have additionally been used in column chromatography. However, rather soft immobilizates from cross-linked antibodies had to be mixed with a rigid support in order to prevent compaction of columns. Direct coupling of antibodies to a rigid matrix is therefore to be preferred. Examples reported in literature include the purification of hepatitis A virus (Elkana et al., 1979), measles virus (Njayou and Quash, 1991), rubella virus (Chong and Gillam, 1985), poliovirus (Brown et al., 1979), and tick-borne encephalitis virus (Gresikova et al., 1984). A general problem in using antibodies remains the often very strong bond to antigens. Frequently, the product bound can only be released under very acidic or alkaline conditions, high ionic strength, or by the use of protein denaturants (Table 5.7), which are likely to damage the product. A second disadvantage is that the high selectivity of antibodies may restrict their use to a single vaccine strain. In this case, new antibodies will have to be generated for every strain to be purified.

If the virus surface is glycosylated (mostly the case for enveloped viruses, see Table 5.1), lectin chromatography may be a viable approach. Lectins are sugar-binding proteins with high selectivity for certain sugar moieties (van Damme et al., 1998). A variety of lectins with different specificity can be isolated from plants, which provide a cheap and safe source. Some lectins are, however, considered harmful and should therefore be avoided in process chromatography (Hartley and Lord, 2004; Vasconcelos and Oliveira, 2004). Owing to their affinity toward sugars, lectins are less specific for a certain virus strain but may also bind other glycosylated proteins, resulting in lower purity compared to antibodies. However, lectin chromatography may be applicable to the purification of different strains of a certain virus as long as their glycosylation pattern is similar. A good starting point for the development of whole-virion lectin chromatography operations is the literature on lectin chromatography of viral proteins (see e.g., Hayman et al., 1973; Kristiansen et al., 1983). It has to be noted, however, that results cannot always be transferred one by one (Kristiansen et al., 1983). In particular, the strength of binding may vary because of the different number of interacting sites. Purification of virions with lectin chromatography has been successfully demonstrated for influenza virus from mammalian cell culture (Opitz et al., 2007b). Adsorption kinetics, however, was comparatively low. Moreover, performance strongly dependent on the matrix used (Opitz et al., 2007a)—a phenomenon which is not unique to lectin chromatography. A crucial issue in lectin chromatography is the dependence of glycosylation patterns on the host and, possibly, also cultivation conditions (Schwarzer et al. 2008; Schwarzer et al., 2009). Any changes in upstream processing therefore need to be thoroughly evaluated with respect to their impact on lectin chromatography.

Another very appealing approach for the development of affinity operations is the exploitation of viral receptors or enzymatic affinity. A prominent example is heparan sulfate, which serves as a specific ligand for viral adhesion to the surface of cells (Liu and Thorp, 2002). It is structurally (but not functionally) related to heparin and belongs to the class of glycosaminoglycans. Heparin is known to specifically interact with a multitude of proteins (Conrad, 1998). Both molecular families are linear polymers consisting of uronic acid-(1 → 4)-D-glucosamine repeating disaccharide subunits with varying degree of N and O substitution by sulfate groups (Rabenstein, 2002). Owing to its use in various medical applications, heparin is available in large quantities, and a number of commercial chromatography media exist. Alternatively, the properties of heparin and heparan sulfate have been mimicked by structurally similar sulfated cellulose. Purification of whole virions by heparin chromatography has been investigated for herpes simplex virus (O'Keeffe et al., 1999), hepatitis B and C virus (Zahn and Allain, 2005), retroviruses (Segura et al., 2005; Segura et al., 2007), and adeno-associated virus (Clark et al., 1999). Purification by bead-based chromatography on sulfated cellulose has been reported for measles virus, parainfluenzavirus, herpes simplex virus, and flavivirus, among others (Ohtaki et al., 2011; O'Neil and Balkovic, 1993). Another point of attack could be the affinity of viral receptors such as hemagglutinins present in measles, rabies, and influenza virus (Curtain, 1954) or that of viral enzymes such as neuraminidase.

A rather new yet interesting concept is the specific recognition of molecules by aptamers (Famulok et al., 2007; Hermann and Patel, 2000). Aptamers are single-stranded oligonucleotides, which, similar to antibodies, are able to recognize specific molecular structures. In contrast to antibodies, they can be easily produced in large quantities. The development of aptamers is driven by a process termed *systematic evolution of ligands by exponential enrichment* (SELEX) (Ellington and Szostak, 1990; Tuerk and Gold, 1990). As part of this process, specific aptamers are selected from a synthetic library by AC and subsequently amplified by polymerase chain reaction. Next to various medical and analytical applications, aptamers can also be used for the recognition of viruses (James, 2007). Particular evidence in literature can be found for influenza virus (Gopinath et al., 2006a; Gopinath et al., 2006b; Jeon et al., 2004), vaccina virus (Nitsche et al., 2007), human immunodeficiency virus 1 (Dey et al., 2005), and cytomegalovirus (Wang et al., 2000). Preparative chromatography, however, has not been reported so far.

Despite the plurality of available options, selection of appropriate affinity ligands and subsequent generation of affinity media remains a tedious task. It is therefore to be anticipated that in the future purification of viruses will be facilitated by artificial introduction of affinity tags into vaccine strains. Affinity tags have proven valuable in the purification of recombinant protein already and usually allow for a dramatic simplification of downstream processes (Flaschel and Friehs, 1993; Waugh, 2005). Integration of his-tags and subsequent purification by metal chelate chromatography has been demonstrated for adeno-associated virus (Koerber et al., 2007; Zhang et al., 2002), murine leukemia virus (Ye et al., 2004), and VLPs (Cheng et al., 2001). Remarkably, adeno-associated virus is a naked virus for which integration of additional peptide sequences can easily interfere with the assembly of viral capsids. Concerning enveloped viruses, conservation of the biological function of surface proteins (such as adhesion or fusion activity) should generally be sufficient. In addition to preserving biological function, one has to ensure that tags do not interfere with the function as a vaccine. Otherwise, tags have to be removed again, for example, by autocleavage or cleavage at protease recognition sites (Arnau et al., 2006).

Unfortunately, most of the literature does not provide truly quantitative measures of the initial and final content of impurities before and after AC. Therefore, two articles providing data on product yield and reduction in protein and DNA content were selected for general discussion. In the first example, Ye et al. (2004) showed that by metal chelate chromatography of a his-tagged murine leukemia virus strain, total protein content could be reduced by a factor of 1229 and DNA by a factor of 6800. Virus yield based on infectivity was 56%. Concerning influenza virus, purification by lectin chromatography resulted only in a 4.5-fold reduction in total protein but 1200-fold reduction in DNA (Opitz et al., 2007b). The product yield based on influenza virus HA activity was as high as 97%. Obviously, results from both examples have to be evaluated in their particular context and cannot easily be transferred to other applications. However, they serve to demonstrate the outstanding performance that can often be achieved by AC operations.

5.3 CONCLUSIONS AND OUTLOOK

A variety of methods for the purification of whole virions and viral antigens has been made available over the last decades. Albeit in many cases, implementation remained restricted to laboratory-scale preparations, and suitability for large-scale manufacturing was not addressed. Consequently, availability should not be confused with implementation and widespread use in large-scale manufacturing. Vaccine manufacturers operating in a highly regulated environment tend to be very conservative with respect to the establishment of new separation technologies. Another obstacle is that although the development of new or the improvement of existing methods has been accompanied by a large number of publications, looking at each virus individually, quantitative information remains rather scarce. Only if available literature is combined, a mosaic of the overall picture can be reconstructed, which comprises all the unit operations that are common to protein purification or biochemical engineering in general. The main difficulty remains in combining appropriate unit operations, which is particularly difficult because of the sometimes very different properties of viruses (e.g., enveloped vs naked viruses) and differences in feed streams (e.g., serum-free vs protein-free medium). Although many promising results have been obtained, research was mostly driven empirically. Method development was often carried out only to the point that a method would work for a certain application. In these instances, a general mechanistic understanding was usually not pursued. However, comparatively, little benefit can be derived from such studies when a method is to be transferred to other applications or an existing unit operation has to be scaled or optimized.

A particular issue remains the limited quantitative information in early publications where much of the analytical technology used today had not yet been available. Sometimes, the outcome of experiments was only judged in a qualitative manner, prohibiting evaluation of performance and comparison to other studies. In order to allow for the evaluation of performance based on hard figures, a minimum extend of analytical analyses has to be conducted—at least for the most important process intermediates and the final bulk. As the minimum requirement, at least one measure for the quantity of virus or viral antigen, total protein, and DNA should be reported. In addition, volumes of process fractions should be given such that total quantities and concentrations can be interconverted and concentration factors calculated.

For the quantitation of virus or viral antigens, standardized assays should be used, which are commonly accepted as a measure of potency. A prominent example is the single-radial diffusion test, which is used for the standardization of inactivated influenza vaccines (Williams, 1993; European Pharmacopoeia Commission, 2012c). If the use of these assays is prohibitive (particularly at intermediate processing steps) because of insufficient sensitivity, matrix interference, or low sample throughput, other methods should be chosen that provide at least some degree of correlation with the assay used to determine antigen input for blending. In addition, assays for the quantitation of virus further need to be precise. In particular, historical assay formats often only allow for the estimation of orders of magnitude of virus yields, which is insufficient for use in material balances and evaluation of overall process performance. In addition, if the assay read-out is only discrete, bias in benchmarks calculated from measured values will occur.

Beyond virus quantity, not only characterization of the virus population, but also properties of viral antigens (glycosylation, folding, chemical modification, etc.) would be highly desirable. In the first line, the determination of size distributions for example, by light scattering analysis (Campbell et al., 2004), gel permeation chromatography (Ando et al., 1997), field flow fractionation (Chuan et al., 2008; Giddings et al., 1977; Wei et al., 2007; Yohannes et al. 2011), surface plasmon resonance (Vicente et al., 2011b), or analytical centrifugation (Berkowitz et al.,

2007) provides valuable insights into sample composition. Such information is necessary not only to confirm integrity of virions, but also to judge the degree of contamination by cell debris and the presence of (viral) aggregates. Likewise valuable is the acquisition of isoelectric titration curves (Trilisky and Lenhoff, 2007; Herzer et al., 2003). Such data canbe used not only to derive optimal conditions for electrostatic interaction chromatography or the design of precipitation operations, but also to select appropriate buffers (pH value and ionic strength) that ensure colloidal stability of the viral solution (Floyd and Sharp, 1978; Floyd and Sharp, 1979). Shifts in titration curves further allow to identify chemical modifications (e.g., as the result of inactivation) or molecular association of polyions such as polycations used for the precipitation of host cell DNA or host cell DNA itself.

In addition, a scale and device independent description of experimental procedures should be aimed at. It is in general of little use, if only the rotational speed of a certain peristaltic pump or the dripping frequency of gravitationally operated columns is specified. Moreover, well-established engineering concepts should be applied wherever possible. Since most of the techniques mentioned in this chapter do have their counterparts in chemical engineering, the related theory is usually available. Once again, the characterization of solid separation in centrifuges by sigma theory (Ambler, 1959), concentration polarization (Porter, 1972), and the critical flux concept (Field et al., 1995; Bacchin et al., 2006) in tangential-flow filtration or the general theory of chromatography (Guiochon et al., 2006) shall be named here. Other concepts such as the combined pore blockage cake filtration model (Ho and Zydney, 2000; Palacio et al., 2002) or the SMA formalism (Brooks and Cramer, 1992) have been particularly developed for the field of biochemical engineering. Only if data are analyzed and presented in the context of such formal concepts, a meaningful comparison between different studies and quantitative evaluation of process performance will be feasible. Another important advantage is the amenability to mathematical optimization and rational scale-up (Vicente et al., 2011c).

Advantages of the engineering approach are evident. However, in order to handle increased experimental effort and complexity, it becomes necessary to enhance the efficiency of process development first. While for the demonstration of feasibility a few experiments are usually sufficient, for a fully quantitative description, a large number of systematic experiments are required. Consequently, experimental procedures need to be scaled down, automated, and parallelized in order to produce the required amount of experimental data within reasonable time at acceptable cost. A good example for advances into this direction is preparative chromatography. These days, a variety of screening columns can be bought out of the shelf, and modular chromatography systems are available that can be tailored to individual needs, allowing for fully automated screening of suitable chromatography media. In addition to increasing experimental capacity, shortening of development cycles by appropriate experimental design should be considered. In particular, a priori prediction of viral properties and process behavior should be helpful in identifying initial operating conditions already close to the optimum. Examples that are instructive in this context are the a priori prediction of SMA adsorption isotherms for proteins (Ladiwala et al., 2005) or prediction of hindrance factors for diffusion and convective transport of macromolecules in liquid-filled pores (Deen, 1987).

Finally, the new possibilities disclosed by genetic engineering technology can be expected to have a major impact on the field. Creation of tailor-made viruses (e.g., Neumann et al., 2001) and VLPs (Chackerian, 2007; Ramqvist et al., 2007) has become possible and is currently being explored for a variety of applications. On the one hand, expression of self-assembling VLPs in stable cell lines could reduce the initial burden of impurities and may allow for continuous production of antigens because of the absence of cytopathogenic effect. On the other hand, tags may be engineered into the surface of viruses or VLPs that allow for the development of standardized affinity operations and simplified analytical procedures. It would not be surprising to see a number of virus or VLP platforms evolve in the near future that can be used to generate arbitrary vaccines by genetic insertion of desired antigens. For these platforms, standardized downstream processes could be developed, reducing the task of process development from years to months.

ACKNOWLEDGMENTS

We thank Mattias Bryntesson and Robert Morenweiser for their comments on the manuscript. We are further indebted to Elke Bauch, Kristina Reinhold, and Cornelia Trieb from our library for the order of several hundred articles from libraries all over Germany. Finally, we thank developers of the free citation tool Zotero (http://www.zotero.org), which was used for formatting of references throughout this chapter.

NOMENCLATURE

Symbol	Units	Description
a	m	Diameter of spherical colloid
c	mol/m^3	Bulk liquid phase concentration
c	mol/m^3	Concentration
C_a		Camp number
D	m^2/s	Diffusion coefficient
g	m/s	Gravitational acceleration
$\overline{G}$	/s	Root-mean-square shear rate
J	m/s	Limiting flux
k_1	/s	Rate constant for first order consumption of inactivant
k_2	m^3/mol/s	Rate constant for second order inactivation of virions
K	m^3/g	Mark-Houwink-Sakurada coefficient
K	m^3/mol	Salting-out constant
K		Relative solubility coefficient

K_a		SMA equilibrium constant
K_{av}		Apparent volume distribution coefficient
K_{SEC}		SEC distribution coefficient
L	m	Length of hollow-fiber
L	m	Length of column
M	g/mol	Molecular weight
N_A	/mol	Avogadro's number
q	mol m^3	Stationary phase concentration
$\overline{q}_s$	mol m^3	Stationary phase concentration of exchangeable salt
$\hat{q}_s$	mol m^3	Stationary phase concentration of shielded salt
Q	m^3/s	Volumetric flow rate
r	m	Radius
s	s	Sedimentation coefficient
S	mol m^3	Solubility
S		Degree of inactivation ($\log_{10}$-scale)
t	s	Time
u_s	m/s	Sedimentation velocity
u	m/s	Axial flow velocity
V	m^3	Volume
V_m	m^3	Molecular hydrodynamic volume
X	-/m^3	Number or concentration of infectious virions
z	m	Distance from column inlet (axial coordinate)
α		Mark-Houwink-Sakurada exponent
α		Stoichiometric ratio of DNA and compacting agent
β	mol m^{-3}	Bulk concentration of compacting agent
β		Relative solubility intercept
$\dot{\gamma}_0$	/s	Wall shear rate
δ	m	Diameter of coiled polymer
ϵ	W m^{-3}	Volumetric power dissipation rate
ϵ_r		Relative dielectric constant
(η)	m^3/g	Limiting viscosity number
Λ	mol m^{-3}	Ion capacity
μ		Correction factor
ν	m^2/s	Kinematic viscosity
ν_a		Stoichiometric factor
ρ	kg m^{-3}	Density
σ_a		Steric factor
Σ	m^2	Equivalent area of settling tank
τ	s	Lag-time
Φ		Solute volume fraction
Φ		Phase ratio
ω	rad/s	Angular velocity

ABBREVIATIONS

AC	Affinity chromatography
AIEC	Anion-exchange chromatography
β-PL	β-propiolactone
BEI	Binary ethylenimine
BSA	Bovine serum albumin
CIEC	Cation-exchange chromatography
DEAE	Diethylaminoethanol
DF	Diafiltration
EP	European Pharmacopoeia
FA	Formaldehyde
FMD	Foot and mouth disease
IEC	Ion-exchange chromatography
PEI	Polyethylenimine
UV	Ultraviolet
VLP	Virus-like particle
SEC	Size-exclusion chromatography
SMA	Steric mass-action
TFUF	Tangential-flow ultrafiltration
WHO	World Health Organization

REFERENCES

Abraham A, Sivanadan V, Newman JA, Maheswaran SK. 1984. Rapid purification of avian influenza virus for use in enzyme-linked immunosorbent assay. Am J Vet Res, 45:959–962.

Aizawa M, Tobita Y. Continuous flow type centrifuge having rotor body and core body disposed therein. US patent No. 7144361. 2006.

Albertsson PA. Separation of particles and macromolecules by phase partition. Endeavour 1977;1:69–74.

Ambler CM. The theory of scaling up laboratory data for the sedimentation type centrifuge. J Biochem Microbiol 1959;1:185–205.

Amosenko FA, Svitkin YV, Popova VD, Terletskaya EN, Timofeev AV, Elbert LB, Lashkevich VA, Drozdov SG. Use of protamine sulfate for elimination of substrate DNA in poliovaccines produced on continuous cell lines. Vaccine 1991;9:207–209.

Anderson NG, Burger CL. Separation of cell components in the zonal ultracentrifuge. Science 1962;136:646–648.

Anderson NG, Waters DA, Nunley CE, Gibson RF, Schilling RM, Denny EC, Cline GB, Babelay EF, Perardi TE. K-series centrifuges. I. Development of K-2 continuous-sample-flow-with-banding centrifuge system for vaccine purification. Anal Biochem 1969;32:460–494.

Anderson NG. The zonal ultracentrifuge. A new instrument for fractionating mixtures of particles. J Phys Chem 1962;66:1984–1989.

Anderson NG. Virus isolation in the zonal ultracentrifuge. Nature 1963;199:1166–1168.

Ando S, Tsuge H, Mayumi T. Preparation of influenza virosome vaccine with muramyldipeptide derivative B30-MDP. J Microencapsul 1997;14:79–90.

Andre BR, Champluvier BPS. 2010. Purification of virus or viral antigens by density gradient ultracentrifugation (WO2010089339).

Arita M, Matumoto M. Heat inactivation of measles virus. Jpn J Microbiol 1968;12:121.

Armstrong ME, Giesa PA, Davide JP, Redner F, Waterbury JA, Rhoad AE, Keys RD, Provost PJ, Lewis JA. Development of the formalin-inactivated hepatitis A vaccine, VAQTA from the live attenuated virus strain CR326F. J Hepatol 1993;18:S20–S26.

Arnau J, Lauritzen C, Petersen GE, Pedersen J. Current strategies for the use of affinity tags and tag removal for the purification of recombinant proteins. Protein Expres Purif 2006;48:1–13.

Arscott PG, Li AZ, Bloomfield VA. Condensation of DNA by trivalent cations. 1. Effects of DNA length and topology on the size and shape of condensed particles. Biopolymers 1990;30:619–630.

Atkinson A, Jack GW. Precipitation of nucleic acids with polyethyleneimine and the chromatography of nucleic acids and proteins on immobilised polyethyleneimine. Biochim Biophys Acta 1973;308:41–52.

Babu GJ, Rajamanickam C. An improved method for the isolation of supercoiled plasmid DNA. Curr Sci 1998;74:572–573.

Bacchin P, Aimar P, Field RW. Critical and sustainable fluxes: theory, experiments and applications. J Membr Sci 2006;281:42–69.

Bacchin P, Si-Hassen D, Starov V, Clifton MJ, Aimar P. A unifying model for concentration polarization, gel-layer formation and particle deposition in cross-flow membrane filtration of colloidal suspensions. Chem Eng Sci 2002;57:77–91.

Badmington F, Wilkins R, Payne M, Honig ES. Vmax testing for practical microfiltration train scale-up in biopharmaceutical processing. Biopharm-Technol Buss 1995;8:46.

Bahnemann HG. Inactivation of viral antigens for vaccine preparation with particular reference to the application of the application of binary ethyleneimine. Vaccine 1990;8:299–303.

Baker JP, Katz SL. Childhood vaccine development: an overview. Pediatr Res 2004;55:347–356.

Bandell A, Woo J, Coelingh K. Protective efficacy of live-attenuated influenza vaccine (multivalent, Ann Arbor strain): a literature review addressing interference. Expert Rev Vaccines 2011;10(8):1131–1141.

Bardiya N, Bae JH. Influenza vaccines: recent advances in production technologies. Appl Microbiol Biotechnol 2005;67:299–305.

Barrett PN, Portsmouth D, Ehrlich HJ. Developing cell culture-derived pandemic vaccines. Curr Opin Mol Ther 2010;12(1):21–30.

Bartlett PD, Small G. Beta-propiolactone. IX. The kinetics of attack by nucleophilic reagents upon the alcoholic carbon of beta-propiolactone. J Am Chem Soc 1950;72:4867–4869.

Baruah GL, Venkiteshwaran A, Belfort G. Global model for optimizing crossflow microfiltration and ultrafiltration processes: a new predictive and design tool. Biotechnol Prog 2005;21:1013–1025.

Beck E, Strohmaier K. Subtyping of European foot-and-mouth disease virus strains by nucleotide sequence determination. J Virol 1987;61:1621–1629.

Belfort G, Davis RH, Zydney AL. The behavior of suspensions and macromolecular solutions in cross-flow microfiltration. J Membr Sci 1994;96:1–58.

Bell DJ, Dunnill P. Shear disruption of soya protein precipitate particles and the effect of aging in a stirred tank. Biotechnol Bioeng 1982a;24:1271–1285.

Bell DJ, Dunnill P. The influence of precipitation reactor configuration on the centrifugal recovery of isoelectric soya protein precipitate. Biotechnol Bioeng 1982b;24:2319–2336.

Bell DJ, Hoare M, Dunnill P. The formation of protein precipitates and their centrifugal recovery. In: Fiechter A, editor. *Downstream Processing (Advances in Biochemical Engineering/Biotechnology 26)*. Berlin: Springer; 1983.

Belshe RB, Maassab HF, Mendelman PM. Influenza vaccine—live. In: Plotkin SA, Orenstein WA, editors. *Vaccines*. 4th ed. Phildadelphia: Saunders; 2004. p 371–388.

Belshe RB, Edwards KM, Vesikari T, Black SV, Walker RE, Hultquist M, Kemble G; Connor EM for the CAIV-T Comparative Efficacy Study Group. Live attenuated versus inactivated influenza vaccine in infants and young children. New Engl J Med 2007;356(7):685–696.

Benedictis PD, Beato MS, Capua I. Inactivation of avian influenza viruses by chemical agents and physical conditions: a review. Zoonoses Public Health 2007;54:51–68.

Berkowitz SA, Philo JS. Monitoring the homogeneity of adenovirus preparations (a gene therapy delivery system) using analytical ultracentrifugation. Analytical Biochemistry 362 2007:16–37.

Berthold W, Kempken R. Interaction of cell-culture with downstream purification—a case study. Cytotechnology 1994;15:229–242.

Birkbeck TH, Stephen J. Specific removal of host-cell or vaccinia virus antigens from extracts of infected cells by polyvalent disulphide-linked immunosorbents. J Gen Virol 1970;8:133.

Boeckle. Purification of polyethylenimine polyplexes highlights the role of free polycations in gene transfer. J Gene Med 2004;6:1102–1111.

Boi C, Dimartino S, Sarti GC. Modelling and simulation of affinity membrane adsorption. J Chromatogr A 2007;1162:24–33.

Boutwell RK, Colburn NH, Muckerman CC. In vivo reactions of beta-propiolactone. Ann N Y Acad Sci 1969;163:751–763.

Boychyn M, Doyle W, Bulmer M, More J, Hoare M. Laboratory scaledown of protein purification processes involving fractional precipitation and centrifugal recovery. Biotechnol Bioeng 2000;69:1–10.

Boychyn M, Yim SS, Bulmer M, More J, Bracewell DG, Hoare M. Performance prediction of industrial centrifuges using scale-down models. Bioproc Biosyst Eng 2004;26:385–391.

Boychyn M, Yim SSS, Shamlou PA, Bulmer M, More J, Hoare A. Characterization of flow intensity in continuous centrifuges for the development of laboratory mimics. Chem Eng Sci 2001;56:4759–4770.

Braas G, Searle PF, Slater NK, Lyddiatt A. Strategies for the isolation and purification of retroviral vectors for gene therapy. Bioseparation 1996;6:211–228.

Brandrup J, Immergut EH, Grulke EA. 1999. Viscosity—molecular weight relationships and unperturbed dimensions of linear chain molecules. In: *Polymer Handbook*. 4th ed. New York: Wiley-Interscience. p VII-67.

Brands R, Visser J, Medema J, Palache AM, Scharrenburg GJ. InfluvacTC: a safe Madin Darby canine kidney (MDCK) cell culture-based influenza vaccine. Dev Biol Stand 1999;98:93–100.

Brooks CA, Cramer SM. Steric mass-action ion-exchange: displacement profiles and induced salt gradients. AIChE J 1992;38:1969–1978.

Brown F, Underwood BO, Fantes KH. Purification of poliovirus by affinity chromatography. J Med Virol 1979;4:315–319.

Brown F. Inactivation of viruses by aziridines. Vaccine 2002;20:322–327.

Brument N Morenweiser R, V Blouin, E Toublanc, I Raimbaud, Y Chérel, S Folliot 2002. A versatile and scalable two-step ion-exchange chromatography process for the purification of recombinant adeno-associated virus serotypes-2 and-5. Mol Ther, 6: 678–686.

Brumfield HP, Stulberg CS, Halvorson HO. Purification of mouse poliomyelitis virus by methanol precipitation at low temperatures. Proc Soc Exp Biol Med 1948;68:410–413.

Brusick DJ. Genetic properties of beta-propiolactone. Mutat Res 1977;39:241–256.

Budowsky EI, Friedman EA, Zheleznova NV, Noskov FS. Principles of selective inactivation of viral genome. VI. Inactivation of the infectivity of the influenza virus by the action of beta-propiolactone. Vaccine 1991;9:398–402.

Budowsky EI, Kostyuk GV, Kost AA, Savin FA. Principles of selective inactivation of viral genome. II. Influence of stirring and optical-density of the layer to be irradiated upon UV-induced inactivation of viruses. Arch Virol 1981;68:249–256.

Budowsky EI, Smirnov YA, Shenderovich SF. Principles of selective inactivation of viral genome. VIII. The influence of beta-propiolactone on immunogenic and protective activities of influenza virus. Vaccine 1993;11:343–348.

Budowsky EI, Zalesskaya MA. Principles of selective inactivation of viral genome. V. Rational selection of conditions for inactivation of the viral suspension infectivity to a given extent by the action of beta-propiolactone. Vaccine 1991;9:319–325.

Budowsky EI. Problems and prospects for preparation of killed antiviral vaccines. Adv Virus Res 1991;39:255–290.

Burak Y, Ariel G, Andelman D. Onset of DNA aggregation in presence of monovalent and multivalent counterions. Biophys J 2003;85:2100–2110.

Camp TR, Stein PC. Velocity gradients and internal work in fluid motion. J Boston Soc Civil Eng 1943;30:219–237.

Campbell JN, Epand RM, Russo PS. Structural changes and aggregation of human influenza virus. Biomacromolecules 2004;5:1728–1735.

Carta G, Ubiera AR, Pabst TM. Protein mass transfer kinetics in ion exchange media: measurements and interpretations. Chem Eng Technol 2005;28:1252–1264.

Chackerian B. Virus-like particles-flexible platforms for vaccine development. Expert Rev Vaccines 2007;6:381–390.

Charlton HR, Relton JM, Slater NKH. Characterisation of a generic monoclonal antibody harvesting system for adsorption of DNA by depth filters and various membranes. Bioseparation 1999;8:281–291.

Chen R, Mieyal JJ, Goldthwait DA. The reaction of beta-propiolactone with derivatives of adenine and with DNA. Carcinogenesis 1981;2:73–80.

Chen V, Li H, Fane AG. Non-invasive observation of synthetic membrane processes—a review of methods. J Membr Sci 2004;241:23–44.

Cheng YS, Lee MS, Lai SY, Doong SR, Wang MY. Separation of pure and immunoreactive virus-like particles using gel filtration chromatography following immobilized metal ion affinity chromatography. Biotechnol Prog 2001;17:318–325.

Choe WS, Middelberg APJ. Selective precipitation of DNA by spermine during the chemical extraction of insoluble cytoplasmic protein. Biotechnol Prog 2001;17:1107–1113.

Chong P, Gillam S. Purification of biologically active rubella virus antigens by immunoaffinity chromatography. J Virol Methods 1985;10:261–268.

Choudhary G, Horvath C. 1996. Ion-exchange chromatography. In: *Methods in Enzymology*. San Diego: Academic Press. p 47–82.

Chuan YP, Fan YY, Lua L, Middelberg APJ. Quantitative analysis of virus-like particle size and distribution by field-flow fractionation. Biotechnol Bioeng 2008;99(6):1425–1433.

Chung SF, Wen CY. Longitudinal dispersion of liquid flowing through fixed and fluidized beds. AIChE J 1968;14:857.

Cinatl J, Michaelis M, Doerr HW. The threat of avian influenza A (H5N1). Part IV: development of vaccines. Med Microbiol Immunol (Berl) 2007;196:213–225.

Clark KR, Liu XL, McGrath JP, Johnson PR. Highly purified recombinant adeno-associated virus vectors are biologically active and free of detectable helper and wild-type viruses. Hum Gene Ther 1999;10:1031–1039.

Collin N, de Radiguès X. Vaccine production capacity for seasonal and pandemic (H1N1) 2009 influenza. Vaccine 2009;27(38):5184–5186.

Conrad HE. *Heparin-Binding Proteins*. New York: Academic Press; 1998.

Cordes RM, Sims WB, Glatz CE. Precipitation of nucleic acids with poly(ethyleneimine). Biotechnol Prog 1990;6:283–285.

Cox HR, Vanderscheer J, Aiston S, Bohnel E. The purification and concentration of influenza virus by means of alcohol precipitation. Public Health Rep 1946;61:1682–1683.

Cox RJ, Brokstad KA, Ogra P. Influenza virus: Immunity and vaccination strategies. Comparison of the immune response to inactivated and live, attenuated influenza vaccines. Scand J Immunol 2004;59:1–15.

Craven P, Wahba G. Smoothing noisy data with spline functions—Estimating the correct degree of smoothing by the method of generalized cross-validation. Numer Math 1979;31:377–403.

Crooks AJ, Lee JM, Dowsett AB, Stephenson JR. Purification and analysis of infectious virions and native nonstructural antigens from cells infected with tick-borne encephalitis-virus. J Chromatogr 1990;502:59–68.

Cruz PE, Peixoto CC, Devos K, Moreira JL, Saman E, Carrondo MJT. Characterization and downstream processing of HIV-1 core and virus-like-particles produced in serum free medium. Enzyme Microb Technol 2000;26:61–70.

Curling J. Process chromatography: five decades of innovation. BioPharm Int 2007;10–48.

Curtain CC. The adsorption of influenza virus by haemagglutination inhibitors coupled to powdered cellulose. Br J Exp Pathol 1954;35:255–263.

Cutler T, Wang C, Qin Q, Zhou F, Warren K, Yoon KJ, Hoff SJ, Ridpath J, Zimmermann J. Kinetics of UV254 inactivation of selected viral pathogens in a static system. Appl Microbiol 2011;111(2):389–395.

Czermak P, Grzenia DL, Wolf A, Carlson JO, Specht R, Han B, Wickramasinghe SR. Purification of densonucleosis virus by tangential flow ultrafiltration and by ion exchange membranes. Desalination 2008;224(1–3):23–27.

Darnell MER, Subbarao K, Feinstone SM, Taylor DR. Inactivation of the coronavirus that induces severe acute respiratory syndrome, SARS-CoV. J Virol Methods 2004;121:85–91.

Davis RH, Grant DC. Theory for deadend microfiltration. In: Ho WS, Sirkar KK, editors. *Membrane Handbook*. New York: Chapman & Hall; 1992. p 461–479.

Davis RH. Modeling of fouling of cross-flow microfiltration membranes. Separation Purif Methods 1992;21:75–126.

Dawkins JV. Calibration of separation systems. In: Janca J, editor. *Steric Exclusion Liquid Chromatography of Polymers*. New York: Marcel Dekker Ltd; 1984. p 53–116.

de Bokx PK, Baarslag PC, Urbach HP. Modeling of displacement chromatography using non-ideal isotherms. J Chromatogr 1992;594:9–22.

de Frutos M, Raspaud E, Leforestier A, Livolant F. Aggregation of nucleosomes by divalent cations. Biophys J 2001;81:1127–1132.

de la Cruz MO, Belloni L, Delsanti M, Dalbiez JP, Spalla O, Drifford M. Precipitation of highly-charged polyelectrolyte solutions in the presence of multivalent salts. J Chem Phys 1995;103:5781–5791.

Deen WM. Hindered transport of large molecules in liquid-filled pores. AIChE J 1987;33:1409–1425.

Delsanti M, Dalbiez JPAS, Belloni L, Drifford M. Phase-diagram of polyelectrolyte solutions in presence of multivalent salts. ACS Sym Ser 1994;548:381–392.

Desbat BE, Lancelot . Effect of the β-propiolactone treatment on the adsorption and fusion of influenza A/Brisbane/59/2007 and A/New Caledonia 20/1999 virus H1N1 on a dimyristoylphosphatidylcholine/ganglioside GM3 mixed phospholipids monolayer at the air–water interface. Langmuir 2011;27(22):13675–13683.

DeRouchey . Structural investigations of DNA-polycation complexes. Eur Phys J E Soft Matter 2005;16:17–28.

DeWalt BW, Murphy JC, Fox GE, Willson RC. Compaction agent clarification of microbial lysates. Protein Expr Purif 2003;28:220–223.

Dey AK, Griffiths C, Lea SM, James W. Structural characterization of an anti-gp120 RNA aptamer that neutralizes R5 strains of HIV-1. RNA 2005;11:873–884.

Dickens F, Jones HE. Carcinogenic activity of a series of reactive lactones and related substances. Br J Cancer 1961;15:85.

Divizia M, Santi AL, Pana A. Ultrafiltration: an efficient second step for hepatitis A virus and poliovirus concentration. J Virol Methods 1989;23:55–62.

Dondi F, Cavazzini A, Remelli M, Felinger A, Martin M. Stochastic theory of size exclusion chromatography by the characteristic function approach. J Chromatogr A 2002;943:185–207.

Drager RR, Regnier FE. Application of the stoichiometric displacement model of retention to anion-exchange chromatography of nucleic-acids. J Chromatogr 1986;359:147–155.

Dubois DR, Eckels KH, Ticehurst J, Binn LN, Timchak RL, Barvir DA, Rankin CT, O'Neill SP. Large-scale purification of inactivated hepatitis A birus by centrifugation in non-ionic gradients. J Virol Methods 1991;32:327–334.

Eglon MN, Duffy OM, O'Brien T, Strappe PM. Purification of adenoviral vectors by combined anion exchange and gel filtration chromatography. Journal of Gene Medicine 2009;11(11):978–989.

Eickbush TH, Moudrianakis EN. Compaction of DNA helices into either continuous supercoils or folded fiber rods and toroids. Cell 1978;13:295–306.

Ejima D, Yumioka R, Arakawa T, Tsumoto K. Arginine as an effective additive in gel permeation chromatography. J Chromatogr A 2005;1094:49–55.

Elkana Y, Thornton A, Zuckerman AJ. Purification of hepatitis A virus by affinity chromatography. J Immunol Methods 1979;25:185–187.

Ellington AD, Szostak JW. Invitro selection of RNA molecules that bind specific ligands. Nature 1990;346:818–822.

Epstein J, Rosenthal RW, ESS RJ. Use of gamma-(4-nitrobenzyl)pyridine as analytical reagent for ethylenimines and alkylating agents. Anal Chem 1955;27:1435–1439.

Eriksson KO. Gel filtration. In: Vijayalakshmi MA, editor. *Biochromatography—Theory and Practice*. Taylor and Francis; 2002. p 9–23.

Espinasse B, Bacchin P, Aimar P. On an experimental method to measure critical flux in ultrafiltration. Desalination 2002;146:91–96.

European Pharmacopoeia Commission. Influenza vaccine (whole virion, inactivated). In: *European Pharmacopoeia*. 7th ed. (7.5) Council of Europe; 2012a. p 795–796.

European Pharmacopoeia Commission. Influenza vaccine (whole-virion, inactivated, prepared in cell cultures). In: *European Pharmacopoeia*. 7th ed. (7.5) Council of Europe; 2012b. p 796–798.

European Pharmacopoeia Commission. Influenza vaccine (whole-virion, inactivated, prepared in cell cultures). In: *European Pharmacopoeia*. 7th ed. (7.5) Council of Europe; 2012c. p 567–568.

Fahrner RL, Iyer HV, Blank GS. The optimal flow rate and column length for maximum production rate of protein A affinity chromatography. Bioprocess Eng 1999;21:287–292.

Famulok M, Hartig JS, Mayer G. Functional aptamers and aptazymes in biotechnology, diagnostics, and therapy. Chem Rev 2007;107:3715–3743.

Ferreira GNM, Cabral JMS, Prazeres DMF. Studies on the batch adsorption of plasmid DNA onto anion-exchange chromatographic supports. Biotechnol Prog 2000;16:416–424.

Field RW, Wu D, Howell JA, Gupta BB. Critical flux concept for microfiltration fouling. J Membr Sci 1995;100:259–272.

Flaschel E, Friehs K. Improvement of downstream processing of recombinant proteins by means of genetic engineering methods. Biotechnol Adv 1993;11:31–77.

Floyd R, Sharp DG. Viral aggregation: effects of salts on aggregation of poliovirus and reovirus at low pH. Appl Environ Microbiol 1978;35:1084–1094.

Fontes LVQ, Campos GS, Beck PA, Brandao CFL, Sardi SI. Precipitation of bovine rotavirus by polyethylen glycol (PEG) and its application to produce polyclonal and monoclonal antibodies. J Virol Methods 2005;123:147–153.

Forcic D, Brgles M, Ivancic-Jelecki J, Santak M, Halassy B, Barut M, Jug R, Markusic M, Stancar A. Concentration and purification of rubella virus using monolithic chromatographic support. J Chromatogr B-Analyical 2011;879(13–14):981–986.

Forster GF, Carson E. The concentration of mumps virus. J Infect Dis 1949;85:62–65.

Fortini A, Dijkstra M, Tuinier R. Phase behaviour of charged colloidal sphere dispersions with added polymer chains. J Phys:Condens Matter 2005;17:7783–7803.

Franzreb M, Siemann-Herzberg M, Hobley TJ, Thomas ORT. Protein purification using magnetic adsorbent particles. Appl Microbiol Biotechnol 2006;70:505–516.

Frazatti-Gallina NM, Mourao-Fuches RM, Paoli RL, Silva MLN, Miyaki C, Valentini EJG, Raw I, Higashi HG. Vero-cell rabies vaccine produced using serum-free medium. Vaccine 2004;23:511–517.

Freitas SS, Santos JAL, Prazeres DMF. Optimization of isopropanol and ammonium sulfate precipitation steps in the purification of plasmid DNA. Biotechnol Prog 2006;22:1179–1186.

Freitas TRP, Gaspar LP, Caldas LA, Silva JL, Rebello MA. Inactivation of classical swine fever virus: association of hydrostatic pressure and ultraviolet irradiation. J Virol Methods 2003;108:205–211.

Frigerio NA, Hettinger TP. Protein solubility in solvent mixtures of low dielectric constant. Biochim Biophys Acta 1962;59:228.

Fukuda K, Levandowski RA, Bridges CB, Cox NJ. Inactivated influenza vaccines. In: Plotkin SA, Orenstein WA, editors. *Vaccines*. 4th ed. Phildadelphia: Saunders; 2004. p 339–370.

Gallant SR, Kundu A, Cramer SM. Modeling nonlinear elution of proteins in ion-exchange chromatography. J Chromatogr A 1995;702:125–142.

Gallop RG, Tozer BT, Stephen J, Smith H. Separation of antigens by immunological specificity —use of cellulose-linked antibodies as immunosorbents. Biochem J 1966;101:711.

Galvez GE. Specific adsorption of plant viruses by antibodies coupled to a solid matrix. Virology 1966;28:171.

Gasparini R, Amicizia D, Lai PL, Panatto D. Live attenuated influenza vaccine--a review. J Prev Med Hyg 2011;52(3):95–101.

GE Healthcare. 2007. *Microcarrier Cell Culture Handbook*. Uppsala: GE Healthcare Life Sciences. Available at: http://www.gelifesciences.com.

Genzel Y, Reichl U. Continuous cell lines as a production system for influenza vacines. Expert Rev Vaccines 2009;8(12):1681–1692.

Geeraedts F, Bungener L, Pool J, ter Veer W, Wilschut J, Huckriede A. Whole inactivated virus influenza vaccine is superior to subunit vaccine in inducing immune responses and secretion of proinflammatory cytokines by DCs. Influenza Other Resp 2008;2(2):41–51.

Gerin JL, Anderson NG. Purification of influenza virus in K-II zonal centrifuge. Nature 1969;221:1255–1256.

Gerin JL, Richter WR, Fenters JD, Holper JC. Use of zonal ultracentrifuge systems for biophysical studies of rhinoviruses. J Virol 1968;2:937–943.

Giddings JC, Mallik KL. Theory of gel filtration (permeation) chromatography. Anal Chem 1966;38:997–1000.

Giddings JC, Yang FJ, Myers MN. Flow field-flow fractionation–New method for separating, purifying, and characterizing diffusivity of viruses. Journal of Virology 1977;21(1):131–138.

Goerke A, To B, Lee A, Sagar S, Konz J. Development of a novel adenovirus purification process utilizing selective precipitation of cellular DNA. Biotechnol Bioeng 2005;91:12–21.

Gopinath SCB, Misono TS, Kawasaki K, Mizuno T, Imai M, Odagiri T, Kumar PKR. An RNA aptamer that distinguishes between closely related human influenza viruses and inhibits haemagglutinin-mediated membrane fusion. J Gen Virol 2006a;87:479–487.

Gopinath SCB, Sakamaki Y, Kawasaki K, Kumar PKR. An efficient RNA aptamer against human influenza B virus hemagglutinin. J Biochem (Tokyo) 2006b;139:837–846.

Goyal SM, Hanssen H, Gerba CP. Simple method for the concentration of influenza-virus from allantoic fluid on microporous filters. Appl Environ Microb 1980;39:500–504.

Grandgenett DP, Brackmann K, Green M. Large-scale purification of ribonucleic acid tumor viruses by use of continuous-flow density gradient centrifugation. Appl Microbiol 1973;26:452–454.

Green AA, Hughes WL. Protein fractionation on the basis of solubility in aqueous solutions of salts and organic solvents. In: *Methods in Enzymology I*. New York: Academic Press; 1955. p 67–90.

Green AP, Huang JJ, Scott MO, Kierstead TD, Beaupre I, Gao GP, Wilson JM. A new scalable method for the purification of recombinant adenovirus vectors. Hum Gene Ther 2002;13:1921–1934.

Gregersen J. *Research and Development of Vaccines and Pharmaceuticals from Biotechnology: A Guide to Effective Project Management, Patenting and Product Registra*. John Wiley & Sons; 1994.

Gresikova M, Russ G, Novak M, Sekeyova M. Purification of tick-borne encephalitis virus by affinity chromatography using monoclonal antibody. Acta Virol 1984;28:141–143.

Grove SF, Lee A, Lewis T, Stewart CM, Chen HQ, Hoover DG. Inactivation of foodborne viruses of significance by high pressure and other processes. J Food Prot 2006;69:957–968.

Gruschkau H, Mauler R, Hinz J, Hennessen W. Purification of influenza virus antigens. Sym Ser Immunol Stand 1973;20:79–84.

Grzenia DL, Carlson JO, Ranil Wickramasinghe SR. Tangential flow filtration for virus purification. J Membrane Sci 2008;321(2):373–380.

Gschwender HH, Haller W, Hofschneider PH. Large-scale preparation of viruses by steric chromatography on columns of controlled pore glass. Biochim Biophys Acta 1969;190:460–469.

Guiochon G, Shirazi DG, Felinger A. Fundamentals of preparative and nonlinear chromatography (2nd edition). Academic Press, San Diego, United Sates, 2006.

Guo YF, Cheng AC, Wang M, Zhou Y. Purification of anatid herpesvirus 1 particles by tangential-flow ultrafiltration and sucrose gradient ultracentrifugation. J Virol Methods 2009;161(1):1–6.

Guskey LE, Wolff DA. Concentration and purification of poliovirus by ultrafiltration and isopycnic centrifugation. Appl Microbiol 1972;24:13–17.

Gustincich S, Manfioletti G, Del Sal G, Schneider C, Carninci P. A fast method for high-quality genomic DNA extraction from whole human blood. BioTechniques 1991;11:298.

Hagen A, Aunins J, DePhilips P. Development, preparation, and testing of VAQTA (R), a highly purified hepatitis A vaccine. Bioprocess Eng 2000;23:439–449.

Hagen AJ, Aboud RA, DePhillips PA, Oliver CN, Orella CJ, Sitrin RD. Use of a nuclease enzyme in the purification of VAQTA(R), a hepatitis A vaccine. Biotechnol Appl Biochem 1996a;23:209–215.

Hagen AJ, Oliver CN, Sitrin RD. Optimization of poly(ethylene glycol) precipitation of hepatitis a virus used to prepare VAQTA, a highly purified inactivated vaccine. Biotechnol Prog 1996b;12:406–412.

Hagen AJ, Oliver CN, Sitrin RD. Optimization and scale-up of solvent extraction in purification of hepatitis A virus (VAQTA(R)). Biotechnol Bioeng 1997;56:83–88.

Haller W. Chromatography on glass of controlled pore size. Nature 1965a;206:693–696.

Haller W. Rearrangement kinetics of liquid-liquid immiscible microphases in alkali borosilicate melts. J Chem Phys 1965b;42:686–693.

Harmant P, Aimar P. Coagulation of colloids in a boundary layer during cross-flow filtration. Colloid Surface A 1998;138:217–230.

Hartley MR, Lord JM. Cytotoxic ribosome-inactivating lectins from plants. BBA-Proteins Proteom 2004;1701:1–14.

Hashimoto K, Adachi S, Shirai Y. Continuous desalting of proteins with a simulated moving-bed adsorber. Agric Biol Chem 1988;52:2161–2167.

Hayman MJ, Skehel JJ, Crumpton MJ. Purification of virus glycoproteins by affinity chromatography using lens culinaris phytohemagglutinin. FEBS Lett 1973;29:185–188.

Hebert TT. Precipitation of plant viruses by polyethylene glycol. Phytopathology 1963;53:362.

Heinz FX, Kunz C, Fauma H. Preparation of a highly purified vaccine against tick-borne encephalitis by continuous-flow zonal ultra-centrifugation. J Med Virol 1980;6:213–221.

Hermann T, Patel DJ. Biochemistry—Adaptive recognition by nucleic acid aptamers. Science 2000;287:820–825.

Hermia J. Constant pressure blocking filtration laws—Application to power-law non-newtonian fluids. Trans Inst Chem Eng 1982;60:183–187.

Herzer S, Beckett P, Wegman T, Moore P. Isoelectric titration curves of viral particles as an evaluation tool for ion-exchange chromatography. Life Science News (Amersham Biosciences) 2003;13.

Heyward JT, Klimas RA, Stapp MD, Obijeski JF. Rapid concentration and purification of influenza virus from allantoic fluid. Arch Virol 1977;55:107–119.

Hilfenhaus J, Köhler R, Barth R, Majer M, Mauler R. Large-scale purification of animal viruses in RK-model zonal ultracentrifuge. I. Rabies virus. J Biol Stand 1976a;4:263–271.

Hilfenhaus J, Köhler R, Behrens F. Large-scale purification of animal viruses in the RK-model zonal ultracentrifuge. II. Influenza, mumps and Newcastle disease viruses. J Biol Stand 1976b;4:273–283.

Hilfenhaus J, Köhler R, Gruschkau H. Large-scale purification of animal viruses in RK-model zonal ultracentrifuge. III. Semliki forest virus and vaccinia virus. J Biol Stand 1976c;4:285–293.

Ho CC, Zydney AL. A combined pore blockage and cake filtration model for protein fouling during microfiltration. J Colloid Interface Sci 2000;232:389–399.

Ho CC, Zydney AL. Transmembrane pressure profiles during constant flux. Microfiltration of bovine serum albumin. J Membr Sci 2002;209:363–377.

Hoare M, Narendranathan TJ, Flint JR, Heywood-Waddingtion D, Bell DJ, Dunnill P. Disruption of protein precipitates during shear in couette-flow and in pumps. Ind Eng Chem Fund 1982;21:402–406.

Hofmeister F. Zur Lehre von der Wirkung der Salze (About regularities in the protein precipitating effects of salts and the relation of these effects with the physiological behaviour of salts). Arch Exp Pathol Phar 1887;24:247–260.

Hong SP, Yoo WD, Putnak R, Srivastava AK, Eckels KH, Chung YJ, Rho HM, Kim SO. Preparation of a purified inactivated Japanese encephalitis (JE) virus vaccine in Vero cells. Biotechnol Lett 2001;23:1565–1573.

Hoopes BC, McClure WR. Studies on the selectivity of DNA precipitation by spermine. Nucleic Acids Res 1981;9:5493–5504.

Horak D, Babic M, Mackova H, Benes MJ. Preparation and properties of magnetic nano- and microsized particles for biological and environmental separations. J Sep Sci 2007;30:1751–1772.

Howard MK, Kistner O, Barret PN. Pre-clinical development of cell culture (Vero)-derived H5N1 pandemic vaccines. Biol Chem 2008;389(5):569–577.

Hu JZ, Ni YY, Drymann BA, Meng XJ, Zhang C. Purification of porcine reproductive and respiratory syndrome virus from cell culture using ultrafiltration and heparin affinity chromatography. J Chromatogr A 2010;1217(21):3489–3493.

Hulskotte EGJ, Dings MEM, Norley SG, Osterhaus ADME. Chemical inactivation of recombinant vaccinia viruses and the effects on antigenicity and immunogenicity of recombinant simian immunodeficiency virus envelope glycoproteins. Vaccine 1997;15:1839–1845.

Hutchinson N, Bingham N, Murrell N, Farid S, Hoare M. Shear stress analysis of mammalian cell suspensions for prediction of industrial centrifugation and its verification. Biotechnol Bioeng 2006;95:483–491.

Igarashi A, Fukuoka T, Sasao F, Surimarut S, Fukai K. Purification of Japanese encephalitis virus grown in BHK21 and Singh's Aedes Albopictus cells by polyethylene glycol precipitation. Biken J 1973;16:67–73.

Iskander J, Broder K. Monitoring the safety of annual and pandemic influenza vacines: lessons from the US experience. Expert Rev Vaccines 2008;7(1):75–82.

Iyer G, Ramaswamy S, Asher D, Mehta U, Leahy A, Chung F, Cheng KS. Reduced surface area chromatography for flow-through purification of viruses and virus like particles. J Chromatogra A 2011;1218(26):3973–3981.

Jain M, Paranandi MR, Roush D, Goklen K, Kelly WJ. Using CFD to understand how flow patterns affect retention of cell-sized particles in a tubular bowl centrifuge. Ind Eng Chem Res 2005;44:7876–7884.

James W. Aptamers in the virologists' toolkit. J Gen Virol 2007;88:351–364.

Janca J. (ed). 1983. *Steric Exclusion Liquid Chromatography of Polymers*. New York: Marcel Dekker Ltd.

Jansons J, Bucens MR. Virus detection in water by ultrafiltration. Water Res 1986;20:1603–1606.

Jendrisak J. The use of polyethyleneimine in protein purification. In: Burgess R, editor. *Protein Purification: Micro to Macro*. New York: Alan R. Liss; 1987. p 75–97.

Jeon SH, Kayhan B, Ben-Yedidia T, Arnon R. A DNA aptamer prevents influenza infection by blocking the receptor binding region of the viral hemagglutinin. J Biol Chem 2004;279:48410–48419.

Jonas E. Salk, John B. Gori. A review of theoretical, experimental, and practical considerations in the use of formaldehyde for the inactivation of poliovirus. Annals of the New York Academy of Sciences 1960;83:609–637.

Josefsberg JO, Buckland B. Vaccine process technology. Biotechnol Bioeng 2012;109(6):1443–1460.

Kalbfuss B, Genzel Y, Wolff M, Zimmermann A, Morenweiser R, Reichl U. Harvesting and concentration of human influenza A virus produced in serum-free mammalian cell culture for the production of vaccines. Biotechnol Bioeng 2007a;97:73–85.

Kalbfuss B, Wolff M, Geisler L, Tappe A, Wickramasinghe R, Thom V, Reichl U. Direct capture of influenza A virus from cell culture supernatant with Sartobind anion-exchange membrane adsorbers. J Membr Sci 2007b;299:251–260.

Kalbfuss B, Wolff M, Morenweiser R, Reichl U. Purification of cell culture-derived human influenza a virus by size-exclusion and anion-exchange chromatography. Biotechnol Bioeng 2007c;96:932–944.

Kalbfuss-Zimmermann B, Seidel-Morgenstern A, Reichl U. Size-exclusion chromatography as a linear transfer system—exemplified for the purification of human influenza virus. J Chromatogr B 2008;873(1):102–112.

Kaludov N, Handelman B, Chiorini JA. Scalable purification of adeno-associated virus type 2, 4, or 5 using ion-exchange chromatography. Hum Gene Ther 2002;13:1235–1243.

Kanarek AD, Tribe MGW. Concentration of certain myxoviruses with polyethylene glycol. Nature 1967;214:927.

Karger A, Bettin B, Granzow H, Mettenleiter TC. Simple and rapid purification of alphaherpesviruses by chromatography on a cation exchange membrane. J Virol Methods 1998;70:219–224.

Käsermann F, Wyss K, Kempf C. Virus inactivation and protein modifications by ethyleneimines. Antiviral Res 2001;52:33–41.

Kato T, Tokuya T, Takahashi A. Comparison of poly(ethylene oxide), pullulan and dextran as polymer standards in aqueous gel chromatography. J Chromatogr 1983;256:61–69.

Keitel WA, Atmar RL. Preparing for a possible pandemic: influenza A/H5N1 vaccine development. Curr Opin Pharmacol 2007;7:484–490.

Kemp G. Process development—when to start, where to stop. In: Subramanian G, editor. *Bioseparation and Bioprocessing: A Handbook.* 2nd ed. Wiley-VCH; 2007. p 798.

Kempken R, Preissmann A, Berthold W. Assessment of a disc stack centrifuge for use in mammalian cell separation. Biotechnol Bioeng 1995;46:132–138.

Kim HS, Chung YJ, Jeon YJ, Lee SH. Large-scale culture of hepatitis A virus in human diploid MRC-5 cells and partial purification of the viral antigen for use as a vaccine. J Microbiol Biotechnol 1999;9:386–392.

Kim JS, Akeprathumchai S, Wickramasinghe SR. Flocculation to enhance microfiltration. J Membr Sci 2001;182:161–172.

King AM, Underwood BO, McCahon D, Newman JW, Brown F. Biochemical identification of viruses causing the 1981 outbreaks of foot and mouth disease in the UK. Nature 1981;293:479–480.

King DJ. Evaluation of different methods of inactivation of Newcastle disease virus and avian influenza virus in egg fluids and serum. Avian Dis 1991;35:505–514.

Kistner O, Barrett PN, Mundt W, Reiter M, Schober-Bendixen S, Dorner F. Development of a mammalian cell (Vero) derived candidate influenza virus vaccine. Vaccine 1998;16:960–968.

Klembala M, Szekacs I. Further simplification of purification procdure of influenza virus on barium sulphate. Nature 1965;205:828.

Knipe DM, Howley PM, editors. *Fields Virology.* 4th ed. Philadelphia: Lippincott Williams & Wilkins; 2001.

Knudsen HL, Fahrner RL, Xu Y, Norling LA, Blank GS. Membrane ion-exchange chromatography for process-scale antibody purification. J Chromatogr A 2001;907:145–154.

Koerber JT, Jang JH, Yu JH, Kane RS, Schaffer DV. Engineering adeno-associated virus for one-step purification via immobilized metal affinity chromatography. Hum Gene Ther 2007;18:367–378.

Konz JO, Lee AL, Lewis JA, Sagar SL. Development of a purification process for adenovirus: Controlling virus aggregation to improve the clearance of host cell DNA. Biotechnol Prog 2005;21:466–472.

Kramberger P, Peterka M, Boben J, Ravnikar M, Strancar A. Short monolithic columns—a breakthrough in purification and fast quantification of tomato mosaic virus. J Chromatogr A 2007;1144:143–149.

Kristiansen T, Sparrman M, Heller L. Towards a subunit influenza vaccine prepared by affinity chromatography on immobilized lectin. J Biosci 1983;5:149–155.

Kröber T, Knöchlein A, Eisold K, Kalbfuss–Zimmermann B, Reichl U. DNA Depletion by precipitation in the purification of cell culture-derived influenza vaccines. Chemical Engineering & Technology 2010;33(6):941–959.

Kroner KH, Kular MR. Extraction of enzymes in aqueous 2-phase systems. Process Biochem 1978;13:7.

Kwon DY, Vigneswaran S, Fane AG, Ben AR. Experimental determination of critical flux in cross-flow microfiltration. Sep Purif Technol 2000;19:169–181.

Labrou N, Clonis YD. The affinity technology in downstream processing. J Biotechnol 1994;36:95–119.

Ladipo JL, Zoeten GA. Utilization of glutaraldehyde cross-linked antibodies in purification of a plant virus. Virology 1971;46:567.

Ladiwala A, Rege K, Breneman CM, Cramer SM. A priori prediction of adsorption isotherm parameters and chromatographic behavior in ion-exchange chromatography. Proceedings of the National Academy of Sciences of America 2005;102(33):11710–11715.

RA, Krug RM. Orthomyxoviridae: the viruses and their replication. In: Knipe DM, Howley PM, editors. *Fields Virology*. 4th ed. Philadelphia: Lippincott Williams & Wilkins; 2001. p 1487–1531.

Lamm O. Die Differentialgleichung der Ultrazentrifugierung. Ark Mat. Astr Fys 1929; 21B:1–4.

Larghi OP, Nebel AE. Rabies virus inactivation by binary ethylenimine: new method for inactivated vaccine production. J Clin Microbiol 1980;11:120–122.

Lauffer MA, Carnelly HL. Thermal destruction of influenza a virus hemagglutinin. 1. The kinetic process. Arch Biochem 1945;8:265–274.

Lauffer MA, Wheatley M. Destruction of influenza A virus infectivity by formaldehyde. Arch Biochem 1949;23:262–270.

Leberman R. Isolation of plant viruses by means of simple coacervates. Virology 1966;30:341.

Lebowitz J, Lewis MS, Schuck P. Modern analytical ultracentrifugation in protein science: a tutorial review. Protein Sci 2002;11:2067–2079.

Lekkerkerker HN, Poon WC, Pusey PN. Phase-behavior of colloid plus polymer mixtures. Europhys Lett 1992;20:559–564.

Lewis GD, Metcalf TG. Polyethylene-glycol precipitation for recovery of pathogenic viruses including hepatitis A virus and human rotavirus from oyster, water and sediment samples. Appl Environ Microbiol 1988;54:1983–1988.

Li H, Fane AG, Coster HGL, Vigneswaran S. Direct observation of particle deposition on the membrane surface during crossflow microfiltration. J Membr Sci 1998a;149:83–97.

Li ZG, Gu YS, Gu TY. Mathematical modeling and scale-up of size-exclusion chromatography. Biochem Eng J 1998b;2:145–155.

Liebhaber H, Gross PA. Structural proteins of rubella virus. Virology 1972;47:684.

Lis JT. Fractionation of DNA fragments by polyethylene glycol induced precipitation. In: Grossman L, Moldave K, editors. *Nucleic Acids Part I*. New York: Academic Press; 1980. p 347–353.

Liu J, Thorp SC. Cell surface heparan sulfate and its roles in assisting viral infectious. Med Res Rev 2002;22:1–25.

Loa CC, Lin TL, Wu CC, Bryan TA, Thacker HL, Hooper T, Schrader D. Purification of turkey coronavirus by Sephacryl size-exclusion chromatography. J Virol Methods 2002;104:187–194.

Loewinger M, Katz E. Ultraviolet-irradiated vaccinia virus recombinants, exposing HIV-envelope on their outer membrane, induce antibodies against this antigen in rabbits. Viral Immunol 2002;15:473–479.

LoGrippo GA. Partial purification of viruses with an anion-exchange resin. Proc Soc Exp Biol Med 1950;74:208–211.

Lubansky AS, Yeow YL, Leong YK, Wickramasinghe SR, Han BB. A general method of computing the derivative of experimental data. AIChE J 2006;52:323–332.

Lucas D, Rabiller-Baudry M, Michel F, Chaufer B. Role of the physico-chemical environment on ultrafiltration of lysozyme with modified inorganic membrane. Colloid Surface A 1998;136:109–122.

Lycke E. Studies of the inactivation of poliomyelitis virus by formaldehyde. Arch Ges.Virusf 1958;8:267–284.

Maiorella B, Dorin G, Carion A, Harano D. Cross-flow microfiltration of animal cells. Biotechnol Bioeng 1991;37:121–126.

Manning GS. Molecular theory of polyelectrolyte solutions with applications to electrostatic properties of polynucleotides. Q Rev Biophys 1978;11:179–246.

Maranga L, Rueda P, Antonis AFG, Vela C, Langeveld JPM, Casal JI, Carrondo MJT. Large scale production and downstream processing of a recombinant porcine parvovirus vaccine. Appl Microbiol Biotechnol 2002;59:45–50.

Maybury JP, Hoare M, Dunnill P. The use of laboratory centrifugation studies to predict performance of industrial machines: Studies of shear-insensitive and shear-sensitive materials. Biotechnol Bioeng 2000;67:265–273.

Maybury JP, Mannweiler K, Titchener-Hooker NJ, Hoare M, Dunnill P. The performance of a scaled down industrial disc stack centrifuge with a reduced feed material requirement. Bioprocess Eng 1998;18:191–199.

Mazzone HM. *CRC Handbook of Viruses: Mass-Molecular Weight Values and Related Properties*. Boston: CRC Press; 1998.

McAleer WJ, Hurni W, Wasmuth E, Hilleman MR. High-resolution flow zonal centrifuge system. Biotechnol Bioeng 1979;21:317–321.

McCombs RM, Rawls WE. Density gradient centrifugation of rubella virus. J Virol 1968;2:409–414.

Melander W, Horvath C. Salt effects on hydrophobic interactions in precipitation and chromatography of proteins—interpretation of lyotropic series. Arch Biochem Biophys 1977;183:200–215.

Melnick J. Virus inactivation: Lessons from the past. Dev Biol Standards 1991;75:29–36.

Merck Patent GmbH. Continuous method for separating substances according to molecular size. International patent WO 00/37156. 2000.

Miller GL, Lauffer MA, Stanley WM. Electrophoretic studies on PR8 influenza virus. J Exp Med 1944;80:549–559.

Miller HK, Schlesinger RW. Differentiation and purification of influenza virus by adsorption on aluminum phosphate. J Immunol 1955;75:155–160.

Mizutani H. A simple method for purification of influenza virus. Nature 1963;198:109–110.

Mizutani T. Adsorption chromatography of biopolymers on porous glass. J Liq Chromatogr 1985;8:925–983.

Mollerup JM. The thermodynamic principles of ligand binding in chromatography and biology. J Biotechnol 2007;132:187–195.

Montagnon BJ, Fanget B, Vincent-Falquet JC. Industrial-scale production of inactivated poliovirus vaccine prepared by culture of vero cells on microcarrier. Rev Infect Dis 1984;6:S341–S344.

Montagnon BJ, Fanget BJ. Process for the large-scale production of a vaccine against poliomyelitis and the resulting vaccine. US patent No. 4525349. 1985.

Moore D, Dowhan D. Manipulation of DNA. In: Ausubel FM, Brent R, Kingston RE, Moore DD, Seidman JG, Smith JA, Struhl K, editors. *Current Protocols in Molecular Biology*. Wiley; 2007. p 59.

Morenweiser R. Downstream processing of viral vectors and vaccines. Gene Ther 2005;12:S103–S110.

Morgeaux S, Tordo N, Gontier C, Perrin P. Beta-propiolactone treatment impairs the biological activity of residual DNA from BHK-21 cells infected with rabies virus. Vaccine 1993;11:82–90.

Mori S, Barth HG. *Size Exclusion Chromatography*. Berlin: Springer; 1999.

Moyer AW, Sharpless GR, Davies MC, Winfield K, Cox HR. Methanol precipitation of influenza virus. Science 1950;112:459–460.

Muller RH, Rose HM. Concentration of influenza virus (PR-8 strain) by a cation-exchange resin. Proc Soc Exp Biol Med 1952;80:27–29.

Murphy JC, Wibbenmeyer JA, Fox GE, Willson RC. Purification of plasmid DNA using selective precipitation by compaction agents—A scaleable method for the liquid-phase separation of plasmid DNA from RNA. Nat Biotechnol 1999;17:822–823.

Nagano H, Yagyu K, Ohta S. Purification of infectious bronchitis coronavirus by sephacryl S-1000 gel chromatography. Vet Microbiol 1989;21:115–123.

Nathanson N, Langmuir AD. The Cutter incident: Polyomyelitis following formaldehyde-inactivated poliovirus vaccination in the United States during the spring of 1955. I. Background. American Journal of Hygiene 1963;78(1):16–28.

Nayak DP, Lehmann S, Reichl U. Downstream processing of MDCK cell-derived equine influenza virus. J Chromatogr B 2005;823:75–81.

Neurath AR, Wiktor TJ, Koprowski H. Density gradient centrifugation studies on rabies virus. J Bacteriol 1966;92:102–106.

Neumann G, Kawaoka Y. Reverse genetics of influenza virus. Virology 2001;287(2):243–250.

Nicoletti VG, Condorelli DF. Optimized PEG method for rapid plasmid DNA purification—high yield from midi-prep. BioTechniques 1993;14:532.

Nitsche A, Kurth A, Dunkhorst A, Pänke O, Sielaff H, Junge W, Muth D, Scheller F, Stöcklein W. One-step selection of Vaccinia virus-binding DNA aptamers by MonoLEX. BMC Biotechnol 2007;7:48.

Njayou M, Quash G. Purification of measles virus by affinity chromatography and by ultracentrifugation—a comparative study. J Virol Methods 1991;32:67–77.

Offit PA. The Cutter incident, 50 years later. New England Journal of Medicine 2005;352(14):1411–1412.

O'Keeffe RS, Johnston MD, Slater NKH. The affinity adsorptive recovery of an infectious herpes simplex virus vaccine. Biotechnol Bioeng 1999;62:537–545.

O'Neil PF, Balkovic ES. Virus harvesting and affinity-based liquid chromatography—a method for virus concentration and purification. Biotechnology 1993;11:173–178.

O'Riordan CR, Lachapelle AL, Vincent KA, Wadsworth SC. Scaleable chromatographic purification process for recombinant adeno-associated virus (rAAV). J Gene Med 2000;2:444–454.

Okuda K, Itoh K, Miyake K, Morita M, Ogonuki M, Matrui S. Purification of Japanese encephalitis-virus vaccine by zonal centrifugation. J Clin Microbiol 1975;1:96–101.

Opitz L, Lehmann S, Zimmermann A, Reichl U, Wolff MW. Impact of adsorbents selection on capture efficiency of cell culture derived human influenza viruses. J Biotechnol 2007a;131:309–317.

Opitz L, Salaklang J, Buttner H, Reichl U, Wolff MW. Lectin-affinity chromatography for downstream processing of MDCK cell culture derived human influenza A viruses. Vaccine 2007b;25:939–947.

Ohtaki N, Takahashi H, Kaneko K, Gomi Y, Ishikawa T, Higashi Y, Todokoro M, Kurata T, Sata T, Kojima A. Purification and concentration of non-infectious West Nile virus-like particles and infectious virions using a pseudo-affinity cellufine sulfate column. J Virol Methods 2011;174(1–2):131–135.

Ozaki Y, Diwan AR, Takizawa M, Melnick JL. Chromatography of poliovirus on calcium phosphate and its application to identification of vaccine progeny strains. J Bacteriol 1965;89:603.

Palacio L, Ho CC, Zydney AL. Application of a pore-blockage—cake-filtration model to protein fouling during microfiltration. Biotechnol Bioeng 2002;79:260–270.

Paredes G, Makart S, Stadler J, Mazzotti M. Simulated moving bed operation for size exclusion plasmid purification. Chem Eng Technol 2005;28:1335–1345.

Paul RW, Morris D, Hess BW, Dunn J, Overell RW. Increased viral titer through concentration of viral harvests from retroviral packaging lines. Hum Gene Ther 1993;4:609–615.

Peixoto C, Ferreira TB, Carrondo MJT, Cruz PE, Alves PM. Purification of adenoviral vectors using expanded bed chromatography. J Virol Methods 2006;132:121–126.

Peixoto C, Sousa MFQ, Silva AC, Carrondo MJT, Alves PM. Downstream processing of triple layered rotavirus like particles. J Biotechnol 2007;127:452–461.

Pelta J, Livolant F, Sikorav JL. DNA aggregation induced by polyamines and cobalthexamine. J Biol Chem 1996;271:5656–5662.

Pepper DS. A chromatographic procedure for the purification of influenza virus. J Gen Virol 1967;1:49–55.

Perardi TE, Leffler RA, Anderson NG. K-series centrifuges. II. Performance of K-2 rotor. Anal Biochem 1969;32:495–511.

Perrin P, Morgeaux S. Inactivation of DNA by beta-propiolactone. Biologicals 1995;23:207–211.

Peterka M, Strancar A, Banjac M, Kramberger P, Maurer E, Muster T. Method for influenza virus purification. International patent No. WO/2008/006780 A1. 2008.

Podgornik A, Jancar J, Mihelic I, Barut M, Strancar A. . Acta Chim Slov 2010;57(1):1–8.

Pollard M, Connolly J, Fromm S. The precipitating effect of methanol on viruses. Proc Soc Exp Biol Med 1949;71:290–293.

Polson A. Purification and aggregation of influenza virus by precipitation with polyethylene-glycol. Prep Biochem 1974;4:435–456.

Polson A. A theory for the displacement of proteins and viruses with polyethylene-glycol (reprinted from Preparative Biochemistry, Vol. 7, Pg. 129, 1977). Prep Biochem 1993;23:31–50.

Porath J, Flodin P. Gel filtration: a method for desalting and group separation. Nature 1959;183:1657–1659.

Porschke D. Dynamics of DNA condensation. Biochemistry 1984;23:4821–4828.

Porter MC. Concentration polarization with membrane ultrafiltration. Ind Eng Chem Prod RD 1972;11:234.

Potschka M. Size exclusion chromatography of DNA and viruses: properties of spherical and asymmetric molecules in porous networks. Macromolecules 1991;24:5023–5039.

Price CA. *Centrifugation in Density Gradients*. New York: Academic Press; 1982.

Purchas DB, Sutherland K. *Handbook of Filter Media*. 2nd ed. Elsevier Advanced Technology; 2002.

Pyke AT, Phillips DA, Chuan TF, Smith GA. Sucrose density gradient centrifugation and cross-flow filtration methods for the production of arbovirus antigens inactivated by binary ethylenimine. BMC Microbiol 2004;4:3.

Rabenstein DL. Heparin and heparan sulfate: structure and function. Nat Prod Rep 2002;19:312–331.

Rabiller-Baudry M, Chaufer B, Aimar P, Bariou B, Lucas D. Application of a convection-diffusion-electrophoretic migration model to ultrafiltration of lysozyme at different pH values and ionic strengths. J Membr Sci 2000;179:163–174.

Rabiller-Baudry M, Chaufer B. Small molecular ion adsorption on proteins and DNAs revealed by separation techniques. J Chromatogr B 2003;797:331–345.

Race E, Stein CA, Wigg MD, Baksh A, Addawe M, Frezza P, Oxford JS. A multistep procedure for the chemical inactivation of human immunodeficiency virus for use as an experimental vaccine. Vaccine 1995;13:1567–1575.

Ramqvist T, Andreasson K, Dalianis T. Vaccination, immune and gene therapy based on virus-like particles against viral infections and cancer. Expert Opin Biol Ther 2007;7:997–1007.

Raspaud E, Chaperon I, Leforestier A, Livolant F. Spermine-induced aggregation of DNA, nucleosome, and chromatin. Biophys J 1999;77:1547–1555.

Raspaud E, de la Cruz MO, Sikorav JL, Livolant F. Precipitation of DNA by polyamines: a polyelectrolyte behavior. Biophys J 1998;74:381–393.

Reimer CB, Baker RS, Newlin TE, Havens ML, van Frank RM, Storvick WO, Miller RP. Comparison of techniques for influenza virus purification. J Bacteriol 1966a;92:1271–1272.

Reimer CB, Baker RS, Newlin TE, Havens ML. Influenza virus purification with the zonal ultracentrifuge. Science 1966b;152:1379–1381.

Reimer CB, Baker RS, van Frank RM, Newlin TE, Cline GB, Anderson NG. Purification of large quantities of influenza virus by density gradient centrifugation. J Virol 1967;1:1207–1216.

Reinsch CH. Smoothing by spline functions. Numer Math 1967;10:177.

Roberts JJ, Warwick GP. Reaction of beta-propiolactone with guanosine, deoxyguanylic acid and RNA. Biochem Pharmacol 1963;12:1441.

Rodrigues T, Carvalho A, Carmo M, Carrondo MJT, Alves PM, Cruz PE. Scaleable purification process for gene therapy retroviral vectors. J Gene Med 2007;9:233–243.

Rodrigues T, Carvalho A, Roldao A, Carrondo MJT, Alves PM, Cruz PE. Screening anion-exchange chromatographic matrices for isolation of onco-retroviral vectors. J Chromatogr B 2006;837:59–68.

Round JJ, Liptak RA, McGregor WC. Continuous-flow ultracentrifugation in preparative biochemistry. Ann N Y Acad Sci 1981;369:265–274.

Rudin A, Hoegy HL. Universal calibration in GPC. J Polym Sci 1972;A1(10):217–235.

Rueda P, Fominaya J, Langeveld JPM, Bruschke C, Vela C, Casal JI. Effect of different baculovirus inactivation procedures on the integrity and immunogenicity of porcine parvovirus-like particles. Vaccine 2000;19:726–734.

Sakata M, Nakayama M, Fujisaki T, Morimura S, Kunitake M, Hirayama C. Chromatographic removal of host cell DNA from cellular products using columns packed with cationic copolymer beads. Chromatographia 2005;62:465–470.

Salk JE. The immunzing effect of calcium phosphate adsorbed influenza virus. Science 1945;101:122–124.

Salt DE, Hay S, Thomas OR, Hoare M, Dunnill P. Selective flocculation of cellular contaminants from soluble proteins using polyethyleneimine— a study of several organisms and polymer molecular-weights. Enzyme Microb Technol 1995;17:107–113.

Sartory WK, Halsall HB, Breillat JP. Simulation of gradient and band propagation in centrifuge. Biophys Chem 1976;5:107–135.

Saxena A, Tripathi BP, Kumar M, Shahi VK. Membrane-based techniques for the separation and purification of proteins: an overview. Adv Colloid Interface Sci 2009;145(1–2):1–22.

Schnabel R, Langer P. Controlled-pore glass as a stationary phase in chromatography. J Chromatogr 1991;544:137–146.

Scholtissek C. Stability of infectious influenza A viruses at low pH and at elevated temperature. Vaccine 1985;3:215–218.

Schu P, Mitra G. Ultrafiltration membranes in the vaccine industry. In: Wang WK, editor. *Membrane Separations in Biotechnology*. New York: Marcel Dekker, Inc.; 2001. p 225–241.

Schubert PF, Finn RK. Alcohol precipitation of proteins—The relationship of denaturation and precipitation for catalase. Biotechnol Bioeng 1981;23:2569–2590.

Schwarzer J, Rapp E, Reichl U. N-glycan analysis by capillary gel electrophoresis—profiling influenza A virus hemagglutinin N-Glycosylation during vaccine production. Electrophoresis 2008;29(20):4203–4214.

Schwarzer J, Rapp E, Hennig R, Genzel Y, Jordan I, Sandig V, Reichl U. Glycan analysis in cell culture-based influenza vaccine production: influence of host cell line and virus strain on the glycosylation pattern of viral hemagglutinin. Vaccine 2009;27:4325–4336.

Schwinge J, Neal PR, Wiley DE, Fletcher DF, Fane AG. Spiral wound modules and spacers—review and analysis. J Membr Sci 2004;242:129–153.

Segura MD, Kamen A, Garnier A. Downstream processing of oncoretroviral and lentiviral gene therapy vectors. Biotechnol Adv 2006;24:321–337.

Segura MD, Kamen A, Lavoie MC, Garnier A. Exploiting heparin-binding properties of MoMLV-based retroviral vectors for affinity chromatography. J Chromatogr B 2007;846:124–131.

Segura MD, Kamen A, Trudel P, Garnier A. A novel purification strategy for retrovirus gene therapy vectors using heparin affinity chromatography. Biotechnol Bioeng 2005;90:391–404.

Shapiro JT, Leng M, Felsenfeld G. Deoxyribonucleic acid-polylysine complexes—structure and nucleotide specificity. Biochemistry 1969;8:3219.

Sheffield FW, Smith W, Belyavin G. Purification of influenza virus by red-cell adsorption and elution. Br J Exp Pathol 1954;35:214–222.

Shukla AA, Yigzaw Y. Modes of preparative chromatography. In: Shukla AA, Etzel MR, Gadam S, editors. *Process scale Bioseparations for the Biopharmaceutical Industry*. Boca Raton: CRC Press; 2007. p 179–225.

Simonet J, Gantzer C. Inactivation of poliovirus 1 and F-specific RNA phages and degradation of their genomes by UV irradiation at 254 nanometers. Appl Environ Microbiol 2006;72:7671–7677.

Singhvi R, Schorr C, OHara C, Xie LZ, Wang DIC. Clarification of animal cell culture process fluids using depth microfiltration. Biopharm Technol Bus 1996;9:35–41.

Smith RH, Ding CT, Kotin RM. Serum-free production and column purification of adeno-associated virus type 5. J Virol Methods 2003;114:115–124.

Smrekar F, Ciringer M, Peterka M, Podgornik A, Strancar S. Purification and concentration of bacteriophage T4 using Q1 monolithic chromatographic supports. J Chromatogr B 2007;861:177–180.

Sokol F, Kuwert E, Wiktor TJ, Hummeler K, Koprowski H. Purification of rabies virus grown in tissue culture. J Virol 1968;2:836.

Sokolov NN, Zhukova TY, Heinman VY, Alexandrova GI, Smorodintsev AA. Purification and concentration of influenza-virus. I. Preservation of infectivity of influenza-virus during purification and concentration by gradient centrifugation. Arch Ges Virusforsch 1971;35:356–363.

Song BJ, Katial RK. Update on side effects from common vaccines. Curr Allergy Asthma Rep 2004;4:447–53.

Sonnenfeld A, Thömmes J. Expanded bed adsorption for capture from crude solution. In: Shukla AA, Etzel MR, Gadam S, editors. *Process Scale Bioseparations for the Biopharmaceutical Industry*. Boca Raton: CRC Press; 2007. p 59–81.

Specht R, Han BB, Wickramasinghe SR, Carlson JO, Czermak P, Wolf A, Reif OW. Densonucleosis virus purification by ion exchange membranes. Biotechnol Bioeng 2004;88:465–473.

Srivastava AK, Putnak JR, Lee SH, Hong SP, Moon SB, Barvir DA, Zhao B. A purified inactivated Japanese encephalitis virus vaccine made in vero cells. Vaccine 2001;19:4557–4565.

Stanley WM. The precipitation of purified concentrated influenza virus and vaccine on calcium phosphate. Science 1945;101:332–335.

Stegeman G, Kraak JC, Poppe H, Tijssen R. Hydrodynamic chromatography of polymers in packed columns. J Chromatogr A 1993a;657:283–303.

Stegeman G, Kraak JC, Poppe H. Dispersion in packed-column hydrodynamic chromatography. J Chromatogr 1993b;634:149–159.

Stephen J, Gallop RG, Smith H. Separation of antigens by immunological specificity—use of disulphide-linked antibodies as immunosorbents. Biochem J 1966;101:717.

Storhas W. *Bioreaktoren und periphere Einrichtungen*. Braunschweig/Wiesbaden: Vieweg; 1994.

Sweet C, Stephen J, Smith H. Purification of influenza viruses using disulphide-linked immunosorbents derived from rabbit antibody. Immunochemistry 1974a;11:295–304.

Sweet C, Stephen J, Smith H. The behavior of antigenically related influenza-viruses of differing virulence on disulfide-linked immunosorbents. Immunochemistry 1974b;11:823–826.

Tang JX, Wong SE, Tran PT, Janmey PA. Counterion induced bundle formation of rodlike polyelectrolytes. Ber Bunsen Phys Chem 1996;100:796–806.

Thomas DN, Judd SJ, Fawcett N. Flocculation modelling: a review. Water Res 1999;33:1579–1592.

Timm EA, McLean IW, Kupsky CH, Hook AE. The nature of the formalin inactivation of poliomyelitis virus. J Immunol 1956;77:444–452.

Tomita S, Asahara T. Study on the purification of influenza virus vaccine—filtration of formalin-inactivated influenza virus with Sepharose 6B. Kitasato Arch Exp Med 1971;44:185–196.

Toplin I, Sottong P. Large-volume purification of tumor viruses by use of zonal centrifuges. Appl Microbiol 1972;23:1010–1014.

Transfiguracion J, Jaalouk DE, Ghani K, Galipeau J, Kamen A. Size-exclusion chromatography purification of high-titer vesicular stomatitis virus G glycoprotein-pseudotyped retrovectors for cell and gene therapy applications. Hum Gene Ther 2003;14:1139–1153.

Transfiguracion J, Jorio H, Meghrous J, Jacob D, Kamen A. High yield purification of functional baculovirus vectors by size exclusion chromatography. J Virol Methods 2007;142:21–28.

Trettin DR, Doshi MR. Limiting flux in ultrafiltration of macromolecular solutions. Chem Eng Commun 1980;4:507–522.

Trilisky EI, Lenhoff AM. Sorption processes in ion-exchange chromatography of viruses. J Chromatogr A 2007;1142:2–12.

Trilisky EI, Lenhoff AM. Flow-dependent entrapment of large bioparticles in porous process media. Biotechnol Bioeng 2009;104(1):127–133.

Trudel M, Marchessault F, Payment P. Purification of infectious rubella virus by gel filtration on Sepharose 2B compared to gradient centrifugation in sucrose, sodium metrizoate and metrizamide. J Virol Methods 1981;2:141–148.

Trudel M, Payment P. Concentration and purification of rubella-virus hemagglutinin by hollow fiber ultrafiltration and sucrose density centrifugation. Can J Microbiol 1980;26:1334–1339.

Trudel M, Trepanier P, Payment P. Concentration and analysis of labile viruses by hollow fiber ultrafiltration and ultracentrifugation. Process Biochem 1983;18:2–9.

Tsvetkova EA, Nepomnyaschaya NM. Principles of selective inactivation of a viral genome—comparative kinetic study of modification of the viral RNA and model protein with oligoaziridines. Biochemistry Moscow 2001;66:875–884.

Tuerk C, Gold L. Systematic evolution of ligands by exponential enrichment—RNA ligands to bacteriophage T4 DNA polymerase. Science 1990;249:505–510.

Turkova J. Affinity chromatography. In: Vijayalakshmi MA, editor. *Biochromatography—Theory and Practice*. London: Taylor and Francis; 2002. p 142–224.

Vajda BP. Concentration and purification of viruses and bacteriophages with polyethylene-glycol. Folia Microbiol (Praha) 1978;23:88–96.

Valeri A, Gazzei G, Botti R, Pellegrini V, Corradeschi A, Soldateschi D. One-day purification of influenza A and B vaccines using molecular filtration and other physical methods. Microbiologica 1981;4:403–412.

Valeri A, Gazzei G, Morandi M, Pende B, Neri P. Large-scale purification of inactivated influenza vaccine using membrane molecular filtration. Experientia 1977;33:1402–1403.

van Damme EJ, Peumans WJ, Pusztai A, Bardocz S. *Handbook of Plant Lectins: Properties and Biomedical Applications*. West Sussex: John Wiley & Sons; 1998.

van Reis R, Leonard LC, HSU CC, Builder SE. Industrial-scale harvest of proteins from mammalian cell culture by tangential flow filtration. Biotechnol Bioeng 1991;38:413–422.

van Reis R, Zydney A. Bioprocess membrane technology. J Membr Sci 2007;297:16–50.

Vasconcelos IM, Oliveira JTA. Antinutritional properties of plant lectins. Toxicon 2004;44:385–403.

Vicente T, Sousa MF, Peixoto C, Mota JP, Alvesa PM, Carrondo MJ. Anion exchange membrane chromatography for purification of rotavirus-like particles. J Membr Sci 2008;311(1–2):270–283.

Vicente T, Peixoto C, Alves PM, Carrondo MJT. Modeling electrostatic interactions of baculovirus vectors for ion-exchange process development. J Chromatogr A 2010a;1217(24):3754–3764.

Vicente T, Mota JPB, Peixoto C, Alves PM, Carrondo MJT. Modeling protein binding and elution over a chromatographic surface probed by surface plasmon resonance. J Chromatogr A 2010b;1217(13):2032–2041.

Vicente T, Roldao A, Peixoto C, Carrondo MJT, Alves PM. Large-scale production and purification of VLP-based vaccines. J Invertebr Pathol 2011a;107:S42–S48.

Vicente T, Faber R, Alves PM, Carrondo MJT, Mota JPB. Impact of ligand density on the optimization of ion-exchange membrane chromatography for viral vector purification. Biotechnol Bioeng 2011b;108(6):1347–1359.

Vicente T, Mota JPB, Peixoto C, Alves PM, Carrondo MJT. Rational design and optimization of downstream processes of virus particles for biopharmaceutical applications: current advances. Biotechnol Adv 2011c;29(6):869–878.

Volkening JD, Spatz SJ. Purification of DNA from the cell-associated herpesvirus Marek's disease for 454 pyrosequencing using micrococcal nuclease digestion and polyethylene glycol precipitation. Journal of Virological Methods 2009;157(1):55–61.

Vollhardt KP, Schore NE. 1999a. *Heterocyclen*. In: *Organische Chemie*. Wiley-VCH.

Vollhardt KP, Schore NE. 1999b. *Reaktionen von oxacyclopropanen*. In: *Organische Chemie*. Wiley-VCH.

Wahlund PO, Gustavsson PE, Izumrudov VA, Larsson PO, Galaev IY. Precipitation by polycation as capture step in purification of plasmid DNA from a clarified lysate. Biotechnol Bioeng 2004;87:675–684.

Walin L, Tuma R, Thomas GJ, Bamford DH. Purification of viruses and macromolecular assemblies for structural investigations using a novel ion-exchange method. Virology 1994;201:1–7.

Wang CH, Tschen SY, Flehmig B. Antigenicity of hepatitis A virus after ultra-violet inactivation. Vaccine 1995;13:835–840.

Wang J, Jiang H, Liu FY. In vitro selection of novel RNA ligands that bind human cytomegalovirus and block viral infection. RNA 2000;6:571–583.

Waugh DS. Making the most of affinity tags. Trends Biotechnol 2005;23:316–320.

Wei Z, Mcevoy M, Razinkov V, Polozova A, Li E, Casas–Finet J, Tous GI, Balu P, Pan AA, Mehta H, Schenerman MA. Biophysical characterization of influenza virus subpopulations using field flow fractionation and multiangle light scattering: Correlation of particle counts, size distribution and infectivity. Journal of Virological Methods 2007;144(1–2):122–132.

WHO Technical Report Series. Recommendations for the production and control of influenza vaccine (inactivated). WHO Technical Report Series, No. 927. 2005.

Widom J, Baldwin RL. Cation-induced toroidal condensation of DNA studies with Co3 + (NH3)6. J Mol Biol 1980;144:431–453.

Wiktor TJ, Fanget BJ, Fournier P, Montagnon BJ. Process for the large-scale production of rabies vaccine. US patent No. 4664912. 1987.

Wilson RW, Bloomfield VA. Counter-ion induced condensation of deoxyribonucleic acid—a light-scattering study. Biochemistry 1979;18:2192–2196.

Williams MS. Single-radial-immunodiffusion as an in-vitro potency assay for human inactivated viral vaccines. Veterinary Microbiology 1993;37(3–4):253–262.

Winona LJ, Ommani AW, Olszewski J, Nuzzo JB, Oshima KH. Efficient and predictable recovery of viruses from water by small scale ultrafiltration systems. Can J Microbiol 2001;47:1033–1041.

Wolf B, Berman S, Hanlon S. Structural transitions of calf thymus DNA in concentrated LiCl solutions. Biochemistry 1977;16:3655–3662.

Wolff MW, Reichl U. Downstream processing of cell culture-derived virus particles. Expert Rev Vaccines 2011;10(10):1451–1475.

Wood JM, Robertson JS. From lethal virus to life-saving vaccine: developing inactivated vaccines for pandemic influenza. Nature 2004;2:842–847.

Wu CX, Soh KY, Wang S. Ion-exchange membrane chromatography method for rapid and efficient purification of recombinant baculovirus and baculovirus gp64 protein. Hum Gene Ther 2007;18:665–672.

Wu DX, Howell JA, Field RW. Critical flux measurement for model colloids. J Membr Sci 1999;152:89–98.

Xie Y, Mun SY, Kim JH, Wang NHL. Standing wave design and experimental validation of a tandem simulated moving bed process for insulin purification. Biotechnol Prog 2002;18:1332–1344.

Yamamoto KR, Alberts BM, Lawhorne L, Treiber G. Rapid bacteriophage sedimentation in presence of polyethylene glycol and its application to large-scale virus purification. Virology 1970;40:734.

Yamamoto S, Nakanishi K, Matsuno R. *Ion-Exchange Chromatography of Proteins*. New York: Marcel Dekker; 1988.

Yamamoto S, Nomura M, Sano Y. Predicting the performance of gel filtration chromatography of proteins. J Chromatogr 1990;512:77–87.

Ye KM, Jin S, Ataai MM, Schultz JS, Ibeh J. Tagging retrovirus vectors with a metal binding peptide and one-step purification by immobilized metal affinity chromatography. J Virol 2004;78:9820–9827.

Yigzaw Y, Piper R, Tran M, Shukla AA. Exploitation of the adsorptive properties of depth filters for host cell protein removal during monoclonal antibody purification. Biotechnol Prog 2006;22:288–296.

Yohannes G, Jussila M, Hartonen K, Riekkola ML. Asymmetrical flow field-flow fractionation technique for separation and characterization of biopolymers and bioparticles. J Chromatogr A 2011;1218(27):4104–4116.

Zahn A, Allain JP. Hepatitis C virus and hepatitis B virus bind to heparin: purification of largely IgG-free virions from infected plasma by heparin chromatography. J Gen Virol 2005;86:677–685.

Zelic B, Nesek B. Mathematical modeling of size exclusion chromatography. Eng Life Sci 2006;6:163–169.

Zeman LJ, Zydney AL. *Microfiltration and Ultrafiltration—Principles and Applications*. New York: Marcel Dekker; 1996.

Zhang HG, Xie JF, Dmitriev I, Kashentseva E, Curiel DT, Hsu HC, Mountz JD. Addition of six-His-tagged peptide to the C terminus of adeno-associated virus VP3 does not affect viral tropism or production. J Virol 2002;76:12023–12031.

Zhang YJ, Cremer PS. Interactions between macromolecules and ions: the Hofmeister series. Curr Opin Chem Biol 2006;10:658–663.

Zhilinskaya IN, Sokolov NN, Golubev DB, Ivanova NA, Elsaed LH. Isolation of A2/Singapore/57 influenza virus V and S antigens by isoelectric focusing. Acta Virol 1972;16:436.

Zhong GM, Guiochon G. Analytical solution for the linear ideal model of simulated moving bed chromatography. Chem Eng Sci 1996;51:4307–4319.

Zhong GM, Guiochon G. Fundamentals of simulated moving bed chromatography under linear conditions. Adv Chromatogr 1998;39:351–400.

Zoran G. *Linear Dynamic Systems and Signals*. New Jersey: Upper Saddle River; 2003.

Zydney AL, Ho CC. Scale-up of microfiltration systems: fouling phenomena and V-max analysis. Desalination 2002;146:75–81.

6

PROTEIN SUBUNIT VACCINE PURIFICATION

Yan-ping Yang and Tony D'Amore

Sanofi Pasteur, Toronto, Ontario, Canada

6.1 INTRODUCTION

Protein antigens are key components of prophylactic vaccines against infectious diseases. Most of these protein antigens are currently produced from native or recombinant heterologous organisms. As a subunit vaccine product, the target protein must be separated from its host cell impurities, such as host cell proteins, nucleic acids, and lipids. If impurities are detected, they must be removed, identified, and/or proven to be harmless. In addition to purity, the protein product in its final formulation must exist in a conformation where it is able to elicit protective immune responses. The manufacturing process must be able to produce the same quality of product each time (i.e., demonstrate consistency). This requires the use of very robust purification processes. A method that works exquisitely in a research laboratory may fail in the production floor where it must be scaled up and reproduced each time.

Analogous to the downstream purification in biotech or biopharmaceutical companies, the vaccine industry has benefited from the recent progresses made in protein purification technology development or improvement, including disposable technology, membrane technology, high throughput process development, process automation, and process data tracking and analysis. The concept of platform technology developed from monoclonal antibody (MAb) purification to facilitate process development, validation, and technology transfer is equally valuable for the purification of a protein subunit vaccine product.

Vaccine Development and Manufacturing, First Edition.
Edited by Emily P. Wen, Ronald Ellis, and Narahari S. Pujar.

This chapter reviews the methods, technologies, and processes used in protein subunit purification to support vaccine production and manufacturing. It first evaluates several purification technologies, including chromatographic adsorbents, suspended adsorption technology, and filtration/membrane technology, with regards to subunit vaccine purification. Then, it discusses the various aspects of vaccine purification, from process development, process scale up, process definition studies, process economy, to process automation. Some of the key technical issues encountered during the protein subunit vaccine purification are also discussed. In addition, the current status and future application of process analytical technology (PAT) in subunit vaccine purification are explored. At the end, it provides an outlook for protein purification in the vaccine industry and aims to shed light on the much anticipated evolutions of downstream purification technologies on the horizon.

6.2 PURIFICATION TECHNOLOGIES—APPLICATIONS IN PROTEIN SUBUNIT VACCINE PURIFICATION

6.2.1 Process Steps of Protein Purification

Purification of protein subunit vaccines employs many generic techniques, with considerations of their feasibility in scale-up manufacturing. The following three main process steps in protein purification are equally applicable to protein subunit vaccine purification.

6.2.1.1 Capturing Capturing serves as a gross purification step of the target protein from its host cell environment and provides the product in a relatively concentrated form. Selectivity and capacity represent two important considerations in developing effective purification processes. For example, the purification of a protein from *Escherichia coli* with a ratio of product to host cell impurities of 1:1,000,000 requires a capture step with high capacity and selectivity. The capturing step not only concentrates the protein target, but also separates the product from the crude solution, which likely contains proteases. At this stage of purification, ion-exchange adsorbents are commonly used, either in a suspended adsorption or in a packed column chromatography mode. This is mainly because of a wide range of adsorbent selections available and the relative ease of operations. Affinity chromatography (e.g., Protein A) has been commonly used as the capturing step in many MAb purification processes because of its high selectivity and the similar characteristics among different MAbs. However, the affinity approach has not commonly been adopted in protein subunit vaccine purification, partly because of the unfavorable balance between cost (in search of specific affinity ligands) and benefit (each protein product is unique).

6.2.1.2 Intermediate Purification This step of purification may involve more than one method, including an ionic exchanger (usually with a different chemistry if the ionic exchanger is also used in the capturing step), hydrophobic interaction (HIC), ceramic hydroxyapatite (CHT) chromatography, or a combination of these.

The criteria for method selection are based on chromatographic adsorbents that would provide high resolution and good recovery.

6.2.1.3 ***Polishing*** The purpose of this step is to remove minor impurities (e.g., host cell proteins, host cell nucleic acids, and endotoxins) from a reasonably pure preparation. Capacity is usually irrelevant at this stage, but selectivity (for impurity removal) is crucial. Besides conventional chromatography using adsorbents described in the "intermediate purification," membrane technology or potential affinity chromatography may play an important role at this stage. Size-exclusion chromatography (SEC) is commonly used in protein purification at laboratory scale but is not practically suitable in large-scale production, particularly in the initial capturing step. However, at the polishing stage, the product is in a relatively concentrated form and at a smaller volume. SEC may be considered as a polishing tool, if desired.

Some general applications of the various chromatographic adsorbents in the three stages of protein subunit vaccine purification are summarized in Table 6.1. However, it must be recognized that each recombinant or native protein is unique, and as such, prediction on the best methods or combinations is difficult to make and oftentimes must be made empirically.

6.2.2 Chromatographic Adsorbents

The application of commonly used chromatographic adsorbents in protein subunit vaccine purification is described in the following sections.

6.2.2.1 ***Ionic Exchanger*** Ionic exchangers are suitable for all three steps of protein purification. By choosing different buffers with specific pH ranges, the same protein can adsorb to either anion exchangers (which bind negatively charged molecules) or cation exchangers (which bind positively charged molecules). Most protein purification is performed on anion exchange columns because most proteins are negatively charged at physiological pH values (pH 6–8). To release the proteins in the order of binding tenacity, one can either increase the salt concentration or change the pH.

TABLE 6.1 Applications of Chromatographic Adsorbents in Protein Subunit Vaccine Purification

Chromatographic Adsorbents	Capturing	Intermediate	Polishing
Ionic exchange	+++	+++	+++
Hydrophobic interaction	+	+++	+++
Hydroxyapatite	+	+++	+++
Size exclusion	+	+	+
Affinity	CS	CS	++

+++: most commonly used.
++: can be used.
+: not preferred.
CS: case specific.

Raising the salt concentration, however, is by far the most commonly used approach in vaccine protein purification, as it is the easiest to control.

6.2.2.2 Hydrophobic Interaction Hydrophobic interaction is most commonly used in the intermediate purification or polishing step of protein purification and not during the initial capturing step. This is because a high salt concentration is required to expose the hydrophobic regions of the protein to the surface, and this is usually achieved by adding salt (e.g., NaCl or ammonia sulfate) directly to the sample. In the crude extract, high salt concentration may easily cause precipitation of other proteins, dragging the product into the precipitates, which results in low product yield. In the intermediate purification or the polishing step, the column beads are coated with hydrophobic fatty acid chains, which interact with the hydrophobic areas of proteins that are exposed to high salt concentrations. The column is eluted with decreasing concentrations of salt in the buffer. The protein is usually eluted in low ionic strength, and it is ready for the next purification step without further buffer exchange.

6.2.2.3 Hydroxyapatite Chromatography Hydroxyapatite adsorbent is a form of calcium phosphate used in the chromatographic separation of biomolecules and is considered to be a "mixed-mode" ion-exchange plus metal affinity adsorbent. It has proven to be an effective purification mechanism in a variety of processes, providing selectivity and complementary to more traditional ion-exchange techniques. Ceramic hydroxyapatite (a spherical, macroporous form of hydroxyapatite produced by Bio-Rad) has often been a choice of chromatographic adsorbent selection in the purification of subunit protein vaccine (Sanofi Pasteur, unpublished observations).

6.2.2.4 Size-Exclusion Chromatography Although SEC is commonly used in research laboratories for protein purification, it is not considered a method of choice in large-scale purification of protein subunit vaccines, particularly at the early capturing stage or the intermediate purification step. This is mainly because of its limitation in capacity and resolution.

A packed-bed column chromatography is the most common method used in protein purification where chromatographic adsorbents are involved. However, the potential for using a suspended adsorption approach in large-scale protein purification processes should not be ignored.

6.2.3 Suspended Adsorption Technology

Although the use of suspended adsorbents in bioprocessing has been known for decades, the true value of this simple technology has not been fully explored. Using any of the existing chromatographic adsorbents available in the market, in combination with a reaction container such as a vertical cylinder or a stirred tank reactor, product capture by adsorption/deadsorption can be achieved without any prior clarification step. The simplicity of the process is astounding, and the savings in time and cost can be impressive. Using suspended chromatographic adsorbents, in a single process step, the solids are removed from the product, as are impurities, and the partially purified product is concentrated (Quinones-GarcaI et al., 2001). This combination of clarification, purification, and concentration makes this technology very attractive for vaccine purification process development.

6.2.3.1 ***Expanded Bed Adsorption*** The use of expanded bed adsorption (EBA) for the purpose of capturing biological products from crude feedstock has been described in literature (Blank et al., 2001; Santambien et al., 2003; Valdes et al., 2003). As shown in Figure 6.1, the EBA system essentially consists of a chromatography column, which is fed in an up-flow mode at a flow velocity sufficiently high to keep the adsorbent particles floating. While the adsorbent particles remain floating at their specific location in the column, the liquid feed flows through the column in near-plug-flow mode. While particles and unbound feed components freely pass between the suspended adsorbents, the product of interest will bind to the adsorbent and, thereby, be separated from the starting material. The application of EBA technology at the pilot scale for protein subunit vaccine capturing and purification has been demonstrated (Sanofi Pasteur, unpublished observations).

6.2.3.2 ***Fluidized Bed Adsorption*** Fluidized bed adsorption is, in part, EBA and, in part, adsorption in a stirred tank. This approach has been used in the biotechnology industry for many years, mainly to recover antibiotics from fermentation broth. Gilliot et al. described a large-scale process for the capture of immunomycin from a Streptomyces culture (Gilliot et al., 1990). While the equipment used for EBA and

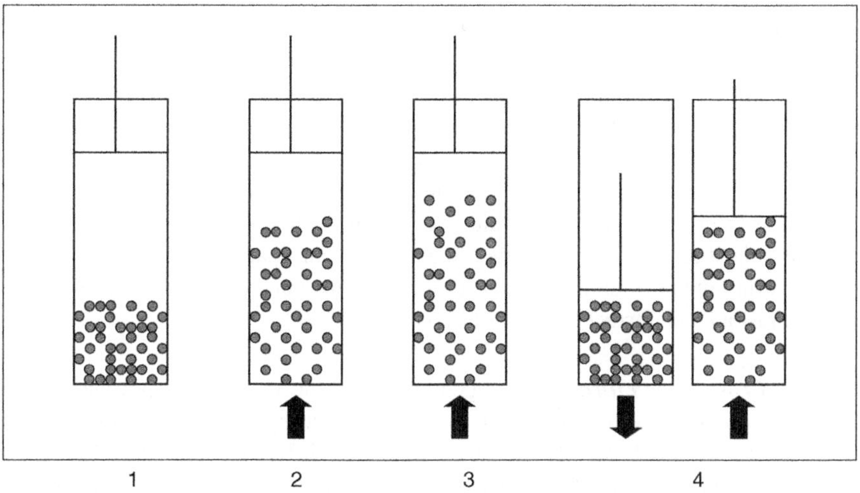

Figure 6.1 Principle of expanded bed adsorption (EBA) technology. (i) Sedimented adsorbent before start-up, (ii) equilibration in expanded mode, (iii) sample application and washing in expanded mode, (iv) target molecule elution in packed or expanded mode, regeneration and cleaning in place in expanded mode.

fluidized bed adsorption is essentially the same, the channeling and turbulent flow pattern observed in fluidized bed contactors results in extensive forward and back mixing and is very different from the plug-flow-like liquid flow pattern achievable in expanded bed systems. In addition, recycling of the feed is frequently required to extend the contact time of product and resin, in order to achieve acceptable product recoveries. This results in increased processing time.

6.2.3.3 Stirred Tank Adsorption Stirred tank adsorption was used very early in bioprocessing for the recovery of biologics from crude extracts such as serum (Brummelhuis, 1980). Most of these processes were run in a batch adsorption mode. While many of the product capture processes by stirred tank adsorption are still performed in batch mode, semicontinuous operations may be achieved easily, from a technical point of view, by separation (settling and sieving) of the spent feed fluids from the particulate adsorbents and replacement by new feed material. The simplicity of the stirred tank adsorption technique is intriguing, and this technique has huge potential in bioprocessing. All the elements of this technique have been well studied and documented, including fluid patterns of viscous and nonviscous suspensions in stirred tanks, stirrer types, cooling and heating methods, and adsorption kinetics. (Luyben and Tramper, 2004; Verschuren et al., 2004).

6.2.4 Filtration and Membrane Technology

Filtration and membrane technology has gained wide acceptance as an important manufacturing step in many of the process lines in the biopharmaceutical and the vaccine industries. For the purification of a protein subunit vaccine, this technology has been used routinely in the clarification, product concentration, buffer exchange, and polishing steps.

6.2.4.1 Depth Filter Technology Depth filtration for the removal and clarification of mammalian or *E. coli* cell debris has played an increasingly important role in bioprocesses and vaccine manufacturing. The most common application of depth filtration is to produce a cell-free fluid stream with high target molecule yield and to provide a clarified material for further downstream purification. The use of depth filtration during the purification process to remove unwanted precipitate has also been noted (Prashad and Tarrach, 2006; Sutherland, 2008).

6.2.4.2 Cross-Flow Filtration Tangential flow filtration (TFF) is a pressure-driven separation process that uses membranes to separate components in a liquid solution or suspension on the basis of their size and charge differences. In TFF, the fluid is pumped tangentially along the surface of the membrane. An applied pressure serves to force a portion of the fluid through the membrane to the filtrate side. Membrane-based TFF unit operations have been used in many stages of protein purification, including clarification, product concentration, and buffer exchange. Thus, this technology has become an integral part of the protein subunit vaccine purification process.

6.2.4.3 Membrane Adsorbers Microporous membrane adsorbers were originally developed as a means of avoiding the disadvantages in the diffusion limitation of conventional chromatographic gels. In theory, they were to improve the chromatographic kinetics and velocity of protein purification. Although advances have been made in recent years in the development of new membrane adsorbers by various vendors, few success stories have been noted regarding the use of membrane adsorbers in the purification of proteins among the biopharmaceutical and vaccine industries. This is mainly due to a limited selection of membrane binding chemistries, sometimes nonmatching construction hardware, insufficient flow distribution, as well as lower surface-to-bed volume ratios leading to lower binding capacities of membrane adsorbents than that with chromatographic beads. Membrane adsorbers have become more popular, however, in the polishing step of protein purification, for the removal of trace impurities, such as endotoxins, DNA, host cell proteins, or viruses. The pros and cons of using a packed-bed column chromatography versus membrane technology have been discussed previously (Knudsen et al., 2001; Table 6.2).

TABLE 6.2 Pros and Cons of Packed-Bed Column Chromatography Versus Membrane Technology

	Pros	Cons
Packed-bed column chromatography	• Unlimited scalability • Many choices of different adsorbents • Mature technology	• Limited flow rate can be used (binding is diffusion controlled) • Binding capacity depending on flow rate for limited throughput • Usually has lower binding capacity for large molecules such as DNA or virus • Complex operation (column packing required)
Membrane chromatography	• High flow rate (convective flow) • Binding capacity independent of flow rate for high throughput • May have higher binding capacity for large molecules such as DNA or virus • Simple operation (no column packing required) • Single disposable unit available • Superior for impurity removal when product is in the flow-through	• Limited absolute binding capacity in terms of bed volume • Limited choice of membrane chemistry commercially available • Limited application in binding-elution mode because of the limitation on the absolute binding capacity

6.3 PURIFICATION PROCESS DEVELOPMENT AND SCALE-UP FOR PROTEIN SUBUNIT VACCINE

6.3.1 Purification Process Development

A purification process is first developed as a small-scale process. In the capturing, intermediate purification, and final polishing steps, chromatographic adsorbents are commonly used (see Section 6.2—purification technology). For each of the purification steps, yield and purity are analyzed to assess the efficiency of the purification process. This information will facilitate decisions on process improvement, as well as potentially reduce the number of purification steps. The following figure summarizes the general approach to purification process development for protein subunit vaccines (Sanofi Pasteur; Fig. 6.2).

Other steps that may be used in purification but not specified in the process map are described in the following section.

6.3.1.1 Benzonase Digestion of Nucleic Acids It is commonly used in viral subunit protein purification before separation technologies but may not be necessary for bacterial/recombinant proteins. Benzonase concentration at 5–25 μg/ml performed at either room temperature or 2–8°C has proven to be effective in the digestion of host cell DNA (Sanofi Pasteur, unpublished observations).

6.3.1.2 Concentration and Buffer Exchange It is commonly used during clarification (preparing materials for downstream purification), between purification steps (preparing materials for the next separation step), and after purification has been completed (preparing material for the next formulation step). TFF has been the most useful technology for concentration and buffer exchange.

6.3.1.3 Endotoxin Removal Endotoxin is a group of polysaccharides derived from *E. coli* cell wall and is pyrogenic if injected in humans in significant quantity. The purification process needs to ensure a satisfactory removal of endotoxin. Endotoxin comprises highly negatively charged molecules (pI = 2–3) with high hydrophobicity. Ion-exchange chromatography steps are efficient in removing the endotoxin. For the HIC column (e.g., Phenyl-Sepharose HP), the endotoxin is usually eluted at the end of the elution gradient (i.e., without salt), at which point the highest elution power is generated for highly hydrophobic molecules, such as endotoxin.

6.3.1.4 Residual Host Cell DNA Removal DNA molecules are highly negatively charged and retained strongly on anion exchange columns (e.g., Q-Sepharose HP) and the hydroxyapaptite column (CHT Type I). Thus, an anion exchange column plus a hydroxyapatite column with appropriate elution conditions is a good combination for DNA removal.

6.3.1.5 Polishing Step Using Membrane Technology In the event that residual DNA or endotoxin levels are still unsatisfactory after the selected separation technologies, inclusion of a membrane step at this point in the purification sequence would

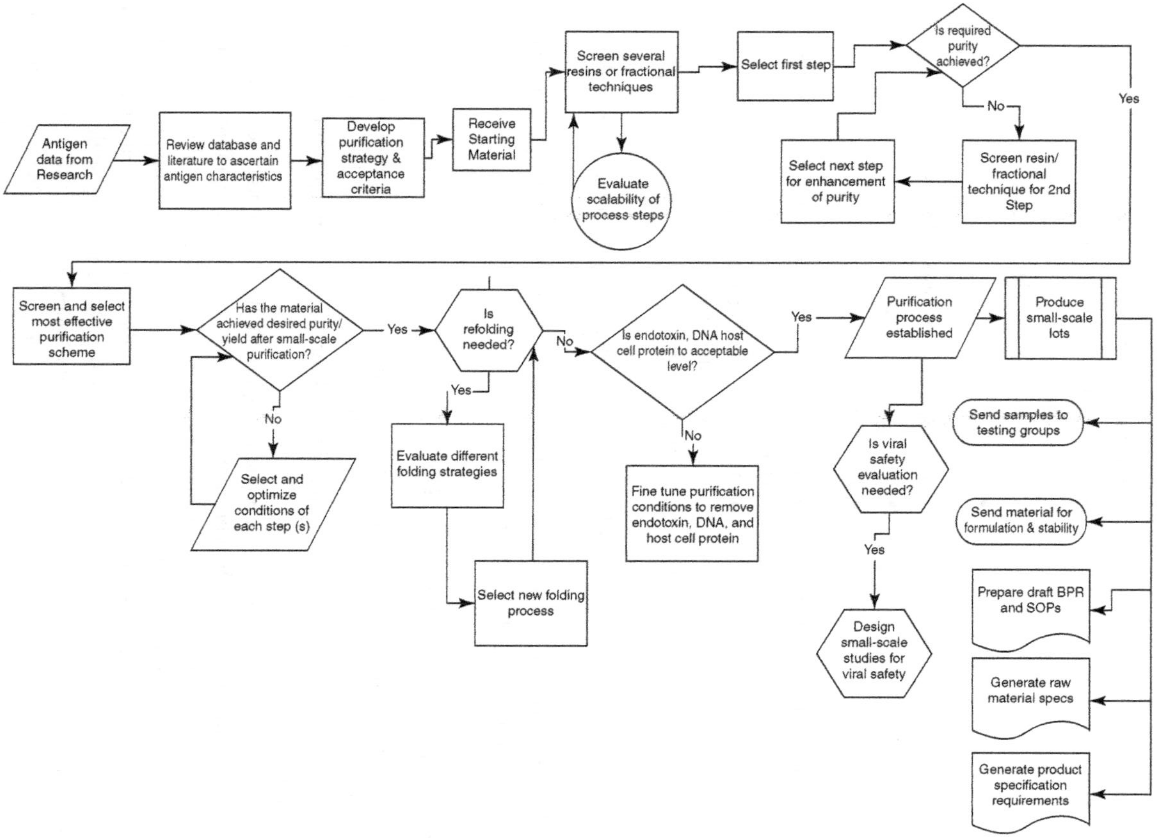

Figure 6.2 Process map for downstream purification process development

TABLE 6.3 Points to Consider in Process Development

Process Aspect	Points to Consider
Technical feasibility	• Reliable, easy to operate, cost-effective
Scalability	• Suitable for manufacturing technologies • Scale meets market demand • Reproducibility • Product yield vs. production cost • Time
Raw materials	• Safe sourced to minimize BSE risk • QC tested and released • USP or EP grade
Test and characterization	• To support process change or scale-up (product comparability) • Well-characterized products to support regulatory submission

be an option. Both Sartorius and Pall Corp. manufacture Q membrane units that are suitable for this purpose.

The points listed in Table 6.3 should be considered when developing a purification process for protein subunit vaccine.

6.3.2 Purification Process Scale-Up

Once the purification process is optimized at laboratory scale, the process is scaled up to pilot scale (e.g., 200-l fermentor or bioreactor scale). With this, a number of adjustments may be required for scalability and for improving process efficiency and economy.

Chromatographic columns are scaled proportionally by keeping several factors constant, including column height, linear flow rate, and chromatographic adsorbent binding capacity. The column diameter, volumetric flow rate, and total loading material are increased proportionally. The TFF operation is also scaled up proportionally according to the membrane surface area. After this, the product purity and purification yield should be comparable to what was obtained at the laboratory scale.

If any discrepancy between pilot and laboratory scales occurs, further investigation is carried out at both scales to fine-tune the operation conditions. Once the pilot-scale process is finalized, preclinical materials at the pilot scale are produced and compared with that from the laboratory-scale process with regard to product purity, process yield, endotoxin level, residual DNA level, and other release testing criteria.

Biochemical, biophysical, and immunological characterizations of products are performed to support process development, stability analysis, and potency evaluation.

An understanding of the primary structure and confirmation of antigens and any tendency toward self-association or degradation can help in correlating structure with functional properties, particularly immunogenicity, and may provide structural parameters of stability. Oftentimes, the biochemical nature of the protein or antigen being purified becomes problematic in scale-up. For example, product degradation, loss of immunogenicity, or potency, all of which may be difficult to predict. Under these circumstances, specific conditions need to be worked out empirically.

Once pilot scale-up runs are completed, a development report for the pilot-scale purification is prepared with all the testing results and summary. A batch production record (BPR), which describes the process steps, operation conditions, and in some cases, product specifications is drafted before clinical lot production under the current Good Manufacturing Practices (cGMP).

6.3.2.1 Process Map The general process map of scale-up purification is summarized in Figure 6.3 (Sanofi Pasteur).

6.3.2.2 Maximizing Processing Data From Development to Manufacturing In the biopharmaceutical or the vaccine industry, product development life cycles typically range from 5 to 8 years (Reichert, 2003). The long lag times between development and industrialization make it difficult for companies to seemingly track data and learn from past experience (Morris et al., 2005). In recent years, there has been increasing competitive pressure in driving the need for faster and more effective development and production processes. However, progress toward these goals is often hindered by the complexity and variability of biological product manufacturing. Many companies are now looking for solutions that would speed progress from laboratory to pilot-scale manufacture and promote cost-effective production processes. One such strategy is to have an effective data management tool or system that could capture process and facility data throughout the product life cycle, enabling early views of project costs and facility fit.

There have been many advances in software development to address data capture, data analysis, and feedback control in the manufacturing of biologics. For example, tailored for vaccine production, the Pertinence software helps users to understand what works and what does not during the production process (Halley, 2006). Through detailed analysis of batch data, the software facilitates reaching the highest yields, best-quality production, and optimal set up. Recently, a UK biotech consortium initiated a collaborative development effort to address data management issues (Hill and Sinclair, 2007). The proposed outcome was a data model, based on the ISA-88 Standard for Batch Control, to capture process and facility data throughout the product life cycle. This data framework may simplify process scale up and facilitate technology transfer from process development to manufacturing. Another example is the Discoverant software developed by Aegis. The software provides users with interactive access to all types of process development and manufacturing data in existing electronic data collection systems and on paper records. This, integrated with data analysis, trending and reporting capabilities, aims to reduce process variability, improve yields, and reduce batch failures.

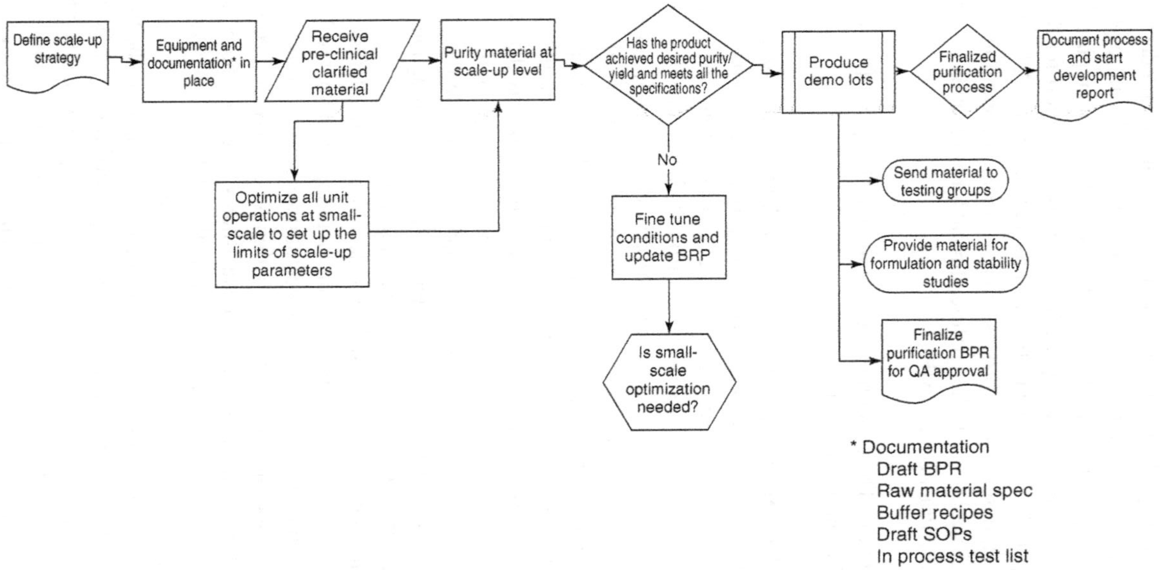

Figure 6.3 Process map of downstream purification scale-up.

There are clear benefits of using data management tools for process development and the industrialization of vaccines. For example, the system could help to maintain process control and identify the root cause of atypical performance in a timely manner. Data capturing and analysis at an early stage of process development could serve to facilitate technology transfer from pilot scale to manufacturing. The system also allows on-demand access to data from all manufacturing systems (raw materials, in-process, and final product) and provides integrated analysis and reporting capabilities. This also assists with compliance requirements, as documentation on process development, process validation, and process control are standardized, which streamlines reporting to regulatory agencies.

6.4 PROCESS DEFINITION STUDIES

Once the purification process is developed and ready to be scaled up to a pilot scale, it is important to demonstrate process robustness and identify critical operating parameters (so called *process definition studies*) before the process industrialization and process transfer to manufacturing. One tool used in process definition studies is experimental design.

6.4.1 Experimental Design

Experimental design is a method that studies the impact of several variables on the process simultaneously using statistical design analyses. Experimental design has been applied to the pharmaceutical and biopharmaceutical industries for many years, especially in the field of testing method validation (Torbeck and Branning, 1996). The main advantage of experimental design is that several variables can be studied simultaneously. More importantly, the study has the ability to predict if there is any interaction between the parameters that will have an additive or offset effect on the process output. The information obtained from the experimental design studies for the unit operations in the manufacturing process is also valuable to the process validation group on the critical process parameters and ranges. The studies carried out with experimental design will improve the overall understating of the manufacturing process, contribute to a shortened timeline for process development, and facilitate the technology transfer to manufacturing.

Experimental design to study the downstream purification process has been widely applied to biological products in both pharmaceutical companies, such as Abbott Laboratories and GlaxoSmithKine, as well as biotechnology companies such as Amgen, Genetech, and IDEC Pharmaceuticals (Table 6.4). Experimental design has been used in typical critical unit operations in the purification process, such as the chromatography step. It has also been applied to other downstream purification unit operations, such as protein folding studies and aqueous two-phase partition studies (Table 6.4). In addition to assessing the impact of variables on the purity and purification yield by experimental design studies, other important information can also be obtained, including the screening of chromatography resins (Cunningham et al., 2003), process sensitivity to different resin lots (Baillargeon et al., 2003), and impurity clearance

TABLE 6.4 Examples of Experimental Design Studies for Downstream Purification Unit Operations

Unit Operation in Downstream Processing	CompanyReferences
Anion exchange chromatography (AEC)	Sanofi Pasteur[a]
	Genetics Institute (Kelley et al., 1997; Leonard et al. 1998)
Cation exchange chromatography (CEC)	Sanofi Pasteur[a]
	Genetech, Inc. (Breece et al., 2002a; Breece et al., 2002b)
Hydrophobic interaction chromatography (HIC)	Sanofi Pasteur[a]
	Amgen Inc. (Hart, 2002)
	Abbott Laboratories (Baillargeon et al., 2003)
Ceramic hydroxyapatite (CHT), type I	Sanofi Pasteur[a]
Protein-A affinity chromatography	IDEC Pharmaceuticals (Cunningham et al., 2003)
Immobilized metal affinity chromatography (IMAC)	Genetics Institute (Leonard et al., 1998)
Aqueous two-phase partition	Genentech Inc. (Hart et al., 1995)
Protein refolding	Avecia Biotechnology (Liddell, 2002)
	Columbia University (Chen and Gouaux, 1997; Armstrong et al., 1999)
Precipitation	GlaxoSmithKline (Eon-Duval et al., 2003)

[a]Unpublished observations.

(DNA, host cell protein, and chromatography ligand) (Leonard et al, 1998; Breece et al., 2002a; Breece et al., 2002b).

In the following section, several points that need to be considered while using experimental design are discussed.

6.4.1.1 Selection of Unit Operations Downstream process in vaccine purification comprises multiple unit operations, such as batch adsorption, column chromatography, and filtration. The selection of the unit operation for experimental design studies is typically based on the importance of the unit operation itself and previous scientific understanding of each unit operation. The focus of process definition is usually put on the most important parameters in the most critical unit operations. Each experimental design study is often limited to one unit operation, while the previous and following unit operations are performed at set points.

6.4.1.2 Selection of Parameters and Ranges for Study Initial selection of parameters and ranges that will be used in experimental design studies is based on scientific theory, previous experience with the process, and manufacturing precision. For example, if the pH of a purification buffer can be prepared within ± 0.1 pH units, the study range of ± 0.2 pH units may be justified. Other considerations included the total number of parameters to be evaluated, as the number of experiments will increase exponentially when a full factorial design is applied.

6.4.1.3 Full Factorial Design Versus Fractional Factorial Design Typically, there are two different applications of experimental design that can be used in downstream purification process development. The first one is a low-resolution (Resolution III) fractional factorial design to study many variables (>five variables) at the same time with a limited number of experiments. The range of variables used is often broad. This type of study is able to identify important variables for further evaluation (Kelly, 2000). The screening application of experimental design may be applied at any stage of the purification development process for vaccine antigens.

The second application is a higher resolution (Resolution IV or V) fractional factorial design or a full factorial design to study the impact of key variables on the process output and to define the operation ranges for future process validation studies (Kelly, 2000). The ranges of the variables may be narrowed down on the basis of the initial screening experiments. These high resolution studies would provide important information for process validation studies. Their initiation is, therefore, usually at the later stage of phase II clinical trial, as adopted by Amgen (Seely and Seely, 2003). At this stage, the manufacturing scale is usually scaled up to the final commercial scale, and the manufacturing process is nearly fixed.

6.4.1.4 Scaled-Down Model Since the experimental design studies have multiple runs, they are usually carried out with a properly scaled down model of the unit operation, such as the chromatography step (Sofer, 1996). Most unit operations in the downstream process are amenable to scaled down models, with certain exceptions, such as TFF (Parenteral Drug Association, 1992). In such a case, full-scale studies or statistical analyses of historical data would be required (Martin-Moe et al., 2000).

6.4.1.5 Testing Method Before performing the robustness study for purification unit operations, the required testing needs to be determined and the corresponding testing methods should be established. There are many process outputs that may be measured for purification unit operations, such as purity, yield, host cell protein or DNA clearance, endotoxin removal, and virus inactivation and removal. (Winkler, 2000). The required testing should be preselected before experimentation.

6.4.2 Case Study

Experimental design was implemented in downstream purification process definition studies for several bacterial-derived recombinant protein antigens (Sanofi Pasteur, unpublished data). The following is an example of how factorial design was applied to define the operating parameters in a unit operation, Q-Sepharose fast flow chromatography. In this study, we evaluated the robustness of a protein subunit vaccine purification process unit using experimental design. The Q-Sepharose chromatography step was identified as a critical unit operation in the process. An experimental design software, Fusion Pro, was used in this study with a scale-down model. As shown in Table 6.5, three parameters (pH and salt concentrations in wash and elution, respectively), each at three levels, were evaluated. Using fractional factorial design, only 11 experiments were needed as compared to 27 with standard design.

TABLE 6.5 Quantitative Analysis of Product Loss by RP-HPLC for Robustness Study on Q-Sepharose Fast Flow Column

Exp#	pH	Wash NaCl (mM)	Elution NaCl (mM)	Wash Loss (%): Wash Loss (%)	Wash Loss (%): 1st CV Elution (%)	Elution Loss (%): Elution Tail (%)	Elution Loss (%): Strip (%)	Overall Yield (%)
1	7.20	30	100	0.7	0.2	1.3	5.5	57
2	7.00	30	100	0.3	0.1	2.3	5.1	47
3	7.20	20	110	0.2	0.1	0.5	5.1	58
4	6.80	20	110	0.6	0.0	1.8	5.2	55
5	7.00	30	100	0.8	0.6	0.7	5.9	58
6	6.80	30	100	0.6	0.1	1.9	6.7	46
7	7.00	40	90	13.6	9.7	1.8	1.7	36
8	6.80	40	90	10.0	3.9	1.1	7.3	34
9	7.20	40	90	16.0	10.3	0.7	7.5	33
10	7.00	30	100	0.4	0.8	0.6	6.1	57
11	7.00	20	110	0.6	0.1	0.8	4.6	60

On the basis of the analysis using Fusion Pro (Table 6.5; Fig. 6.4), the results clearly indicated that a range of pHs from 6.8 to 7.2 had no major impact on the product yield. However, significant product loss occurred when the salt concentration had reached 40 mM in the wash buffer. A preferred operating range of salt concentrations (NaCl) in the wash buffer was found to be between 20 and 30 mM. Under these conditions, a product yield of approximately 55% can be expected. These conditions appeared robust because it would not be difficult to control the salt concentration in the wash buffer (i.e., 25 mM as a set point, 20–30 mM will have a ±20% margin on the set point). Similarly, the desired salt concentration in the elution buffer was also

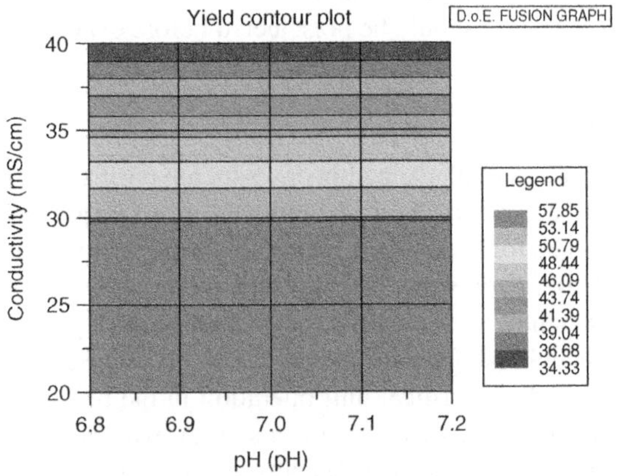

Figure 6.4 Fusion Pro analysis of the effect of pH and wash conductivity on the purification yield on Q-Sepharose FF column.

easy to control (100 mM set point, 90–110 mM will have a ±10% margin on the set point), as the accuracy for buffer conductivity at the manufacturing scale is ±5%.

6.5 PROCESS ECONOMY AND AUTOMATION

6.5.1 Purification Technology Development to Address Process Challenges and to Improve Process Economy

As with any other downstream bioprocessing activity, the purification of protein antigens faces many challenges. The downstream purification process is a very complex, technically demanding, and often unpredictable process, with inherent complexities, such as high initial volume and low target protein titer. The increasing regulatory requirement (product quality and comparability, process consistency, and reproducibility) has added even more challenges to the already complex process. The cost of downstream processing for biological products may be as high as until 75% of the overall manufacturing costs. To increase productivity and process economy, downstream purification is clearly the target for improvement. In the following section, several areas that may potentially impact the downstream process efficiency and productivity are discussed.

6.5.1.1 Platform Technology In recent years, the approach of platform technology has become more popular in many large biopharmaceutical companies for dealing with process development to the ultimate process design (Jagschies et al., 2006; Sofer and Chirica, 2006; Grönberg et al., 2007; Eppink et al., 2007). Platform technologies are standard sets of unit operations, conditions, and methods applied to molecules of a given class. The use of platform technology has allowed for rapid and economical product development from the R&D to commercialization (Jagschies et al., 2006). The most common example is for MAb purification (Grönberg et al., 2007), as these represent a relatively homogeneous group of molecules. The use of platform technology approach has allowed some companies to reduce the need for process alteration before full manufacturing scale-up. Some of the benefits of using a platform technology include (i) facilitating rapid and economical process development and scale-up, potentially allowing evaluation of a larger number of product candidates and speed to market entry, (ii) reducing validation effort by using modular validation, (iii) providing familiarity with a process that may result in more robust processes and better technology transfer from process development to manufacturing, and (iv) using established vendors for raw materials and standardized waste disposal procedures. The bottom line benefit of this is cost and time savings.

The concept of platform technology can also be applied to the purification of protein antigens. Although most vaccine target molecules are heterogeneous in nature (e.g., each protein molecule is unique), it is not unrealistic to identify some common elements among the protein targets produced in the same host system, such as *E. coli*. For example, anion exchange chromatography is commonly used in the purification of recombinant proteins produced in *E. coli*. Most protein candidates have acidic isoelectric points, typically less than 6, so they bind to the anion exchangers under neutral pH and low conductivity conditions. This can potentially be developed into a standard unit operation for the initial capturing step to remove host cell impurities. The unit operation may be applied (with modifications) to other proteins that are produced using the same host system. In addition, many recombinant proteins are produced as inclusion bodies in *E. coli*. With this, there is a potential for developing a unit operation to standardize inclusion body extraction (i.e., to remove host cell impurities) and solubilization. This approach could potentially accelerate process development, scale-up, and technology transfer, resulting in significant savings in manpower and investment. However, protein refolding may need to be addressed on a case-by-case basis to achieve a final purified and properly folded molecule.

6.5.1.2 Single-Use, Disposable Technology In recent years, there has been an increasing trend toward the use of disposable technologies by biopharmaceutical manufacturers (Hardy, 2006; Boehm et al., 2009). This is no surprise, considering that the increased volume and diversity of biopharmaceutical products are causing manufacturers to design their facilities on the basis of shorter production runs with multiple changeovers. Meeting such demands requires greater operational flexibility. Advantages of using disposables include reducing downtime for cleaning, sterilization, and process engineering, as well as improved equipment lead time and process utility requirements that meet quality and compliance standards (Terry and Thor, 2006). The use of disposable component decreases capital costs and cost of goods and labor, improves operability and flexibility, and optimizes utilization of space (LoMonaco and Rumsey, 2006; Zhou et al., 2007).

As compared to the other areas of manufacturing, the incorporation of disposable systems into downstream processing has been relatively slow (DePalma, 2007). Chromatography and membrane filtration are the main techniques used in downstream purification. In recent years, there has been aggressive campaigning by vendors on the use of membrane technologies in replacing column chromatography. However, many major biopharmaceutical companies have been reluctant to adapt to this approach, mainly because of a limited selection of membrane binding chemistries and lower binding capacities of membrane adsorbers compared to that with chromatographic beads. In contrast, in the area of membrane filtration, the approach of single-use membrane in the process has been increasingly accepted for downstream purification to avoid cleaning validation. In vaccine production, the closest use of disposable systems for downstream purification are single-use disposable bags for buffer or intermediate product storage, single-use depth filters for product clarification, disposable sterile connectors, and disposable membrane adsorption chromatography for the polishing step (removal of endotoxin, DNA, or host cell proteins).

The savings in capital investment with building a facility equipped with disposable bioproduction systems and the reduction of overall manufacturing cost while using disposable technology have been documented (Terry and Thor, 2006). However, unlike many biotech companies in which the push is for quick turnaround and changeover to accommodate multiple products, vaccine manufacturers usually have relatively stable product lines that require continuous supplies. The use of disposable systems to meet short-term production facility needs is, therefore, less justified. In contrast, the advantages of using disposable technology in new vaccine process development have been well recognized where multiple new products awaits clinical development and testing. Without the option of disposable technology replacement, the equipment changeover or cleaning validation could be time-consuming or become a bottleneck.

6.5.1.3 Simulated Moving-Bed Liquid Chromatography or Continuous Chromatographic Process The use of "fixed-bed" chromatographic methods is paramount in purifying products of acceptable purity in the biopharmaceutical and vaccine industries. A major challenge for chromatography is in scale up. When processes move out of the laboratory or pilot scale and into a production setting, the "fixed-bed" nature of traditional column-based systems usually exhibits some constraints, including (i) inefficient use of the entire adsorbent bed, (ii) the large consumption of desorbent (e.g., buffer with higher salt), (iii) the diluted states of the separated components, and (iv) the increased technical challenges associated with large column operations (e.g., packing and cleaning). As the productivity in upstream processes continues to improve, materials to be processed at the downstream purification phase become larger. This results in significant increases in downstream purification cost and space/facility requirement.

To overcome this bottleneck, there have been attempts at developing continuous chromatography systems for the purification of biomolecules. One such system is the simulated moving-bed chromatography (SMB) (Imamoglu, 2002). The concept of SMB is based on the "moving" column bed chromatography principle but without actually moving the adsorbents (Finnfeeds et al., 2004; Wankat, 2004). In an SMB system, the chromatographic adsorbent layers are separated into several smaller columns, each connected to form a circular loop. With this, each column has its own openings for the feeding and drawing of fluids. The columns are connected to inlet and outlet manifolds through on/off valves. Instead of moving the columns, the various valves are opened and closed to simulate the movement. The feed mixtures are introduced successively along with the direction of desorbent flow, and the separated components are removed in a continuous manner from its respective withdrawal point (Fig. 6.5). With SMB systems, a larger volume of material can be processed because of higher per column capacity and less use of buffers as compared to the fixed-bed chromatography systems. In addition, the separated products have higher product concentration, which may reduce the need of a further concentration step.

The concept of SMB is not new. It has been reported that a continuous chromatography process improved separation efficiency and production capacity for small molecules (e.g., glucose and fructose) at industrial scale (Subramani et al., 2003). However, its application has been limited to the separation of two fractions and is still premature for the purification of biologicals, where processing materials are usually much more complex. As the design of SMB is more complex, these would add additional technical challenges in meeting the ever-increasing requirements in

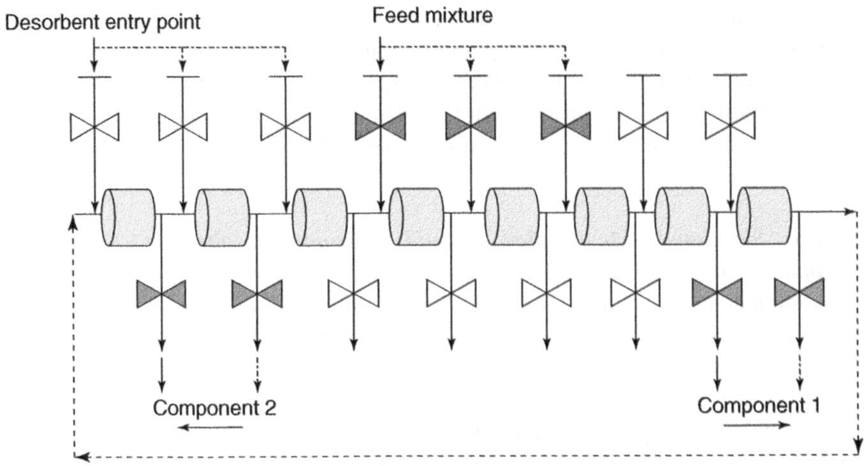

Figure 6.5 Schematic presentation of simulated moving-bed chromatography (SMB) set-up.

equipment and process validation imposed by regulatory agencies. As a result, the overall cost associated with capital investment and operation would likely increase. Although it has shown some promise, the application of SMB technology in subunit vaccine purification is not expected to have an impact in the near future for the reasons described previously.

Recently, a continuous chromatographic process for MAb purification using the multicolumn countercurrent solvent gradient purification process (MCSGP) has been documented (Strohlein et al., 2007). There have been indications that the MCSGP process may increase the productivity (i.e., purification efficiency) by a factor of 10 and reduce the solvent requirement by 90% as compared to the conventional MAb purification process (i.e., batch chromatography with Protein A). The potential of the MCSGP process in the purification of proteins from other complex biological mixtures remains to be demonstrated.

6.5.2 High Throughput and Automation in Purification Process Development and Operation

Process automation is an attractive "buzz" word in today's bioprocessing environment because much attention is being placed on high throughput, cutting-edge technologies and technical competitiveness. With rapid advances in computer technology and robotic system development, some laborious laboratory work can now be replaced by automated instrumentation. The advantage of an automated system is more than just the saving of manpower or reduction in tedious experimental operations. The combination of sophisticated instrumentation and comprehensive data capture and analysis provides the potential to increase output and process efficiency, enhance process control and reproducibility, strengthen data tracking and documentation, and ultimately reduce overall operational costs. Several applications of high throughput process development and automation in downstream purification are discussed in the following section.

6.5.2.1 Multiwell Plate and Miniaturized Columns Microtiter plates have been used for many years in analytical research and clinical diagnostic laboratories to facilitate the high throughput of samples. The speed, accuracy, and efficiency of these activities are often further enhanced using robotic systems that can dispense and aspirate relevant fluids, as well as manipulate multiple plates, simultaneously. In recent years, the application of 96-well microplates and/or miniaturized columns (in 20–600 μl range) in combination with robotics for the rapid screening of chromatographic adsorbents has been documented (Charlton et al., 2006; Friedle, 2008; Hubbuch and Willimann, 2008; Yang, 2012).

Today, a wide range of chromatographic adsorbents has been made available by several manufacturers. Current screening methods for chromatographic adsorbents often include either miniscale batch adsorption or miniaturized column chromatography in a 96-well format. To reduce the burden of tedious or time-consuming manipulations, robotic liquid handling systems have been developed to provide an automated and high throughput screening tool for the identification of promising chromatographic adsorbents and preliminary optimization of chromatographic buffer conditions.

6.5.2.2 Protein Chip Technology The ProteinChip® system comprises biochip arrays and a mass spectrometry-based analytical system integrated with computer software to analyze captured proteins (Brenac et al., 2004). Each array is composed of an aluminum strip on which eight small (~2 mm diameter) "chip" surfaces are affixed. The geometry is such that the chips have the same spacing as the wells in a standard 96-well microplate. The materials on the chip spots are analogous to chromatographic adsorbents. These include the following: ion-exchange (Q type anion and CM type cation), immobilized metal affinity capture (IMAC), HIC, and affinity, each containing eight spots that can bind proteins or peptides from complex mixtures. The spots can then be subjected to buffer washes and elution steps analogous to the approaches used in conventional column chromatography. With rapid microscale chromatographic fractionation followed by detection accomplished through mass spectroscopy, the instrument can be used for the development of protein purification strategies, including selection of chromatographic adsorbents and the optimization of chromatography conditions.

The protein chip technology (SELDI protein chip from CIPHERGEN) has been applied to facilitate the purification process development for several recombinant vaccine antigens (Sanofi Pasteur). As shown in Figure 6.6, a target antigen was tested on a Q-type strong anion exchanger using ProteinChip system. An optimum binding pH of 7.5–8 was found for the target antigen, which can be further eluted at pH 7.5 containing 200 mM NaCl. These conditions were in good agreement with the column chromatography methods using Q-Sepharose. Only 2 days were required for this process development, including all of the extensive screening and optimization

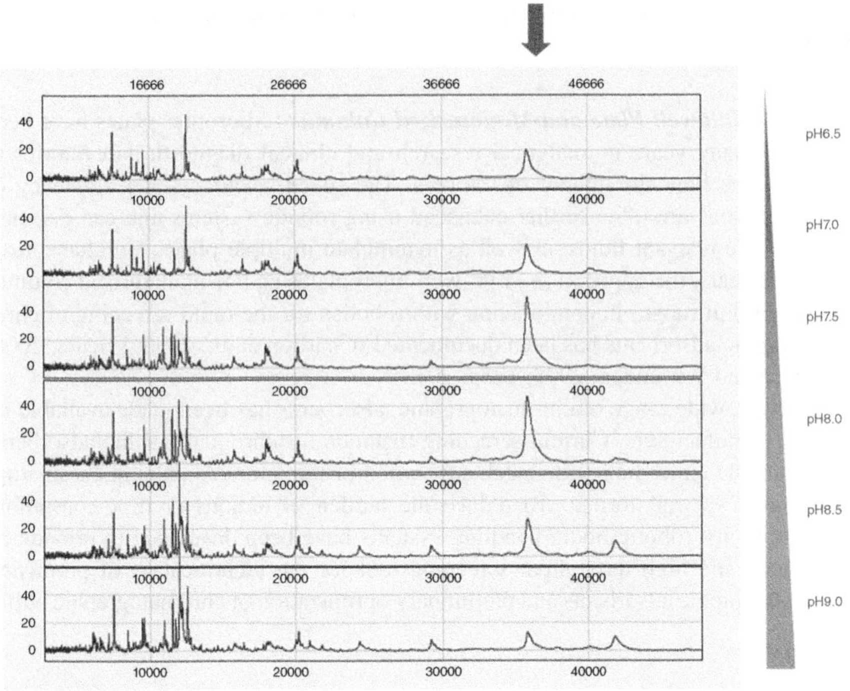

Figure 6.6 pH dependence of target antigen binding to Q-type ProteinChip: the arrow highlights the peak size of the target protein (these results are similar to those found with Q-Sepharose chromatography).

studies. Conventional approaches would have required in the range of 7 weeks of development (i.e., tested on batches or columns).

6.5.2.3 Robotic Liquid Handling System Robotic liquid handling systems (a class of devices that includes automated pipetting systems, as well as microplate washers) have been commonly used in analytical laboratories for years (such as enzyme-linked immunosorbent assay (ELISA)). The robots dispense sample liquids in tubes or wells and are often integrated as automated injection modules. These labor-saving devices offer precision on sample preparation for high throughput screening and sequencing. In recent years, the application of robotic liquid-handling devices in purification process development (e.g., chromatography media scouting) is gaining momentum (Friedle, 2008; Wiendahl et al., 2008; Lye et al., 2009; Yang, 2012).

Tecan Freedom EVO® protein chromatography workstation is one such robotic system available today (Hubbuch and Willimann, 2008; Lye et al., 2009). It is an automated liquid-handling robot with flexible and modular design to suit user's needs. The system consists of two major components: liquid handling arm (LiHa) and robotic manipulator arm (RoMa). LiHa contains eight stainless steel needles to carry out all liquid aspiration and dispensing functions. RoMa is responsible for moving objects from one place to another over the deck. To perform the chromatography function, a shaker and vacuum are also needed to carry out experiments in 96-well filter plates in a batch absorption mode. Te-chrom and Te-shuttle are specially designed for carrying out column chromatography experiments in miniaturized robotic columns. This approach enables fully automated and parallel chromatography, with significant savings on experimental time and materials.

6.5.2.4 Microfluidic Electrophoresis The full benefit of automation and high throughput in purification process development can only be realized when the high throughput analytical testing is in place. The conventional protein analytical methods (e.g., sodium dodecyl sulfate polyacrylamide gel electrophoresis (SDS-PAGE)) became a bottleneck when dealing with a large number of samples. When the volume, speed, and accuracy are paramount, microfluidic electrophoresis technology presents a good alternative.

The LabChip® GX II (Caliper) is one of the microfluidic electrophoresis systems in the market (Caliper LifeSciences Application note 401, 2009). One key component of the instrument is the chip that contains a network of miniaturized microfabricated channels, through which fluids and chemicals are moved to perform experiments. The instrument and software control the movement of fluids via pressure or voltage, and an integrated optical system detects the signals. Each sample acquisition time is less than 40 s, and the instrument can analyze 96 protein samples in less than an hour, eliminating throughput bottlenecks and improving efficiency. The data management suite also allows users to visualize results via an electropherogram or virtual gel view or be exported into a spreadsheet format for further analysis.

6.5.2.5 Case Study Studies were performed to evaluate the feasibility and benefit of applying high throughput technology in the experimental design study of a bacterial protein in support of the development of a protein subunit vaccine (Sanofi Pasteur). In this example, a set of 24 experiments (from experimental design) was performed in parallel using the conventional chromatography system AKTA Explorer (GE Healthcare) with 50-ml packed columns and the robotic Freedom EVO150 (Tecan) with 600-μl RoboColumns™ (Atoll). The results from both systems were analyzed for purity, yield, and step recovery using SDS-PAGE analysis (Bio-Rad) and LabChip® GX II (Caliper) micorfluidic electrophoresis, respectively. A fit model was obtained, which generated a similar trend for the critical operating parameters obtained between the conventional and high throughput approach. However, significant savings on operation time and materials were achieved using the high throughput system. As shown in Table 6.6, it required about 2 months to complete the studies under the conventional approach, whereas only 8 days were required with the application of a high throughput system (Yang, 2012).

6.5.2.6 In-Line Buffer Dilution A typical purification process for proteins requires, on average, 10–20 different buffers. Buffer volume can range from 50 to several hundred liters, depending on the scale. The current paradigm for buffer preparation is to premix and store buffers in tanks. Most of the buffers used in the

TABLE 6.6 Significant Time Saving Using High Throughput System Over Conventional Approach

Equipment Used	Conventional Approach	High Throughput System
Chromatography	AKTA Explorer, 50 ml column	TECAN, 600 μl Rocolumn (Atoll)
Analysis	SDS-PAGE, HPLC	Labchip GXII (96 well), UPLC

Days Required On the basis of 24 Studies)	Conventional Approach	High Throughput System
For experimental runs	50 d	6 d
For sample analysis	8 d	2 d
Total # of days required	58 d	8 d

purification process are of low salt concentration, which can be easily concentrated by 10- to 100-folds. The use of buffer concentrates and in-line dilution technologies will reduce the buffer hold and preparation tank size and result in space/equipment size reduction in both process and utility areas.

Buffer concentrates, coupled with disposable systems can reduce capital and operational investments. Several vendors produce portable, computer-controlled blending and dilution skids of different capacities that are able to accurately and repeatedly dilute concentrates, using piped-in water for injection (WFI), to any desired final blend (Matthews, 2006; Walker, 2006). In addition to the benefits of reducing space/equipment requirements, the in-line buffer dilution technology also provides an excellent application of PAT. With this system, appropriate sensors measure the blend and dilution accuracy in real time. These signals are then used in a two-part control strategy to instantly adjust the blend to compensate for any variability in the concentrate feed and release the precise blend to the process. In this way, continuous validation and real-time release are achieved. The elimination of numerous storage tanks and other equipment enables a 10× or greater increase in capacity from the existing floor space. To implement in-line buffer dilution technology, it is important to understand the potential for pH, conductivity, and temperature shift during buffer dilution. Process robustness related to the accuracy of buffer concentration must be carefully examined as well. In addition, the potential corrosive impact associated with the use of concentrated buffer should not be overlooked.

6.6 APPLICATION OF PROCESS ANALYTICAL TECHNOLOGY IN PROTEIN PURIFICATION

The quality of a pharmaceutical and/or biological product is typically demonstrated by an array of laboratory tests that are performed after completion of manufacturing, and as such, it is too late to make corrections if a batch is out of specification. Both the industry and regulatory agencies have realized that this is not an efficient and cost-effective system to deliver new quality therapeutics to patients in a timely manner. To address these issues, a series of guidelines have been published by FDA and ICH since 2002 with the aim to build a "Quality by Design" (QbD) framework (Rathore and Winkle, 2009). Under the QbD paradigm, product quality is ensured by process understanding and control based on sound science and quality risk management. Through systematic identification and characterization of critical quality attributes and critical process parameters, all critical sources of variability are identified, explained, and controlled by the process. Product quality attributes can then be accurately and reliably predicted over the process design space. Operating within an approved design space is not considered as a change and therefore will not require further regulatory reviews. QbD encourages the use of new technologies, particularly PAT, which advances end-of-manufacturing laboratory testing to in-process, near-line tests, that can monitor and control processes in real time (Rathore and Winkle, 2009; Rathore, 2009; Wu et al., 2011).

According to the Center for Drug Evaluation and Research (CDER) of FDA, PAT is "a system for designing, analyzing, and controlling manufacturing through timely measurements (i.e., during processing) of critical quality and performance attributes of raw and in-process materials and processes with the goal of ensuring final product quality" (FDA Guidance for Industry, 2004). This approach is used to understand and control the manufacturing process because "quality cannot be tested into products; it should be built-in or should be by design." This PAT initiative has been largely embraced by the biopharmaceutical and vaccine industries as demonstrated by a surge in the number of conferences and publications on this subject in recent years (Francois et al., 2009; Rathore et al., 2010; Read et al., 2010).

6.6.1 The PAT Initiatives

The PAT initiative was created by the CDER branch of the US FDA in 2002 and was aimed at providing guidance for employing analytical techniques for producing small molecule pharmaceutical products (FDA Guidance for Industry, 2004). In recent years, PAT processes have become an established tool to promote and improve quality and production efficiencies in the pharmaceutical manufacturing process. The successes of early implementation in small molecule manufacturing processes have led early adopters to explore PAT techniques and processes for potential use in biopharmaceutical products (Larson et al., 2003; Larson and Lam, 2004). It has been demonstrated that the same PAT technology used in traditional pharmaceutical manufacturing can be employed in the manufacturing of biologics with the same positive effect (Rathore et al., 2006; Francois et al., 2009; Rathore et al., 2010; Read et al., 2010). To that end, FDA is now focusing its PAT initiative on biologics manufacturing through its Center for Biologics Evaluation and Research (CBER) and PAT offices (FDA Guidance for Industry, 2004).

Successful PAT programs are defined by a carefully combined application of statistical process control and use of on-line (diverted sample), in-line (inserted probe), at-line (production area testing), or off-line (laboratory testing) instrumentation, capable of measuring key parameters of the manufacturing system in real time.

Downstream processing applications are a specific target for the implementation of PAT processes because this production stage is where the desired product is separated from the complex production matrix, concentrated, identified, quantified, and collected for final processing and formulation.

6.6.2 Current PAT Applications in Downstream Purification Process

A typical protein purification process consists of multiple unit operations, including, but not limited to, column chromatography and membrane filtration. It is important to understand the impact of each purification step on the overall product quality and process consistency. The PAT requirements for each step may be different, and the critical quality attributes of each step needs to be identified. Traditional chemical analyses (e.g., SDS-PAGE, Western blot, and protein assay) during downstream purification manufacturing operations have been performed in off-line laboratories. With the availability of chromatography control instruments and filtration units, many in-line measurements, including UV, conductivity, pH, pressure, and flow rate can be obtained. A summary of major steps in protein purification and their corresponding monitoring systems are shown in Table 6.7.

The purpose of PAT initiatives is to move analytical laboratory functions close to the manufacturing process and improve manufacturing efficiencies and product quality. This can be accomplished by providing real-time support and control of manufacturing processes through analysis of the process stream coupled with statistical process control and tight feedback control loops.

In considering PAT for the downstream process of a biological product, it is important to realize the major differences between an upstream and a downstream process. The cycle time for an upstream step is usually counted in days or hours (e.g., bioreactor or fermentation process), whereas that for a downstream unit operation

TABLE 6.7 Major Steps in Purification and their Corresponding Monitoring

Step	In-Line Monitoring	Off-Line Monitoring
Homogenization/ clarification	Pressure	Viscosity, SDS-PAGE, HPLC
Centrifugation	Speed, centrifugal force, temperature,	SDS-PAGE, HPLC
Viral inactivation	Temperature, duration, (inactivation agent), (virus)	Viral clearance test
Benzonase treatment	Temperature, agitation, duration	DNA content (pico green or qPCR), residual benzonase
Tangential flow filtration	Conductivity, flux, TMP, shear, UV, and concentration factor	pH, conductivity, SDS-PAGE, HPLC
Chromatography	OD, pH, conductivity, pressure, flow rate	pH, conductivity, SDS-PAGE, HPLC

(e.g., fractionation on column chromatography) is based on minutes. In addition, unlike the upstream process, where only a few outputs are expected (e.g., OD or cell mass, and titers of the target molecule), a downstream process produces multiple outputs, including product purity, product yield, residual DNA, host cell impurities, residual endotoxin, and viral clearance. This cycle time requirement (usually <10–15 min) and the need to separate, identify, and characterize the desired product in an often complex matrix, therefore, require precise and high speed instrumentation with high accuracy, reproducibility, and resolving power. The combination of these requirements places limits for on-line PAT instrumentations during the downstream purification. For instance, near-infrared spectroscopy, mass spectroscopy, and liquid chromatography, all of which have been demonstrated as powerful tools in upstream on-line PAT applications, are not suitable for downstream on-line monitoring.

6.6.3 New Downstream Technology Development to Support PAT Implementation

The primary analyses required for downstream processing are molecular identification, quantification, and qualification. The most powerful and useful analytical techniques to consider for such downstream processing in the PAT context are spectroscopy and analytical scale separation methods that can characterize products on a molecular basis. As compared to upstream, the progress of incorporating versatile technologies into PAT on-line applications for vaccine downstream purification has lagged behind because of the reasons described previously.

The use of high performance liquid chromatography (HPLC) as an on-line analytical tool for downstream purification process of proteins has been documented (Cooley, 2003). However, the main drawback of this technique for process characterization appears to be related to the complexity of fully automated HPLC systems and their attendant control processes. These include column switching, fast column equilibration, and high flow systems, all of which are strategies used to reduce cycle times (Barringer, 2006). Recently, there have been new developments for on-line bioanalytical technologies aimed at identification and quantification (GPA1000 Process Analyzer, Groton Biosystems). With a wide range of selections available for in-line, at-line, and off-line analyzers to support purification process control and feedback, the additional benefit of using an on-line analyzer awaits further demonstration.

6.7 DOWNSTREAM PURIFICATION—AN OUTLOOK

In biopharmaceutical industry, downstream processing has recently become a hot topic, with special attention being focused on its constraints and potential bottlenecks (Gottschalk, 2006; Langer, 2007; Pytlik, 2009; Bolton et al., 2011). This is because for over the past 10 years, there have been dramatic improvements of upstream productivity in both mammalian cell culture and bacterial fermentation process (Wurm, 2004; Sofer and Chirica, 2006). Some experts have claimed that the best is yet to come. However, as compared to the increased upstream productivity, improvements

TABLE 6.8 Impact of Increased Upstream Productivity on Downstream

Factors	Upstream	Downstream
Equipment size	Unchanged	Increase
Buffer/media consumption	Unchanged	Increase
Space requirement	Unchanged	Increase
Process time	Unchanged	Increase
Production cost	Unchanged or decreased	Increase

made in downstream purification have not been as impressive. Results from a recent survey of 352 biomanufacturers and CMOs conducted by BioPlan Associates, Inc. indicated that a significant number of companies (68.5%) experienced at least some degree of capacity bottleneck in their facility as a result of downstream process. When asked about where improvements could reduce capacity bottlenecks, the majority (51.4%) expressed needs of "developing better downstream purification technologies" (BioPlan Associates Inc., 2011). Another interesting viewpoint from a 2007 publication (Jagschies and O'Hara, 2007) stated that the true bottleneck is not due to the purification technology available today but related to the inflexibility of available facilities and process designs, regulatory hurdles, and the difficulties in predicting future demands. In any case, as manufacturing bottlenecks shift to downstream processes, the demand for innovation and workable solution in downstream processing has become increasingly clear (Houlton, 2011; Langer, 2011). Many in the industry are asking how to translate upstream success into downstream cost reductions and production improvements.

6.7.1 Impact of Increased Upstream Productivity on Downstream

While upstream and downstream processes may face similar challenges in process scale-up (such as equipment and space requirement, buffer/media consumption, process time, and production cost), the impact of increased productivity is very different on downstream as compared to upstream. This is because the upstream productivity is mainly driven by biological efficiencies. When microbes produce more products per unit of volume space, many upstream scale-up factors remain unchanged, and the relative production cost is most likely to decrease (Table 6.8). In contrast, for a downstream process, productivity is largely driven by engineering efficiencies. Therefore, any increase in biomass produced by upstream would require proportional increases in equipment size, buffer consumptions, space requirement, process time, and production cost for downstream (Table 6.8). While upstream continues to push the limit of microbial systems to increase productivity, downstream scale-up processes are often restricted by its physical requirements, such as equipment size or facility space. To anticipate and overcome this potential downstream bottleneck issue, many suppliers are capitalizing on this opportunity and offering alternative technical solutions.

6.7.2 Current Trends—Suppliers Offer Alternative Technical Solutions

6.7.2.1 Improved Column Design and Packing Chromatography continues to be an essential technology used during the purification of proteins. It is technically feasible to run very large-scale chromatography columns. However, big columns tend to add more technical challenges in terms of column packing, unpacking, and cleaning. To tackle these issues, suppliers have offered various solutions. For example, chromatography columns with improved design and packing have now become available. Packing motors and bed height indicators are offered to deliver constant packing speed for reproducible packing. New designs are being introduced to make column unpacking easier and column cleaning-in-place feasible (e.g., Bio-Rad, GE Healthcare, PALL Life Sciences). In addition, the availability of transfer devices makes it easier for moving chromatography media and cleaning solution between tanks and large columns.

6.7.2.2 New Chromatographic Adsorbents for More Selectivity and Higher Productivity Improvements in upstream feed titers translate into the need for improvements in downstream processing productivity. It has been noted that suppliers continue to develop "second-generation" chromatographic adsorbents with higher flow velocity and binding capacity and with enhanced stability to harsh cleaning and sanitization conditions (Sofer and Chirica, 2006; Sievers, 2011). By combining speed, binding capacity, and reusability features in chromatographic adsorbents, an overall productivity and process economy in downstream can be enhanced.

To create novel interactions and enhance resolution with column chromatography, some suppliers have invented new chromatographic adsorbents having beads with more than one binding chemistry. This has been achieved by introducing new interactions (e.g., HIC) on a media with already one primary interaction (e.g., ionic exchange) to produce multimodal (e.g., GE Healthcare) or mixed-mode (e.g., PALL Life Sciences) chromatographic adsorbents. Such new adsorbents provide a broader base for selection and may allow users to more successfully separate proteins that have very similar properties.

6.7.2.3 Single-Use, Disposable System Is Entering Mainstream of Bioprocessing As discussed in Section 6.5, single-use, disposable systems have been widely accepted for bioprocessing. In the purification of a protein subunit vaccine, the main applications of disposable systems include single-use disposable bags for buffer or intermediate product storage, single-use depth filters for product clarification, disposable sterile connectors and clean room technology, disposable membrane adsorption chromatography for the (polishing) removal of endotoxin, DNA, or host cell proteins, and pre-packed columns (RepliGen) or Ready to Process disposable columns (GE Healthcare) for purification. To continue pushing disposable systems into the mainstream of bioprocessing, suppliers are actively developing new materials that would ensure better mechanical integrity of the disposable systems, reduce sources of leaks, contamination, and product loss because of protein adsorption. Other areas of disposable system development pursued by suppliers include new sensor technology, validation of sensors, and integration of sensors into process control systems (Wong, 2007). Single-use sensors are currently available but are new to bioprocess requirements. The challenge will be to demonstrate sensors that are not adversely affected by sterilization required for bioprocessing.

6.7.3 Innovative Technologies in Protein Purification

6.7.3.1 Continuous Process In recent years, continuos process has attracted lots of attention in the field of biomanufacturing, which is reflected by the significant number of industrial and academic researchers who are actively involved in the development of continuous bioprocessing systems (Cooney and Konstantinov, 2014). These efforts are further encouraged by guidance expressed in recent FDA conference presentations (Woodcock, 2011, 2014). The advantages of continuous process include reduced equipment size, flexible production scale, high volumetric productivity, consistent product quality, streamlined process flow, low cycle times and reduced capital cost.

Today, various small- and pilot-scale continuous chromatography systems are offered by several equipment manufacturers, such as Novasep, Tarpon, Semba, GE Healthcare, and ChromaCon, etc. In addition to these sophisticated systems, the idea of a continuous chromatography system using a disposable Rotary Drum Filter presented by Steadfast Equipment Inc. also looks intriguing (Kossik, 2003). The design combines conventional batch adsorption, disposable filter, and the concept of chromatography in a continuous mode. The process starts in a batch adsorption tank containing feed material and chromatographic beads. The separation of product from impurities is achieved through a series of steps, including (i) continuously feeding the adsorbed bead suspension into a disposable rotary drum filter, a continuous solid/liquid separation device, (ii) the unbound impurities in the supernatant are removed, (iii) the beads with bound product are pumped to a tank containing deadsorption buffer, (iv) separation of the eluted product from beads is achieved in the same manner in a second disposable rotary drum filter (Fig. 6.7). Although a number of considerations must be accounted for before using this technology as a continuous chromatography system, the idea of having a chromatography system that can be operated in a simple, continuous, and disposable mode, and that can potentially process large amounts of feed material using a relatively small device, holds great promise.

6.7.3.2 Closed System Unlike upstream processes, where microbes or cells are cultured in a closed sterile environment, most downstream purification processes are open operations. With increasing regulatory scrutiny toward well-controlled processes and quality products, there is a desire to move downstream separation processes toward closed systems, particulary in the continuous capturing and/or column chromatography where the process could be run in weeks or months. Although this approach does not completely eliminate the need for a final sterile filtration step, a closed downstream process would reduce risks of bioburden and contamination of purified products, and thereby enhance product quality. With

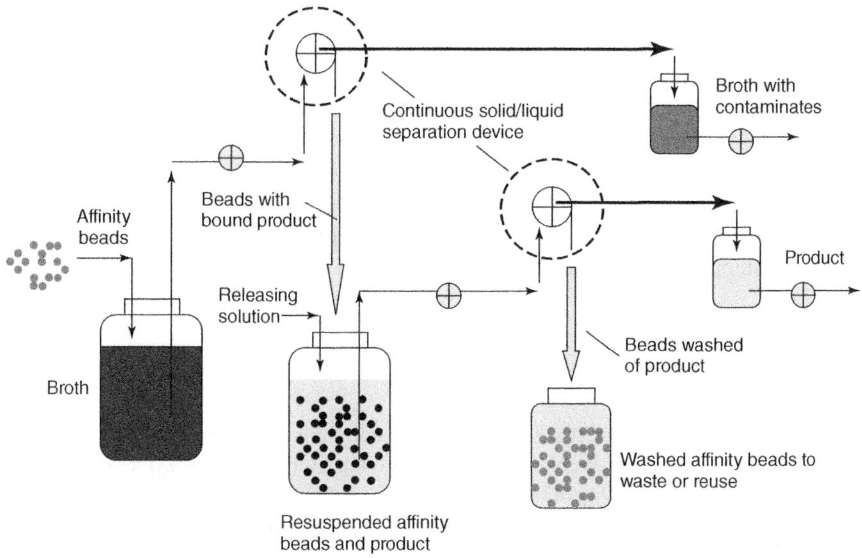

Figure 6.7 Continuous protein purification system centered on the use of disposable continuous solid/liquid separation device (Kossik, 2003). Reproduced with permission from John Kossik, Steadfast Equipment Inc.

rapid technology advancements in disposable bag technologies, sterile connectors, tube welders, single-use filters, membranes, and columns, a completely closed downstream purification process connecting the upstream harvest to the further downstream of product formulation and filling is waiting to be explored.

6.7.4 Protein Subunit Vaccine Purification—Outlook

A clear trend in protein purification is to develop simple, automated, and scalable processes with the least numbers of unit operations possible. Continued efforts are made to combine steps (e.g., combining clarification and capturing steps into one using suspended adsorption technology), to reduce the need for staging tanks or hold-up volumes between unit operations through system connections (i.e. continuous processing), and to apply standardized unit operations (platform technology) in polishing (e.g., removal of DNA, virus, or endotoxin). Any new technology development or innovative solution to support this goal would greatly advance the field.

Process understanding is the key toward a well-controlled and reproducible process in protein subunit vaccine purification, which eventually leads to the path of QbD. Process analytical technology will, no doubt, play an important role in helping us to reach this goal. Although many in-line, off-line, and at-line tools are available for the implementation of PAT in purification, an innovative, easy-to-use, and effective online sensor or device that enables real-time purification process measure and feedback requires further development.

There is a clear desire in vaccine purification to use computer software to effectively capture and analyze processing data, to identify areas for improvement in productivity and process economy at an earlier stage, and to facilitate technology transfer from process development to industrialization. The benefits of using computer-assisted data analysis, decision-making, and technology transfer are only to be realized further in the years to come.

Over the coming years, the development and integration of these new technologies in downstream purification will greatly enhance the productivity, quality, consistency, and cost effectiveness for vaccine development and production.

REFERENCES

Armstrong N, Lencastre AD, Gouaux E. A new protein folding screen: application to the ligand binding domains of a glutamate and kainite receptor and to lysozyme and carbonic anhydrase. Prot Sci 1999;8:1475–1483.

Baillargeon MW, Ross D A, Eisenhauer D, and Lundell EO. 2003. Hydrophobic interaction chromatography: determination of critical process parameters using design of experimental methodology. The 225th American Chemical Society (ACS) National Meeting; March 23–27; New Orleans, LA. 2003.

Barringer G. Downstream process optimization opportunities using on-line and at-line PAT instrumentation. BioPharm Int 2006;June Suppl:38–41.

BioPlan Associates Inc. Eighth annual report and survey of biopharmaceutical manufacturing capacity and production. BioPlan Associates, Inc. 2011 ISBN 978-1-934106-21-1. 2011.

Blank GS, Zapata G, Fahrner R, Milton M, Yedinak C, Knudsen H, Schmelzer C. Expanded bed adsorption in the purification of monoclonal antibodies: a comparison of process alternatives. Bioseparation 2001;10:65–71.

Boehm J, Dixit M, Hodge G, Jagschies G, Krishnan M, Martin J. Single-use bioprocessing equipment. BioPharm Int Suppl 2009;Sep 18. Available at: http://www.biopharminternational.com/biopharm/Biopharm+Business/Single-Use-Bioprocessing-Equipment/ArticleStandard/Article/detail/627768.

Bolton GR, Violand BN, Wright RS, Sun S, Sunasara KM, Waltson K, Coffman JL, Gallo C, Godavarti R. Addressing the challenges in downstream processing today and tomorrow. BioPharm Int Suppl 2011;24(4):s8–s15.

Breece TN, Gilkerson E, Schmelzer C. Validation of large-scale chromatographic processes, Part 1: case study of neuleze capture on Macroprep High-S. BioPharm Int 2002a;5:6–20.

Breece TN, Gilkerson E, Schmelzer C. Validation of large-scale chromatographic processes, Part 2: results from the case study of neuleze capture on Macroprep High-S. BioPharm Int 2002b;7:35–42.

Brenac V, Santambien P, Egrot C. RC-SELDI-MS: ProteinChip® platform expression monitorint, impurity tracking. Ciphergen BioSepra Process division. 2004.

Brummelhuis HGJ. Preparation of the prothrombin complex. In: Curling JM, editor. *Methods of Plasma Protein Fractionation*. London: Academic Press; 1980. p 117–128.

Caliper LifeSciences Application note 401. A novel approach to automated high-throughput protein enrichment and characterization. LCGX-AP-401. 2009.

Charlton H, Galarza B, Leriche K, Jones R. Chromatography process development using 96-well microplate formats. BioPharm Int 2006;June suppl:20–42.

Chen G-Q, Gouaux E. Overexpression of a glutamate receptor (GluR2) ligand binding domain in *Escherichia coli*: Application of a novel protein folding screen. Proc Natl Acad Sci U S A 1997;94:13431–13436.

Cooley RE. 2003. Utilizing PAT to monitor and control bulk technology processes; March 4; Eli Lilly and Co: University of Michigan Pharmaceutical Engineering Seminars; 2003.

Cooney C, and Konstantinov K. Continuous bioprocessing. White paper 4. MIT-CMAC International Symposium on Continuous Manufacturing of Pharmaceuticals. Available at: http://iscmp.mit.edu/white-papers.

Cunningham E, Myers D, Bork C, and Conley L. Evaluating chromatography process variability using design of experiments. The 225th American Chemical Society (ACS) National Meeting; March 23–27; New Orleans, LA, 2003.

DePalma A. Disposables win downstream acceptance. Gen Eng News 2007;27(3):34–36.

Eon-Duval A, Gumbs K, Ellett C. Precipitation of RNA impurity with high salt in a plasmid DNA purification process: use of experimental design to determine reaction conditions. Biotech Bioeng 2003;83:544–553.

Eppink M, Schreurs R, Gijsen A, Verhoeven K. Downstream processing: platform technology for developing purification processes. BioPharm Int 2007;20(3):44–50.

FDA Guidance for Industry. PAT—A framework for innovative pharmaceutical development, manufacturing, and quality assurance. Available at: www.fda.gov/cder/OPS/PAT.html. 2004.

Finnfeeds F, Paananen H, Kuisma J, Heikkila H, Ravanko V, Lewandowski J, Karki A. A simulated moving bed system and process. Publication Number: WO/2004/076021. 2004.

Francois K, Streefland M, Vangenechten R, Hammendorp L. Integration of PAT in biopharmaceutical research: a case study. Pharm Technol (online) 2009;July 33(7).

Friedle J. Chromatography media scouting. Euro Biotech News 2008;7(5–6):41–42.

Gilliot FP, Gleason C, Wilson JJ, Zwarick J. Fluidized bed adsorption for whole broth extraction. Biotechnol Prog 1990;6:370–375.

Gottschalk U. The renaissance of protein purification. BioPharm Int 2006;June suppl:8–9.

Grönberg A, Monié E, Murby M, Rodrigo G, Wallby E, Johansson HJ. A Strategy for developing a monoclonal antibody purification platform. BioProcess Int 2007;5:48–54.

Halley F. 2006. Pertinence offers solutions to maximize vaccine production. General manager Frederic Halley talks to Pharma DD. Excluisive conference coverage. PHarma DD Track Discovery and Development, August. 2006.

Hardy J. Considerations for use of disposable technology in contract manufacturing. Biopharmaceutical Manufacturing Development Summit; 6–7 December 2006; Orlando, FL; Westborough, MA: IBC Life Sciences; 2006.

Hart R. Use of statistically designed experiments in developing a purification process for a family of monoclonal antibodies. IBC's 3rd International Conference on Recovery & Purification; November 18–19; San Diego; 2002.

Hart RA, Ogez JR, Builder SE. Use of multifactorial analysis to develop aqueous two–phase systems for isolation of non-native IGF-I. Bioseparation 1995;5:113–121.

Hill C, Sinclair A. Process development: maximizing process data from development to manufacturing. BioPharm Int 2007;20:38–42.

Houlton S. A world of innovation. BioProcess Int 2011;9(6):10–14.

Hubbuch J, Willimann E. Chromatography on Tecan Freedom EVO® robotic workstations. BioProcess Int Indust Yearbook 2008:104–105.

Imamoglu S. Simulated moving bed chromatography (SMB) for application in bioseparation. Adv Biochem Eng Biotechnol 2002;76:211–231.

Jagschies G, O'Hara A. Debunking downstream bottleneck myth. Genetic Eng Biotech News 2007;27(14):62–64.

Jagschies G, Gronberg A, Bjorkman T, Lacki K, Johansson HJ. Technical and economical evaluation of downstream processing options for monoclonal antibody (Mab) production. BioPharm Int 2006;June Suppl:10–19.

Kelly BD. Establishing process robustness using designed experiments. In: Sofer G, Zabriskie DW, editors. *Biopharmaceutical Process Validation*. New York: Marcel Dekker; 2000. p 29–59.

Kelley BD, Jennings P, Wright R, Briasco C. Demonstrating process robustness for chromatography purification of a recombinant protein. BioPharm Int 1997;10:36–47.

Knudsen HL, Fahrner RL, Xu Y, Norling LA, Blank GS. Membrane ion-exchange chromatography for process-scale antibody purification. J Chromatogr A 2001;907(1–2):145–154.

Kossik J. New continuous chromatography options in the manufacturing of biopharmaceuticals. PREPTECH 2003 Process Scale Separation Technology in the Manufacturing of (Bio)-Pharmaceuticals; July 7–9; Germany: Dorint Hotel, Quellenhof, AACHEN; 2003.

Langer ES. Downstream production challenges in 2007. BioProcess Int 2007;6:22–28.

Langer ES. Alleviating downstream process bottlenecks. Genetic Eng Biotech News 2011; 31(13):1.

Larson TM, Lam H. Process analytical technology in biopharmaceutical production: past successes and future challenges. J Process Anal Technol 2004;1:20–22.

Larson TM, Davis J, Lam H, Cacia J. Use of process data to assess chromatographic performance in production-scale protein purification columns. Biotechnol Prog 2003;19: 485–492.

Leonard MW, Sefton L, Costigan R, Shi L, Hubbard B, Bonam D, Kelly BD, Foster B, Charlebois T. Validation of the recombinant coagulation factor IX purification process for the removal of host cell DNA. In: Kelly BD, Ramelmeier RS, editors. *Validation of Biopharmaceutical Manufacturing Processes*. ACS Symp Ser No. 698. Washington DC: American Chemical Society; 1998. p 55–68.

Liddell JM. 2002. Refolding process development—doing more with less. IBC's 3rd International Conference on Recovery & Purification, November 18–19; San Diego; 2002.

LoMonaco J, Rumsey T. The economics of single-use systems: a media prep ROI analysis. BioProcess Int 2006;4:64–68.

Luyben KCAM, Tramper J. Optimal design for continuous stirred tank reactors in series using Michaelis-Menten kinetics. Biotechnol Bioeng 2004;24:1217–1220.

Lye G, Hubbuch J, Schroeder T, Willimann E. Shrinking the costs of bioprocess development. BioProcess Int 2009;Oct Suppl:2–5.

Martin-Moe S, Ellis J, Coan M, Victor R, Savage J, Bogren N, Leng B, Lee C, Burnett M, Montgomery P. Validation of critical process input parameters in the production of protein pharmaceutical products: a strategy for validating new processes or revalidating existing processes. PDA J Pharma Sci Technol 2000;54:315–319.

Matthews T. Inline dilution of buffer concentrates and bioprocess bags: an integrated approach. Biopharmaceutical Manufacturing Development Summit; 6–7 December 2006; Orlando, FL. Westborough, MA: IBC Life Sciences; 2006.

Morris K, Venugopal S, Eckstut M. Making the most of drug development data. PharmaManufacturing 2005;4(10):16–23.

Parenteral Drug Association. Industry perspective on the validation of column-based separation process for the purification of proteins. J Parenteral Sci and Technol 1992;46:87–97.

Prashad M, Tarrach K. Depth filtration: cell clarification of bioreactor offloads. Filtr Sep 2006;43(7):28–30.

Pytlik W.. Downstream processing: bottleneck purification process. BIOPRO Baden-Württemberg GmbH; July 30; 2009.

Quinones-GarcaI I, Rayner I, Rayner I, Levison PR, Dickson N, Purdom G. Performance comparison of suspended bed and batch contactor chromatography. J Chromatogr A 2001;908:169–178.

Rathore AS. Roadmap for implementation of quality by design (QbD) for biotechnology products. Trends Biotechnol 2009;27(9):546–53.

Rathore AS, Winkle H. Quality by design for biopharmaceuticals. Nat Biotechnol 2009; 27(1):26–34.

Rathore AS, Bhambure R, Ghare V. Process analytical technology (PAT) for biopharmaceutical products. Anal Bioanal Chem 2010;398(1):137–154.

Rathore AS, Sharma A, Chilin D. Applying process analytical technology to biotech unit operations. BioPharm Int 2006;19:48–57.

Read EK, Park JT, Shah RB, Riley BS, Brorson KA, Rathore AS. Process analytical technology (PAT) for biopharmaceutical products: Part I. concepts and applications. Biotechnol Bioeng 2010;105(2):276–284.

Reichert JM. Trends in development and approval times for new therapeutics in the United States. Nature Reviews Drug Discovery 2003;2(9):695–703.

Santambien P, Voute N, Schapman A, Ravault V, Boschetti E. Effective protein capture in fluidized-bed mode with zirconia-based beads. BioProcess Int 2003;10:46–59.

Seely JE, Seely RJ. A rational, step-wise approach to process characterization. BioPharm Int 2003;8:24–34.

Sievers D. Chromatographic purification in downstream processing: new sorbents and membranes for process chromatography. BioProcess Int Industry Yearbook 2011–2012. 2011;9(7):74–76.

Sofer G. 1996. Validation: ensuring the accuracy of scaled-down chromatography models BioPharm Int 10:51-54.

Sofer G, Chirica LC. Improving productivity in downstream processing. BioPharm Int 2006;19:48–55.

Strohlein G, Aumann L, Muller-Spath T, Tarafder A, Morbidelli M. The multicolumn countercurrent solvent gradient purification process. Biopharm Int 2007;Feb Suppl 10:42–48.

Subramani HJ, Hidajat K, Ray SK. Optimization of simulated moving bed and varicol processes for glucose-fructose separation. Chem Eng Res Design 2003;81:549–567.

Sutherland K. Filtration overview: a close look at depth filtration. Filtr Sep 2008;45(8):25–28.

Terry JW and Thor G. Biodisposables utility and technological advances. D&MD publications; 2006.

Torbeck LD, Branning RC. Designed experiments—a vital role in validation. Pharm Technol 1996;6:108–114.

Valdes R, Gomez L, Padilla S, Brito J, Reyes B, Alvarez T, Mendoza O, Herrera O, Ferro W, Pujol M, Leal V, Linares M, Hevia Y, Garcia C, Mila L, Garcia O, Sanchez R, Acosta A, Geada D, Paez R, Luis Vega J, Borroto C. Large-scale purification of an antibody directed against hepatitis B surface antigen from transgenic tobacco plants. Biochem and Biophys Res Commun 2003;308:94–100.

Verschuren ILM, Wijers JG, Keurentjes JTF. Effect of mixing on product quality in semibatch stirred tank reactors. AlChE J 2004;47:1731–1739.

Walker J. In-line buffer dilution: the "killer App" for process analytical technology. BioProcess Int 2006;4:66.

Wankat PC. Systems and processes for performing separations using a simulated moving bed apparatus. US patent 6740243. May 25 2004.

Wiendahl M, Schulze Wierling P, Nielsen J, Fomsgaard Christensen D, Krarup J, Staby A, Hubbuch J. High throughput screening for the design and optimization of chromatographic processes—miniaturization, automation and parallelization of breakthrough and elution studies. Chem Eng Technol 2008;31(6):893–903.

Winkler ME. Purification issues. In: Sofer G, Zabriskie DW, editors. *Biopharmaceutical Process Validation*. New York: Marcel Dekker; 2000. p 143–155.

Woodcock J. FDA-the next 25 years. AAPS Oct 2011. Available at: http://www.aaps.org/Career_Center/Professional_Development/2011_AAPS_Annual_Meeting_and_Exposition_Webcasts/

Woodcock J. Modernizing Pharmaceutical Manufacturing—Continuous Manufacturing as a Key Enabler. MIT-CMAC International Symposium on Continuous Manufacturing of Pharmaceuticals, May 20–21, 2014. Available at: http://iscmp.mit.edu/white-papers.

Wong R. Conceiving a totally disposable process for upstream and downstream processing. Sixth Annual Biological Production Forum. World Trade Group; March 27–28; Berlin, Germany; 2007.

Wu H, White M, Khan MA. Quality-by-Design (QbD): an integrated process analytical technology (PAT) approach for a dynamic pharmaceutical co-precipitation process characterization and process design space development. Int J Pharm 2011;405(1–2):63–78.

Wurm FM. Production of recombinant protein therapeutics in cultivated mammalian cells. Nature Biotechnol 2004;22:1393–1398.

Yang YP. Accelerate protein-based vaccine purification development using high throughput technology. BTI's 5th Annual Protein and Peptide Conference 2012; March 23–25; Beijing; 2012.

Zhou JX, Tressel T, Guhan S. Disposable chromatography. BioPharm Int 2007;Feb Suppl 10: 26–35.

7

CONJUGATE VACCINE PRODUCTION TECHNOLOGY

SUDHA CHENNASAMUDRAM AND WILLIE F. VANN

Laboratory of Bacterial Polysaccharides, Office of Vaccine Research and Review, Center for Biologics Evaluations and Research, Bethesda, MD, USA

7.1 CONJUGATE VACCINE PRODUCTION TECHNOLOGY

Many pathogenic bacteria are encapsulated with polysaccharides and require the presence of this capsule for virulence. It has been demonstrated that serum antibody against these polysaccharides is protective against diseases caused by *Haemophilus influenzae, Neisseria meningitidis, Streptococcus pneumoniae,* and *Salmonella typhi*. These observations are the basis for the development of polysaccharide-based vaccines against infectious diseases caused by these encapsulated pathogens. Vaccines against these organisms were first prepared and used as purified polysaccharides and recently as polysaccharides conjugated to a carrier protein. The polysaccharide vaccines currently licensed for use in the United States are listed in Table 7.1. Although polysaccharides were effective in reducing the incidence of disease in adults and are relatively straightforward to be produced as vaccines, they have a number of immunological disadvantages. The problems associated with polysaccharide vaccines have been well described and include the age dependence of the immune response, lack of boosting, and limited persistence of protection. They are not useful as vaccines in the infants and young children (Makela et al., 1977; Parke et al., 1977; Peltola et al., 1977) who are often the population with highest incidence of certain diseases caused by encapsulated pathogens (Fothergill and Wright, 1933).

It is well established that conjugation of polysaccharides or oligosaccharides derived from capsular polysaccharides changes the nature of immune response to the

Vaccine Development and Manufacturing, First Edition.
Edited by Emily P. Wen, Ronald Ellis, and Narahari S. Pujar.

TABLE 7.1 Currently Licensed Polysaccharide Vaccines in the United States

Vaccine	Manufacturer	Composition
PneumoVax	Merck	23 pneumococcal polysaccharides
Menomune	Sanofi	Meningococcal types A, C, Y, W-135 polysaccharides
Typhim Vi	Sanofi	Vi polysaccharide

polysaccharide antigen (Avery and Goebel, 1929). Vaccines prepared on the basis of this concept of conjugation do not have the disadvantages described previously for polysaccharide vaccines. In general, conjugate vaccines induce much higher antibody levels, have greater efficacy, and induce serum bactericidal antibody in infants and children and a booster response.

Consequently, several polysaccharide conjugate vaccines are the subject of public health success stories. Most notable among these are the *H. influenzae* type b conjugates (Robbins et al., 1996) and the heptavalent pneumococcal conjugate vaccine (Lexau et al., 2005; Whitney et al., 2003; Sinha et al., 2007).

Conjugate vaccines against *H. influenzae* type b designed by Schneerson, Barrera, Sutton, and Robbins (Schneerson et al., 1980) consisted of purified Hib polysaccharide coupled to diphtheria toxoid. This polysaccharide conjugate technology was adapted by Connaught for coupling to diphtheria toxoid to develop the first licensed conjugate vaccine against *Haemophilus* disease. Subsequent variation in conjugation procedure by other investigators and pharmaceutical manufacturers lead to the development of four licensed vaccines against *Haemophilus* disease (see Table 7.2). The public health impact of these vaccines was dramatic, resulting in a decrease in the incidence of Hib disease. In an efficacy and safety study performed by Connaught laboratories (Fritzell and Plotkin, 1992), 100,000 infants were evaluated. After three doses, 98% of infants showed antibody response. Significant increase of PRP polyribosyl-ribitol-phosphate, (*H. influenzae* type b capsular polysaccharide) antibody titer after the second and third dose was noted, indicating that immunologic memory was effectively established through the T-cell-dependent behavior of conjugate vaccine.

Conjugate vaccines are chemically complex. Their design is partly based on our knowledge of carbohydrate chemistry and of the immune response to carbohydrate

TABLE 7.2 Hib Conjugate Vaccines Licensed in the United States

Vaccine	Conjugate Composition	Manufacturer
ProHIBit	Hib polysaccharide—Diphtheria toxoid	Connaught
HibTITER	Hib oligosaccharide—CRM197	Lederle-Praxis
ActHIB	Hib polysaccharide—tetanus toxoid	Sanofi Pasteur
PedvaxHIB	Hib polysaccharide—meningococcal outer membrane proteins	Merck

antigens. Analogous to other complex biologics, the consistent manufacture of these products and their predictability are of utmost importance. This consistency in manufacturing affords vaccines that invite confidence in their continued efficacy and makes the review of vaccine manufacturing by regulatory authorities more straightforward. The manufacture of a conjugate vaccine can be divided into four stages: (i) preparation of antigen and carrier protein, (ii) activation of the polysaccharide and/or protein, (iii) coupling for the activated components, and (iv) characterization of intermediates and conjugated drug substance. These stages in the context of licensed protein polysaccharide conjugate vaccines are discussed, while mentioning some vaccines not licensed in the United States to illustrate certain concepts.

7.2 PREPARATION OF ANTIGEN AND CARRIER PROTEIN

Although there has been much work on the development of synthetic routes for bacterial carbohydrate antigens (Hoogerhout et al., 1988; Peeters et al., 1992; Pozsgay, 1998; Thijssen et al., 1998), most conjugate vaccines are prepared from polysaccharides isolated from bacterial cultures. Thus, the bulk polysaccharides previously used to formulate licensed vaccines have been used as feeder stocks for conjugate vaccine synthesis. The polysaccharide is purified to specification suitable for formulation of vaccines. In most cases, the polysaccharide is either used as is or converted to the desired size for use in aqueous solution. In one case, the Hib polysaccharide is converted to an alkylammonium salt to facilitate the activation reaction in a nonaqueous solvent (Marburg et al., 1986).

The carrier protein may be activated before coupling by the introduction of reactive function groups such as thiols or hydrazides. In some cases, the carrier protein is used in the conjugation reaction without prior derivatization.

7.3 POLYSACCHARIDE SIZE

One of the key characteristics of a conjugate vaccine is its size. The size of the conjugate and the oligosaccharide or polysaccharide coupled to the carrier protein appears to be an important determinant of vaccine potency (Dintzis et al., 1989; Paoletti et al., 1992; Szu et al., 1989; Bardotti et al., 2005). The optimal size varies with the conjugate. One advantage of adjusting the size of the starting polysaccharide is that it allows separation of unreacted polysaccharide from the final conjugate. The conjugation product is larger than the size reduced and activated polysaccharide and can usually be separated by size-exclusion chromatography from the unreacted polysaccharide or oligosaccharides. For currently licensed conjugate vaccines, there are three methods in use to reduce the size of the polysaccharide before coupling: (i) acid hydrolysis, (ii) periodate oxidation, and (iii) depolymerization with hydrogen peroxide. Adequate methods for monitoring the depolymerization reaction and termination of the reaction at the desired size should be established when size-reduced polysaccharide is used as an intermediate in conjugate preparation. Negatively charged oligosaccharides are monitored by ion-exchange chromatography (Costantino et al., 1999; Ravenscroft et al., 1999); however, size is most frequently monitored by high-performance liquid chromatography (HPLC) size-exclusion chromatography (Bardotti et al., 2008). Since the HPLC methods are rapid, they can be used to monitor the end point for depolymerization.

Polysaccharides that are size reduced by periodate oxidation are cleaved as a result of the activation process (Anderson et al., 1986). This approach has been used for the synthesis of conjugates prepared with the *H. influenzae type* b (Anderson et al., 1986) and meningococcal group C polysaccharide. In both cases, each oxidation of the repeat unit results in a cleavage of the chain because of the location of vicinal hydroxyls in the repeat unit (see Fig. 7.1). Thus, the chain length is controlled by the stoichiometry of the reaction, that is, ratio of periodate to the repeat unit. A combination of controlling reaction conditions and modern purification techniques can yield a relatively tight range of depolymerized polysaccharide. A second approach is mild acid hydrolysis (Bardotti et al., 2005; Costantino et al., 1999), which can be somewhat selective if the repeat unit contains a linkage that is much more acid labile than its neighboring residues. One disadvantage of this method is the loss of acid labile substituents that may be important for immunogenicity, such as fucose or sialic acid present on branching sites. The presence or absence of these labile groups can be readily detected by NMR (Jones, 2005; Lemercinier and Jones, 1996).

The third method takes advantage of the observation of several investigators that polysaccharides such as dextran or hyaluronan could be degraded by exposure to hydrogen peroxide (Christensen et al., 1996; Miller, 1986). This method is also the activation process for the polysaccharide. These authors observed the appearance of reducing ends in the presence of hydrogen peroxide. One disadvantage of this procedure is the potential for the hydrogen peroxide reactions with saccharides to change in the presence of metals (Christensen et al., 1996; Blattner and Ferrier, 1985; Isbells et al., 1975). Thus, metal ion contaminants have the potential to influence the outcome of the activation reaction. Meningococcal group C polysaccharide has been degraded using this method before conjugation (Cai et al., 2004). These authors used mass spectrometry data to support the suggestion that the meningococcal group C polysaccharide was cleaved by hydrogen peroxide without alteration of the reducing end sialic acid.

Although size reduction of the polysaccharide before activation or conjugation is useful, it is not essential. Some conjugate vaccines have been prepared directly from purified polysaccharide. The first Hib–diphtheria toxoid conjugate, the Hib–tetanus toxoid conjugate, and Hib outer membrane vesicle are prepared from Hib polysaccharide without prior size reduction.

7.3.1 Carrier Protein

Some common carrier proteins used in licensed conjugate vaccines are tetanus toxoid, diphtheria toxoid, diphtheria toxin CRM_{197} (Uchida et al., 1973), and outer membrane proteins of *Neisseria meningtitidis* group B. Diphtheria and tetanus toxoids are attractive as carrier because they are components of licensed vaccines. The bulk

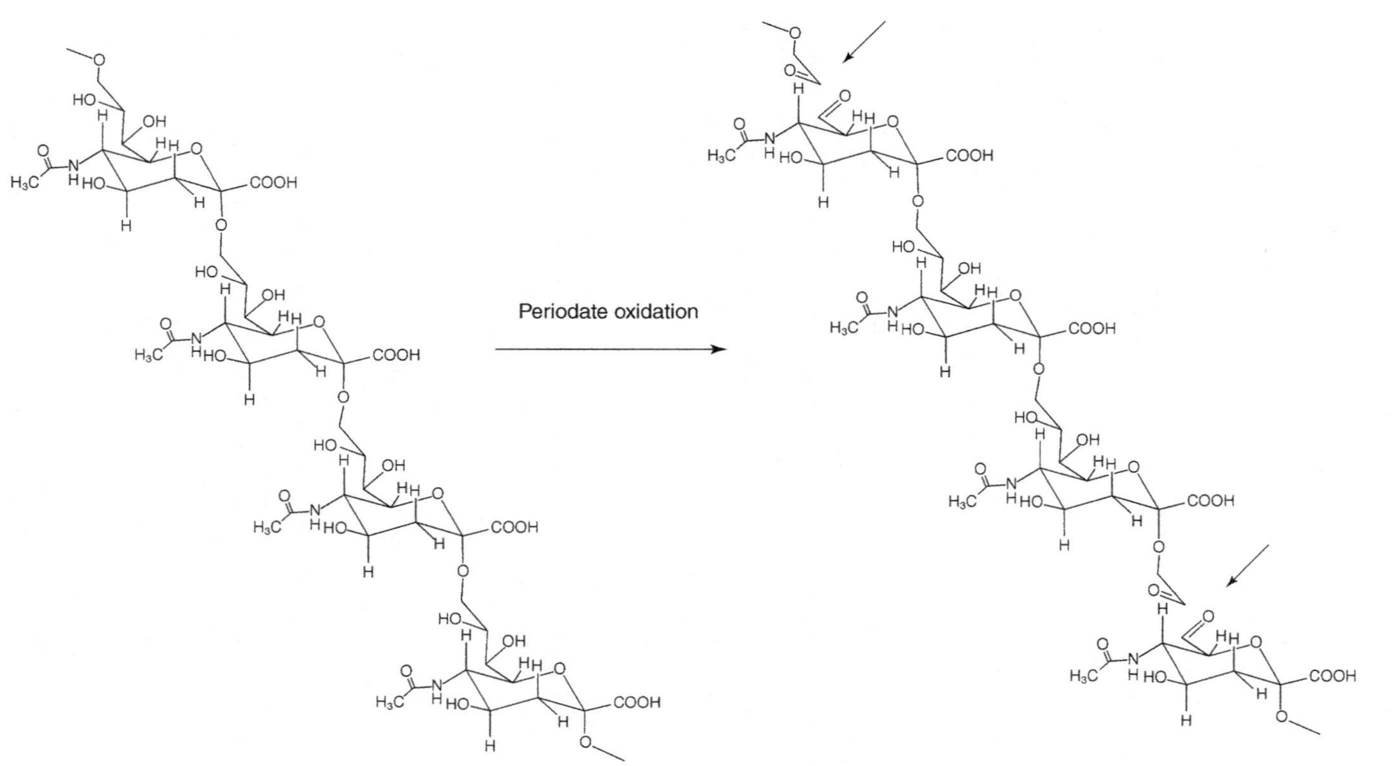

N. meningitidis Group C polysaccharide

Figure 7.1 Activation and cleavage of a polysaccharide by periodate oxidation.

toxoid intermediates of these vaccines are used in some case as starting materials for the preparation of conjugates.

7.3.1.1 Tetanus Toxoid Tetanus toxin, isolated from *Clostridium tetani* has a molecular weight of 150 kDa (Robinson and Hash, 1982). It consists of two polypeptide chains with molecular weights of 53 and 107 kDa, respectively (Matsuda and Yoneda, 1975), which are covalently linked by a disulfide bridge (Krieglstein et al., 1990). Before its use in vaccines, the toxin is converted into nontoxic toxoid by treatment with formaldehyde (Anderson et al., 2007). Tetanus toxoid is used as the carrier protein in the HiB conjugate vaccine, ActHiB. ActHIB is the only licensed vaccine so far to use tetanus toxoid as the carrier protein. Other vaccines with tetanus toxoid as carrier protein are still being evaluated. For example, in a Phase 1 clinical study of meningococcal group A–tetanus toxoid conjugate vaccine, in healthy Indian adults, the vaccine seemed to be safe and immunogenic (Kshirsagar et al., 2007).

7.3.1.2 Diphtheria Toxoid Diphtheria toxin is released extracellularly by *Cornyebacterium diphtheriae* as a single polypeptide chain of 62 kDa (Uchida et al., 1973). It is composed of two fragments, A and B. Both are required in vaccine preparations. Diphtheria toxin is also treated with formaldehyde to make a nontoxic toxoid (Aggerbeck and Heron, 1992). ProHIBit, the first Hib conjugate vaccine licensed in the United States, used diphtheria toxoid as the carrier protein. Diphtheria toxoid is also used as carrier protein in Menactra, a conjugate vaccine against meningococcal serogroups A, C, Y, and W135.

7.3.1.3 Diphtheria Toxin CRM_{197} This protein is a mutant of diphtheria toxin (Rappuoli, 1983; Uchida et al., 1973) with a single missense mutation changing glycine 52 to glutamic acid within the fragment A region of the toxin (Giannini et al., 1984). This nontoxic mutant is antigenically indistinguishable from native toxin and is an advantageous candidate for carrier proteins, as no formaldehyde treatment is needed. CRM_{197} has been shown to be as immunogenic as diphtheria toxoid (Cryz et al., 1980). CRM_{197} is the carrier protein in the Hib conjugate vaccine, HIBTITER, and in the heptavalent pneumococcal conjugate vaccine, Prevnar.

7.3.1.4 Outer Membrane Proteins of* Neisseria meningitidis *Group B The meningococcal outer membrane contains a number of proteins that are divided into five classes on the basis of their molecular weight (Tsai et al., 1981). Frasch et al. showed that monoclonal antibodies against serotype 2 proteins are bactericidal. Class 1 proteins have a molecular weight of approximately 46 kDa. The epitopes on this class of proteins are shared between different serotypes and serogroup strains. Class 2 and 3 proteins are porins and have a molecular weight of 41 kDa (Minetti et al., 1998). They are implicated in pathogenic infection (Tsai et al., 1981). Both these classes of proteins are present as trimers. Different serogroups of meningococcus have either class 2 or class 3 proteins, but not both. Each subunit consists of 16 antiparallel beta strands (Minetti et al., 1998). These proteins are highly stable and withstand harsh conditions such as low pH, elevated temperatures, and the presence of detergents.

Outer membrane protein vesicles are used as carrier proteins in PedvaxHIB. This vaccine is unique among all the other Hib conjugate vaccines, as most infants respond to this vaccine by producing a high level of antibody after the first injection. The Hib vaccines with other carrier proteins such as diphtheria toxoid, $CRM_{197,}$ and tetanus toxoid do not induce as much antibody concentration as PedvaxHIB after the first injection.

The carrier protein preparations that have been detoxified before their use in the conjugate vaccine preparation have chemically modified surface residues. Formaldehyde, which reacts with the epsilon amine of lysine residues, can result in cross-links with amino acids such as lysine and tyrosine (Metz et al., 2004). Thus, protein or peptides present during the detoxification could potentially become cross-linked to the toxoid. In order to avoid cross-linking foreign proteins to the toxoid, it is good practice to purify the toxin before treatment with formaldehyde.

7.4 ACTIVATION AND COUPLING OF POLYSACCHARIDE AND CARRIER PROTEIN

A well-characterized conjugate vaccine has the following characteristics:

1. A defined chemical structure
2. Potency is predictable in relationship to structural characteristics of the protein–polysaccharide conjugate
3. Coupling chemistry is straightforward and efficient
4. No undesirable epitopes are introduced.

There are currently no polysaccharide conjugate vaccines that meet all of these criteria, although some of these criteria are met by all licensed vaccines. The currently available coupling chemistries limit the extent to which a conjugate can be characterized. The following coupling chemistries are or have been used in licensed polysaccharide–protein conjugate vaccines (see Fig. 7.2).

The first licensed Hib conjugate was prepared by cyanylation of Hib polysaccharide. Hydrazide was coupled to the carboxylates of the carrier protein diphtheria toxoid by carbodiimide catalyzed amidation. The activated polysaccharide was then coupled to the carrier protein hydrazide. The resulting conjugate was high molecular weight and induced more antibodies than the free Hib polysaccharide. A variation of this procedure was published by Chu et al. (Chu et al., 1983). In this procedure, the adipic dihydrazide was first introduced into the polysaccharide followed by carbodiimide mediated coupling of the protein to hydrazide Hib polysaccharide. Coupling by the latter procedure was an improvement because the resulting conjugate induced higher levels of antibody in animals. Fewer solubility problems were observed with this conjugation procedure.

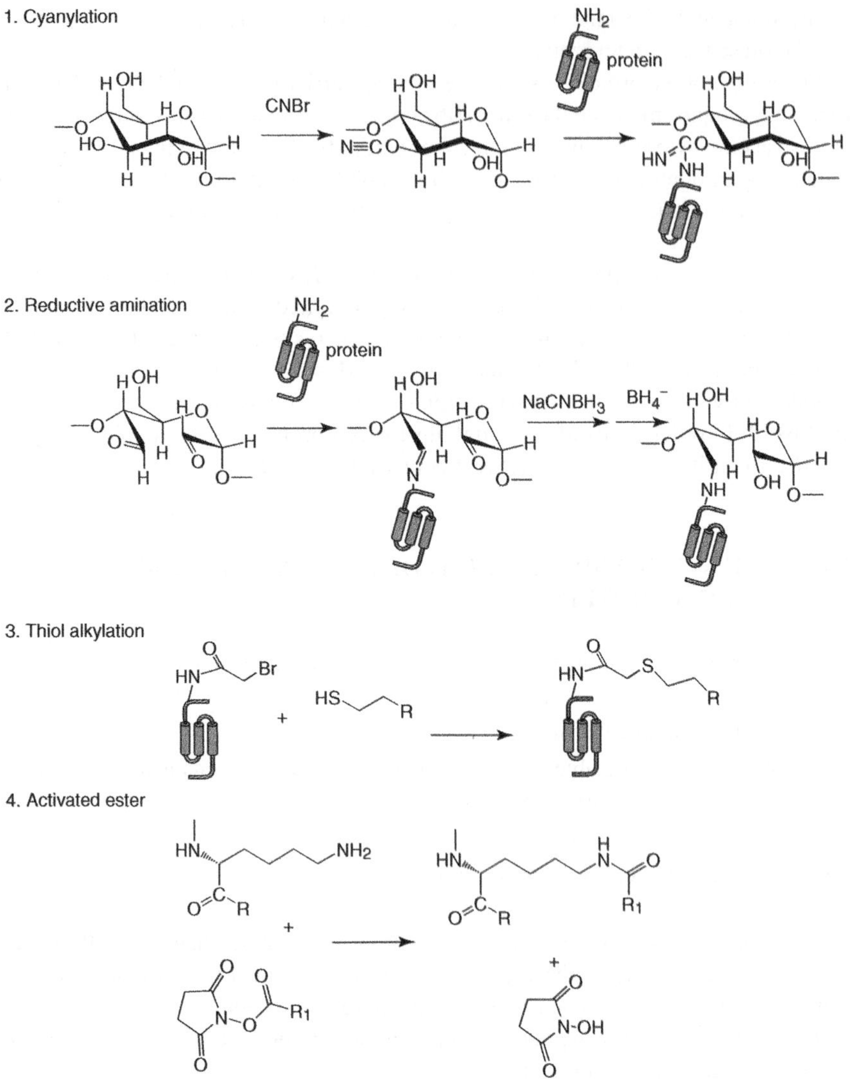

Figure 7.2 Common methods of activation.

The cyanylation procedure has the advantage of being a general method for carbohydrates because it only requires the presence of hydroxyl groups (see Fig. 7.2). Its disadvantage is the instability of the activated intermediate formed during the reaction of polysaccharide hydroxyls with cyanogen bromide (Bartling et al., 1972). In order to maintain a consistently manufactured product, careful attention must be paid to the reaction conditions for activation and coupling of the protein. Cyanoester formation and its subsequent reaction with the ligand to be coupled are performed at higher pH. The high pH required to facilitate the reaction of hydroxyls with cyanogen bromide results in hydrolysis of the cyanoesters and the formation of imidocabonates (Bartling et al., 1972), which are less reactive than cyanoesters, thus creating another variable in the reactivity of the activated polysaccharide. The CNBr activation procedure is seldom used at present. It is being replaced by a reagent cyano-4-dimethylamino pyridinium tetrafluoroborate (CDAP; Kohn and Wilchek, 1983; Lees et al., 1996) that also activates hydroxyls with a cyanoester group. Since the reactions with CDAP are performed at or near neutral pH, the intermediate is more stable to hydrolysis. The coupling of the amino group is carried out under much less alkaline conditions. The coupling efficiency of the CDAP activated polysaccharides is reported to be higher than that obtained by CNBr activation (Lees et al., 1996).

Marburg et al. developed what they termed a bigeneric method (Marburg et al., 1986) of constructing a protein–polysaccharide conjugate. The reaction that was used to couple the activated polysaccharide to the activated protein is the alkylation of a sulfhydryl group (see Fig. 7.2). In this case, the *Haemophilus* or pneumococcal polysaccharide is derivatized with a bromoacyl group. Sulfhydryls are randomly introduced on the surface of the carrier protein that are then allowed to react with the bromoacyl groups on the polysaccharide. The resulting linkage is very stable and formed under very mild conditions. This methodology is the chemical basis for formation of the Hib–Meningococcal outer membrane protein conjugate, Pedvax HIB. The Marburg method is complex and begins with activation in a nonaqueous solvent. The polysaccharide is first converted to an alkylammonium salt dissolved in DMF or DMSO and activated with carbonyldiimidazole. The activated polysaccharide is then reacted with diaminohexane to introduce an amino group. These amino groups are then acylated with bromoacetic acid. The protein component (OMV) is activated by the reaction of amino groups with N-acetylhomocysteine thiolactone. This reaction yields a thiolylated protein, which is then coupled to the bromoacylated polysaccharide.

Perhaps, the most commonly used method of conjugation for the preparation of licensed vaccines is reductive amination (Jennings and Lugowski, 1981; see Fig. 7.2). HibTiter, a diphtheria toxin CRM_{197} conjugate of Hib oligosaccharide, was originally developed by Praxis Biologics. This vaccine is prepared by reductive amination of periodate oxidized Hib with the amino groups on the surface of CRM_{197} (Anderson et al., 1986). A similar methodology was used to prepare a heptavalent pneumococcal polysaccharide CRM_{197} vaccine. This procedure yields a conjugate without the introduction of a linker and thus minimized the introduction of undesirable linkage groups into the resulting conjugate vaccine.

A different approach to reductive amination was used in the synthesis of a meningococcal Group C vaccine. Porro et al. (Porro et al., 1985b) described a procedure using which the reducing end of oligosaccharides is aminated with high concentrations of ammonium salts. These authors used this method to aminate oligosaccharides on pneumococcal 6A (Porro et al., 1985b) and *N. meningitidis* group C capsules (Porro et al., 1985a; Porro et al., 1986). The aminated oligosaccharides were then activated with a N-hydroxylsuccinimide diester of adipic acid as described in Figure 7.2. The aminated oligosaccharides were coupled to the inactive mutant diphtheria toxin CRM_{197} as a carrier protein. Such conjugates were immunogenic in mice. The procedure was used to develop a conjugate vaccine of *N. meningitidis* group C oligosaccharide-diphtheria CRM_{197}. This vaccine is licensed in Canada and Europe.

A problem with all of the procedures described previously is that the overall yield of conjugate drug substance is low. The low yield and complicated coupling procedures are impediments to the development of low cost vaccines based on these technologies. Recently, Lee and Frasch improved on the reductive amination to prepare a meningococcal group A conjugate. In this procedure, the protein carrier is first derivatized with hydrazine (Gudlavalleti et al., 2007) to introduce a large number of hydrazide groups. The polysaccharide is oxidized with periodate (see Fig. 7.1) to introduce aldehyde groups. The hydrazide-activated protein is coupled by mixing with the periodate-oxidized polysaccharide. The use of a hydrazide protein results in a much higher coupling efficiency than that obtained with aliphatic amines or the amine side chains of proteins lysines. This technology was developed as part of a WHO—PATH project for low cost meningococcal vaccines project for the developing world.

Hydroxylamines have also been proposed as alternative nucleophiles for reductive amination. Lees et al. (Lees et al., 2006) described a procedure for introducing aminooxy groups into protein and subsequent coupling of the protein with oxidized pneumococcal polysaccharides. These authors have compared the hydrazide and aminooxy methods using the model substrates dextran and bovine serum albumin. The aminooxy reaction showed a higher degree of conjugate formation in the model system when assayed by HPLC gel filtration.

Perhaps, one of the most innovative recent approaches to conjugate vaccine synthesis is the use of completely synthetic oligosaccharides. This procedure has the advantage of control of structure and high yields. Verez-Bencomo and Roy developed a method (Verez-Bencomo et al., 2004) to prepare repeat structures of the *H. influenzae* type B capsule. Since the oligosaccharides were completely synthetic, the options for adjusting the coupling chemistry and size were greater than that for oligosaccharide derived from native polysaccharides. Synthetic oligosaccharide containing an average of eight repeat units was prepared on a 100-g scale in high yield (80%). The azide-containing arm on the oligosaccharide was used to attach a maleimide linker. The maleimide-linked oligosaccharides were coupled to thiolated tetanus toxoid in good yield.

7.4.1 Removal of Residual Active Sites

After the conjugation reaction is completed, unreacted active sites remaining must be removed to alleviate the possibility of covalent reactions *in vivo*. The choice of deactivation methods is a function of the conjugation procedure. Reactive aldehydes remaining after reductive amination are typically removed by reduction with sodium borohydride (see Fig. 7.2). Residual cyanoesters and imidocarbonates resulting from

CNBr activation are deactivated by the addition of an excess of small molecule amines. Residual alkyl halides are deactivated by the addition of excess thiols such as cysteine.

7.5 CHARACTERIZATION OF THE CONJUGATE

Perhaps, one of the most critical steps in the manufacture of a conjugate is the characterization of the conjugate. The technology used for this characterization has evolved over the years. In general, animal assays are not used for routine analysis of polysaccharide conjugate vaccines. Instead, the consistency of manufacture of a particular vaccine is evaluated by a battery of physicochemical tests whose limits have been set on the basis of lots of vaccine used in clinical trials. For this reason, the physicochemical method of evaluation must be chosen with care to reflect parameters that are important for the induction of protective antibodies. There are two levels of characterization required as follows: (i) in-depth analysis to validate the process and serve as a resource during the history of the vaccine and (ii) characterization to insure potency and manufacturing consistency, such as in process and release test.

7.5.1 Proof of Conjugation

Proof of conjugation can be established using several methods. An increase in the apparent size of the carrier protein or both polysaccharide and protein on size-exclusion chromatography is usually an indicator that a conjugation reaction has occurred. SDS-PAGE of the conjugate mixture also shows a dramatic change in migration of the carrier protein. After conjugation, the carrier protein usually migrates as a smear or does not enter the gel. In cases where the oligosaccharide is directly coupled to the protein by reductive amination, a unique amino acid residue is generated. The presence of such residues in conjugate acid hydrolysates is proof of covalent conjugation. Similarly, the bigeneric conjugate approach of Marburg also yields a unique amino acid on acid hydrolysis of the conjugates prepared using this method.

7.5.2 Free Polysaccharide

Free polysaccharide is probably one of the more difficult parameters to measure because of the problems of separating conjugated polysaccharide from free polysaccharide. Separation of oligosaccharide intermediates from conjugates can be accomplished by size-exclusion chromatography. Hib conjugates prepared from polysaccharide have been separated from free polysaccharide by hydrophobic interaction chromatography on reverse phase resins in at least one case. In this instance, the method takes advantage of the tendency of protein to bind to C-18 resins under hydrophobic interaction chromatography conditions, whereas charged polysaccharides do not. Thus, any polysaccharide linked to a protein would bind. The unbound polysaccharide is measured using colorimetric assays. Guo et al. described a method on the basis of acid precipitation of Hib–tetanus toxoid conjugates in the presence of deoxycholate (Guo et al., 1998; Lei et al., 2000a). Polysaccharides do not precipitate under these conditions. This method has also been applied to the analysis of meningococcal polysaccharide conjugate vaccines (Lei et al., 2000b).

7.5.3 Degree of Derivatization

The degree of derivatization is a function of the method chosen for conjugation. In many cases, the number of functional groups can be measured using a colorimetric assay. When the polysaccharide is activated by periodate oxidation, the measure of derivatization is concentration of aldehydes generated. Typically, these residues are measured using the Park Johnson reaction (Park and Johnson, 1949). The addition of hydrazide groups to either protein or polysaccharide is measured with TNBS (Habeeb, 1966). The Marburg method uses NMR to determine the degree of derivatization of Hib polysaccharide with diaminobutane groups (Marburg et al., 1986). The introduction of thiols into protein or polysaccharides is determined using a reaction of Ellman's reagent with free thiols (Ellman, 1959).

7.5.4 Degree of Conjugation

The degree of conjugation, also referred to as *covalency*, is a critical parameter associated with the potency and consistency of a conjugate vaccine. Ideally, this should be measured using a unique property resulting from the conjugation reaction. The Hib oligosaccharide–CRM_{197} conjugate contains a hydroxyethyl lysine residue for oligosaccharide aldehyde reductive aminated to the carrier protein (Seid et al., 1989). The Marburg method yields an S-carboxymethylhomocysteine for polysaccharide-active site coupled to the outer membrane protein (Marburg et al., 1986). Since some methods of conjugation do not yield such unique markers, the degree of conjugation is inferred from other parameters, such the ratio of polysaccharide to protein in a high molecular weight fraction containing conjugate. The results from this method should be interpreted with care because unreacted saccharide is frequently not easily separated from conjugate by size-exclusion methods and nature of the conjugation may not be straightforward.

7.5.5 Molecular Size

Molecular size is an important measurement for the conjugate and for the in-process polysaccharide or oligosaccharide intermediates as described previously in the polysaccharide size section. Most conjugates of licensed conjugate vaccines are very large, and, traditionally, their size has been related as a size-exclusion partition coefficient, Kd, on a Sepharose 4B column. The same chromatographic approach was used to estimate the size of polysaccharide vaccines. Both conjugate and polysaccharide vaccines that were licensed and tested in clinical trials used Kd values as a specification for molecular size. Typically, the position of the peak was determined using refractive index, colorimetric assay, or ELISA. Multiangle laser light scattering is being used as a detection system on size-exclusion chromatography (Bardotti et al., 2008). The advantage of this method is that a more quantitative estimate of size and polydispersity can be obtained. Care must be taken, however, in transitioning between these methods because most of the clinical experience has been with the Kd specification conjugate vaccines.

7.5.6 Concentration of Residual Active Sites

The Marburg method is designed such that a unique residue is generated when an active site is deactivated. Reactive bromoacetamide residues are capped with N-acetylcysteamine. Hydrolysis of the capped conjugate yields the unique amino acid S-carboxymethyl cysteamine for each active site not involved in a conjugation linkage (Marburg et al., 1986).

7.5.7 Residual Reactants and Reagents

Conjugation chemistry uses and generates some toxic chemicals and by-products. These by-products of conjugation are removed by inactivation and ultrafiltration in the manufacturing production. It is essential that validated assays be used to verify the removal of these compounds. NMR has been a valuable tool for the detection of contaminants in intermediates during the manufacturing process. Polysaccharides used in conjugation can be contaminated with antifoam agents that were used in the fermentation process or phenol residue from purification or culture inactivation procedures. These types of compound are readily detected in H-NMR spectra of the polysaccharide (Jones, 2005).

7.6 FUTURE DIRECTIONS

The sophistication of polysaccharide–protein conjugate vaccine manufacturing has evolved during the last 20 years with our understanding of their efficacy and safety profile. Nevertheless, there remain several challenges to producing more effective, economical, and predictable conjugate vaccines. Among these challenges are (i) more efficient coupling methodologies, (ii) greater selection of carrier proteins, and (iii) rapid and accurate methods of characterization. These challenges are very much linked to our understanding of the structures that are critical in eliciting the desired immune response. The current repertoire of reactions used to couple saccharides to protein carriers is rather limited and does not reflect the available chemical space in carbohydrate or organic chemistry to the field. This limited repertoire slows the creative development of vaccines. Only with an increase in long-term scientific research effort can this situation improve. While "click chemistry" in its present state may not be suitable for vaccine synthesis, it demonstrates the feasibility and utility of highly efficient aqueous coupling reactions (Kolb et al., 2001). Metabolic engineering is another approach that has the potential to improve the economy of conjugate synthesis by having several of the critical steps for conjugate synthesis performed *in vivo* (Fort et al., 2005).

The development of increasingly complex multivalent conjugate vaccines has resulted in an increased demand for specific and sensitive methods of quantitation and characterization of the component antigens. This will become more important as the valence of the vaccines increases. Rate nephelometry is currently being applied to this problem (Lee, 1983). Microarray and quantum dots (Yang and Li, 2006) are examples of newer technologies that have potential for providing solutions to this problem of measuring multiple antigens in a rapid and sensitive manner.

The "800-lb gorilla" in the room is the carrier protein. The use of the diphtheria and tetanus toxoid as carrier proteins and immunogens in multivalent vaccines has a potential for serious immunological consequences. It has been postulated that the use of the same carrier in multiple instances can cause interference, immune tolerance (Schutze et al., 1989; Schutze et al., 1985), or may not enhance immunogenicity of some vaccine components (McCool et al., 1999). Researchers have therefore sought to develop alternative carriers such as *Haemophilus* protein D (Akkoyunlu et al., 1997), *Neisseria* outer membrane proteins, and *Pseudomonas* exoprotein A (Fattom et al., 1990) to name a few. How these alternative carriers will be used and whether more than one carrier can be used in a single multivalent vaccine are issues yet to be resolved.

REFERENCES

Aggerbeck H, Heron I. Detoxification of diphtheria and tetanus toxin with formaldehyde. Detection of protein conjugates. Biologicals 1992;20:109–115.

Akkoyunlu M, Melhus A, Capiau C, van Opstal O, Forsgren A. The acylated form of protein D of *Haemophilus influenzae* is modre immunogenic than the nonacylated form and elicits an adjuvant effect when it is used as a carrier conjugated to polyribosyl ribitol phosphate. Infect Immun 1997;65(12):5010–5016.

Anderson MT, Jorgensen SB, Wilhelmsen SE, Petersen JW, Hojrup P. Investigation of the detoxification mechanism of formaldehyde treated tetanus toxin. Vaccine 2007;25:2213–2227.

Anderson PW, Pichichero ME, Insel RA, Betts R, Eby R, Smith DH. Vaccines consisting of periodate-cleaved oligosaccharides from the capsule of *Haemophilus influenzae* type b coupled to a protein carrier: structural and temporal requirements for priming in the human infant. J Immunol 1986;137(4):1181–1186.

Avery OT, Goebel WF. Chemo-immunological studies on conjugated carbohydrate-proteins. J Exp Med 1929;50:533–550.

Bardotti A, Averani G, Berti F, Berti S, Carinci V, D'Ascenzi S, Fabbri B, Giannini S, Giannozzi A, Magagnoli C, Proietti D, Norelli F, Rappuoli R, Ricci S, Costantino P. Physicochemical characterisation of glycoconjugate vaccines for prevention of meningococcal diseases. Vaccine 2008;26(18):2284–2296.

Bardotti A, Averani G, Berti F, Berti S, Galli C, Giannini S, Fabbri B, Proietti D, Ravenscroft N, Ricci S. Size determination of bacterial capsular oligosaccharides used to prepare conjugate vaccines against Neisseria meningitidis groups Y and W135. Vaccine 2005;23(16):1887–1899.

Bartling GJ, Brown HD, Forrester LJ, Koes MT, Mather AN, Stasiw RO. A study of the mechanism of cyanogen bromide activation of cellulose. Biotechnol Bioeng 1972;14(6):1039–1044.

Blattner R, Ferrier RJ. Effects of iron, copper, and chromate ions on the oxidative degradation of cellulose model compounds. Carbohydr Res 1985;138:73–82.

Cai X, Lei QP, Lamb DH, Shannon A, Jacoby J, Kruk J, Kensinger RD, Ryall R, Zablackis E, Cash P. LC/MS characterization of meningococcal depolymerized polysaccharide group C reducing endgroup and internal repeating unit. Anal Chem 2004;76(24):7387–7390.

Christensen BE, Myhr MH, Smidsrod O. Degradation of double-stranded xanthan by hydrogen peroxide in the presence of ferrous ions: comparison to acid hydrolysis. Carbohydr Res 1996;280(1):85–99.

Chu C, Schneerson R, Robbins JB, Rastogi SC. Further studies on the immunogenicity of *Haemophilus influenzae* type b and pneumococcal type 6A polysaccharide-protein conjugates. Infect Immun 1983;40(1):245–256.

Costantino P, Norelli F, Giannozzi A, D'Ascenzi S, Bartoloni A, Kaur S, Tang D, Seid R, Viti S, Paffetti R, Bigio M, Pennatini C, Averani G, Guarnieri V, Gallo E, Ravenscroft N, Lazzeroni C, Rappuoli R, Ceccarini C. Size fractionation of bacterial capsular polysaccharides for their use in conjugate vaccines. Vaccine 1999;17(9–10):1251–1263.

Cryz SJ Jr, Welkos SL, Holmes RK. Immunochemical studies of diphtherial toxin and related nontoxic mutant proteins. Infect Immun 1980;30(3):835–846.

Dintzis RZ, Okajima M, Middleton MH, Greene G, Dintzis HM. The immunogenicity of soluble haptenated polymers is determined by molecular mass and hapten valence. J Immunol 1989;143(4):1239–1244.

Ellman GL. Tissue sulfhydryl groups. Arch Biochem Biophys 1959;82(1):70–77.

Fattom A, Schneerson R, Szu SC, Vann WF, Shiloach J, Karakawa WW, Robbins BJ. Synthesis and immunologic properties in mice of vaccines composed of Staphylococcus aureus type 5 and type 8 capsular polysaccharides conjugated to Pseudomonas aeruginosa exotoxin A. Infect Immun 1990;58(7):2367–2374.

Fort S, Birikaki L, Dubois MP, Antoine T, Samain E, Driquez H. Biosynthesis of conjugatable saccharidic moities of GM2 and GM3 gangliosides by engineered *E. coli*. Chem Commun 2005;20:2558–2560.

Fothergill LD, Wright JJ. Relation of age incidence to the bactericidal power of blood against the causal organism. Immunol 1933;24:273–284.

Fritzell B, Plotkin S. Efficacy and safety of a *haemophilus influenza* type b capsular polysaccharide-tetanus protein conjugate. J Pediatr 1992;121:355–362.

Giannini G, Rappuoli R, Ratti G. The amino-acid sequence of two non-toxic mutants of diphtheria toxin: CRM45 and CRM197. Nucl Acids Res 1984;12(10):4063–4069.

Gudlavalleti SK, Lee CH, Norris SE, Paul-Satyaseela M, Vann WF, Frasch CE. Comparison of *Neisseria meningitidis* serogroup W135 polysaccharide-tetanus toxoid conjugate vaccines made by periodate activation of O-acetylated, non-O-acetylated and chemically de-O-acetylated polysaccharide. Vaccine 2007;25(46):7972–7980.

Guo YY, Anderson R, McIver J, Gupta RK, Siber GR. A simple and rapid method for measuring unconjugated capsular polysaccharide (PRP) of *Haemophilus influenzae* type b in PRP–tetanus toxoid conjugate vaccine. Biologicals 1998;26(1):33–38.

Habeeb AF. Determination of free amino groups in proteins by trinitrobenzenesulfonic acid. Anal Biochem 1966;14(3):328–336.

Hoogerhout P, Funke CW, Mellema JR, van Boeckel CA, Evenberg D, Poolman JT, Lefeber AWM, van der Marel GA, van Boom JH. Synthesis of fragments of the capsular polysaccharide of *Haemophilus influenzae* type b II. Synthesis and structural analysis of fragments comprising two and three repeat units. J Carbohydr Chem 1988;7:399–416.

Isbells HS, Parks EW, Naves RG. Degradation of reducing sugars and related compounds by alkaline hydrogen peroxide in the presence and absence of iron and magnesium salts. Carbohydr Res 1975;45(1):197–204.

Jennings HJ, Lugowski C. Immunochemistry of groups A, B, and C meningococcal polysaccharide-tetanus toxoid conjugates. J Immunol 1981;127(3):1011–1018.

Jones C. NMR assays for carbohydrate-based vaccines. J Pharm Biomed Anal 2005;38(5):840–850.

Kohn J, Wilchek M. 1-Cyano-4-dimethylamino pyridinium tetrafluoroborate as cyanylating agent for covalent attachment of ligand to polysaccharide resins. FEBS Lett 1983;154:209–210.

Kolb HC, Finn MG, Sharples KB. Click chemistry: diverse chemical function from a few good reactions. Angew Chem Int Ed Engl 2001;40(11):2004–2021.

Krieglstein K, Henschen A, Weller U, Habermann E. Arrangement of disulfide bridges and positions of sulfhydryl groups in tetanus toxin. Eur J Biochem 1990;188:39–45.

Kshirsagar N, Mur N, Thatte U, Gogtay N, Viviani S, Préziosi M-P, Elie C, Findlow H, Carlone G, Borrow R, Parulekar V, Plikaytis B, Kulkarni P, Imbault N, LaForce FM. Safety, immunogenicity, and antibody persistence of a new meningococcal group A conjugate vaccine in healthy Indian adults. Vaccine 2007;25(Suppl 1):A101–A107.

Lee CJ. The quantitative immunochemical determination of pneumococcal and meingococcal capsular polysaccharides by light scattering rate nephelometry. J Biol Stand 1983;11(1):55–64.

Lees A, Nelson BL, Mond JJ. Activation of soluble polysaccharides with 1-cyano-4-dimethylaminopyridinium tetrafluoroborate for use in protein-polysaccharide conjugate vaccines and immunological reagents. Vaccine 1996;14(3):190–198.

Lees A, Sen G, LopezAcosta A. Versatile and efficient synthesis of protein-polysaccharide conjugate vaccines using aminooxy reagents and oxime chemistry. Vaccine 2006;24(6):716–729.

Lei QP, Lamb DH, Heller R, Pietrobon P. Quantitation of low level unconjugated polysaccharide in tetanus toxoid-conjugate vaccine by HPAEC/PAD following rapid separation by deoxycholate/HCl. J Pharm Biomed Anal 2000a;21(6):1087–1091.

Lei QP, Shannon AG, Heller RK, Lamb DH. Quantification of free polysaccharide in meningococcal polysaccharide–diphtheria toxoid conjugate vaccines. Dev Biol (Basel) 2000b;103:259–264.

Lemercinier X, Jones C. Full 1H NMR assignment and detailed O-acetylation patterns of capsular polysaccharides from *Neisseria meningitidis* used in vaccine production. Carbohydr Res 1996;296:83–96.

Lexau CA, Lynfield R, Danila R, Pilishvili T, Facklam R, Farley MM, Harrison LH, Schaffner W, Reingold A, Bennett NM, Hadler J, Cieslak PR, Whitney CG. Changing epidemiology of invasive pneumococcal disease among older adults in the era of pediatric pneumococcal conjugate vaccine. JAMA 2005;294(16):2043–2051.

Makela PH, Peltola H, Kayhty H, Jousimies H, Pettay O, Ruoslahti E, Sivonen A, Renkonen OV. Polysaccharide vaccines of group A Neisseria meningtitidis and *Haemophilus influenzae* type b: a field trial in Finland. J Infect Dis 1977;136(Suppl):S43–S50.

Marburg S, Jorn D, Tolman RL, Arison B, McCauley J, Kniskern PJ, Hagopian A, Vella PP. Bimolecular chemistry of macromolecules:synthesis if bacterial polysaccharide conjugates with *Neisseria meningitidis* membrane protein. J Am Chem Soc 1986;108:5282–5287.

Matsuda M, Yoneda M. Isolation and purification of two antigenically active, "complementary" polypeptide fragments of tetanus neurotoxin. Infect Immun 1975;12:1147–1153.

McCool TL, Harding CV, Greenspan NS, Schreiber JR. B- and T-cell immune responses to pneumococcal conjugate vaccines: divergence between carrier- and polysaccharide-specific immunogenicity. Infect Immun 1999;67(9):4862–4869.

Metz B, Kersten GF, Hoogerhout P, Brugghe HF, Timmermans HA, de Jong A, Meiring H, ten Hove J, Hennink WE, Crommelin DJ, Jiskoot W. Identification of formaldehyde-induced modifications in proteins: reactions with model peptides. J Biol Chem 2004;279(8):6235–6243.

Miller AR. Oxidation of cell wall polysaccharides by hydrogen peroxide: a potential mechanism for cell wall breakdown in plants. Biochem Biophys Res Commun 1986;141(1):238–244.

Minetti CASA, Blake MS, Remeta DP. Characterization of the structure, function, and conformational stability of PorB class 3 protein from *Neisseria meningitidis*. A porin with unusual physicochemical properties. J Biol Chem 1998;273(39):25329–25338.

Paoletti LC, Kasper DL, Michon F, DiFabio J, Jennings HJ, Tosteson TD, Wessels MR. Effects of chain length on the immunogenicity in rabbits of group B Streptococcus type III oligosaccharide-tetanus toxoid conjugates. J Clin Invest 1992;89(1):203–209.

Park JT, Johnson MJ. A submicrodetermination of glucose. J Biol Chem 1949;181(1): 149–151.

Parke JC Jr, Schneerson R, Robbins JB, Schlesselman JJ. Interim report of a controlled field trial of immunization with capsular polysaccharides of *Haemophilus influenzae* type b and group C *Neisseria meningitidis* in Mecklenburg county, North Carolina (March 1974-March 1976). J Infect Dis 1977;136(Suppl):S51–S56.

Peeters CC, Evenberg D, Hoogerhout P, Kayhty H, Saarinen L, van Boeckel CA, van der Marel GA, van Boom JH, Poolman JT. Synthetic trimer and tetramer of 3-beta-D-ribose-(1–1)-D-ribitol-5-phosphate conjugated to protein induce antibody responses to *Haemophilus influenzae* type b capsular polysaccharide in mice and monkeys. Infect Immun 1992;60(5):1826–1833.

Peltola H, Kayhty H, Sivonen A, Makela H. *Haemophilus influenzae* type b capsular polysaccharide vaccine in children: a double-blind field study of 100,000 vaccines 3 months to 5 years of age in Finland. Pediatrics 1977;60(5):730–737.

Porro M, Costantino P, Fabbiani S, Pellegrini V, Viti S. A semi-synthetic glycoconjugate antigen prepared by chemical glycosylation of pertussis toxin by a meningococcal group C oligosaccharide hapten. Dev Biol Stand 1985a;61:525–530.

Porro M, Costantino P, Viti S, Vannozzi F, Naggi A, Torri G. Specific antibodies to diphtheria toxin and type 6A pneumococcal capsular polysaccharide induced by a model of semi-synthetic glycoconjugate antigen. Mol Immunol 1985b;22(8):907–919.

Porro M, Costantino P, Giovannoni F, Pellegrini V, Tagliaferri L, Vannozzi F, Viti S. A molecular model of artificial glycoprotein with predetermined multiple immunodeterminants for Gram-positive and Gram-negative encapsulated bacteria. Mol Immunol 1986;23(4):385–391.

Pozsgay V. Synthesis of glycoconjugate vaccines against *Shigella dysenteriae* type 1. J Org Chem 1998;63(17):5983–5999.

Rappuoli R. Isolation and characterization of *Corynebacterium diphtheriae* nontandem double lysogens hyperproducing CRM197. Appl Environ Microbiol 1983;46(3):560–564.

Ravenscroft N, Averani G, Bartoloni A, Berti S, Bigio M, Carinci V, Costantino P, D'Ascenzi S, Giannozzi A, Norelli F, Pennatini C, Proietti D, Ceccarini C, Cescutti P. Size determination of bacterial capsular oligosaccharides used to prepare conjugate vaccines. Vaccine 1999;17(22):2802–2816.

Robbins JB, Schneerson R, Anderson P, Smith DH. The 1996 Albert Lasker Medical Research Awards. Prevention of systemic infections, especially meningitis, caused by *Haemophilus influenzae* type b. Impact on public health and implications for other polysaccharide-based vaccines. JAMA 1996;276(14):1181–1185.

Robinson JP, Hash JH. A review of the molecular structure of tetanus toxin. Mol Cell Biochem 1982;48:33–44.

Schneerson R, Barrera O, Sutton A, Robbins JB. Preparation, characterization, and immunogenicity of *Haemophilus influenzae* type b polysaccharide-protein conjugates. J Exp Med 1980;152(2):361–376.

Schutze MP, Deriaud E, Przewlocki G, LeClerc C. Carrier-induced epitopic suppression is initiated through clonal dominance. J Immunol 1989;142(8):2635–2640.

Schutze MP, Leclerc C, Jolivet M, Audibert F, Chedid L. Carrier-induced epitopic suppression, a major issue for future synthetic vaccines. J Immunol 1985;135(4):2319–2322.

Seid RC Jr, Boykins RA, Liu DF, Kimbrough KW, Hsieh CL, Eby R. Chemical evidence for covalent linkages of a semi-synthetic glycoconjugate vaccine for *Haemophilus influenzae* type B disease. Glycoconj J 1989;6(4):489–498.

Sinha A, Levine O, Knoll MD, Muhib F, Lieu TA. Cost-effectiveness of pneumococcal conjugate vaccination in the prevention of child mortality: an international economic analysis. Lancet 2007;369(9559):389–396.

Szu SC, Li XR, Schneerson R, Vickers JH, Bryla D, Robbins JB. Comparative immunogenicities of Vi polysaccharide-protein conjugates composed of cholera toxin or its B subunit as a carrier bound to high- or lower-molecular-weight Vi. Infect Immun 1989;57(12):3823–3827.

Thijssen MJ, van Rijswijk MN, Kamerling JP, Vliegenthart JF. Synthesis of spacer-containing di- and tri-saccharides that represent parts of the capsular polysaccharide of *Streptococcus pneumoniae* type 6B. Carbohydr Res 1998;306(1–2):93–109.

Tsai CM, Frasch CE, Mocca LF. Five structural classes of major outer membrane proteins in *Neisseria meningitidis*. J Bacteriol 1981;146:69–78.

Uchida T, Pappenheimer AM Jr, Greany R. Diphtheria toxin and related proteins. I. isolation and properties of mutant proteins serologically related to diphtheria toxin. J Biol Chem 1973;248(11):3838–3844.

Verez-Bencomo V, Fernandez-Santana V, Hardy E, Toledo ME, Rodriguez MC, Heynngnezz L, Rodriguez A, Baly A, Herrera L, Izquierdo M, Villar A, Valdes Y, Cosme K, Deler ML, Montane M, Garcia E, Ramos A, Aguilar A, Medina E, Torano G, Sosa I, Hernandez I, Martinez R, Muzachio A, Carmenates A, Costa L, Cardoso F, Campa C, Diaz M, Roy R. A synthetic conjugate polysaccharide vaccine against *Haemophilus influenzae* type b. Science 2004;305(5683):522–525.

Whitney CG, Farley MM, Hadler J, Harrison LH, Bennett NM, Lynfield R, Reingold A, Cieslak PR, Pilishvili T, Jackson D, Facklam RR, Jorgensen JH, Schuchat A. Decline in invasive pneumococcal disease after the introduction of protein–polysaccharide conjugate vaccine. N Engl J Med 2003;348(18):1737–1746.

Yang L, Li Y. Simultaneous detection of *Escherichai coli* O157:H7 and *Salmonella typhimurium* using quantum dots as fluorescence labels. Analyst 2006;131(3):394–401.

Velez-Pimentel V, [illegible] S, Hardy L, [illegible] G, Rodriguez M, [illegible] A, Herrera L, [illegible] M, [illegible] A, [illegible] K, [illegible] H, Martinez M, [illegible] P, [illegible] A, [illegible] M, [illegible] J, Martinez K, [illegible] A, [illegible] A, Cossart [illegible] (2007) [illegible] genome sequencing [illegible]. Science [illegible]

Wheeler [illegible] (2008) [illegible] Mattioli [illegible] Klitgord [illegible] Riddihough [illegible] the interaction of [illegible] proteins [illegible] Nucleic Acids Res [illegible]

[illegible]

8

STABILIZATION AND FORMULATION OF VACCINES

TIMOTHY S. PRIDDY AND C. RUSSELL MIDDAUGH

Department of Pharmaceutical Chemistry, University of Kansas, Lawrence, KS, USA

8.1 INTRODUCTION

Many, if not most, vaccine formulations that are currently in use were originally developed using a largely empirical approach on the basis of immune responses in animal models. With significant time and effort, empirical approaches have proven to be effective for most current vaccines, but many of these have not been formulated to achieve optimum stability. Most of these successes were achieved without any detailed knowledge of the effects of physicochemical stress on the structure of the antigen. A recently developed systematic method offers the promise of a more direct approach to optimize formulation development. This approach has several advantages, including improvement in the chemical and physical stability of the antigen that is necessary to extend shelf-life and the enhancement of immunogenicity to decrease effective dosage, among others.

Many factors that are fundamental to achieving improved stability in vaccine formulations are ultimately determined by the structural characteristics of the antigenic biomolecules. In this chapter, some general guidelines for the development of a comprehensive approach for the stabilization and formulation of vaccines are provided; one that employs a rational, systematic platform for the characterization of the physicochemical properties of the antigenic components of vaccines, as well as other biopharmaceuticals. In addition, examples of the power of this methodology

Vaccine Development and Manufacturing, First Edition.
Edited by Emily P. Wen, Ronald Ellis, and Narahari S. Pujar.

are provided, and evidence of recent successes as well as future developments of the approach is presented.

8.2 AN EXAMPLE OF A MODERN VACCINE CHARACTERIZATION STRATEGY

The formulation development of early vaccines was almost entirely empirical compared to modern standards. The consequences of this lack of understanding of the structure and composition of past vaccines resulted in a number of problems that could have probably been avoided if better characterization methods had been available (Ferran, 1885; Bornside, 1981). In this chapter, the merits of including a comprehensive structural analysis of target antigens as a vital phase of the formulation process, especially with regard to vaccine stability, are described. To this end, we argue that it is advantageous to employ a diverse battery of biophysical testing methods to assess the physicochemical characteristics of antigens at all structural levels. The use of high throughput instrumentation permits this process to be rapid, precise, and thorough and allows for acquisition of the large amounts of data that are required for comprehensive structural analyses. This process employs diverse data sets to provide an indicator of discrete structural states of the antigen, as they are induced by a variety of environmental perturbations. In practice, once a structurally stable form of an antigen is identified, additional physical and chemical conditions can be modified, to investigate differential effects on the antigen. The intent is to ultimately improve the intrinsic structural integrity of the antigen by adding excipients, or by modifying solution conditions to extend product shelf-life and viability. This approach to improve the integrity of the structurally favored form of antigens is a clear advancement over the empirical trial-and-error formulation schemes of the past. In this chapter, only the consideration of solution physical stability is discussed.

8.2.1 Measurable Physicochemical Characteristics

Vaccines are formulated to stimulate a protective immune response, while minimizing the potential for negative side-effects on exposure to the recipient. Most vaccines are grouped according to the nature of the antigen. Examples include attenuated or killed pathogens, natural or recombinant proteins or their assemblies, polysaccharides, or DNA plasmids encoding appropriate proteins. Each has intrinsic benefits and limitations from numerous perspectives that affect their purification, storage, deliverability, and immunogenicity. A variety of factors contributes to a drug's overall stability and effectiveness, and most importantly, virtually all are highly structure dependent. Thus, focus on structural change appears to be a reasonable approach, although the ever-present possibility of failure to detect key, and possibly quite subtle, structurally disruptive events provide an ever-present limitation to consider.

The nature of the structural characterization of vaccines varies with the level of complexity of the antigen. This fundamentally is the case because the antigen may be a simple protein such as a toxoid, which is much less complex than a whole virus and even simpler than an entire bacterium. The complexity of the antigen then dictates the type and number of analyses that will be performed to characterize its structure. Fortunately, the antigenic components of interest are actually of only a few types, including proteins, nucleic acids, lipids, and polysaccharides and their complexes. In actual vaccine formulations, these antigens may be present in a relatively impure state and must therefore be further purified for the types of analyses described in the following section. This presents less of a problem than might first be imagined, however, because the results obtained with the purified antigen (namely, the identification of stabilizers, their optimal concentration, and use in combination) can still be directly implemented in the final, more heterogeneous vaccine formulation.

The stability of vaccine components in solution is a direct function of a number of environmental conditions that ultimately contribute to the measurable physicochemical properties of the critical biomolecules. Most significant are solution pH, ionic strength, redox potential, and temperature, all of which often contribute directly to the stability of macromolecules. In addition, more pharmaceutical variables such as agitation and freeze/thaw stress, as well as surface activity, may all play key roles in formulation considerations. Because many of the processes that contribute to a vaccine antigen's stability are largely nonequilibrium, strict thermodynamics considerations do not generally apply. Rather, a "stable" vaccine is simply thought of in terms of a formulation that maintains its native biological activity and/or immunogenicity until it can be administered. In essence, the "stability of a pharmaceutical product may be defined as the capability of a particular formulation in a specific container/closure system, to remain within its physical, chemical, microbiological, therapeutic, and toxicological specifications" (Vadas, 1995).

Solution pH contributes to both the chemical and physical stability of biomolecules. Chemical effects are manifest through acid- or base-catalyzed as well as oxidation reactions, among others. This includes the hydrolysis of peptide bonds or deamidation of glutamine and asparagine side chains in proteins as well as the oxidation of a variety of other amino acid side chains (Song et al., 2001). Solution pH can also affect the rate of glycosidic bond cleavage between the nucleotide bases and the deoxyribose backbone of DNA (Middaugh et al., 1998). These bases are also subject to a variety of oxidation and other reactions. Physical effects of pH include alterations in solubility based on the degree of protonation of ionizable groups, which may also affect interactions that are crucial to proper domain folding and/or both intermolecular and intramolecular contacts among and within multimeric complexes. More uniquely, pH can also affect the rate of enzymatic activity of live and attenuated, bacterial or viral vaccines, such as the intrinsic endonuclease activity that was a serious concern with the oral polio vaccine (Newman et al., 1995; Newman et al., 1996).

The ionic strength of solutions can dramatically affect the solubility of biomolecules. At lower ionic strength (e.g., <0.2), Debye-Hückel charge sharing tends to increase solubility, whereas decreases in solubility are typically seen at higher ionic strength because of the well-known salting-out effect (with the exception of chaotropic salts). Ionic strength can also shift the osmotic balance and promote membrane lysis of enveloped viruses and whole-cell bacterial vaccines. Ionic strength may also contribute favorably to the stability of vaccines by maintaining the overall repulsive forces between molecules, inhibiting aggregation and precipitation.

The effects of temperature on the stability of vaccines can be disruptive at both extremes. As harmful as increased temperature can be to all but a select few classes of biological molecules that are used in vaccines, freezing may also be destructive as seen in the case of diphtheria, pertussis, tetanus, and polio vaccines (WHO, 1980; WHO, 2000). The thermolability of biological molecules is often a very problematic degradative factor for vaccines outside of rigorously controlled environments. For this reason, temperature studies are usually considered essential to a comprehensive biophysical characterization scheme. More importantly, however, temperature studies are used as an accelerated stability stress to identify specific processes that may be responsible for the destabilization of antigen, whether they are from aggregation, viral capsid dissociation, protein secondary or tertiary structure rearrangements, or other temperature-dependent processes. The long-standing and ever-present question concerning temperature-based accelerated stability studies is their relevance to lower temperature storage conditions. Are those 20–60°C temperatures that are often tested accelerating pharmaceutically irrelevant degradation pathways? Experience tells us that this is not usually the case, but this certainly does occur and must always be kept in mind when attempting to interpret data from such studies.

8.2.2 Empirical Phase Diagrams

A more detailed description of a complex macromolecular system can be obtained by combining a series of measurements that provides information about multiple aspects of its structure. Comparing, contrasting, and overlaying relevant data sets can assist in characterizing overall structure from numerous perspectives, although the interpretation of multiple data sets can become quite complicated, occasionally leading to significant misinterpretation. One way to at least partially obviate such problems is through the use of multidimensional vector analysis-based methods such as that of the empirical phase diagram (EPD). For a detailed description of the mathematics behind EPDs, please see Kueltzo et al., 2003a and Fan et al., 2005. Briefly, EPDs are constructed by combining raw data from a number of physical measurements at regular increments of selected parameters, such as temperature and pH. Each discrete parameter combination (e.g., T and pH) is associated with a set of variables (*a, b, c, d, … n*) representing results from the chosen techniques. When combined, the ordered variables create a single summation vector that is represented by a color (or shade of gray, Fig. 8.1), where a change in color, or shade of gray, in the EPD that creates an apparent phase boundary is interpreted as a change in the physical structure of the molecule. EPDs can assist the analyst in the selection of an appropriate methodology and combination of assay conditions to assess the structural stability of antigenic components of vaccines in the subsequent phase of formulation development in which the effects of stabilizers are measured and evaluated. Data from virtually any experimental technique that permits control of both thermal and temporal parameters can be incorporated into an EPD.

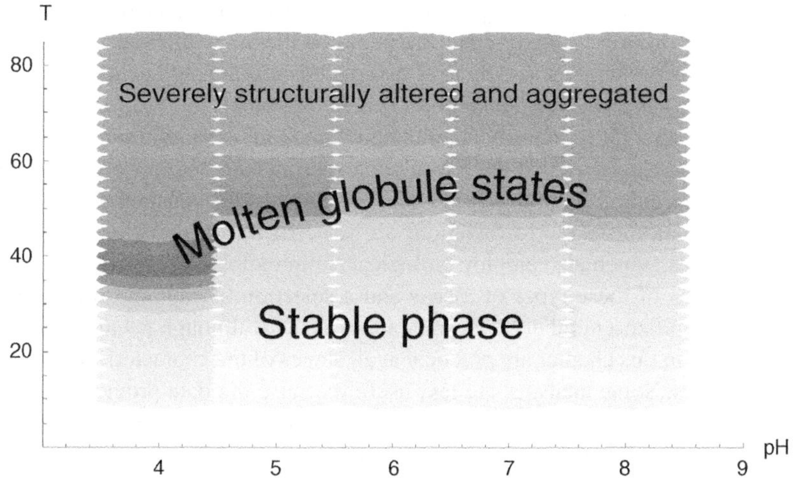

Figure 8.1 Empirical phase diagram, EPD, for recombinant ricin toxin A-chain generated using CD molar ellipticity at 208 nm, ANS fluorescence, and intrinsic Trp fluorescence intensity data. Descriptions of the three general structural states of the protein are defined by the boundaries of the shaded regions. Similar structural states of the protein are characterized among the variable solution conditions tested (*e.g.*, temperature (T) as a function of pH) within regions of the EPD that are similarly shaded. (Reprinted with permission of Wiley-Liss, Inc. and the American Pharmacists Association).

8.3 A COMPREHENSIVE APPROACH TO VACCINE FORMULATION IN PRACTICE

The comprehensive approach to biophysical characterization of vaccines proposed in this chapter involves four iterative steps. First, the types of analyses to be performed are selected. The selection criteria depend on the type of antigen being characterized, that is, whether they are proteins, viruses, bacteria, or nucleic acids. A certain amount of *a priori* knowledge of the system may permit the investigator to select the appropriate wavelength to use for protein or nucleic acid secondary structure analyses by circular dichroism (CD), Fourier transform infrared spectroscopy (FTIR), or an appropriate class of fluorescent dyes for binding analyses if the antigen is a globular protein, lipid, or nucleic acid. Second, analyses are performed as a function of selected environmental variables (temperature, pH, etc.), and the data from individual techniques are processed and incorporated into an EPD. Apparent phase boundaries are then identified and provide possible solution conditions to be used as a starting point for the assay(s) used to search for stabilizers. For example, potential combinations of pH and temperature near the boundary of two apparent phases that are not too far from solution conditions that may be feasible for a final formulation are typically selected. Third, the raw data that contributed to the construction of the EPD are reviewed to assist in assay selection. For instance, in the case of a protein antigen, if intrinsic tryptophan fluorescence and CD data indicate very little change in a boundary region, while the effective diameter (D_{eff}) measured using dynamic light scattering (DLS) is substantially increased, light scattering might be the assay of choice for stabilizer screening. Fourth, excipient screening of compounds that are both generally regarded as safe (GRAS) and possibly some non-GRAS compounds are used in the selected assay(s) in an attempt to identify stabilizing compounds or a mixture of stabilizing compounds that can be used in the formulation. Through an iterative process focused on antigen concentration, solution pH as well as excipient concentration and their use in combination, several formulations are selected for examination in long-term stability studies, which also employ biological (immunological) assays.

Descriptions of these types of assays and a selection of examples of successful attempts to stabilize a number of vaccines are presented, although not all of the methods discussed in this chapter are practical at all stages of the characterization process for all antigens. Some analyses are less useful because the data provided cannot be directly incorporated into EPDs or they are not currently available in high throughput format. They may become useful, however, when employed during the final stages of analysis when a final characterization of the vaccine antigen is required.

8.3.1 Hydrodynamic and Calorimetric Studies

Analysis of the overall structure and stability of molecules that are used as vaccine antigens includes characterization of a number of macromolecular properties such as their overall dimensions, net charge, diffusion characteristics, and conformational alteration temperatures. The net charge on macromolecules can often be related to their solution behavior. Protein-based vaccines are usually formulated at a pH that is away from their isoelectric point (pI) where solubility is typically at minimum and association behavior at maximum. These phenomena can be assessed by isoelectric focusing (IEF) using gels or capillaries and zeta potential analyses. Zeta potential measurements using phase analysis light scattering, a particularly powerful technique, calculate the electrophoretic mobility of particles of colloidal dimensions as detected by light scattering in an alternating electromagnetic field (McNeil-Watson et al., 1998) and can be performed in solution over a wide range of conditions at varying temperatures and pH. This is an advantage over IEF, in which the pI of the naked particle is measured in the presence of an artificially formed pH gradient. Zeta potential analysis permits comparison of the diffusion characteristics of macromolecules and their complexes as a direct function of pH and ionic strength simultaneously, which is critical for selecting optimal buffer conditions.

Particle size can be measured using a number of techniques, including size-exclusion high performance liquid chromatography (SE-HPLC), static light scattering, DLS, and analytical ultracentrifugation (AUC). DLS and SE-HPLC are currently the sizing techniques that are most easily applied to high throughput analyses of vaccines because of their current availability in a high throughput format as well as their resolving power and ability to provide a measure of polydispersity. For example, the data shown in Figure 8.2 illustrates DLS studies of an adenovirus type 5 vector used in several experimental DNA vaccines in the presence of sucrose as a stabilizer. Data are shown from 25 to 75°C with measurements of three important

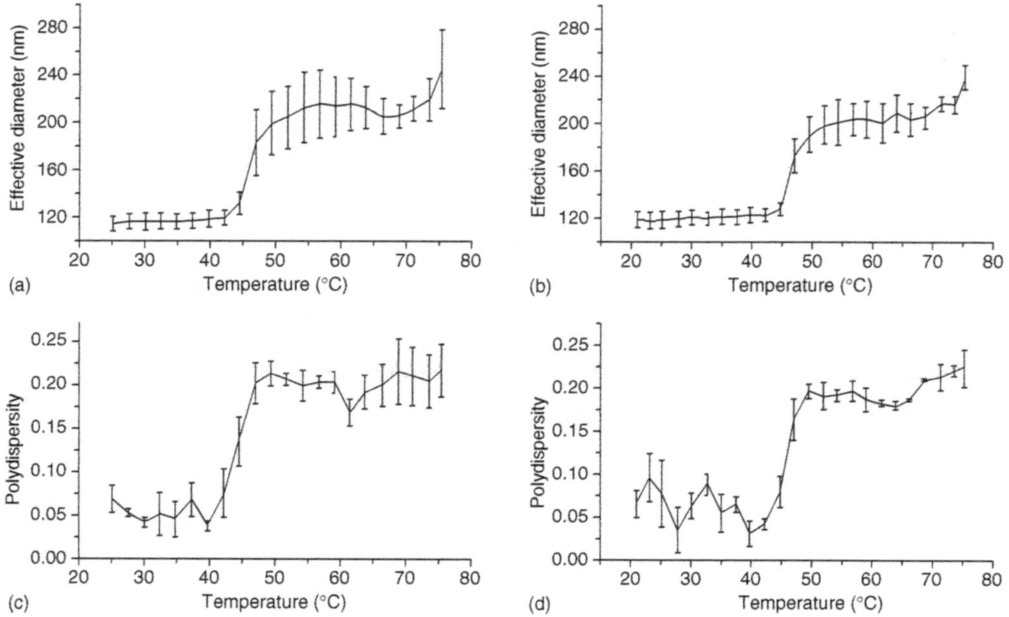

Figure 8.2 Adenovirus quaternary structure/aggregation. Effective diameter of Ad was followed as a function of temperature using DLS. (a) (2% sucrose) and (b) (10% sucrose). Polydispersity index as a function of temperature (c) (2% sucrose) and (d) (10% sucrose). Intensity of scattered light at an angle of 90° as a function of temperature (°C). Panel (e) (2% sucrose) and (f) (10% sucrose). (Reprinted with permission of Wiley-Liss, Inc. and the American Pharmacists Association).

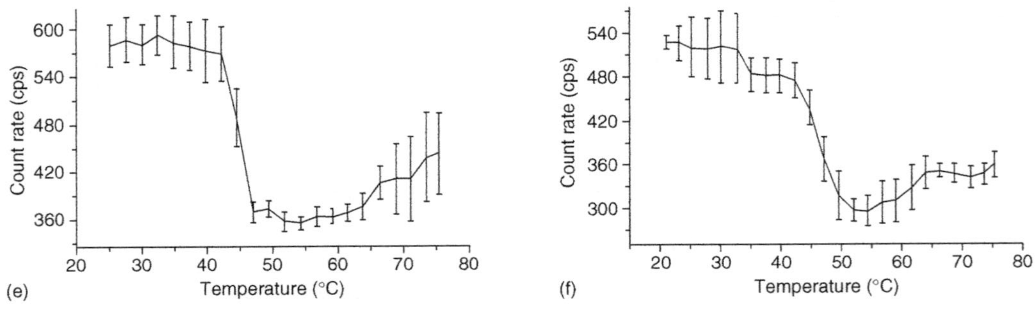

Figure 8.2 *(Continued)*

hydrodynamic characteristics (Rexroad et al., 2003). First, the particle effective diameter (D_{eff}) is the diameter of a solid sphere of uniform density having the same diffusion characteristics of the particles being measured. Second, the polydispersity index (PDI) is a unitless measure of the width of the intensity-weighted diffusion coefficient distribution. Highly monodisperse solutions are characterized as having PDIs near zero. Third is the static light scattering intensity, which is directly proportional to the hydrodynamic mass of the particles in solution. Rapid simultaneous measurements of the particle size, number distribution, and static intensity are particularly information rich and can be collected in seconds to minutes by DLS in a microtiter-based format. As a component of the comprehensive structural analyses of Ad5 by Rexroad et al., valuable information characterizing the physical effects of thermal perturbation on the quaternary arrangement of the virus was obtained by DLS. In this case (Fig. 8.2), DLS data combined with that from other techniques indicated that temperature-induced inactivation, or loss of infectivity of Ad5, is the result of a combination of structural alterations that occur throughout a greater range of temperatures than was previously recognized. The effects of sucrose on the virus's structural stability were also well described by these measurements (Rexroad et al., 2003).

Although a number of methodologies can be used to describe select types of structural transitions as a function of temperature, differential scanning calorimetry (DSC) directly measures heat capacity changes, which can be used to calculate the melting temperatures (T_m) of biomolecules. If transitions are reversible, enthalpies and entropies can also be calculated. In a DSC experiment, the heat capacity of the contents of a sample chamber is measured relative to that of a reference material. With modern instruments, this can be performed under high pressure and in a high throughput mode to measure T_ms of macromolecular complexes and viruses with multiple T_ms at temperatures until, and greater than, 120°. Using this approach, one can easily measure the effects of pH and temperature (Fig. 8.3; Ausar et al., 2006) or the effect of the presence of potential excipients on everything from recombinant proteins to viral vaccine preparations to DNA-based vaccines and determine which component in a maromolecular complex is being perturbed by a particular excipient or altered solution condition. In the case of the comprehensive structural analysis of Norwalk virus-like particles (NV-VLP), calorimetric measurements revealed at least three important physical characteristics (Fig. 8.3). First, overall thermal unfolding of the NV-VLPs comprises two events, one major and one minor. Second, the observed thermal transitions are pH dependent. Third, the thermal transition of the C-terminal P-domain corresponds to the major transition of the entire NV-VLP (Ausar et al., 2006). Insight into the thermal unfolding temperatures of the entire NV-VLP and the P-domain specifically can be used to stabilize this vaccine antigen.

8.3.2 Tertiary Structure

The tertiary structure of vaccine components can often be analyzed by spectroscopic methods. These include, among others, second-derivative ultraviolet (UV) absorption, intrinsic tryptophan fluorescence, and fluorescent dye binding

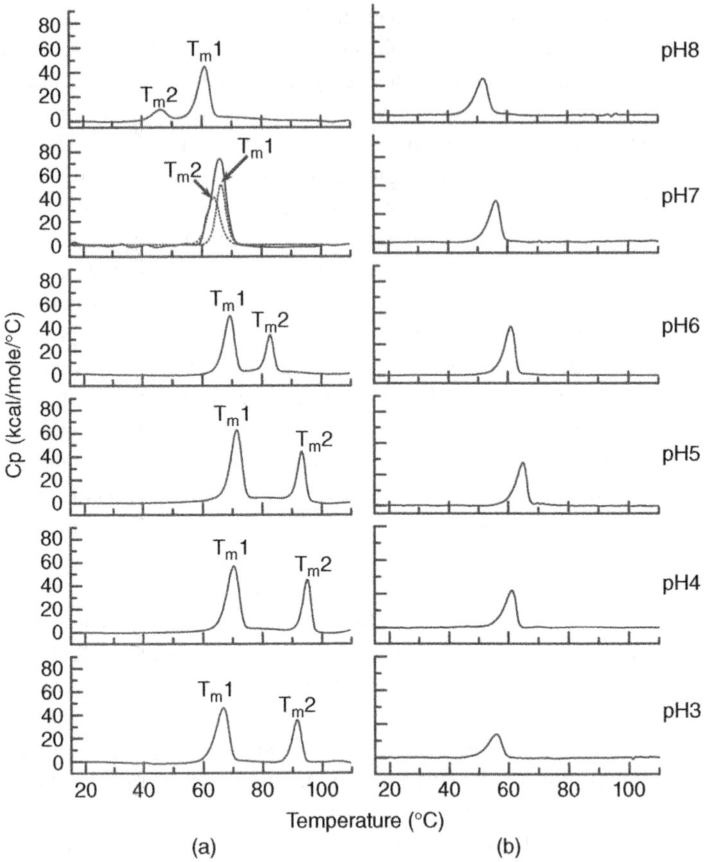

Figure 8.3 DSC analysis of intact NV-VLPs and the isolated P-domain of VP1 as a function of pH. DSC analysis was used to measure temperature-induced phase transitions indicative of VP1 unfolding at the indicated pH values. Thermograms represent the analyses of intact NV-VLPs (panel A) and the isolated P-domain of VP1 (panel B) over a range of 10–110°C. The data shown are representative of three experiments. This research was originally published in The Journal of Biological Chemistry © the American Society for Biochemistry and Molecular Biology.

assays. Second-derivative UV absorption spectroscopy simultaneously monitors discrete populations of the aromatic side chain chromophores of proteins (Mach and Middaugh, 1994). Spectral properties of the Phe, Tyr, and Trp chromophore side chains are very sensitive to their local environments. As such, the wavelength positions of second-derivative minima of the far-UV spectra of proteins can be resolved for Phe, Tyr, and Trp on the basis of their sensitivity to solvent exposure and provide a relative measure of protein tertiary structure (Fig. 8.4A). Altered tertiary arrangements of proteins are then indicated using red- or blue-shifted second-derivative minima (Fig. 8.4B–D). Such data can be used to trace pH (Ausar

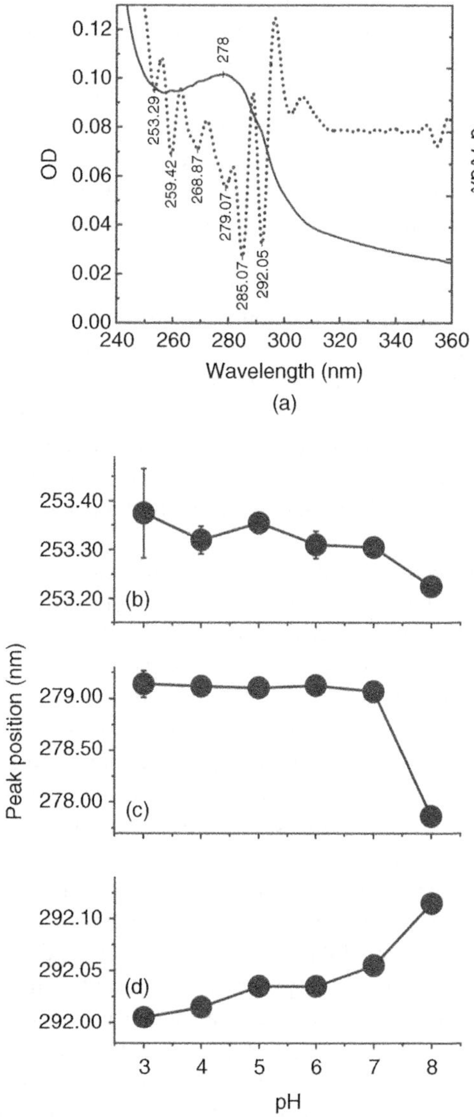

Figure 8.4 Second-derivative UV absorbance studies of NV-VLPs. (A), UV zero order (solid line) and second-derivative (dotted line) absorbance spectra of NV-VLPs at pH 7. The position of the wavelength minima of phenylalanine (B), tyrosine (C), and tryptophan (D) minima is plotted as a function of pH at 10°C (n=3). OD, optical density. This research was originally published in The Journal of Biological Chemistry © the American Society for Biochemistry and Molecular Biology.

et al., 2006) and temperature-dependent (Peek et al., 2007a) transitions that occur in protein-containing vaccine formulations. Proteins that contain multiple Phe, Tyr, and Trp residues are readily amenable to second-derivative UV analysis. For example, chromophore-rich viral vaccines in which the local environments of the UV-active side chains are presumed to be similarly arranged among the quasiequivalent subunits of the icosahedral capsid are susceptible to such analysis. As such, the induction of any temperature, pH, or concentration-dependent perturbations that occur may become amplified to produce very informative and reproducible wavelength shifts. The second-derivative UV absorption analyses presented by Ausar et al. (Ausar et al., 2006) indicate that the tertiary structure of NV-VLP is disrupted at alkaline pH but stabilized by acidic environments, corroborating previous observations. The functional relevance for the low pH stability of NV-VLPs is related to the physiological extremes that these particles are exposed to during passage through the gastrointestinal tract of the host. These should be among the key considerations when attempting to develop a structurally stable vaccine formulation for Norwalk virus. Similarly, changes in the UV spectra of nucleic acid containing formulations such as viral or DNA-based vaccines can be used in a related manner (Braun et al., 2001).

Intrinsic Trp fluorescence can also be used to aid in the assessment of the tertiary structure stability of proteins that contain tryptophan. Trp side chains are highly sensitive to their environment, as evidenced by shifts in the wavelength of maximum emission (λ_{max}) and change in emission intensity (Harrington et al., 2006; Brandau et al., 2007; Joshi et al., 2007). In general, a blue-shifted λ_{max} suggests a structural change in which one or more of a protein's indole side chains moves into a more apolar environment (Demchenko, 1986). Blue shifts are often seen in aggregating systems as well because of side chain burial. Conversely, red-shifted fluorescence spectra are typically seen when indole side chains become more exposed to the aqueous solvent driving events such as protein unfolding.

Fluorescent dye binding may also be sensitive to the tertiary structure arrangement of proteins (Schneider et al., 1979; Kueltzo et al., 2003; Fan et al., 2007), nucleic acids (Rexroad et al., 2003), and lipid bilayers (Cheng et al., 1999; Garcia Fernandez et al., 2004). Depending on the type of dye, probes such as 1-anilionaphthalene-8-sulfonate (ANS) (Schneider et al., 1979) are selective for the presence of features such as apolar regions and to a lesser extent surface-charged sites. More specific types of interactions such as intermolecular β-sheets are commonly detected using either Congo Red or one of the Thioflavine dyes (Vassar and Culling, 1959; Klunk et al., 1989; Guntern et al., 1992; LeVine, 1999). Dyes that intercalate between the stacked bases of double-stranded regions of DNA and RNAs or within their major and minor grooves are used to assess the relative thermal stability of the double-stranded regions of nucleic acids. Common examples of these types of dyes and their utility as probes of nucleic acids are propidium-iodide (Rexroad et al., 2006) and those of the TOTO-class (Rexroad et al., 2003). Probes of lipid bilayers are discussed in the following section in the context of bacterial vaccines.

8.3.3 Secondary Structure

Protein and nucleic acid secondary structure content and stability can also be measured using spectroscopic methods. Among those most commonly used are CD and FTIR spectroscopies. CD measures the difference in the absorption of left and right circularly polarized light (usually expressed as an intrinsic property by normalization to concentration as ellipticity). The backbone amide bonds of peptides are the chromphores used for protein far-UV CD and the bases in nucleic acids. Different types of secondary structure for both proteins and nucleic acids display distinct spectral characteristics that allow them to be identified and are used to monitor the maintenance of structure as it is perturbed by environmental stress such as pH and temperature (Harn et al., 2007; Peek et al., 2007a). Induced CD in dyes that bind to polysaccharides can also be used to probe the structure of polysaccharide-based vaccines (unpublished results). Although primarily a solution-based technique, CD can be used at very high concentrations using short pathlength cuvettes (Harn et al., 2007).

FTIR is also a common probe of the secondary structure of both proteins and nucleic acids. There is inherently more information present in the amide-I band of the infrared spectrum of proteins than that found in the far-UV CD spectrum of proteins, although the discrete infrared (IR) bands are strongly overlapped and are obscured by the strong water signal. There are, however, simple methods to increase the resolution of FTIR analyses (e.g., Fourier deconvolution and derivative analysis), as well as to eliminate the effect of water using subtraction techniques (Susi and Byler, 1983; Byler and Susi, 1986; Susi and Byler, 1986). The versatility of FTIR sampling methods such as transmittance, diffuse reflectance (DIR), or attenuated total reflectance (ATR) lend flexibility to this approach by allowing analysis of solid, crystalline, or lyophilized powders by DIR, in addition to emulsions, suspensions, and liquids by ATR or transmittance, with the added ability of temperature control for each. Accurate secondary structure estimation can be made using the aforementioned methods, although somewhat higher concentrations are typically necessary for solution-based sampling compared to CD analyses. The second-derivative spectra presented in Fig. 8.5 illustrate the concentration-dependent effects on the secondary structure of a pharmaceutical monoclonal antibody preparation using transmittance and ATR data collection methods (Harn et al., 2007). Similarly, the signals from the DNA bases, sugars, and phosphate groups can be clearly resolved in the infrared and used for structural analyses (Choosakoonkriang et al., 2001; Braun et al., 2003; Choosakoonkriang et al., 2003). Furthermore, lipid methylene groups are detectable using FTIR and can be used to determine various aspects of their conformational features (Lobo et al., 2002).

8.3.4 Dynamic Characteristics

The fact that the macromolecules that constitute vaccines are not static entities is becoming increasingly apparent in the analyses of the structure and stability of these systems. There are currently only a limited number of methods that can

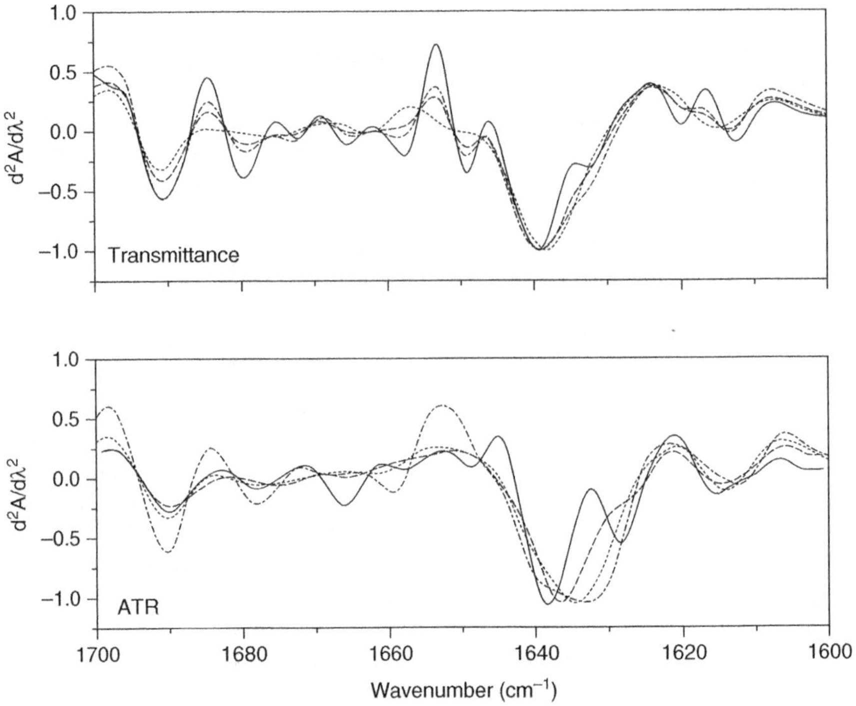

Figure 8.5 Second-derivative FTIR spectra of monoclonal antibodies. (A) Representative second-derivative FTIR spectra of MAb 1 obtained using transmittance sampling geometry. (B) Representative second-derivative FTIR spectra of MAb 1 obtained using ATR sampling geometry (—) 10 mg/ml, (– –) 100 mg/ml, (_ _ _) 140 mg/ml, (–_-) 190 mg/ml. (Reprinted with permission of Wiley-Liss, Inc. and the American Pharmacists Association).

assess dynamic internal motions of biomolecules that adequately balance the speed, resolution, and sampling versatility necessary for routine analysis. Currently, hydrogen-deuterium (H-D) exchange can be measured using a variety of methods, including NMR, mass spectrometry, and two-dimensional correlation FTIR spectroscopy. For example, the latter has revealed differential pH-dependent H-D exchange rates in a therapeutic monoclonal antibody preparation (Kamerzell and Middaugh, 2007). Fluorescence anisotropy in which rotational correlation times of chromophores are determined is also useful for this purpose. Other methods such as ultrasonic spectroscopy and pressure perturbation DSC enable the investigation of the rigidity or flaccidity of biomolecules in solution (Kamerzell et al., 2006). Elasticity, density, and internal fluctuations of macromolecules can be determined by ultrasonic velocity in which the degree of attenuation of ultrasonic waves varies according to the compressibility of the molecules present in the solution. These characteristics can be used to define the elastic modulus of biomolecules and their complexes. Conversely, the coefficient of thermal expansion (α) is related to the compressibility of biomolecules and can be measured using pressure perturbation DSC, wherein the heat that is produced or absorbed when pressure is applied to molecules in solution can be used to obtain α. Although the complex relationship between flexibility and stability is not well understood, it is becoming increasingly apparent that dynamic motions of biomolecules contribute to this property and will need to be included in more comprehensive structural analyses of the stability of vaccines.

8.3.5 Whole-Cell Bacterial and Viral Vaccines (Killed and Live-Attenuated)

Descriptions of structural analyses of vaccines from the preceding sections have been in large part relevant to the studies of purified components. A large number of vaccines, however, contain whole-cell bacterial species or viruses in live-attenuated or killed form. This can present severe complications from the perspective of assay design and data interpretation on the basis of the inherent structural complexities of these multicomponent systems. Live or killed bacteria and viruses contain at minimum a mixture of protein and nucleic acids and, in many cases, an unknown combination of proteins, nucleic acids, polysaccharides, lipids, and other small molecule chromophores, especially in the case of bacteria. Perhaps surprisingly, however, structurally sensitive methods can still be employed to provide information that can be used in formulation development. Obviously, a much more cautious approach is necessary in the interpretation of data from such studies. Most importantly, it will be necessary to recognize that it may not be possible to attribute changes in the target parameters to specific molecular events. Rather, they are simply employed as correlates of stability. For example, chromatography or light scattering techniques can still be used to assess the macromolecular arrangement or aggregation state of biological particles, alterations in which may produce reductions or losses in immunogenicity. In addition, highly reproducible spectroscopic characteristics of bacteria and viruses can be obtained by CD, FTIR, Raman, fluorescence, and other techniques. The large library of extrinsic fluorescent probe molecules, which has proven quite useful for characterizing the structural state of purified macromolecules, can also be used to label bacteria and viruses to indirectly monitor their structure. Many of the various classes of fluorescent molecules exhibit sufficient differential interaction with proteins, nucleic acids, and lipids to be used for this purpose. For example, such molecules can be used to sense any number of physicochemical states of vaccine antigens, such as the apolar nature of protein components with ANS, the single- or double-stranded nature of nucleic acids using either propidium-iodide or ethidium-bromide, the intracellular or endosomal redox state of bacterial organelles with dihydrofluoresceins, or intermolecular β-sheet interactions of capsid proteins detected by Thioflavine T or S, among others. Within a class of fluorescent probes, their altered fluorescence is a general indicator of any number of specific macromolecular phenomena, and as we again emphasize, require caution on the part of the analyst when interpreting one's observations. Thus, we generally believe that it is best not to attribute to any probe a specific underlying mechanism altering fluorescence spectra. Rather, such changes should be employed as nonspecific measures of stability as described in the following section. In preliminary studies, we have found that the best probes of bacterial stability are those of membrane integrity, although this generalization requires extensive further confirmation.

8.3.6 Construction of Empirical Phase Diagrams

Once an adequate amount of complementary data from at least three different techniques has been accumulated for a particular vaccine over a significant temperature range and for a number of solution conditions (temperature, pH, ionic strengths, concentration, etc.), these data can be combined to construct an EPD (Fig. 8.1). The usual strategy for the construction of a phase diagram is to include a number of experimental techniques that sample multiple structural phenomena, that is, dynamic, quaternary, tertiary, and secondary structure. This ensures that one does not rely on only a single physical phenomenon, and as a result, unwittingly skew stability information. For example, it would not be recommended to rely on the results of an EPD that contains data from three techniques sensitive to protein tertiary structure alone (e.g., second-derivative UV absorbance, fluorescent dye binding, and intrinsic Trp fluorescence). Such reliance would almost certainly neglect hydrodynamic, secondary, and dynamic components of macromolecular, viral, or cellular structure and their contributions to the overall stability of the antigen.

A major benefit of using EPDs is that it permits one to observe the results of a number of studies that describe more than one structural characteristic of the antigen simultaneously, thus facilitating a qualitative description of stable, intermediate, or highly disrupted states (Fig. 8.1) of biomolecules as separate forms that are fundamentally defined by empirical data. Discrete colored phases and apparent phase boundaries are the prominent features of EPDs. In practice, from the EPD presented in Figure 8.1, an analytical method, temperature, and pH combination were selected to assay the structural stability of recombinant ricin toxin-subunit A (rRTA) to develop a high throughput screening assay, which was then used to identify potential stabilizers (Peek et al., 2007a). Using this approach, the apparent phase boundary at pH 6 and 45°C was determined to reflect aggregation and could be sensitively monitored by simple turbidity (optical density) measurements. On further turbidity analyses in the presence of potential stabilizers, a handful of compounds were observed to inhibit aggregation of rRTA. These included sucrose, glycerol, lactose, and arginine. Although effective at preventing aggregation, most of these compounds improved the thermostability as detected by CD and fluorescence to only a limited extent. The exception was glycerol (50%), which increased the T_m of rRTA by 17°C (Peek et al., 2007a). This was used as the basis for a successful formulation of a previously unstable vaccine (Peek et al., 2007a).

8.3.7 Excipient Screening

Potential excipients are usually screened for use in pharmaceutical formulations on the basis of their established history of safety and effectiveness throughout a range of concentrations (Powell et al., 1998). They are generally selected from the so-called GRAS list of compounds and polymers (Powell et al., 1998). Compounds that are used as excipients occupy several classes of chemical families. Some are as simple as monovalent or divalent salts, whereas others are of slightly greater complexity such as citrate and malate. Sucrose, trehalose, dextrose, and other saccharides have frequently shown great utility as stabilizers in addition to their functional relatives, the dextrans and cyclodextrins. Amino acids such as glycine and lysine as well as high molecular weight gelatins are also used. Several select groups of nonionic and ionic detergents as well as a variety of high molecular weight polymers have also frequently been found to be effective stabilizers.

Usually, only a small number of such compounds will be found to have a significant stabilizing effect on a vaccine. Each class of compounds typically has a general mechanism of stabilization. As a group, salts most often act through their ability to produce charge shielding, increasing solubility, or reducing interactions between macromolecules. In addition, they can stabilize the phosphodiester backbone of vaccines that contain DNA or RNA. Sucrose, trehalose, and related sugars have shown to be thermoprotective stabilizers of numerous vaccines, including the recent improvement to the anthrax vaccine formulations (Jiang et al., 2006). The protective effect of high concentrations of sugars (Sola-Penna and Meyer-Fernandes, 1998; Kaushik and Bhat, 2003) and amino acids is thought to be provided by a preferential hydration effect (Timasheff and Inoue, 1968; Inoue and Timasheff, 1972; Timasheff, 1993). Nonspecific binding of charged polymers can also stabilize protein structure and protect them from thermal perturbation (Derrick et al., 2007; Fan et al., 2007; Kamerzell et al., 2007). For example, polyanions are thought to bind to positively charged exposed surfaces of proteins, thus stabilizing native states (Jones et al., 2004; Salamat-Miller et al., 2006; Salamat-Miller et al., 2007).

8.3.8 Characterizing Adjuvanted Vaccine Formulations

An important component of many vaccines such as those employing recombinant proteins is the adjuvant. Adjuvants are used to increase the effectiveness of vaccines by enhancing the immune response to the antigenic component. There are numerous agents known to induce an increased immune response that are used as adjuvants, but in many cases, an imbalance between safety and effectiveness has precluded their widespread use, especially in humans. For example, the effectiveness of many recombinant vaccines may show increased mammalian immune stimulatory responses in the presence of a nucleic acid adjuvant. Case in point, the bacterially derived CpG motif that is greater than 20 times more common in bacteria than in humans (Krieg et al., 1995; Klinman et al., 1996) can be used for this purpose. Another bacterially derived compound, lipopolysaccharide A (lipid A), of gram-negative bacteria exerts a strong adjuvant effect but displays some toxicity (Johnson et al., 1956), although the monophosphoryl A derivative of lipid A has proven to be much less so, facilitating its effective use in humans (Rudbach et al., 1990). Plant-derived saponins exhibit strong adjuvanticity but are also often reactogenic, which has so far precluded their use in human vaccines, although the less toxic saponin derivative QS21 is much less toxic and appears useable in humans (Kensil et al., 1991; Kensil et al., 1995). Various water-in-oil and oil-in-water adjuvants have been examined as well, with less toxic forms looking quite promising (Freund et al., 1937; Edelman, 1980; Edelman, 2002). The only compounds, however, that are currently approved for use as adjuvants in human vaccines in the United States are aluminum salts, most commonly aluminum hydroxide (Alhydrogel®) and aluminum phosphate (Adju-phos®).

Although the mode of action that confers the increased immune stimulatory effect by aluminum salt adjuvants is not known, there are three widely discussed potential mechanisms (Gupta et al., 1995; Gupta, 1998; Lindblad, 2004). The first idea is that the adjuvant creates a depot effect at the site of injection, which causes gradual release of the antigen to stimulate long-term presentation to the immune system. Second, the size and particulate nature of the adjuvant facilitate uptake by the cellular components of the immune system to increase antigen presentation efficiency. And third, the adjuvant–antigen component stimulates cytokine production.

A recently proposed mechanism by which aluminum salt adjuvants enhance the immune response to vaccines is that the adsorbed antigen is destabilized through a potential combination of increased electrostatic and hydrophobic interactions at the antigen–adjuvant binding surface. Such potential structural disruptions may facilitate antigen processing (Jones et al., 2005). Thus, it has become increasingly recognized that the effects of such surface adsorption needs to be characterized. Recent studies using model proteins and potential vaccine candidates have examined the physical effects of adsorption and binding efficiency of aluminum salt adjuvants (Jones et al., 2005; Peek et al., 2007b). These studies and others generally find (with a few exceptions) that the adsorbed proteins are less stable when bound to aluminum salt adjuvants in either the absence or presence of stabilizers than when they are present in solution (Jones et al., 2005; Peek et al., 2007b). Interestingly, EBA-175 RII-NG (a malaria vaccine candidate; Peek et al., 2006) was shown to be slightly more thermostable when bound to Adju-phos compared to Alhydrogel using both DSC and intrinsic tryptophan fluorescence, suggesting differential interaction mechanisms (Peek et al., 2007b). In support of using a structure-based approach to the formulation of vaccines, the conclusion from this set of studies (Fig. 8.6) was that although the proteins were less stable when bound to adjuvant, the compounds that were identified as potential stabilizers in solution also stabilized the protein when adsorbed to adjuvant (Jones et al., 2005; Peek et al., 2006).

On the basis of studies such as these, a general approach to the formulation of proteins in the presence of aluminum salt adjuvants can be proposed. Initially, binding isotherms of the protein to the adjuvant need to be obtained over a range of solution conditions (i.e., pH and solute concentration) within the limitation that the amount of aluminum salt needs to be minimized (e.g., <0.8 mg/dose). Ideally, the structure and thermal stability of the antigen should be characterized on the adjuvant's surface. Common methods for this purpose include intrinsic fluorescence (possibly in a front-face mode), FTIR, and DSC. Using these methods, stability should then be optimized, typically using temperature as an environmental stress, through variation in solutes with due care for reduction in surface binding induced by solutes. Alternatively, the antigen can be removed from the surface after incubation under appropriate conditions of time and temperature. Although proteins can often be removed from the surface of aluminum salts by dissolution of the adjuvant by high concentration of citrate or salt or low pH, use of agents such as detergents (e.g., SDS) or chaotropic compounds (urea and guanidine-HCl) requires caution owing to their intrinsic protein structure disrupting properties. Use of the latter at low concentrations may, however, be possible. A problem that is sometimes encountered with the use of aluminum hydroxide involves the increase in pH at

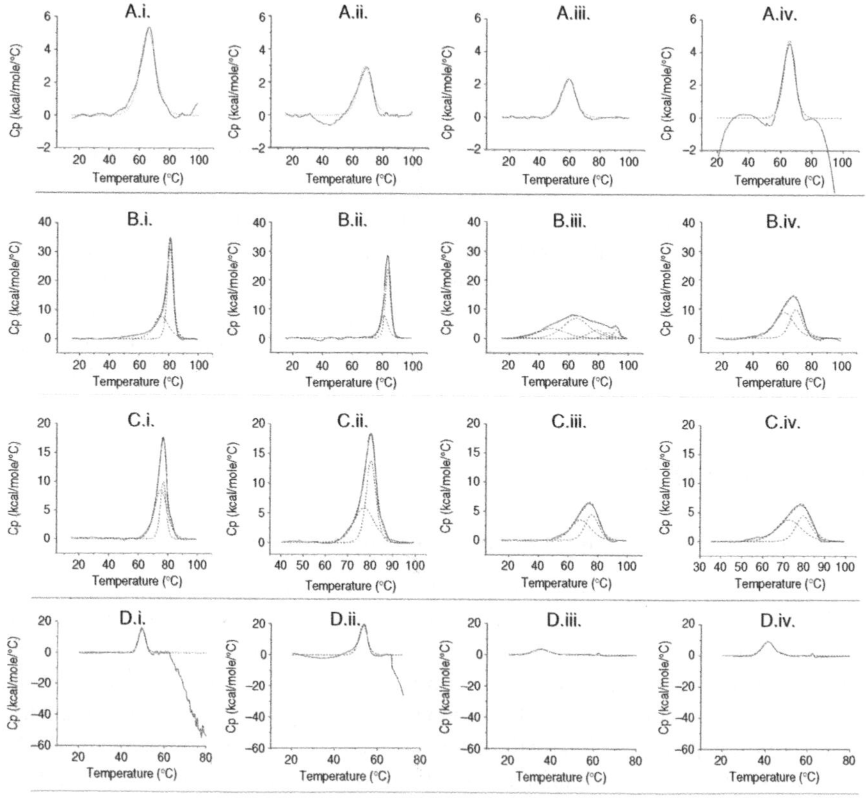

Figure 8.6 Thermograms and peak fits (dashed line) obtained by differential scanning calorimetry. Data sets for (A) lysozyme, (B) BSA, (C) ovalbumin, (D) rRTA, and (E) EBA-175 RII-NG. The stability of the protein was evaluated in solution (i), in the presence of a stabilizer (ii), adsorbed to an aluminum salt adjuvant (iii), and adsorbed to an aluminum salt adjuvant in the presence of a stabilizer (iv). In the case of EBA-175 RII-NG, the stability was evaluated in solution (i), in the presence of sucrose (ii), adsorbed to Adju-Phos1 (iii), adsorbed to Alhydrogel1 (iv), adsorbed to Adju-Phos1 in the presence of sucrose (v), and adsorbed to Alhydrogel1 in the presence of sucrose (vi). (Reprinted with permission of Wiley-Liss, Inc. and the American Pharmacists Association).

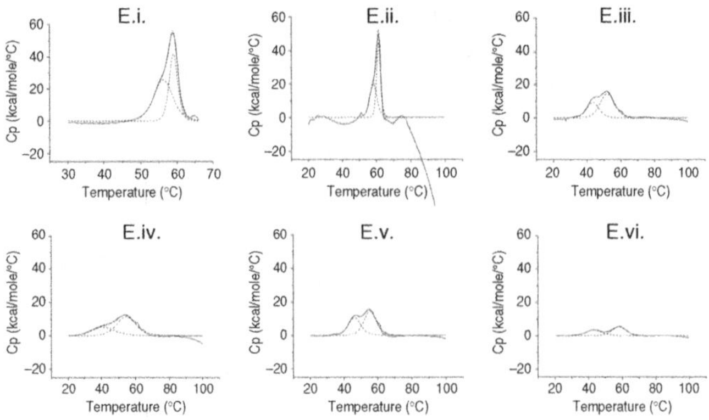

Figure 8.6 (*Continued*)

its surface because of the attraction of basic hydroxyl anions (Wittayanukulluk et al., 2004). This can lead to acceleration of deamidation reactions. This effect can often be minimized by the use of low concentration of phosphate to reduce surface pH (Wittayanukulluk et al., 2004). Thus, the general rule that one uses aluminum hydroxide with acidic proteins and aluminum phosphate with basic ones is not absolute, and it may be worthwhile to test both adjuvants. Similar interaction studies between other adjuvants and antigens should also be performed, although only limited information exists concerning such phenomenon (Jorgensen et al., 2004).

8.4 CONCLUSIONS

8.4.1 Future Prospects for Twenty First Century Vaccine Formulations

It seems highly likely that focus on the physical and chemical aspects of vaccine formulation will continue to increase. As mentioned previously, studies of the dynamic properties of proteins and nucleic acids and their relationship to stability are currently a leading candidate for such advances. Similarly, more emphasis on the chemical stability of vaccine components will surely occur, although we have not discussed this topic in this chapter. It is already the case that events such as oxidation and deamidation can be directly analyzed at high resolution using HPLC coupled to MS-detection. Can this be applied to something as complex as a virus, which contains multiple components? Preliminary studies of a variety of molecular complexes employing multidimensional chromatographic techniques coupled to advanced spectrometric methods suggest that this is quite possible (van Duijn et al., 2006; Benesch et al., 2007). We have also seen increased use of panels of monoclonal antibodies to map neutralizing epitopes, and we can expect this approach to increase in scope and intensity. The current use of only GRAS libraries for excipient selection seems likely to be relaxed as well. Could all of these lead to a substantial reduction in the use of biologically based assays during the formulation (and possibly even the vaccine release) process? Certainly for preformulation and early formulation work, this is already the case. As our analytical methods for large molecules and their complexes continue to improve, this appears a reasonable and important goal.

8.4.2 Strengths of a Rational Comprehensive Characterization Approach

Employing a systematic approach to vaccine formulation on the basis of structural considerations rather than immunogenicity in animal models offers a number of advantages. High throughput instrumentation is readily available and permits a rapid picture of structural lability to be built using a wide variety of environmental stresses. Because the basic structural elements are shared among active ingredients of vaccines, whether they are protein, nucleic acid, carbohydrate, or lipid based, the methods used are generally similar and are transferable from one type of vaccine to another. The rapid data collection rate of modern instruments facilitates the process of rapid excipient screening as well. One can easily test the effects all of the compounds that are available and immediately analyze the entire formulation space available, rather than indiscriminately exclude a class of compounds because of limited time or resources. Understanding structure as it relates to the stability of vaccines increases the potential that the product can be stored, transported, and administered to the patient anywhere in the world and that it will be done so in a safe, pure, and highly immunogenic form. That this approach appears to frequently work for fairly complex systems may at first appear surprising but simply follows from the predominance of only one or a few major degradation pathways in most vaccines.

REFERENCES

Ausar SF, Foubert TR, Hudson MH, Vedvick TS, Middaugh CR. Conformational stability and disassembly of Norwalk virus-like particles. Effect of pH and temperature. J Biol Chem 2006;281:19478–19488.

Benesch JL, Ruotolo BT, Simmons DA, Robinson CV. Protein complexes in the gas phase: technology for structural genomics and proteomics. Chem Rev 2007;107:3544–3567.

Bornside GH. Jaime Ferran and preventive inoculation against cholera. Bull Hist Med 1981;55:516–532.

Brandau DT, Joshi SB, Smalter AM, Kim S, Steadman B, Middaugh CR. Stability of the *Clostridium botulinum* type A neurotoxin complex: an empirical phase diagram based approach. Mol Pharm 2007;4:571–582.

Braun CS, Jas GS, Choosakoonkriang S, Koe GS, Smith JG, Middaugh CR. The structure of DNA within cationic lipid/DNA complexes. Biophys J 2003;84:1114–1123.

Braun CS, Kueltzo LA, Middaugh CR. Ultraviolet absorption and circular dichroism spectroscopy of nonviral gene delivery complexes. Methods Mol Med 2001;65:285–317.

Byler DM, Susi H. Examination of the secondary structure of proteins by deconvolved FTIR spectra. Biopolymers 1986;25:469–487.

Cheng KH, Virtanen J, Somerharju P. Fluorescence studies of dehydroergosterol in phosphatidylethanolamine/phosphatidylcholine bilayers. Biophys J 1999;77:3108–3119.

Choosakoonkriang S, Wiethoff CM, Anchordoquy TJ, Koe GS, Smith JG, Middaugh CR. Infrared spectroscopic characterization of the interaction of cationic lipids with plasmid DNA. J Biol Chem 2001;276:8037–8043.

Choosakoonkriang S, Wiethoff CM, Koe GS, Koe JG, Anchordoquy TJ, Middaugh CR. An infrared spectroscopic study of the effect of hydration on cationic lipid/DNA complexes. J Pharm Sci 2003;92:115–130.

Demchenko AP. *Ultraviolet Spectroscopy of Proteins*, Rev. and enl. translation of the Russian ed. Berlin: Springer-Verlag. New York; 1986. p x–312.

Derrick T, Grillo AO, Vitharana SN, Jones L, Rexroad J, Shah A, Perkins M, Spitznagel TM, Middaugh CR. Effect of polyanions on the structure and stability of repifermin (keratinocyte growth factor-2). J Pharm Sci 2007;96:761–776.

Edelman R. Vaccine adjuvants. Rev Infect Dis 1980;2:370–383.

Edelman R. The development and use of vaccine adjuvants. Mol Biotechnol 2002;21:129–148.

Fan H, Ralston J, Dibiase M, Faulkner E, Middaugh CR. Solution behavior of IFN-beta-1a: an empirical phase diagram based approach. J Pharm Sci 2005;94:1893–911.

Fan H, Vitharana SN, Chen T, O'Keefe D, Middaugh CR. Effects of pH and polyanions on the thermal stability of fibroblast growth factor 20. Mol Pharm 2007;4:232–240.

Ferran J. Sur la prophylaxie du cholera au moyen d'injections hypodermiques des cultures pures du bacile-virgule. CR Acad Sci Paris 1885;101:147–149.

Freund J, Casals J, Hosmer EP. Sensitization and antibody formation after injection of tubercle bacilli and paraffin oil. Proc Soc Exp Biol Med 1937;37:509–513.

Garcia Fernandez MI, Ceccarelli D, Muscatello U. Use of the fluorescent dye 10-N-nonyl acridine orange in quantitative and location assays of cardiolipin: a study on different experimental models. Anal Biochem 2004;328:174–180.

Guntern R, Bouras C, Hof PR, Vallet PG. An improved thioflavine S method for staining neurofibrillary tangles and senile plaques in Alzheimer's disease. Experientia 1992;48:8–10.

Gupta RK. Aluminum compounds as vaccine adjuvants. Adv Drug Deliv Rev 1998;32:155–172.

Gupta RK, Rost BE, Relyveld E, Siber GR. Adjuvant properties of aluminum and calcium compounds. Pharm Biotechnol 1995;6:229–248.

Harn N, Allan C, Oliver C, Middaugh CR. Highly concentrated monoclonal antibody solutions: direct analysis of physical structure and thermal stability. J Pharm Sci 2007;96:532–546.

Harrington A, Darboe N, Kenjale R, Picking WL, Middaugh CR, Birket S, Picking WD. Characterization of the interaction of single tryptophan containing mutants of IpaC from *Shigella flexneri* with phospholipid membranes. Biochemistry 2006;45:626–636.

Inoue H, Timasheff SN. Preferential and absolute interactions of solvent components with proteins in mixed solvent systems. Biopolymers 1972;11:737–743.

Jiang G, Joshi SB, Peek LJ, Brandau DT, Huang J, Ferriter MS, Woodley WD, Ford BM, Mar KD, Mikszta JA. Anthrax vaccine powder formulations for nasal mucosal delivery. J Pharm Sci 2006;95:80–96.

Johnson AG, Gaines S, Landy M. Studies on the O antigen of *Salmonella typhosa*. V. Enhancement of antibody response to protein antigens by the purified lipopolysaccharide. J Exp Med 1956;103:225–246.

Jones LS, Peek LJ, Power J, Markham A, Yazzie B, Middaugh CR. Effects of adsorption to aluminum salt adjuvants on the structure and stability of model protein antigens. J Biol Chem 2005;280:13406–13414.

Jones LS, Yazzie B, Middaugh CR. Polyanions and the proteome. Mol Cell Proteomics 2004;3:746–769.

Jorgensen L, Van de Weert M, Vermehren C, Bjerregaard S, Frokjaer S. Probing structural changes of proteins incorporated into water-in-oil emulsions. J Pharm Sci 2004;93:1847–1859.

Joshi SB, Kamerzell TJ, McNown C, Middaugh CR. The interaction of heparin/polyanions with bovine, porcine, and human growth hormone. J Pharm Sci 2007;97:1368–1385.

Kamerzell TJ, Middaugh CR. Two-dimensional correlation spectroscopy reveals coupled immunoglobulin regions of differential flexibility that influence stability. Biochemistry 2007;46:9762–9773.

Kamerzell TJ, Joshi SB, McClean D, Peplinskie L, Toney K, Papac D, Li M, Middaugh CR. Parathyroid hormone is a heparin/polyanion binding protein: binding energetics and structure modification. Protein Sci 2007;16:1193–1203.

Kamerzell TJ, Unruh JR, Johnson CK, Middaugh CR. Conformational flexibility, hydration and state parameter fluctuations of fibroblast growth factor-10: effects of ligand binding. Biochemistry 2006;45:15288–15300.

Kaushik JK, Bhat R. Why is trehalose an exceptional protein stabilizer? An analysis of the thermal stability of proteins in the presence of the compatible osmolyte trehalose. J Biol Chem 2003;278:26458–26465.

Kensil CR, Patel U, Lennick M, Marciani D. Separation and characterization of saponins with adjuvant activity from *Quillaja saponaria* Molina cortex. J Immunol 1991;146:431–437.

Kensil CR, Wu JY, Soltysik S. Structural and immunological characterization of the vaccine adjuvant QS-21. Pharm Biotechnol 1995;6:525–541.

Klinman DM, Yi AK, Beaucage SL, Conover J, Krieg AM. CpG motifs present in bacteria DNA rapidly induce lymphocytes to secrete interleukin 6, interleukin 12, and interferon gamma. Proc Natl Acad Sci USA 1996;93:2879–2883.

Klunk WE, Pettegrew JW, Abraham DJ. Quantitative evaluation of congo red binding to amyloid-like proteins with a beta-pleated sheet conformation. J Histochem Cytochem 1989;37:1273–1281.

Krieg AM, Yi AK, Matson S, Waldschmidt TJ, Bishop GA, Teasdale R, Koretzky GA, Klinman DM. CpG motifs in bacterial DNA trigger direct B-cell activation. Nature 1995;374:546–549.

Kueltzo LA, Osiecki J, Barker J, Picking WL, Ersoy B, Picking WD, Middaugh CR. Structure-function analysis of invasion plasmid antigen C (IpaC) from *Shigella flexneri*. J Biol Chem 2003;278:2792–2798.

LeVine H 3rd. Quantification of beta-sheet amyloid fibril structures with thioflavin T. Methods Enzymol 1999;309:274–284.

Lindblad EB. Aluminum compounds for use in vaccines. Immunol Cell Biol 2004;82:497–505.

Lobo BA, Rogers SA, Choosakoonkriang S, Smith JG, Koe G, Middaugh CR. Differential scanning calorimetric studies of the thermal stability of plasmid DNA complexed with cationic lipids and polymers. J Pharm Sci 2002;91:454–466.

Mach H, Middaugh CR. Simultaneous monitoring of the environment of tryptophan, tyrosine, and phenylalanine residues in proteins by near-ultraviolet second-derivative spectroscopy. Anal Biochem 1994;222:323–331.

McNeil-Watson F, Tscharnuter W, Miller J. A new instrument for the measurement of very small electrophoretic mobilities using phase analysis light scattering (PALS). Colloids Surf A Physicochem Eng Asp 1998;140:53–57.

Middaugh CR, Evans RK, Montgomery DL, Casimiro DR. Analysis of plasmid DNA from a pharmaceutical perspective. J Pharm Sci 1998;87:130–146.

Newman JF, Tirrell S, Ullman C, Piatti PG, Brown F. Stabilising oral poliovaccine at high ambient temperatures. Vaccine 1995;13:1431–1435.

Newman JF, Tirrell S, Ullman C, Piatti PG, Brown F. Stabilising oral poliovaccine at high ambient temperatures. Dev Biol Stand 1996;87:103–111.

Peek LJ, Brandau DT, Jones LS, Joshi SB, Middaugh CR. A systematic approach to stabilizing EBA-175 RII-NG for use as a malaria vaccine. Vaccine 2006;24:5839–5851.

Peek LJ, Brey RN, Middaugh CR. A rapid, three-step process for the preformulation of a recombinant ricin toxin A-chain vaccine. J Pharm Sci 2007a;96:44–60.

Peek LJ, Martin TT, Elk Nation C, Pegram SA, Middaugh CR. Effects of stabilizers on the destabilization of proteins upon adsorption to aluminum salt adjuvants. J Pharm Sci 2007b;96:547–557.

Powell MF, Nguyen T, Baloian L. Compendium of excipients for parenteral formulations. PDA J Pharm Sci Technol 1998;52:238–311.

Rexroad J, Evans RK, Middaugh CR. Effect of pH and ionic strength on the physical stability of adenovirus type 5. J Pharm Sci 2006;95:237–247.

Rexroad J, Wiethoff CM, Green AP, Kierstead TD, Scott MO, Middaugh CR. Structural stability of adenovirus type 5. J Pharm Sci 2003;92:665–678.

Rudbach JA, Cantrell JL, Ulrich JT, Mitchell MS. Immunotherapy with bacterial endotoxins. Adv Exp Med Biol 1990;256:665–676.

Salamat-Miller N, Fang J, Seidel CW, Assenov Y, Albrecht M, Middaugh CR. A network-based analysis of polyanion-binding proteins utilizing human protein arrays. J Biol Chem 2007;282:10153–10163.

Salamat-Miller N, Fang J, Seidel CW, Smalter AM, Assenov Y, Albrecht M, Middaugh CR. A network-based analysis of polyanion-binding proteins utilizing yeast protein arrays. Mol Cell Proteomics 2006;5:2263–2278.

Schneider AS, Middaugh CR, Oldewurtel MD. Role of bound water in biological membrane structure: fluorescence and infrared studies. J Supramol Struct 1979;10:265–275.

Sola-Penna M, Meyer-Fernandes JR. Stabilization against thermal inactivation promoted by sugars on enzyme structure and function: why is trehalose more effective than other sugars? Arch Biochem Biophys 1998;360:10–14.

Song Y, Schowen RL, Borchardt RT, Topp EM. Effect of 'pH' on the rate of asparagine deamidation in polymeric formulations: 'pH'-rate profile. J Pharm Sci 2001;90:141–156.

Susi H, Byler DM. Protein structure by Fourier transform infrared spectroscopy: second derivative spectra. Biochem Biophys Res Commun 1983;115:391–397.

Susi H, Byler DM. Resolution-enhanced Fourier transform infrared spectroscopy of enzymes. Methods Enzymol 1986;130:290–311.

Timasheff SN. The control of protein stability and association by weak interactions with water: how do solvents affect these processes? Annu Rev Biophys Biomol Struct 1993;22:67–97.

Timasheff, S.N., and Inoue, H. 1968. Preferential binding of solvent components to proteins in mixed water—organic solvent systems. Biochemistry 7: 2501–2513.

Vadas EB. *Stability of Pharmaceutical Products*. Philadelphia: Philadelphia College of Pharmacy; 1995. p 639–647.

van Duijn E, Simmons DA, van den Heuvel RH, Bakkes PJ, van Heerikhuizen H, Heeren RM, Robinson CV, van der Vies SM, Heck AJ. Tandem mass spectrometry of intact GroEL-substrate complexes reveals substrate-specific conformational changes in the trans ring. J Am Chem Soc 2006;128:4694–4702.

Vassar PS, Culling CF. Fluorescent stains, with special reference to amyloid and connective tissues. Arch Pathol 1959;68:487–498.

WHO. Expanded Programme on Immunization. Heat stability of vaccines. Wkly Epidemiol Rec 1980;55:252–254.

WHO. Proper handling and reconstitution of vaccines avoids programme errors. Vaccines and Biologicals Update 34; 2000.

Wittayanukulluk A, Jiang D, Regnier FE, Hem SL. Effect of microenvironment pH of aluminum hydroxide adjuvant on the chemical stability of adsorbed antigen. Vaccine 2004;22:1172–1176.

9

LYOPHILIZATION IN VACCINE PROCESSES

ALEXIS WASSERMAN
Merck & Co., West Point, PA, USA

RANJIT SARPAL
Amgen, Thousand Oaks, CA, USA

BRET R. PHILLIPS
Merck & Co., West Point, PA, USA

9.1 INTRODUCTION

Lyophilization, or freeze-drying, is a stabilizing process in which a solution is frozen and the water/solvent is removed from the solid state through sublimation and desorption processes. This process is used throughout the pharmaceutical/biotechnology industry in order to raise the allowed product storage temperature, increase shelf life, and/or minimize the impact of temperature excursions during shipping and storage. The topic of lyophilization has been discussed extensively in the literature (Jennings, 2002; Constantino, 2004).

Although freeze-drying is commonly used for a variety of pharmaceutical and biological products, this chapter focuses on the process as it applies to vaccines. The chapter has been broadly divided into the following subsections:

1. Overview of the filling and lyophilization process, the advantages and disadvantages of lyophilization, and the use of lyophilization in vaccine manufacturing.

Vaccine Development and Manufacturing, First Edition.
Edited by Emily P. Wen, Ronald Ellis, and Narahari S. Pujar.

2. Formulation development for lyophilized products, including excipient selection and component selection.
3. Lyophilization theory, including treatment of freezing and primary and secondary drying.
4. Commercial-scale freeze-dryer equipment and design, including discussions on product defects.

Throughout this chapter, various case studies drawn from vaccine lyophilization process development and commercial-scale manufacturing are presented.

9.1.1 Lyophilization Process Summary

Lyophilization is best considered in the context of the overall manufacturing process. Its place in this process is depicted in Figure 9.1. The active bulk vaccine is mixed with the appropriate diluent and excipients. These ingredients are added in proper proportion to dilute the product to its target potency and provide an optimal excipient concentration for product stability during both processing and long-term storage.

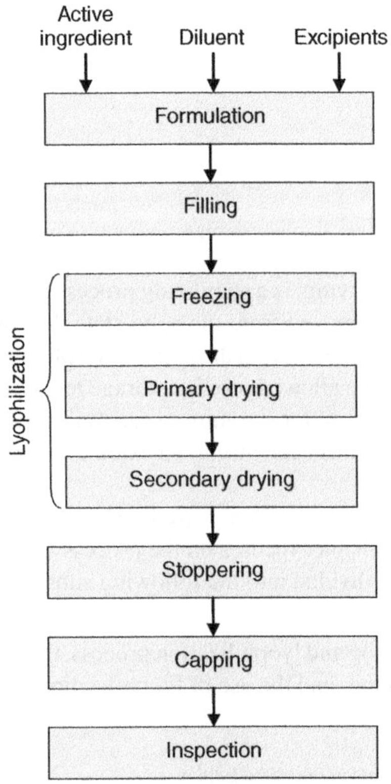

Figure 9.1 Process flow diagram of formulation, filling, lyophilization, and finishing process.

As water is by far the most predominant solvent used to formulate vaccine products, the focus of these discussions will be the lyophilization of aqueous solutions. After this step, the product is filled into vials, which are then partially stoppered. These partially stoppered vials proceed to lyophilization, which consists of three main steps: freezing, primary drying, and secondary drying. During the freezing step, the liquid product is frozen to below its glass transition temperature, T'_g. In primary drying, the lyophilizer chamber pressure is lowered, and the ice crystals are removed via sublimation. During secondary drying, the lyophilizer shelf temperature is raised, and the excipient bound, noncrystallized water is desorbed. After secondary drying, the vacuum is broken by introducing head space gas into the lyophilizer chamber until it reaches the desired pressure, at which time the vials are stoppered. If the vials are stoppered under partial vacuum, the chamber pressure is then raised to atmospheric pressure. The vials are subsequently unloaded, sealed, and inspected.

9.1.2 Benefits of Lyophilization

Compared to a vaccine in the aqueous phase, the freeze-dried solid state cake demonstrates significantly slower degradation kinetics. This stabilization allows the product to be stored at warmer temperatures than would otherwise be possible.

Many vaccines are simply not stable in solution, even under refrigerated conditions (2–8°C). Even for more stable solutions, the stability may be such that the allowed shelf life of the product, the time between when the product is manufactured until it must be used, is too restricting for commercial distribution and use. Similarly, limiting a vaccine to frozen storage conditions (i.e., <-20°C) also greatly limits its commercial availability, as the infrastructure for shipping and storing a vaccine under frozen conditions is mostly limited to the United States. In these cases, lyophilization is the only viable means for making such a vaccine product commercially available. Although most lyophilized vaccines still require storage under refrigerated conditions, the infrastructure for managing the supply chain under refrigerated conditions is readily available in the United States, Europe, and throughout most of the developed world.

9.1.3 Drawbacks of Lyophilization

Although lyophilization results in a more stable product, it has several significant drawbacks.

In comparison to a liquid state product, a lyophilized product not only requires the same formulation, filling equipment, and processing steps, but also requires the additional unit operation of freeze-drying, as well as the unique equipment required to inspect the appearance of the lyophilized cake. Not only does this add significant time to the overall manufacturing process, but also it is costly in terms of both utility and capital expenses. Owing to its complex nature, manufacturing issues related to both the lyophilization equipment and process are also commonly encountered during routine commercial manufacturing.

Lyophilization also requires far more effort and time during process/product development than a liquid state product. Significantly more effort is generally required during the scale-up phase; the heat transfer properties and variability of bench or pilot-scale equipment are not necessarily equivalent to the commercial-scale lyophilizers.

Other concerns relate to the effect of the lyophilization process on the vaccine, as many vaccines experience significant potency loss during the freeze-drying process. There is also an additional sterility risk associated with the handling of partially stoppered vials before lyophilization.

In addition to the added complexity of the manufacturing process, lyophilized products require a methodology for inspecting the freeze-dried vials. Manual inspection procedures are costly, time consuming, and can be very challenging to validate. Automated inspection systems have a high capital cost, and the equipment is very complex in its operation and on-going performance maintenance. Lyophilized products also require several additional release tests for attributes such as residual moisture and product reconstitution time. These lyophilization-specific needs add to the cost of the product and to the overall manufacturing cycle time.

Lyophilized products are reconstituted with a diluent before administration, which presents a further drawback. From a vaccine manufacturing perspective, diluent is in effect an additional product, resulting in additional cost. This in turn requires additional storage capacity for the manufacturer, distributor, and the end user. Finally, the vaccine administrator must take the extra step of reconstitution before administering the vaccine, resulting in additional work to the immunization process.

Finally, the packaging equipment required for a lyophilized product is complex and expensive. The lyophilized product may need to be copackaged with a diluent, syringe, and needle. If the diluent has been prefilled into syringes, even further complexity is added, as packaging equipment must be specialized in order to be compatible with both vials and prefilled syringes.

9.1.4 Use of Lyophilization in the Vaccine Industry

For all of the reasons discussed previously, a lyophilized product is only pursued when a stable liquid form cannot be successfully developed. This is the case for many vaccine products. A brief survey of lyophilized vaccines is presented in Table 9.1. Owing to the biophysical and biochemical nature of these products, stable liquid formulations are not feasible. However, it is important to note that the scope of lyophilized products is not limited to biological entities. There are many examples of small molecule pharmaceuticals that also require a lyophilized stable formulation to provide the shelf life and storage conditions necessary to make it a commercially viable product.

9.1.5 Desired Characteristics of a Lyophilized Product

9.1.5.1 Stability The fundamental goal of lyophilization is to produce a stable product, specifically in those cases where a stable liquid formulation cannot be

TABLE 9.1 Some Marketed Lyophilized Vaccines

Vaccine	Target	Vaccine Type	Manufacturer
Varilrix®	Chicken pox	Attenuated live virus	GlaxoSmithKline
VARIVAX®	Chicken pox	Attenuated live virus	Merck
ActHIB®	*Haemophilis influenza* B	Polysaccharide–protein conjugate	Sanofi Pasteur
Hiberix®	*Haemophilis influenza* B	Polysaccharide–protein conjugate	GlaxoSmithKline
M-M-R® II	Measles, mumps, rubella	Attenuated live virus	Merck
Priorix®	Measles, mumps, rubella	Attenuated live virus	GlaxoSmithKline
ProQuad®	Measles, mumps, rubella, chicken pox	Attenuated live virus	Merck
ACWY Vax®	Meningitis	Polysaccharide	GlaxoSmithKline
Menomune®	Meningitis	Polysaccharide	Sanofi Pasteur
IMOVAX®	Rabies	Inactivated virus	Sanofi Pasteur
RabAvert®	Rabies	Inactivated virus	Novartis
Rotarix®	Rotavirus	Attenuated live virus	GlaxoSmithKline
ZOSTAVAX®	Shingles	Attenuated live virus	Merck
BCG vaccine SSI	Tuberculosis	Attenuated live bacteria	Statens Serum Institut
YF-VAX®	Yellow fever	Attenuated live virus	Sanofi Pasteur

developed. Stability is determined through long-term studies in which the product is maintained at the required storage conditions for a period equal to or exceeding the desired product shelf life, typically 18–36 months. At defined intervals throughout this duration, the product is tested for attributes such as potency, percent residual moisture, pH, appearance, and reconstitution time—the time required for the lyophilized product to dissolve in the prescribed diluent. Accelerated stability studies, in which the product is exposed to warmer conditions relative to the intended storage condition, are used to provide a more rapid estimation of product stability, as well as to provide data that can be used to support temperature excursions that occur during product sealing and inspection, packaging, shipping, and distribution to the end user.

9.1.5.2 Moisture The stability of the vaccine product may be strongly dependent on the moisture of the final product. The general rule is that stability is improved as lower moisture levels are achieved. Vaccine products typically have a moisture specification falling within the range of 0–5%. However, this rule is not necessarily based on an extensive database, as generating such data is not only very challenging from a technical point of view, but also extremely time-consuming and costly. As discussed in the case study presented in the following section, for some biological products, it is also possible that extremely low moisture levels may not be optimal.

Case Study 1—Stability For a varicella vaccine formulation, it was found that increased moisture correlated with better lyophilization yield and better product stability. Three lyophilization cycles were used as follows: one with drying for 8 h at 0.47 m Bar pressure, one with drying for 14 h at 0.14 m Bar pressure, and one with drying for 48 h at <0.07 mM bar pressure. The 8-h drying cycle resulted in 6–8% residual moisture, the 14-h cycle in 2–7% residual moisture, and the 48-h cycle in 0.5–1.5 % residual moisture. The 8-h drying cycle resulted in final product with a higher initial vaccine titer and with improved long-term stability as compared to the other two cycles (Bennett et al., 1992). This case demonstrates that within a certain range, it is possible to overdry, resulting in reduced potency and stability.

9.1.5.3 Appearance One indicator of successful lyophilization is product cake appearance. Lyophilization resulting in an elegant pharmaceutical appearance is generally preferred and, in some markets, expected. Ideally, the lyophilized cake has a smooth surface without cracks, is neither shrunken nor pulling away from the sides of the vial, and is consistent in color and sheen across all surfaces.

9.1.5.4 Reconstitution The vaccine administrator reconstitutes the vaccine using the prescribed sterile diluent. Rapid reconstitution with minimal effort leading to a visually clear solution is expected. Deviations from typical reconstitution times may be indicative of an incomplete lyophilization.

9.1.6 Economic Considerations in Lyophilization Process Development

In the competitive world of vaccines, speed to the marketplace can be the deciding factor for hundreds of millions of dollars in product revenue. Once commercialized, the reliability of the process and equipment plays a crucial role in the management of that supply chain and associated revenue stream.

As stated previously, the capital cost of a lyophilization manufacturing facility is much greater than that for a liquid state product because of the additional equipment required to perform the freeze-drying step. In addition, the time required to build and start up a lyophilization manufacturing facility is greater than that required for a liquid filling facility because of the complexity of both the process and the equipment.

The scale-up issues that may be encountered are typically far more complex than those associated with a liquid state product. A pilot-scale freeze-dryer may have one-tenth the capacity of a commercial-scale unit, and a bench-scale freeze-dryer may have only one-hundredth the capacity of the commercial-scale unit. There are known instances where issues encountered during the scale-up of the lyophilization process have resulted in many months of delay to product commercialization. As mentioned previously, such a delay has the potential to result in significant lost revenue.

9.2 FORMULATION

Before discussing the fundamental principles of lyophilization, it is important to first describe the impact that the formulation has on lyophilization and vaccine stability. Different excipients will confer specific stability attributes on the product. Although some excipients may provide outstanding long-term stability, they may pose inherent problems for the successful development of the lyophilization process. In addition, the final blend of excipients and active vaccine product must result in the desired pH and tonicity. The formulation must also protect the product during the freezing and lyophilization steps in order to minimize vaccine potency loss across these processes. For these reasons, the formulation must be carefully developed. Further discussions on this subject are presented in the following section.

9.2.1 Considerations in Excipient Selection

The fundamental goal of lyophilizing a vaccine is to ensure that potency is adequately maintained over the desired shelf life at storage temperatures acceptable to the marketplace. For a vaccine, the shelf life is typically 18–36 months. In the United States, infrastructure and shipping logistics normally allow for the commercialization of vaccines requiring storage at −20°C or below. However, for the rest of the developed world, shelf-life storage conditions must be at or above refrigerated temperatures, 2–8°C. As discussed previously, the product must also be able to withstand short-term temperature excursions that occur during product capping and inspection, packaging, shipping, and distribution to the end user.

The selection of the appropriate excipients is necessary to confer both physical and biochemical stability to the vaccine under consideration. Biochemical stability needs to be optimized not only for the shelf life and temperature excursion conditions experienced by the final lyophilized dosage form as described previously, but also for the product while it is in solution before freezing, during freezing (cryopreservative), during lyophilization (lyoprotectant), and again before administration while the product is in solution after reconstitution. These considerations are further discussed in the following section.

The stability of the formulation before freezing can have a very significant impact on the manufacturing process and product cost. There are examples of lyophilized vaccine products whose stability in the liquid phase before freezing and lyophilization is such that it makes economic sense to allow a full day for this step, enough time to fill an entire manufacturing-scale lyophilizer (see the following section). There are many other examples of lyophilized vaccine products whose stability in the liquid phase before freezing is such that it is necessary to limit the duration of this step to several hours, therefore limiting the amount of vials that can be filled to perhaps only one-third or even one-fourth of the commercial freeze-dryer capacity. In these instances, the choice can be made to continue processing with only a partially loaded freeze-dryer—a significant impact to plant capacity—or formulate and fill additional vaccine lots until the freeze-dryer is full. The second scenario has a significant impact on manufacturing complexity, including segregation logistics associated with having multiple lots in the same lyophilizer, as well as a significant impact on product cost, as each of the independent formulations required to maximize the capacity of the lyophilizer, in some cases three or four, requires independent product quality testing. On the basis of these discussions, the advantage of developing a formulation that provides not only the necessary shelf-life stability but also a "stable" liquid formulation is readily apparent.

Similarly, the biochemical and biophysical properties of the formulation must also be such that minimal damage to the vaccine occurs during the freezing and lyophilization steps. Vaccine potency loss during freeze-drying can be significant. However, with a careful evaluation of excipients and excipient concentration, potency yields across lyophilization can be greatly improved without negatively impacting final product stability. Studies have suggested that for some vaccine formulations, a slight change in the excipient concentration in the formulation can reduce the vaccine potency loss across freeze-drying by half without negatively impacting either the stability of the formulation in the liquid phase or that of the final freeze-dried product.

In addition to the biochemical stability concerns discussed previously, the formulation must also ensure the physical stability and integrity of the lyophilized cake. As the actual mass of vaccine in the formulation mixture is normally extremely low, the formulation must include a bulking agent to provide mechanical strength to the lyophilized cake. During the freeze-drying process, this mechanical strength prevents the cake from collapsing in on itself (discussed in the following section). Mannitol is one commonly chosen bulking agent to meet this need. As collapse of the vaccine structure may also occur because of osmotic dehydration, solution tonicity must also be considered during formulation development.

On the basis of all of these complexities, the formulation development of lyophilized vaccines requires a unique and carefully chosen set of excipients.

9.2.2 Excipients and Glass Transition Temperature

In order to ensure optimal lyophilization performance, it is important to avoid excipients that lower the T_g' or collapse temperature, T_c, of the frozen product. Both T_g' and T_c are material properties of the glassy amorphous phase that was created during the freezing process. The amorphous phase comprises the noncrystallized excipients and water in the frozen matrix.

The T_g' is defined as the temperature below which the molecular mobility of the amorphous phase, consisting of bound water, vaccine, and the vaccine excipients, approaches zero. T_g' is typically determined using differential scanning calorimetry (DSC).

T_c is typically a few degrees centigrade higher than the T_g'. If T_c is exceeded during lyophilization, gross defects in the cake appearance may be observed. While vaccine potency may be sensitive to exceeding T_g', the cake appearance may not be affected during lyophilization until T_c is exceeded. T_c is most often determined using freeze-drying microscopy.

For best results, it is best to carry out primary drying below T_g'. The T_g' of some commonly used excipients are presented in Table 9.2 (Levine and Slade, 1988). Because T_g' and T_c are generally close to each other, the two terms and associated values are commonly used interchangeably.

As the product temperature approaches the T_g', the viscosity in the amorphous phase can change several orders of magnitude over a relatively small temperature span. It is for this reason that the product temperature must be kept below the T_g' during the freeze-drying process. If the product is allowed to warm above this temperature, the increase in product mobility (decrease in viscosity) may result in collapse of the product because of changes in the structure of the amorphous phase. Owing to the high concentration of excipients in the amorphous phase, this product mobility may also result in (significant) vaccine potency loss. The need to maintain a lower product temperature during lyophilization results in longer freeze-drying cycles, increased product cost, and a reduced plant capacity.

Similarly, some vaccine formulations can experience unacceptable potency loss during the freezing process. Specifically, these potency losses occur during the time interval beginning when the ice crystallizes and ending when the product is cooled

TABLE 9.2 Some Commonly Chosen Excipients and their T_g' (Levine and Slade, 1988)

Excipient	T_g' (°C)
Mannitol	−40
Sorbitol	−43.5
Trehalose	−29.5
Sucrose	−32
Lactose	−28

to below the T_g'. When the water molecules crystallize, the vaccine is exposed to a greatly increased excipient concentration and associated pH shift. Because the amorphous phase retains molecular mobility above the T_g', the exposure of vaccine product to the conditions experienced during the freezing process has the potential to greatly impact potency. In order to minimize the exposure of the vaccine to these conditions during the freezing process, very sensitive vaccine formulations are flash-frozen at cryogenic temperatures. Such freezing requires complex equipment and additional unit operations, further complicating the overall manufacturing process. This is described in further detail in a later section.

Inorganic salts that are typically used to optimize tonicity and/or provide liquid stability are also known to lower the T_g' (Her et al., 1995). As discussed previously, the need to maintain a lower product temperature during lyophilization results in longer freeze-drying cycles, increased product cost, and reduced plant capacity.

Case Study 2—Formulation During the formulation development of a varicella-zoster-virus vaccine, it was found that sugar functioned as an effective cryopreservative, whereas other excipients such as glutamate or albumin were not effective. Electron micrographs showed enveloped viral particles for freeze-dried vaccine formulations containing sugar. In contrast, electron micrographs of freeze-dried vaccine formulations without sugar showed had no enveloped particles. The potency yield across the lyophilization step was high for formulations containing sugar and low for formulations that did not contain sugar. It was further hypothesized that sugar may help retain some residual moisture, which in turn may improve vaccine stability of the final product (Grose, 1981).

9.3 FILLING

The vast majority of vaccines are filled into vials. However, a few products filled into syringes are under development. For the sake of simplicity, this chapter focuses on the vaccine development and manufacturing in glass vials alone.

9.3.1 Vials

9.3.1.1 Vial Selection As stated previously, most lyophilized vaccines are filled into glass tubing or molded vials. The fill depth in a vial greatly determines the lyophilization cycle efficiency, as well as the quality of the finished lyophilized product. An increase in fill depth corresponds to a greater distance through which mass transfer must occur during lyophilization and therefore to an increased cycle time and potentially poor product quality. The fill depth can be decreased by selecting an appropriate vial diameter size or by altering the fill volume. A fill depth of approximately 0.5–1 cm typically results in an efficient lyophilization process with good product quality.

Vial sizes cannot be too large, as this will lead to difficulties in manufacturing capacity, as well as in storage capacity. By increasing the vial diameter, the number of vials per shelf decreases, thus decreasing the capacity of the freeze-dryer. However, the reduced lyophilization cycle time and the improved product quality may offset these concerns. The balance between vial diameter and fill depth must be appropriately considered.

9.3.1.2 Vial Preparation Relative to a liquid state product, a lyophilized product introduces one unique consideration in regards to vial preparation. Owing to the temperature sensitivity of the vaccine in its prelyophilized liquid state, if a depyrogenation tunnel is used, it may be necessary to cool the vials to an extent greater than what is normally achieved in the cooling zone. In these instances, depyrogenation equipment with added cooling zones may be required.

9.3.2 Stoppers

9.3.2.1 Stopper Selection The primary goal in stopper selection is to choose a stopper that will provide adequate container closure to ensure product sterility and protection from moisture during long-term storage. The chemical compatibility of a lyophilized product with a stopper is generally not a concern, as there is no liquid phase present during long-term storage and storage of the product after reconstitution and before administration is typically limited on the scale of hours.

The physical properties and geometry of the stopper must also be considered during the selection process. Some potential problems include the following:

1. Stoppers twinning or clumping to other stoppers before partial stoppering.
2. Stoppers falling out of the vial before lyophilization.
3. Stoppers failing to fully stopper or seat at the conclusion of lyophilization.
4. Stoppers sticking to the underside of the lyophilization shelf at the conclusion of stoppering.

For facilities where the lyophilizer is loaded and unloaded manually, stopper sticking to the underside of the shelf can be managed during the unloading process. For facilities that use automated loading/unloading systems, steps must be taken to eliminate the potential for stoppers to stick to the underside of the lyophilizer shelf. Avoidance of this problem can be achieved either by designing the underside of the lyophilizer shelves with a textured finish or by choosing a stopper that is specifically designed to minimize this tendency.

Stoppers are available in several different materials of construction, geometries, and coatings. Most stoppers used for biopharmaceuticals are made from chlorobutyl rubber. A vent is necessary in the underside of the stopper in order to allow the water vapor to escape during lyophilization. This vent can exist in a variety of shapes, and in recent years, vendors have optimized the design to minimize stopper twinning/clumping.

9.3.2.2 ***Stopper Processing*** Processing of uncoated stoppers includes washing, siliconization, and sterilization. Silicone is used to lubricate the stoppers, which allows the processing of stoppers through the mechanical equipment and placement into the vial to proceed more readily. Alternatively, some stoppers are manufactured with a polymer coating that eliminates this need. After sterilization, it is important to dry the stoppers thoroughly, removing any water that is absorbed by the stopper during washing. Failure to fully desorb water from the stopper can potentially impact long-term stability, as residual stopper moisture may escape to the vial headspace and ultimately be absorbed by the lyophilized cake.

Stopper processing can be achieved using a variety of methods and equipment. Stoppers can be washed and siliconized, if required, in one process, and then sterilized and dried in a steam autoclave. In this case, the washed and siliconized stoppers are placed into moisture-permeable bags for sterilization and drying. If a product is moisture sensitive, it may be necessary to transfer the moisture-permeable bag into another bag in which the moisture permeability is negligible. Alternatively, stoppers can be washed, siliconized, if required, and sterilized in one unit operation designed specifically for this purpose. This approach allows for a much tighter control of the residual moisture in the stopper and provides added sterility assurance.

9.3.3 Vial/Stopper Compatibility

The container-closure integrity of vial and stopper is dependent on the appropriate fit between the vial inner diameter (ID) and stopper outer diameter (OD) dimensions. A tight interface between the vial and stopper can lead to stopper pop up before capping. However, a loose interface between vial ID and stopper OD can lead to the stopper sliding loosely into the vial. Both of these defects can lead to loss of vacuum and of stabilizing gas. In addition, this presents an increased sterility risk if the stoppered vials are not processed through classified Grade A area before or during capping. If stopper pop up does indeed occur, appropriate in-line technologies that can detect popped or raised stoppers must be implemented before capping to eliminate such defects.

9.3.4 Filling Process

As briefly described previously, vial preparation is normally integrated with the filling line. The vials are sterilized, depyrogenated, cooled, and transferred to the filling machine. At manufacturing scale, several filling needles, operating in parallel, are used to simultaneously fill multiple vials. The volume of vaccine solution dispensed into each vial is precisely controlled to ensure that the appropriate dosage is ultimately delivered to the patient. Appropriate in-process controls, whether off-line or in-line, are used to measure and control fill weights. The filled vials are then transferred to the stoppering station, where the stoppers are partially inserted.

9.3.4.1 ***Freeze-Dryer Loading*** During loading, the temperature of the lyophilizer shelf may be controlled from ambient to sub-T_g' temperatures. The required loading temperature is dependent on the stability of the vaccine solution and its specific freezing requirements. The vials may be loaded into the lyophilizer manually, semi-automatically, or in a fully automated manner. Depending on the manufacturing logistics, the filled vials may be placed onto a tray, which is then placed on the lyophilizer shelf. The tray bottom, however, creates an additional resistance to heat flow between the lyophilizer shelf and the product, resulting in prolonged cycle times. In addition, if the trays do not sit perfectly flat on the freeze-dryer shelf (i.e., warped tray bottom), there will be heterogeneity in the rate of heat transfer to the vials throughout the cabinet, potentially impacting product quality. On the basis of these arguments, it is recommended that facilities be designed and operated such that tray bottoms are not required. This can be achieved either by using trays with removable bottoms or by designing a facility with an automated loading/unloading system. Automated loading/unloading employs robotic systems that manage all vial movements from the time the stopper is partially seated through the unloading of the freeze-dryer. These systems typically bunch vials in discreet subsets, normally equal to the load of one full lyophilizer shelf. After filling and partial stoppering, these systems allow the appropriate number of vials to accumulate and then transport the vials, as a single pack, to the lyophilizer where they are loaded on to the appropriate shelf.

As the loading process continues, thermocouples or wireless temperature data loggers may be inserted into a select few vials. This allows for the monitoring of product temperature during the lyophilization process. During development trials at both bench and full scale, such temperature data can be invaluable in helping to evaluate the appropriateness of the cycle, as well as to provide additional data to support observations made during inspection of the final product. Where possible, it is recommended to position thermocouple-containing vials at various locations throughout the cabinet—with particular emphasis on the known hot and cold spots—such that the range of heat transfer rates experienced by the vials throughout the entire cabinet can be observed and evaluated.

The use of thermocouples during normal commercial manufacturing is typically unnecessary, and in the case of automated loading systems, practically impossible. If product temperature monitoring is required during routine production, the thermocouple wires are placed only in the front section of the lyophilizer. This is due to the inaccessibility of the product at deeper locations within the shelf and the need to minimize any sterility risk associated with an operator reaching over vials to place thermocouples in the deeper locations. To obtain product temperature data across different areas of the shelf, it is recommended to use wireless data loggers that can be inserted in specific locations of the vial pack.

Depending on where thermocouple-containing vials are placed inside the lyophilizer, different temperature profiles will be observed. This is due to the fact that vials on the edge of each shelf experience more radiant heat from the walls compared to those situated at the center of the shelf. Depending on the lyophilizer design, locations near the door, in front of the condenser, on the corners of the upper and lower shelves may also be areas of lesser or greater heat transfer. Such edge effects are typically less pronounced in the commercial-scale equipment in comparison to the laboratory-scale lyophilizers. In addition, the placement of the thermocouples in the vials may also influence the data—the thermocouple may be touching the inside wall of the vial and thus may be influenced by the temperature of the glass, the weight, and pull of the wire may slightly tilt the vial off the shelf surface, reducing the rate of heat transfer to the vial, or the thermocouple may simply not be fully immersed into the product.

Case Study 3—Loading In one study, it was found that the method of loading product into the lyophilizer resulted in an increased incidence of product collapse. This was believed to be due to inadvertent temperature cycling when the door of the lyophilizer was opened and closed during the course of loading each shelf. In this study, the product was cryogenically flash-frozen before loading. The manufacturing-scale lyophilizer had a full-sized door. When all shelves of the lyophilizer were first raised and product was loaded into the chamber beginning on the top shelf, a relatively low incidence of product collapse was observed, although the incidence was slightly higher in the top of the cabinet. When the shelves were instead compressed in the bottom of the cabinet and indexed upward as product was loaded, the incidence of collapse was substantially higher. The amount of vials containing collapsed product correlated with the observed temperature cycling during the loading process. The data suggest that the shelf positioning and opening–closing movement of the lyophilizer door during loading allowed room temperature air to enter the precooled lyophilizer, raising the product temperature of the product on the shelves to above the T'_g. It was hypothesized that this temperature cycling changed the ice crystal structure of the frozen product, leading to an increased incidence of product collapse. It was further hypothesized that the cause of the product collapse was decreased surface area within the lyophilized cake, which lead to a decreased rate of water desorption in the secondary drying process (Wallen et al., 2009).

9.4 LYOPHILIZATION

As described in previous sections, lyophilization occurs in three distinct phases—freezing and primary and secondary drying. A schematic representation of the three steps is presented in Figure 9.2. Plotted on the x-axis is the time required to complete three phases of lyophilization. The primary y-axis is temperature, used to describe the shelf, product, and condenser temperature. The secondary y-axis is chamber pressure.

9.4.1 Freezing

In the first stage of lyophilization, a liquid formulation is frozen to a temperature below its T'_g. The importance of the freezing step cannot be overemphasized, as not only does it have the potential to detrimentally impact vaccine potency, but it also determines the structure of the frozen product and therefore the vapor transport kinetics and the efficiency of the subsequent sublimation step. This structure is reflected as a fossil in the dried cake and can be examined through techniques such as scanning electron and optical microscopy.

Freezing can be accomplished in several ways, most typically on the lyophilizer shelf. In this scenario, the product chamber is maintained at atmospheric pressure. Throughout the loading process and depending on the construction of the lyophilizer and the operational logistics of the facility, the condenser may or may not be operating during this step. The shelf temperature can be either precooled to −45 to −60°C (near the lower limit of most commercially available freeze dryers) or cooled to this range once all vials have been loaded into the freeze-dryer. In the latter case, the vial loading most often occurs on shelves set to a temperature above 0°C.

As discussed previously, owing to the unique characteristics of some vaccines, freezing vials on precooled shelves or by reducing shelf temperature after all vials have been loaded may result in significant and unacceptable damage to the vaccine. In these instances, it may be necessary to freeze the vials outside the lyophilizer in a separate cryogenic freezer. This significantly reduces the time from when ice first crystallizes until the frozen solution is cooled to below the T_g'.

Additional discussions on shelf freezing, cryogenic freezing, and annealing are presented in the following section.

9.4.1.1 Freezing on the Lyophilizer Shelf—Slow to Intermediate Freezing Rates

The freezing curve is shown in Figure 9.2. As product and process consistency are critical in vaccine manufacturing and as subtle differences in freezing can impact freeze-drying, it is recommended that freezing be accomplished by gradual reduction of the shelf temperature at a controlled rate (i.e., 0.5°C/min) rather than by a step change in shelf temperature. Once the target shelf temperature is reached, it is advisable to hold this temperature for a few hours to ensure that all vials have equilibrated.

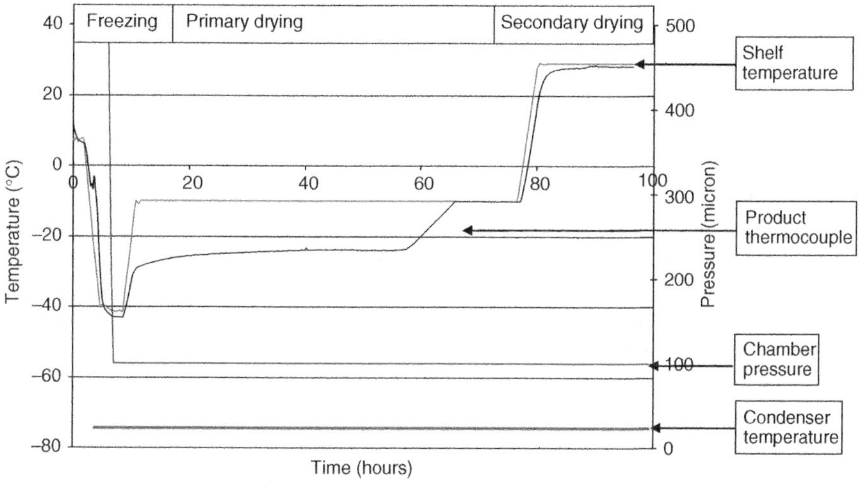

Figure 9.2 Schematic description of a typical lyophilization cycle.

The size of ice crystals in the frozen product is determined by the freezing conditions—both the rate of freezing as well as the degree of supercooling. Supercooling is defined by the difference between the nucleation temperature and the equilibration freezing temperature. This concept is discussed further in the following sections. Product frozen at a slow rate should yield large ice crystals. However, if the degree of supercooling is high, it can offset the effect of slow freezing and may lead to small ice crystals. This is typically seen when freezing on the lyophilizer shelf. Conversely, if a sample is frozen at a fast rate, the size of ice crystals should be smaller. However, if the degree of supercooling is smaller, this can offset the effect of fast freezing and may lead to large ice crystals. This is typically seen when freezing under cryogenic conditions.

Freezing of vials on the lyophilizer shelf occurs primarily by conductive heat transfer. During this process, the temperature of the vaccine solution decreases below the equilibrium freezing point before ice crystallization. Supercooling is the presence of unfrozen liquid at temperatures below the equilibrium freezing temperature of the liquid. Ice nucleation leads to a biphasic separation consisting of the majority of water in the form of ice crystals as one phase and a second glassy amorphous phase consisting of the active vaccine product and the noncrystallized excipients and bound water. Since the degree of supercooling is relatively large for complex vaccine media when frozen on the lyophilizer shelf, the size of ice crystals is expected to be small relative to freezing at cryogenic conditions. As heat removal predominantly occurs from the bottom surface of the vial, the freezing front starts from the vial bottom and advances upward, resulting in a general vertical alignment of the ice crystals. The vaccine and excipients concentrate in between the ice crystals, resulting in an exposure of the vaccine to very high concentrations of excipients (Pikal, 1990). As mentioned previously, exceeding T_g' during primary drying can lead to mobility in the glassy state, which in turn can cause significant potency loss without necessarily impacting cake appearance.

9.4.1.2 Annealing Annealing is a process that is sometimes used to improve the primary drying rate, improve product homogeneity, and/or crystallize solution components. This process consists of one or more cycles in which product frozen to below the T_g' is warmed to a temperature above the T_g' but below the equilibration freezing point and then subsequently cooled back to below the T_g'. As components are mobile within the frozen matrix above the T_g', rearrangement of components may occur, including excipient crystallization. Smaller ice crystals may aggregate into larger ones through a phenomenon called *Ostwald ripening*. These larger ice crystals sublime more quickly during primary drying because of the decreased surface area and therefore may decrease the time necessary for primary drying.

Annealing can improve batch homogeneity by removing variability introduced during the freezing process. The temperature at which freezing actually occurs is not identical in each vial; this difference leads to variability of the ice crystal structure of the frozen product. The gradual warming and cooling of the annealing process create a frozen matrix, which is consistent across all vials.

Annealing can also be used to ensure the crystallization of certain excipients or other small molecules. For some formulations, crystallization of excipients may be required. The crystallization of excipients, and in some cases, active small molecule pharmaceuticals, depends on the kinetics of freezing. Fast freezing rates may trap crystallizable materials in metastable states that eventually crystallize during either drying or product storage, potentially impacting product quality. Typically, slow cooling rates, <0.1°C/min, are required for excipient crystallization. Alternatively, annealing can be used to ensure complete crystallization (Lu and Pikal, 2004). In this case, it is necessary to raise the temperature of the frozen product to above the crystallization temperature of the specific molecule during the annealing process.

Although annealing can be useful for ensuring crystallization, not all products benefit from crystallization. Crystallization of buffers can lead to large pH shifts, which in turn may impact product potency and/or stability. Although the annealing process has been successfully demonstrated for small molecule pharmaceuticals, the effect of annealing on biological products may be more complicated and is generally not employed for vaccine freeze-drying.

9.4.1.3 Freezing Outside the Lyophilizer—Fast Freezing Rates For vaccines that require quick or flash freezing at cryogenic temperatures, specially designed freezers that have the ability to cool to −100°C may be required. Such low temperatures are typically obtained using liquid nitrogen. After freezing, the frozen vials are transported to the lyophilizer shelves that have been precooled to below the T_g' of the product. Before initiating the drying cycle, the vials must be allowed time to equilibrate to the shelf temperature.

Freezing in cryogenic freezers occurs predominantly by convective means through the sides and bottom of the vial. Additional cooling is provided by conductive heat transfer, primarily from the bottom of the vial to the surface on which the vial is sitting. As the cooling occurs from all sides of the vial, the ice crystals are formed and grown in a random manner. Although the freezing occurs at much faster rates compared to conventional shelf-freezing methods, the degree of supercooling is much less because of uniform cooling of the vial. Consequently, the size of the ice crystals is much bigger than that of those formed under shelf-freezing conditions.

Flash freezing is only employed when absolutely necessary. This unique process step not only further complicates an already complex process, but also adds additional sterility assurance concerns as well as increases the utility and capital cost of the manufacturing facility.

9.4.2 Primary Drying

During primary drying, ice crystals are removed from the frozen solution via sublimation. This is achieved by establishing a low vacuum, typically <200 mTorr and by keeping the product temperature at or below the T_g'. Once the ice crystals are removed, a porous structure of the formulation solids is created. The rate of primary drying is dependent on the size of ice crystals formed during the freezing process, the shelf temperature, and the chamber pressure.

The primary drying step is illustrated in Figure 9.2. In this example, once the product is equilibrated below −40°C, the chamber pressure is decreased to a vacuum pressure of 100 mTorr. After the vacuum is established, the shelf temperature is increased to −10°C at a controlled rate, providing the necessary energy to sublime the water from the solid to the gaseous phase. A notable temperature difference exists between the shelf-temperature set point and the actual product temperature because of the heat input required for the solid-to-gaseous phase change. This phenomenon is known as *evaporative cooling*. Once all of the ice crystals have been sublimed, there is no more evaporative cooling. The product temperature then rises and equilibrates with the shelf temperature as shown in Figure 9.2. The temperature of the product during primary drying is dependent on both the shelf temperature and the chamber pressure.

9.4.2.1 Product Temperature During Primary Drying Although warmer temperatures allow primary drying to proceed more quickly, it is critical that the product temperature not exceed the T_c of the partially dried product. If this temperature is exceeded, viscous flow of components is permitted, and the product structure formed during the freezing step will collapse. This collapse may result in high residual moisture levels and an undesirable product appearance. Therefore, the primary drying temperature must be developed to ensure product quality, while maximizing the rate of primary drying.

9.4.2.2 Chamber Pressure During Primary Drying The lyophilizer chamber pressure plays an important role in determining the product temperature during the primary drying process. Chamber pressure must therefore be developed in tandem with the shelf temperature in order to ensure that the product remains below the T_c, while optimizing the primary drying rate. The chamber pressure must be below the vapor pressure on the drying edge of product temperature in order to provide a driving force for sublimation to occur.

The gas in the freeze-drying chamber transfers energy to the product. At the nanoscale, molecular conductive heat transfer occurs via collisions of gas molecules with the vial and then subsequently with the product. As the chamber pressure is increased, there are more molecules available to transfer energy to the product, thus increasing the overall rate of sublimation. The relationship between the product–air interface temperature versus the ice vapor pressure is given in Table 9.3.

9.4.3 Secondary Drying

The purpose of secondary drying is to remove the noncrystalline moisture trapped in the amorphous phase to a level acceptable for the long-term stability of the product. The secondary drying phase is depicted in Figure 9.2. The residual water is desorbed from the product at elevated temperatures, typically room temperature or warmer. Within the pressure ranges typically employed for freeze-drying of biological products, the rate of secondary drying is not strongly dependent on pressure (Pikal et al.,

TABLE 9.3 Vapor Pressure of Ice as a Function of Temperature (Constantino, 2004)

Temperature (°C)	Vapor Pressure (μM of Hg)
0	4579
−10	1950
−20	776
−30	286
−40	96.6
−50	29.8
−60	8.08
−70	1.94

1989). The chamber pressure is often maintained at the same set point as used for primary drying.

After primary drying, the shelf temperature is gradually raised to the secondary drying shelf temperature set point. If the rate of temperature increase is too aggressive, microcollapse may occur. This collapse may not be visibly evident and may result in higher-than-desired final product moistures. During process development, it is desirable to measure the T_g' of the cake during the course of secondary drying. These data can provide much insight into developing effective and efficient secondary drying parameters.

The secondary drying plateau temperature is a function of the desired final product moisture content and the desorption isotherms associated with the particular formulation. In order to achieve the desired moisture level, the appropriate selection of shelf temperature is critical.

9.4.4 Stoppering and Headspace

After the completion of the lyophilization cycle, the vacuum is broken by introducing air into the chamber, typically an inert gas such as argon or nitrogen. After the appropriate pressure is achieved, normally within the range of 7–11 psia, the lyophilized vials are stoppered by collapsing the lyophilizer shelves. Stoppering the vials under a slight vacuum provides a "void" volume to allow for the addition of the diluent into the vial during reconstitution and minimizes the propensity for foaming to occur during reconstitution. In extreme cases, the vials may be stoppered at full vacuum. This is again to facilitate the reconstitution process and reduce foaming. For some products, the presence of a specific headspace gas is essential for the long-term stability of the product. After stoppering, the shelves are raised to allow removal of the vials from the lyophilizer. If the product is not immediately unloaded, the shelf temperature is often reduced to refrigerated or frozen temperatures to minimize any additional degradation of the product.

9.4.5 Inspection

After stoppering, the vials are unloaded from the lyophilizer. They are capped and then inspected for defects. Product inspection can occur either manually or through the use of automated equipment.

Automated inspection machines comprise a series of lights and digital cameras, which capture images of the container and product from various angles. These images are analyzed by the computer software for various defects.

Defects fall into several general categories: components, filling, and cake physical appearance. Defective components may include a missing stopper, a damaged or missing seal, or a cracked vial. Filling defects include high or low fills or product streaks on the inside of the vial. Physical appearance defects include collapse, meltback, broken or cracked cakes, and discoloration/sheen.

As described previously, the root cause for any physical appearance defect is complex and can be caused by one or more events during the freeze-drying process. Investigation into the processing steps of freezing, annealing (if applicable), primary and secondary drying, and even stoppering may be warranted as a result of physical appearance defects. In addition, inadequately prepared components can also contribute to lyophilization defects. As also described previously, products with visible collapse and/or meltback often contain excessive residual moisture, potentially impacting long-term product stability.

9.5 EQUIPMENT

The main parts of the lyophilizer are the product and the condenser chambers. The condenser may be positioned behind, above, or below the chamber, providing flexibility for facility design and infrastructure.

The product chamber contains the shelves on which the vials sit. The inside of each shelf is designed such that the heat transfer fluid, most commonly silicone oil, is channeled and flows in a serpentine pattern through the shelf interior. This design reduces heterogeneity in temperature across the surface of the shelf and therefore helps ensure that all vials are dried at the same rate.

The condenser chamber consists of a number of cooling coils on which the water vapor that is generated during sublimation (primary drying) and desorption (secondary drying) condenses and, because of the low temperatures of the coils, less than −60°C, is immediately cooled to the solid phase, resulting in a build-up of ice on the coils.

As stated previously, silicone oil is the fluid most commonly used to circulate through the lyophilizer shelves. Silicone oil may also be used as the coolant in the condenser coils. Silicone oil has been traditionally cooled using a series of compressors and is heated via electrical elements. The compressors and electrical heater are appropriately balanced to achieve the appropriate temperature. The properties of the silicone oil, in combination with compressor capacity, result in a practical minimum temperature limit of approximately −65°C. Silicone oil is also commonly used in the condenser coils.

In more recent years, however, and in recognition of the expense associated with compressor maintenance, many suppliers and firms have opted to use liquid nitrogen in the condenser. In this case, liquid nitrogen is introduced into the coils and, on absorbing heat from the water vapor condensing, cooling, and crystallizing on the outside of the coils, evaporates and is allowed to freely vent to the atmosphere. One distinct advantage of liquid-nitrogen-cooled condensers is that the silicone oil used to flow through the shelves can be cooled by liquid nitrogen via heat exchanger, thus eliminating the need for mechanical compressors and their associated cost of maintenance.

Connecting the product and condense chambers is a large diameter pipe. Connected to the condenser chamber is a series of vacuum pumps, which are used to establish the low freeze-drying pressures throughout the entire system.

9.5.1 Production Scale

The scale or capacity of a lyophilizer is determined by the total surface area of the shelves and by the total amount of water vapor that can be trapped by the condenser. Commercial-scale freeze dryers typically contain 18–22 shelves with a total surface area of approximately 33–50 m^2, large enough to hold 100,000 3 ml vials—a standard commercial vaccine vial. The corresponding condenser capacity ranges from 600 to 800 kg of water and typically far exceeds the capacity needed for a full lyophilizer load.

9.5.2 Laboratory Scale

Bench-scale lyophilizers can have as little as two shelves, a total surface area of approximately 0.5 m^2 and a condenser capacity of 30 kg. As stated previously, it is not atypical to encounter scale-up difficulties between the laboratory- and commercial-scale freeze dryers.

9.5.3 Scale-Up

Although the basic design of a bench or pilot-scale lyophilizer is the same as that of the full-scale lyophilizer, scale-up concerns must not be underestimated. There are several differences that must be taken into account when moving from one scale to another.

A small scale lyophilizer will contain a larger surface area to volume ratio than a larger unit. This allows for a larger relative contribution of radiant heat from the walls of the drying chamber to the product sitting on the shelves. As a general rule, the vials on the middle of the shelf experience the coolest drying conditions. The vials on the perimeter of the shelf and, perhaps even more so, those vials on the exact corner of each shelf, experience the warmest drying conditions. This is due to the radiant heat effect of the walls of the lyophilizer, in which additional subtleties may be observed near the door or near the upper or lower portions of the cabinet, depending on condenser placement, as well as other design features.

Scale can also play a role in the extent of supercooling. At large scale, vaccines are typically filled into vials using automated equipment in a class 100 environment. However, during small scale development, vials may be manually filled in the open laboratory or in a biosafety cabinet, allowing for more particulate introduction relative to the full-scale manufacturing environment. The presence of particulates can minimize the extent of supercooling at the laboratory scale as compared to the manufacturing scale, resulting in a different ice crystal morphology and thus possibly leading to a difference in performance during subsequent freeze-drying steps.

Case Study 4—Scale-Up Differences in lyophilizer designs and scales mean that lyophilization temperatures, pressures, and times determined at small scale may not be directly applicable at commercial scale. Tsinontides et al. developed operating parameters for a laboratory-scale freeze-dryer and a mathematical model, which, on the basis of those parameters, allowed for the determination of the overall heat transfer coefficient, encompassing the conductive heat transfer between the product vial and the shelf, the radiant heat transfer to the vial, and the convective heat transfer from the air between the shelve and the vial. The model was used to establish manufacturing-scale parameters and to examine the robustness of those parameters. The selected cycle was scaled up successfully using a minimum of manufacturing-scale runs (Tsinontides et al., 2004).

9.6 CONCLUSIONS

This chapter has discussed the importance and interconnections of formulation, processing, equipment, and components within the context of vaccine lyophilization. While providing a broad overview, this chapter also presented considerations unique to vaccines and provided case studies from commercial vaccine lyophilization processes.

The lyophilization of vaccines allows the distribution of otherwise unstable products to markets around the world. However, lyophilization is a complex process. Selection of formulation excipients and primary packaging components and process development, including freezing, primary drying, and secondary drying are all interdependent. Owing to these complexities, relatively long developmental timelines are required, and changes in one aspect can require extensive reoptimization of the process. In addition, lyophilization equipment is expensive, may require extensive maintenance, requires a large amount of factory space, and has a long lead time. The requirement of a reconstituting diluent adds cost to already expensive process. It is for these reasons that a lyophilized product is normally only developed when a liquid stable formulation is not feasible. In these instances, which occur frequently in the vaccine world, formulation development, process development, and facility design must be approached with great care and forethought.

In conclusion, the complexities associated with the development and operation of a commercial-scale lyophilization process cannot be underestimated. However, such operations can be made robust, and meeting this challenge is essential for some products. Ultimately, the implementation of well-developed lyophilization processes helps to ensure the availability of these critical vaccines to the world.

REFERENCES

Bennett PS, Maigetter RZ, Olson MG, Provost PJ, Scattergood EM, Schofield TL. The effects of freeze-drying on the potency and stability of live varicella virus vaccine. Dev Biol Stand 1992;74:215–221.

Constantino HR. In: Pikal MJ, editor. *Lyophilization of Biopharmaceuticals*. Arlington, VA: AAPS Press; 2004.

Grose C. Cryopreservation of varicella-zoster virions without loss of structural integrity or infectivity. Intervirology 1981;15:154–160.

Her L, Deras M, Nail S. Electrolyte-Induced changes in glass transition temperatures of freeze concentrated solutes. Pharm Res 1995;12:768–772.

Jennings TA. *Lyophilization: Introduction and Basic Principles*. Interpharm/CRC; 2002.

Levine H, Slade L. Water as plastizer: physico-chemical aspects of low moisture polymeric systems. Water Sci Rev 1988;3:79–185.

Lu X, Pikal MJ. Freeze-drying of mannitol-trehalose-sodium chloride based formulations: the impact of annealing on dry layer resistance to mass transfer and cake structure. Pharm Dev Technol 2004;9:85–95.

Pikal MJ. Freeze-drying of proteins II: formulation selection. BioPharm 1990;3:26–30.

Pikal MJ, Shah S, Roy ML, Putnam R. The secondary drying stage of freeze drying: drying kinetics as a function of temperature and chamber pressure. Int J Pharm 1989;60:203–217.

Tsinontides SC, Rajniak P, Pham D, Hunke WA, Placek J, Reynolds SD. Freeze drying—principles and practice for successful scale-up to manufacturing. Int J Pharm 2004;280:1–16.

Wallen AJ, Van Ocker SH, Sinacola JR, Phillips BR. The effect of loading process on product collapse during large-scale lyophilization. J Pharm Sci 2009;98:997–1004.

10

STRATEGIES FOR HEAT-STABLE VACCINES

SATOSHI OHTAKE, DAVID LECHUGA-BALLESTEROS, VU TRUONG-LE, AND ERIC J. PATZER

Aridis Pharmaceuticals LLC, San Jose, CA, USA

10.1 INTRODUCTION: IMPORTANCE OF STABLE VACCINES

Historically, vaccines are among the most complex biologicals in the pharmaceutical industry. They consist of live attenuated bacteria and viruses, killed whole-cell bacteria and viruses, subunit vaccines containing proteins and/or carbohydrates, and, more recently, isolated DNA. In order to maximize the immune response, vaccines may also contain complex mixtures of excipients, termed *adjuvants*. Vaccines are most effective in protecting populations at risk when they are broadly administered in widespread vaccination programs, which typically encompass varied geographical settings. For vaccines to survive the logistical complexities of these mass vaccination campaigns, a maximally stable product is required. Among pharmaceuticals, vaccines have the greatest need for stability, and, yet, are among the most difficult to stabilize, leading to a significant challenge for the vaccine developer. The magnitude of this challenge can be judged by the lack of any vaccines on the Centers for Disease Control and Prevention (CDC)–recommended immunization schedule that can withstand long-term storage above refrigerated temperatures (2–8°C). The sensitivity of vaccines to storage temperature is distinctly different from many other biopharmaceutical products in the pharmaceutical industry, the majority of which can be stored at room temperature.

To ensure full potency at time of administration, a vaccine must be able to withstand a robust range of specified storage, handling, and administration conditions.

Vaccine Development and Manufacturing, First Edition.
Edited by Emily P. Wen, Ronald Ellis, and Narahari S. Pujar.

According to regulatory guidelines, the shelf life of vaccines is typically 18–24 months at the designated storage temperature to allow sufficient time for use. This can be a challenging endeavor, especially with live attenuated vaccines that require the preservation of replication-competent organisms. In addition, once removed from its designated storage conditions, each vaccine must retain sufficient stability to allow a convenient interval for handling and administration, typically at room temperature. In outlying regions of developing countries, the facilities to control temperatures are much less readily available, which further underscores the need for a maximally stable vaccine.

Another key issue for vaccines and other complex biologicals is their stability during shipment from the manufacturing site. According to a recent U.S. Army study, up to 15% of monitored vaccine and immunologic drug shipments were subjected to unacceptable temperature excursions (Frank, 1999), which can have a deleterious effect on the potency and efficacy of the vaccine. To address this issue, stable vaccines are needed that can not only survive prolonged storage, but also withstand temperature excursions both above and below 2–8°C during transport and handling.

More recently, the issue of long-term stockpiling of vaccines has gained greater prominence primarily due to the national priority of developing biodefense vaccines. Under these circumstances, it cannot be estimated when, if ever, the vaccine will be used, and so it is desirable to be able to develop vaccines with much longer expiry measured in decades rather than in years. The importance of achieving even a minimally stable biodefense vaccine is illustrated by the example of a second-generation anthrax vaccine that was developed on the basis of purified protective antigen (PA) of *Bacillus anthracis*. It is well known that purified PA is an effective immunogen, which can stimulate a protective immune response. Nevertheless, this vaccine was placed on clinical hold because of instability (Grabenstein, 2008), and ultimately the project was terminated. However, developing a biodefense vaccine with maximum stability remains an important objective, as evidenced by a recent request for proposals for a third-generation PA-based anthrax vaccine, which requires candidate vaccines to have stability for at least 3 years at 35°C or above (see http://grants.nih.gov/grants/guide/notice-files/NOT-AI-07-046.html).

In summary, although there has been a multifaceted approach to the route of administration of vaccines (i.e., oral, subcutaneous, parenteral, intranasal, and oral inhalation), the development of dosage forms has been more limited, as evidenced by the prevalence (>60%) of solution- and suspension-based formulations on the market (see Fig. 10.1). The result is that, more often than not, vaccines in liquid form are not sufficiently stable to allow storage and distribution without refrigeration. Fortunately, the need for heat-stable vaccines has recently been recognized and has fueled new research efforts to develop novel formulation and processing approaches. In this chapter, the current state of the art in vaccine stability is reviewed, and various approaches to produce vaccines with improved stability are discussed.

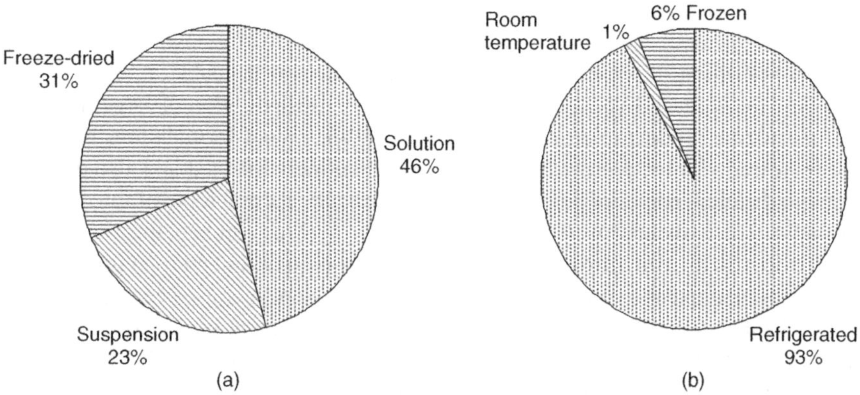

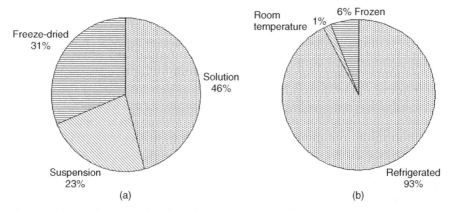

Figure 10.1 Marketed vaccine formulation presentation (a) and storage requirements (b). Despite the increase in the number of freeze-dried formulations (roughly 20 of 79), only one is recommended for room temperature storage. Plots created on the basis of survey by (Costantino, 2004).

10.2 STABILITY OF CURRENT VACCINES

The bioactive ingredient in a vaccine product can be viruses, bacteria, proteins, synthetic peptides, carbohydrates, nucleic acids, or subviral or subcellular particles. A viral particle can be as simple as a naked genome or a genome surrounded by a protein-based protective shell, also known as *a capsid*, to form a nucleocapsid. The nucleocapsid may constitute the virion (the complete viral particle) or may be surrounded by an envelope composed of a lipid bilayer, with enzymes and structural proteins that may or may not be glycosylated. The main challenge in dealing with a formulation of a simple nucleic acid genome in solution is chemical degradation via hydrolysis of glycosidic bonds. For vaccines that are more structurally complex, multiple routes of chemical degradation arise, such as hydrolysis reactions involving both glycosidic and peptide bonds. Viral vaccines are also sensitive, and respond differently, to physical stresses caused by various solvents, pH, ionic strength, or extreme temperatures (heat or cold). These stresses can trigger chemical and/or physical instabilities. These challenges are currently addressed through the development of an effective formulation and storage at low temperature. Furthermore, owing to the multitude of degradation pathways possible in a complex vaccine system, it may be difficult to identify and measure the specific chemical and/or physical instability of importance. Since the instabilities result in bioactivity loss, it is common to perform biological assays that measure the activity of the vaccine, although these assays generally lack precision and are not revealing in terms of molecular causes of bioactivity loss. Thus, from a formulation scientist's perspective, vaccines constitute a formidable challenge, as they encompass a multitude of structural and chemical variations and complexity. This is further complicated by the fact that vaccines are often formulated as a multidisease or a multivalent combination.

Years ago, it was proposed that the ideal vaccine dosage form would combine all childhood vaccines into a single dose, preferably oral, to circumvent painful injections. In addition, the ideal vaccine dosage form would be stable at ambient temperature for at least 3 years to enable storage and transportation of large quantities of the vaccine product (Katkocin and Hsieh, 1999). Liquid formulations have been the preferred vaccine presentation, as it can be routinely injected and also delivered through different routes of administration to mimic the natural route of infection. For example, a recently approved flu vaccine, FluMist^{TM} (MedImmune, Inc.), is administered intranasally as a drop or spray, the first-generation polio and rotavirus vaccines were administered as an oral solution, and measles vaccine has also been administered via oral inhalation in the form of a nebulized mist (Bennett et al., 2002). Furthermore, from the manufacturing perspective, a liquid formulation may be the easiest to implement and is the most cost effective to produce, even in the case of a combination product. A liquid presentation was also thought to be most convenient for the health care provider, as it avoids reconstitution and any other manipulations.

Most vaccines that are presented in liquid form require refrigeration. A survey of common vaccines and their shelf-life stability are shown in Table 10.1. The presence of adjuvants in some vaccines makes them particularly unstable to freezing, thus instability can arise from both low and high temperature excursions, requiring storage conditions to be maintained in a well-controlled temperature range. The existing cold chain distribution and storage infrastructure in developed countries have reduced the need for room-temperature-stable vaccines and, combined with their ease of manufacture, have contributed to the prevalence of liquid vaccine formulations. Although it is clear that the need for heat-stable vaccines is greater in developing world countries, there are also benefits in developed world settings, which include decrease in vaccine wastage from short expiry dating periods and reduction in the cost and complexity of restrictive temperature conditions during storage, handling, and administration of the vaccine by the end user. Alternatively, vaccines in the dried dosage format not only tend to be more stable than their liquid counterparts, but also usually take up less storage space at distribution and vaccination sites. Furthermore, they are less prone to agitation-induced shipping damage and more amendable to fabrication into compact, convenient-to-administer dosage formats, if desired.

Vaccine stability depends on several factors, including the type of formulation (liquid or solid form), the interaction between strains (in the case of multivalent vaccines) or different immunogenic components, and the presence of adjuvants. Furthermore, vaccine stability is strongly dependent on the biochemical property of the labile molecule; toxoid- and polysaccharide-based vaccines are typically the most stable, whereas live attenuated viruses and bacteria tend to be the least stable. In addition, a multicomponent vaccine, whether it comprises various serotypes or strains, invariably demonstrates inferior stability compared to a single-strain product, leading to formulations that tend to be much more complex. A common approach to achieving improved thermal stability in the most difficult cases has been to freeze-dry vaccines,

TABLE 10.1 Storage Conditions and Shelf Life of Common Vaccines

Storage Conditions	Vaccines	Shelf Life and Comments[a]
	DTaP[b] DTPI (not recommended) DT[b] Td	≤18 mo see MCSD[c] (should not be frozen) Diphtheria and tetanus toxoids are stable for years at refrigerated conditions, months at 25°C, several weeks at 37°C, and less than 1 wk at 45°C. Whole-cell pertussis and adjuvant are relatively stable at 2–8°C (approx. 2 yr) but susceptible to freezing. Combinations containing acellular pertussis are stable 2–3 yr at 2–8°C. Adsorbed toxoids should never be frozen. Twenty-four hours freezing at −3°C of both acellular and whole-cell pertussis antigens in a DTP formulation has been reported to reduce the immunogenic response in a murin model.
Refrigerated conditions 2–8°C (35.6–46.4°F) NOT to be frozen (potency reduced or destroyed)	Cholera (not recommended by WHO)	2–3 yr see MCSD (use immediately after reconstitution; should not be frozen) An oral killed whole-cell vaccine is stable for 3 yr if kept in the refrigerator at 2–8°C. Live oral CVD103 HgR vaccine has also been developed, and an effective cold chain is likely to be needed. The bacteria must be protected from stomach acids with buffer, and the product must be administered immediately after reconstitution.
	All hepatitis[b]	≤2 yr see MCSD (reconstituted ≤24 h; should never be frozen) The vaccine is stable for up to 4 yr at temperatures of 2–8°C, for months at 20–25°C, for weeks at 37°C, and for days at 45°C. As with other vaccines adsorbed on aluminum salts, freezing of HepB vaccine may cause a significant reduction of potency. The freezing point of HepB vaccine is approximately −0.5°C. Aluminum hydroxide or aluminum phosphate is used as adjuvant in the case of three of the products (Merck, GSK, and Sanofi-Pasteur); the Berna vaccine uses a liposome adjuvant. The aluminum adjuvanted vaccines should not be frozen. Both the Merck and the GSK products retain potency for

(*continued*)

TABLE 10.1 (*Continued*)

Storage Conditions	Vaccines	Shelf Life and Comments[a]
		2 yr at 2–8°C. GSK vaccine (Havrix) upon release and following storage for 15 mo under refrigerated condition demonstrated no loss of immunogenicity upon storage at 37°C for up to 3 wk. Merck vaccine (VAQTA) did not differ in its stability profile at the recommended storage temperature if stored at 37°C for 12 mo.
Refrigerated conditions 2–8°C (35.6–46.4°F) NOT to be frozen (potency reduced or destroyed)	All Hib conjugate	≤3 yr see MCSD (reconstituted ≤6 h; liquid Hib should never be frozen) Preliminary results suggest that the lyophilized Hib vaccine (tetanus toxoid conjugate vaccine containing purified polyribosyl-ribitolphosphate capsular polysaccharide, PRP-T) is stable under refrigerated condition for 36 mo and at 25°C for at least 24 mo. Liquid monovalent Hib or liquid DTP-Hib vaccines are stable under refrigerated condition for 24 mo. In a multidose formulation, liquid Hib and DTP-Hib vaccines may be used in a subsequent session, even if they have been opened. Lyophilized Hib maintained its release specifications for 36 mo at 2–8°C, for 24 mo at 25°C, and for 1 mo at 37°C, while the reconstituted form was stable for only 5 d at 37°C. Synthetic liquid Hib vaccine is stable at 2–8°C for more than 18 mo, and at 37°C for 3 mo.
	Influenza	≤1 yr see MCSD Influenza vaccines can be either inactivated or live attenuated. There are several vaccines produced by different manufacturers, and they vary in stability. Most products are stable for 2 yr at 2–8°C but seasonal influenza vaccines are valid for 1 yr only because of the need to adapt the vaccine strain to the circulating field virus. The potency of the individual virus vaccine components can decline at varying rates. A refrigerator-stable intranasal formulation has been developed in the USA (Flumist, MedImmune).
	MMR or individual component vaccines	1–2 yr see MCSD (protect from light to avoid virus inactivation; may be frozen but diluent should NOT be frozen, can be kept at room temperature; discard reconstituted vials within 8 h)

		Measles vaccines, even those with enhanced thermostability in dry form, quickly lose their potency upon reconstitution if stored at elevated temperatures. Reconstituting vaccine with a warm diluent may be harmful; vaccine reconstituted with the diluent prewarmed to 41°C and then further incubated in the water bath at that temperature lost half of its original potency after half an hour and 0.5–0.7 $\log_{10}$ after 1 h. At 37°C the loss of titer was 0.4–0.5 and 0.8–1.0 $\log_{10}$ after three and 6 h respectively. The enhanced second-generation freeze-dried measles vaccines stored at 37°C for up to 14 d were able to induce seroconversion in seronegative children. Unreconstituted Merck measles vaccine can retain potency for 8 mo at room temperature and 4 wk at 37°C. One day exposure at 54°C induced loss of more than 0.65 $\log_{10}$.
Refrigerated conditions 2–8°C (35.6–46.4°F) NOT to be frozen (potency reduced or destroyed)	Meningococcal	2 yr see MCSD (reconstituted ≤24 h) Stable at 37°C (98.6°F) for 4 d; use reconstituted single-dose vial within 24 h, multidose vials within 5 d. Vaccines from two manufacturers showed significant reduction in potency after exposure to 55°C but not after freeze–thawing cycles. One meningitis C conjugate vaccine with a shelf life of 2 yr at 2–8°C showed retention of potency as detected by a bactericidal or an enzyme linked immunosorbent assay (ELISA) method, as well as integrity of the conjugate on exposure to either 2–8°C or 25°C for up to 36 mo.
	Pneumococcal (polyvalent and conjugated)	≤2 yr 2–8°C see MCSD (should not be frozen) Available as unconjugated polysaccharide and conjugated polysaccharide vaccines. The polysaccharide vaccines contain 23 serotypes dissolved in isotonic saline with either phenol or thiomersal adjuvants with shelf life of 24 mo at 2–8°C and should not be frozen. Polysaccharide components may lose antigenicity upon storage, up to 10% per year. The only currently licensed pneumococcal conjugate vaccine, a 7- or 13-valent vaccine produced by Pfizer, is formulated with aluminum adjuvant, is a liquid, and should be protected from

(continued)

TABLE 10.1 ***(Continued)***

Storage Conditions	Vaccines	Shelf Life and Comments[a]
		freezing. There are differences in the heat stability of BCG (Bacillus Calmette-Guérin) vaccines prepared by different manufacturers from different substrains. It is not clear if these differences are strain dependent or caused by the different lyophilization and stabilization techniques used by the manufacturers, although it is probably the latter. Recently spray dried BCG has been successfully prepared and tested in animal models (Harvard University).
	Poliovirus inactivated (IPV)	≤1 yr 2–8°C see MCSD (do not use vaccine with color, turbidity, or particulate matter) IPV is stable alone or when combined with other components under refrigerated conditions (at least 2 yr) and stable for 1 mo at 25°C and several days at 37°C. It is rapidly inactivated by freezing or exposure to mercury-containing compounds such as thiomersal (or thimerosal).
Refrigerated conditions 2–8°C (35.6–46.4°F) NOT to be frozen (potency reduced or destroyed)	Japanese encephalitis virus	≤1 yr see MCSD (reconstituted <8 h) Formalin-inactivated Japanese encephalitis (JE) vaccines derived from mouse brain (Biken vaccine used in India, Japan, the Republic of Korea, Thailand) and from primary hamster kidney cell culture (used in China). Biken vaccine retains potency after storage in lyophilized form at 4°C for 1 yr, at 22°C for 28 wk, and at 37°C for 4 wk. A freeze-dried JE vaccine presents potency loss of only 4.7% in 52 wk at 4°C, 8.7% in 28 wk at 22°C, and 14% and 24% during 18 wk at 37°C and 40°C respectively. After reconstitution, the vaccine is still stable at 22°C with a 1% drop after 2 wk and 4 wk at 37°C and 40°C, respectively. SA-14-14-2 strain grown in primary hamster kidney cells is stable at 37°C for seven to 10 d, at room temperature for 4 mo, and at 2–8°C for 1.5 yr. After reconstitution, it is stable for 2 h at 23°C. At present this vaccine has limited availability on the international market.

	Plague	See MCSD Vaccine licensed for use in the United States is prepared from *Y. pestis* organisms grown in artificial media, inactivated with formaldehyde, and preserved in 0.5% phenol. A freeze-dried formulation (originally prepared in 1947) stored under vacuum retained immunogenic properties of plague vaccine strain EV, line NIIEG for 30 yr. The subcultures prepared from this strain showed good immunogenic properties which were preserved for 6–10 yr (after three passages in guinea pigs). Even after 30-yr of storage, the stock culture of strain EV, line NIIEG, has been used for the preparation of NIIS live plague vaccine.
Refrigerated conditions 2–8°C (35.6–46.4°F) NOT to be frozen (potency reduced or destroyed)	Rabies (HDCV; PCEV)	≤18 mo see MCSD (reconstituted < 1 h) Human diploid cell vaccine (HDCV) in its lyophilized form retains its potency for at least 3.5 yr at temperatures between 2–8°C and for 1 mo at 37°C. The new vaccines include the following: the purified chicken embryo cell vaccine (PCEV) developed by Chiron Behring in Germany, which was stable for 3 mo at 37°C. New generation vaccines derived from hamster kidney, duck embrio, and Vero cells currently being developed are likely to have much better stability than the former vaccines prepared on neural tissues.
	Typhoid (inactivated and oral)	See MCSD Purified Vi polysaccharide vaccine is a liquid in phenolic isotonic buffer stable up to 6 mo at 37°C and for 2 yr at 22°C, but it should not be frozen. Live oral vaccine contains Ty21, a mutant of *S. typhi*, which should be stored at 4°C. It is available as an enteric-coated capsule that is reconstituted in buffer. Capsules should be stored 2–8°C and protected from light. The shelf life of the lyophilized vaccine is 1 yr at 2–8°C, if aluminum blister has not been opened because its stability is dependent on residual moisture content. Study

(continued)

TABLE 10.1 ***(Continued)***

Storage Conditions	Vaccines	Shelf Life and Comments[a]
		of errors in following prescribing information indicated that about half of them were related to storage under incorrect temperature. Vaccine failures for Swiss travelers have been associated with vaccines that were not kept in a refrigerated state. Prolonged storage at room temperature resulted in progressively lower viable counts over time, although all tested lots evaluated after storage for 7 d at 20°C to 25°C met potency requirements. Three lots of the vaccine stored at 37°C for 12 h also maintained potency.
Refrigerated conditions 2–8°C (35.6–46.4°F) NOT to be frozen (potency reduced or destroyed)	Rotavirus	≤2 yr see MCSD (protect from light, reconstituted ≤1 h at room temperature and ≤4 h when refrigerated) Store at 2–8°C protected from light. Stable for 24 mo between 20 and 25°C in the lyophilized state. An additional vaccine, Rotarix, is available as a live attenuated lyophilized product stable for 3 yr at 2–8°C, can be frozen with 2 yr of stability at −20°C and is also stable for 1 wk at 37°C. A second rotavirus vaccine (Rotateq) was licensed in the United States in 2003. It is a liquid formulation, which requires refrigeration. Recently, spray dried live attenuated rotavirus vaccine powders have been incorporated in a fast dissolving oral thin film (Aridis Pharmaceuticals, LLC)
Freeze conditions <0°C (32°F) Deep freeze conditions: ≤−15°C (5°F)	Varicella	≤18 mo see MCSD (protect from light, reconstituted ≤30 min; diluent should not be frozen) There are three producers of varicella vaccines made in human cells: Merck, GSK, and Biken (distributed by Sanofi-Pasteur). The vaccine is a cell-free virion preparation that generally contains sucrose and buffer salts, and is lyophilized. The lyophilized form can be stored at refrigerator temperature for 1.5 yr or more, but manufacturers suggest storage in freezer.

	Poliovirus, oral (OPV)[d]	≤12 mo at −20°C see MCSD Not approved for use in United States; color changes not important but must remain clear. OPV as supplied by most manufacturers is stable for an extended period at −20°C, for over 6 mo at 2–8°C, and for over 48 h at 37°C. Sorbitol keeps vaccine (not recommended) fluid to −14°C (7 °F): refreezing acceptable (maximum 10 freeze–thaw cycles)
Freeze conditions <0°C (32°F) Deep freeze conditions: ≤−15°C (5°F)	Yellow fever	≤2 yr at −20°C (ship in dry ice; reconstituted ≤1 h) Lyophilized yellow fever vaccine can be safely stored at −20°C (+4 °F) for 2 yr. Should be quickly administered after reconstitution, maintained at 2–8°C, and discarded at the end of the session, not only to preserve potency, but also to minimize risk of contamination of this lyophilized vaccine once reconstituted. Glassification in sugars such as lactose with other excipients including sorbitol, histidine, and alanine have considerably improved the heat stability of lyophilized 17D yellow fever vaccine. Vaccines meeting the WHO stability guidelines are stable after exposure to 37°C for 14 d, and their loss in potency during this exposure is less than 1 $\log_{10}$.

[a]From (Milstein et al., 2006; Galazka et al., 1998).
[b]Discard if contains clumps of material that cannot be suspended with vigorous shaking. May occur with 24 h or longer temperature <2°C (35.6 °F) or >25°C (77 °F).
[c]Manufacturer's cold storage date.
[d]May store unreconstituted vaccine at 2°C.

and in many cases, lyophilized vaccines are resistant to freezing, thus improving the long-term stability. As a result of these early successes, freeze-drying has become the preferred approach toward improving the stability of vaccines in the solid state.

10.3 VACCINE STABILIZATION STRATEGIES

10.3.1 Molecular Protein Engineering Approaches

Thermal stabilization strategies for subunit vaccines encompass a wide array of approaches, from molecular protein engineering to formulation and process optimization. Protein engineering applications include *de novo* protein re-engineering and *in vitro* molecular evolution; the former uses computational design to modify thermally labile sequences (Shah et al., 2007; Vizcarra and Mayo 2005), whereas the latter is used to select variants with higher unfolding temperatures (Wunderlich et al., 2005a). A common strategy for these approaches involves calculating the Gibbs free energy of protein folding for various regions on a protein to optimize Coulombic intra- and inter-molecular interactions of charged residues, thereby increasing the thermodynamic favorability of folding (Wunderlich et al., 2005b). Other molecular strategies include site-specific amino acid addition, such as cysteine, to immobilize the protein to a more stable matrix or stabilizer (Mansfeld et al., 1999), addition of Ca^{2+} binding sites that can increase the alpha-helix content of some proteins leading to enhanced thermal stabilization (Zhang et al., 2007b), addition of charged amino acid residue segments as a way to maintain tertiary protein structures (Nakagawa et al., 2002), and modification of intermolecular disulfide bonds to enhance secondary and tertiary structures (Dey et al., 2006; Garcia et al., 2006). However, although the subunit vaccine candidates that are involved in the aforementioned strategies demonstrated promise, such as the outer surface protein A (OspA) from *Borrelia burgdorferi* (Zhang et al., 2007b), HIV gp160 (Dey et al., 2006; Garcia et al., 2006), and streptococcal protein G (Wunderlich et al., 2005a), these approaches tend to be protein-specific and are still very early in development. Although there have not been any documented cases of molecular engineering modifications of live or virus-like particles (VLPs) that demonstrated improved stability, it is possible that a small change in amino acid sequence in some of the key structural proteins may lead to dramatic differences in thermal stabilities for live vaccines. One example is Gardasil™ (Merck, Inc.), the human papilloma virus vaccine, for which significant differences in vaccine stability among the vaccine serotypes were attributed to the small differences in amino acid structures that led to large changes in the intermolecular contacts that stabilize the L1 proteins and the VLP assembly (Shank-Retzlaff et al., 2006).

10.3.2 Formulation Approaches

The need for an optimal biopharmaceutical formulation is typically driven by a diverse set of factors, including manufacturing and storage requirements, compatibility with specific dosage forms, as well as economic factors and marketing considerations. For vaccines, there is a greater technical challenge to satisfy these requirements, compared to a typical mAb, given that many vaccines are composed of live organisms that are structurally complex and usually very unstable to prolonged storage. One exception worth noting is the specific case of seasonal vaccines, such as influenza, for which the administration cycles and annual strain redevelopment requirements preclude the need for long-term storage. The vaccine changes every year, thus long-term shelf life beyond 1 year is typically unnecessary. The most common approach to stabilize vaccines is through optimization of pharmaceutical formulations and processing conditions. Vaccine formulations are currently produced as liquid, frozen, or dried dosage form, and each presents a different challenge.

Formulation and process-related approaches typically strive to avoid changes to the original molecular makeup of the vaccine. Many vaccines, however, will benefit from a more universal strategy that can be applied across many different vaccines at an earlier stage of production. For example, upstream bulk vaccine manufacturing processes, such as cell culture (or egg) infection or transfection conditions, incubation temperature and time to harvest, and purification conditions can all impact the potency, purity, and quality of the starting material, which in turn will directly affect the stability of the vaccine, irrespective of the formulation selected. In one published study, it was shown that the use of optimal depth filtration and ultrafiltration purification conditions reduced the aggregates of rotavirus-like vaccine particles and other degradation products. The resulting vaccine possessed higher purity and exhibited improved storage stability (Peixoto et al., 2007). For live viral vaccines, the inoculation conditions such as the multiplicity of infection and time and temperature of harvest can significantly impact the starting virus titer and ultimately, the stability of the vaccine. Similarly, for bacterial vaccines, the inoculation and harvesting conditions (e.g., lag, logarithmic, or stationary phase growth) can determine the live-to-dead (or defective) particle ratios and have significant impact on stability (Chiueh et al., 2007). The process stability of a live attenuated bacterial vaccine strain (e.g., *Salmonella typhi* Ty21a) depends markedly on the growth parameters used to produce the vaccine (see Fig. 10.2). The precise mechanism for these differences has not been described, but it is clear that a prudent stabilization strategy involves the optimization of the upstream process manufacturing conditions prior to formulation development.

Despite the abundance of biopharmaceutical products that are manufactured in the liquid form, dry dosage forms will continue to grow, driven by the need for improved thermal stability and the development of cost-effective and market-competitive drug delivery systems. In the last 30 years, the pharmaceutical industry has benefited from the development of drug delivery technologies that have been largely applied to small molecule drugs. More recently, these systems have been applied to more complex molecules such as hormones (e.g., Exubera™, room-temperature-stable inhaled insulin) and vaccines (e.g., FluMist nasal flu vaccine), and examples include implants, controlled release patches, needleless injections, and devices for nasal and oral inhalation delivery. One of the few commercial oral vaccines that has benefited from recent developments in drug delivery technology is Vivotif® (Crucell) typhoid vaccine, which is manufactured as enteric-coated capsules. Vivotif

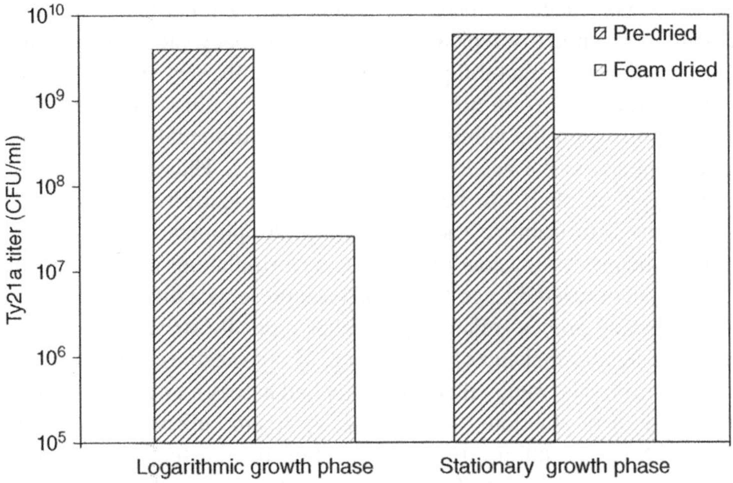

Figure 10.2 The metabolic state of live bacteria vaccines may impact process stability as is demonstrated by the improved desiccation tolerance of Ty21a when isolated at the stationary growth phase. Foam dried Ty21a titer remains within acceptable limits at room temperature for more than 1 year (Chiueh et al., 2007).

is a live attenuated vaccine for oral administration. It consists of gelatin capsules that contain a freeze-dried formulation of Ty21a and are coated with a pH-sensitive polymer to limit the contact of live attenuated bacteria to contacting the stomach acid. However, unlike most solid oral dosage forms, Vivotif capsules need to be refrigerated (2–8°C) and protected from light to ensure prolonged stability.

The contents of several dry vaccines are shown in Table 10.2. The process of preparing this dosage form demonstrates the complexities faced by vaccine manufacturer, attempting to make improvements on existing liquid formulations. The vaccine Ty21a strain is grown in fermenters, under controlled conditions, in a media containing a digest of yeast extract, casein, dextrose, and galactose. Bacteria are collected by centrifugation, then resuspended in a solution containing sucrose, ascorbic acid, and amino acids, and subsequently freeze-dried. The Ty21a-containing freeze-dried solid is then milled, mixed with lactose and magnesium stearate, and filled into gelatin capsules that are coated with an organic polymer, most likely by spraying a polymer solution, to render them resistant to dissolution in the acidic gastric fluid. The enteric-coated capsules are then packaged in blisters for distribution. As is evident from this description, vaccine solid formulations are far more complex in composition and preparation than a liquid formulation, however, the benefits will many times significantly outweigh the production costs. In addition to the marked improvement in shelf life and reduced dependency on cold chain storage requirements, dry formulations have significant advantages in comparison to liquid or frozen formulations in the avoidance of freeze–thaw stress, agitation/shear sensitivity, and container-closure integrity problems. Other benefits of drying generally

TABLE 10.2 Excipients Used in Commercialized Products Including Enveloped and Nonenveloped Viruses, Bacteria, Toxoids, Subunits, and Antigens

Type	Species	Form	Product	Storage	Excipients
Enveloped virus	Measels, rubella, mumps, varicella, vaccinia, Japanese encephalitis	Live attenuated, inactivated[a]	Lyophilized	Refrigerated	Bovine gelatin, fetal bovine serum, formaldehyde, glycine, HEPES, human albumin, hydroylzyed gelatin, mannitol, monosodium L-glutamate, mouse serum protein, neomycin, polysorbate 80, potassium chloride, potassium phosphate, sodium bicarbonate, sodium chloride, sodium phosphate, sorbitol, sucrose, thimerosal, urea
	Varicella-zoster, yellow fever	Live attenuated	Lyophilized	Frozen	Bovine gelatin, EDTA, fetal bovine serum, hydrolyzed gelatin, monosodium glutamate, monosodium L-glutamate, neomycin, potassium chloride, potassium phosphate monobasic, processed gelatin, sodium chloride, sodium phosphate dibasic, sodium phosphate monobasic, sucrose
	Influenza, rabies	Inactivated	Solution, suspension	Refrigerated	Aluminum phosphate, bovine gelatin, formaldehyde, monosodium glutamate, neomycin, octoxynol-10 (TRITON X-100), ovalbumin, phenol red, polymyxin, polysorbate 80, potassium phosphate monobasic, β-propiolactone, sodium phosphate dibasic, sucrose, thimerosal, TNBP, α-tocopheryl hydrogen succinate, Triton N101, WFI
Nonenveloped virus	Rotavirus	Live attenuated	Lyophilized	Refrigerated or room temperature	Amphotericin, citric acid, fetal bovine serum, monosodium glutamate, neomycin, potassium phosphate monobasic, sodium bicarbonate, sodium phosphate dibasic, sucrose

(continued)

TABLE 10.2 *(Continued)*

Type	Species	Form	Product	Storage	Excipients
		Live	Solution	Refrigerated	Cell culture media, fetal bovine serum, poysorbate 80, sodium citrate, sodium hydroxide, sodium phosphate monobasic monohydrate, sucrose
	Hepatitis A, poliovirus	Inactivated	Suspension	Refrigerated	Aluminum hydroxide, aluminum phosphate, amino acids, formaldehyde, formalin, neomycin, 2-phenoxyethanol, phosphate buffer, polymyxin B, polysorbate 20, sodium borate, sodium chloride, sodium hydroxide, streptomycin, WFI
Bacteria	*Mycobacterium Bovis*[b]	Live	Lyophilized	Refrigerated	Ammonium citrate, asparagine, citric acid, glycerin, iron ammonium citrate, lactose, magnesium sulfate, monosodium glutamate, potassium phosphate
	Vibrio cholerae,[c] *Salmonella typhi*[d]	Inactivated	Suspension	Refrigerated	Agar, phenol, sodium chloride
	Salmonella typhi (Ty21a) Vivotif	Live	Oral capsule	Refrigerated	Freeze-dried formulation: sucrose; ascorbic acid; amino acid mixture; mixed with lactose; magnesium stearate
Toxoids, subunits, and antigens	*Haemophilus* b conjugate[e]	N/A	Lyophilized	Refrigerated	Aluminum hydroxide, formaldehyde, lactose, sodium chloride, sucrose

	Tetanus toxoid, *Mycobacterium tuberculosis* protein fraction, *Streptococcus pneumoniae* saccharide antigens, *Salmonella Typhi* surface polysaccharide	N/A	Solution	Refrigerated	Formaldehyde, phenol, polydimethylsiloxane, polysorbate 80, sodium chloride, sodium phosphate dibasic, sodium phosphate monobasic, thimerosal, WFI (pH 7 ± 0.3)
	Tetanus toxoid, Meningococcal polysaccharide diphtheria toxoid conjugate, acellular pertussis, Hepatitis B[f], Lyme disease vaccine[g], Human papillomavirus recombinant vaccine, *Bacillus anthracis*[h]	N/A	Suspension	Refrigerated	Aluminum phosphate, aluminum hydroxide, aluminum potassium sulfate, benzethonium chloride, formaldehyde, gelatin, gluteraldehyde, L-histidine, 2-phenoxyethanol, polysorbate 80, sodium borate, sodium chloride, sodium phosphate, thimerosal, WFI

[a]Only Japanese encephalitis.
[b]Tuberculosis.
[c]Cholera.
[d]Typhoid.
[e]Meningococcal protein conjugate, tetanus toxoid conjugate, *H. influenzae* type b.
[f]Recombinant surface antigen.
[g]Recombinant lipoprotein OspA.
[h]Anthrax vaccine.

include reduced product weight and bulk, improved ease of shipping and distribution, and the possibility of increasing the vaccine titer concentration range on reconstitution using low diluent volume.

10.3.3 Drying Processes to Stabilize Vaccines

In recent years, there has been a surge in research demonstrating the feasibility of alternative drying processes that could improve vaccine stability and, at the same time, produce more flexible dosage presentations than what can be accomplished with conventional methods, which includes refrigerated, or frozen liquid, and freeze-dried formulations.

As mentioned previously, the process selection for vaccines is significantly influenced by the stability requirements and economics of manufacturing implementation. Even for vaccines with projected sales in excess of one billion dollars (e.g., influenza vaccine, pneumococcus vaccine, rotavirus vaccines, and human papilloma virus vaccines), there has been a reluctance to adopt new processes outside of liquid or freeze-drying. The reasons for this are understandable; the cost of developing a new manufacturing process and, more importantly, that of clinical trial retesting with new dosage forms are significant. These are amplified by two factors: vaccines tend to be low profit margin product, and they are typically considered not "well-characterized biologicals" for regulatory purposes, thus requiring large-scale clinical trials to support a process change. As a result, vaccine processes have not evolved beyond what was developed over five decades ago.

In the past 10 years, reports on the improved stability of vaccine formulations by rendering into the solid state have increased significantly. Freeze-drying, spray drying, spray freeze-drying, and foam drying have been shown to possess the potential to become a commercially viable process, which can be used not only to prepare the vaccine into a solid, but also to control powder properties demanded by different drug delivery systems, such as particle size for needleless injections, nasal, or inhalation applications.

Recent comparative studies have also demonstrated that understanding the stresses encountered during drying for each method is necessary to gain insight into formulation, process selection, and process optimization decisions, mainly because the stability of a vaccine in the dry state may be affected differently depending on the dehydration process chosen (see Fig. 10.3). A summary of the drying mechanisms of these alternative drying methods applied to vaccines is described in the following sections.

10.3.3.1 Freeze-drying By far, the most widely used process to dry and stabilize vaccines is freeze-drying. All marketed vaccines that are in a dried format are processed by freeze-drying; these include Bacillus Calmette-Guérin (BCG), measles/mump/rubella (MMR), varicella, *Haemophilus influenza* (Hib), yellow fever, rotavirus (Rotarix^{TM}), meningococcal (MPSV4), and shingles (Burke et al., 1999; Carpenter et al., 2002). Freeze-drying involves three basic thermal processing steps as follows: freezing, ice sublimation (primary drying), and secondary drying.

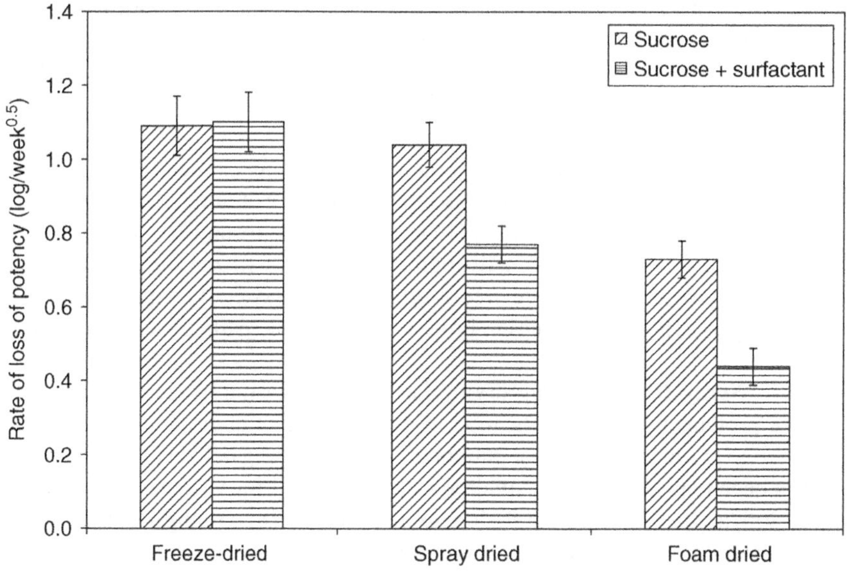

Figure 10.3 Effect of drying process on the stability of live parainfluenza vaccine measured by the magnitude of the rate of decomposition at 25°C of powders made by freeze, spray, and foam drying. In this study, the same formulation containing sucrose and potassium phosphate with or without Pluronics F68 surfactant was used in three different drying methods to generate dry vaccine preparations. The data demonstrated the process-related differences in vaccine solid-state stability and that the role of the protective excipient, surfactant in this case, is clearly dependent on the drying process. Adapted from Abdul-Fattah et al., 2007b.

Freezing is performed in order to crystallize unbound water and to remove the ice via sublimation under vacuum. Primary drying is typically performed at low pressure (typically ≤200 mTorrs) and below the product collapse temperature (T_c). The process ends when the product temperature rises above shelf temperature and/or a decrease in the pressure reading of a Pirani vacuum gauge occurs (Rambhatla et al., 2006; Tang and Pikal, 2004). By the end of this step, nearly 70–80% of water has been removed in the form of ice, while the rest remains in the amorphous phase (Carpenter et al., 1997; Tang and Pikal, 2004). The secondary drying step is conducted at a higher shelf temperature to remove the remaining water (bound water) via evaporation.

Stress factors associated with freeze-drying include ice crystal formation and desiccation-related stress. This stress is particularly challenging for biological materials that contain plasma membranes, including enveloped viruses and bacterial cells (Greiff, 1969). In addition, there are other stresses associated with freezing, such as pH shifts, buffer crystallization (as is the case with sodium phosphate buffer system), cold denaturation, and instability caused by dehydration (Nail et al., 2002; Privalov, 1990; Shalaev et al., 2002). The process of removing hydrogen bonds from the protein surface is known to be stressful, thus, rational selection of stabilizers (lyoprotectants with or without surfactants) and/or process modifications, such as annealing, will be critical to the successful implementation of freeze-drying (Maa and Prestrelski, 2000; Nguyen et al., 2004; Sonner et al., 2002; Webb et al., 2003; Yu et al., 2006).

The freeze-drying process is not without its shortcomings. Freeze-drying has been shown to be ineffective in processing vaccines containing aluminum adjuvant, which is sensitive to freezing; for example, HBsAg vaccine adjuvanted with $Al(OH)_3$ can undergo serious damage and deactivation if it becomes frozen during processing, shipping, or storage. Furthermore, freeze-dried samples generally require further processing (e.g., sieving, jet-milling) in order to produce fine particulates, if required.

10.3.3.2 Spray Drying Spray drying has seen increasing usage as a process to stabilize proteins by rapid vitrification in the presence of amorphous sugars. It has been used to produce particles for pulmonary and nasal drug delivery (Vehring, 2007) and has been explored as a potential processing method for vaccines (Abdul-Fattah et al., 2007a; Baras et al., 2000; Johansen et al., 1998; Truong-Le and Scherer, 2005). In addition to its ability to control powder properties (e.g., particle size, particle morphology, powder density, and surface composition), the key advantages of spray drying are as follows: shorter process cycle time (i.e., more batches per unit time), scalability (i.e., large batch size per unit operation, requiring less number of production units), and the ability to process continuously. Spray drying involves several steps, including atomization, drying, and powder separation/collection. Atomization is a process by which the solution, suspension, or colloidal dispersion is sprayed to micron-sized droplets (1–200 μm) at high velocity. In the drying phase, the spray comes into thermal contact with a heated, dry gaseous stream (such as dry air or nitrogen). The resulting powders are separated from moist gas stream by means of a cyclone, electrostatic precipitator, or bag filter and collected in a holding chamber (collector) (Vehring, 2007).

The atomization step involves not only shear stress but also high surface tension stress due to surface area expansion. While spray drying can be used to produce stable protein powders (Maa et al., 2000; Maa and Prestrelski, 2000; Mumenthaler et al., 1994), certain proteins that during atomization (Yu et al., 2006); exposing proteins to large air–water interface can lead to protein unfolding followed by aggregation. Human growth hormone (hGH) and bovine serum albumin (BSA) are examples of proteins that undergo extensive aggregation during atomization. Surface-related stresses can be mitigated with the addition of surface active excipients (Lechuga-Ballesteros et al., 2008) or specific ions such as zinc (Johnson et al., 1997).

Protein denaturation has been observed during spray drying due to dehydration, thus necessitating the use of excipients to replace the hydrogen bonds previously provided by water (e.g., sugars, polyols, amino acids). Although the drying air temperature may exceed 100°C in normal spray drying conditions, thermal denaturation is most likely not the principal cause of protein damage because the temperature of the

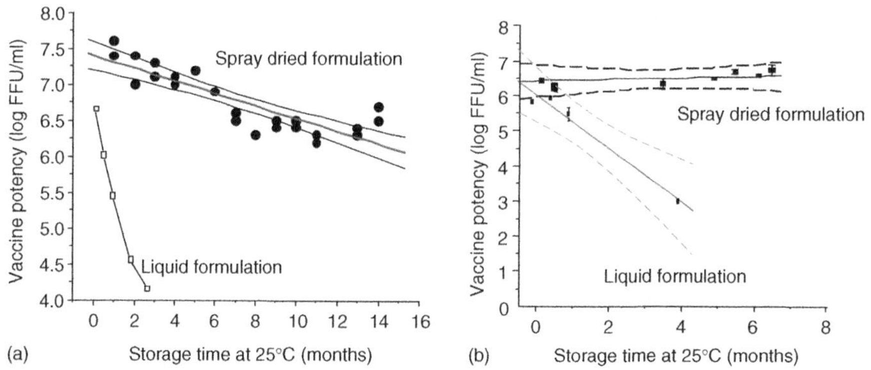

Figure 10.4 Spray dried formulations of live attenuated influenza (a) and live rotavirus (b) vaccines display improved room temperature stability over their liquid counterparts. Under optimal formulation and processing conditions, spray drying can be used to stabilize live virus vaccines for a year or more at 25°C. Influenza vaccine stability data was adapted from Truong-Le, 2004. Rotavirus vaccine stability data is a courtesy of Aridis Pharmaceuticals LLC (San José, CA).

droplet hardly exceeds the wet bulb temperature of water (approx. 40°C) (Vehring, 2007).

Spray drying has been used to dry highly complex biologicals, including live organisms such as live attenuated influenza vaccine and live attenuated rotavirus vaccine, which displayed improved room temperature solid-state stability (see Fig. 10.4). For live bacteria, lower outlet processing temperature has generally been associated with higher viability (Kim and Bhowmik, 1990; Prajapati et al., 1987; Santivarangkna et al., 2007). Spray dried gram-positive *Lactobacillus paracasei* bacteria has been reported to be stable for long periods, if prepared at processing conditions employing low outlet temperature (Desmond et al., 2002). Spray dried antigenic products have been described as far back as 10 years ago (Kay, 1997), and spray drying suspensions of anthrax spores and vegetative cells, such as *Francisella tularensis*, using common off-the-shelf excipients have been reported to form respirable particles (Rhian and Lynch, 2004). Pulmonary delivery of vaccines has also been the subject of recent research, as the robust immune response and protection elicited by pulmonary administration of inactivated influenza vaccine were clinically demonstrated in 1969 (Waldman et al., 1969). Spray dried Fluzone® (Aventis Pasteur), a split subunit vaccine in a phospholipid-based microparticle, demonstrated increased exposure of the bronchial-associated lymphoid tissue in triggering specific immunity compared to that administered parenterally or nasally. A more stable vaccine powder, containing BCG with good aerosolization properties has been successfully prepared by spray drying, using L-leucine as a stabilizer. The viability loss was reduced by two orders of magnitude compared to that processed by freeze-drying (Wong et al., 2007).

10.3.3.3 Spray Freeze-Drying Spray freeze-drying (SFD) is a recently developed drying process that involves elements of spray and freeze-drying. This process has been used to produce free flowing powder of porous, micron-sized, dense particles with a high specific surface area and improved bioavailability. Spray freeze-drying has potential applications ranging from dermal delivery of vaccines using needle-free ballistic injection devices to pulmonary delivery (Maa et al., 2004; Maa et al., 1999; Schiffter 2007; Sonner et al., 2002). The process steps in SFD include atomization, rapid freezing, and primary and secondary drying. As in spray drying, atomization involves spraying or atomizing the formulated solution. However, instead of atomizing into heated gaseous medium, the feedstock is atomized directly into a cryogenic medium in which rapid freezing of droplets takes place to form ice particles (Schiffter, 2007; Weers et al., 2007; Yu et al., 2006). The suspended frozen droplets are collected by sieves or are collected after cryogen has boiled off (Schiffter, 2007). The sample is then transferred to prechilled shelves (typically $\leq -40°C$) of a lyophilizer for subsequent drying. The principle of drying by ice sublimation for this phase of the process is identical to the primary drying step in a conventional freeze-drying process. One advantage with SFD is that sublimation and secondary drying of the frozen particles are more rapid than those associated with conventional freeze-drying due to the expanded surface area of the frozen particles.

SFD was applied to prepare sugar-based high density particles containing an influenza vaccine suitable for epidermal powder immunization. The dry powder retained its stability, potency, and immunogenicity and was successfully tested in a human clinical study delivered with a needleless injection device (Maa et al., 2004). In addition, an engineered powder of influenza vaccine using SFD has demonstrated superior stability over liquid and *in vivo* equivalence to liquid formulation upon nasal administration to rodents (Garmise et al., 2007). The immunogenic potential of influenza subunit antigen was vastly improved in the spray freeze-dried antigen powder compared to the liquid formulation on storage (Amorij et al., 2007a). Powder formulations consisting of the recombinant PA of *B. anthracis* for nasal mucosal delivery has been demonstrated in a rabbit model; spray freeze-dried formulations were prepared at pH 7–8 using trehalose as stabilizer and a CpG-containing oligonucleotide adjuvant. In addition, pulmonary delivery of an inulin-stabilized influenza subunit vaccine prepared by SFD has been shown to induce systemic, mucosal, humoral, as well as cell-mediated immune responses in BALB/c mice. (Amorij et al., 2007b).

10.3.3.4 Foam Drying Air drying refers to evaporative drying at near-atmospheric pressure conditions. In comparison, drying processes in which moisture removal is carried out mainly by evaporation under reduced pressure have a long development history, but they have not been implemented at commercial scale for biopharmaceuticals (Nastaj, 1994). Under certain operating conditions, vacuum drying can result in a foamy, rigid sponge-like cake structure, and hence is referred to as *foam drying*. Besides convection, heat can also be supplied by conduction or radiation (e.g., infrared [IR] and microwave) (Durance et al., 2007), either separately or in various combinations designed to enhance the efficiency in moisture removal.

Since drying is accomplished at ambient or near-ambient temperatures, foam drying is characterized by relatively brief and minimal excursions to extreme temperature regimes. Hybrid vacuum drying technologies, such as microwave vacuum drying and vacuum drying with radiative heating, are also emerging as a commercially viable process to dry foods (Cui et al., 2004; Mongpraneet et al., 2002; Shibata, 2006; Yagi, 1999). Foam drying was successfully used to dry and stabilize formulations of several vaccines well over a half century ago (Abdul-Fattah et al., 2008; Annear, 1956; Annear, 1961; Annear, 1964). Adaptations of Annear's original foam processes have surfaced in recent years using conventional freeze-dryers, which allow for better process controls than the earlier process (Bronshtein, 2004 #51; Mattern et al., 1997; Miller et al., 1998; Pisal et al., 2006; Santivarangkna et al., 2007; Truong-Le, 2006). However, the basic processing features remain the same.

Foam drying can be broken down into primary and secondary drying phases. Primary drying step initiates once the chamber pressure starts to decrease. At this point, evaporation initiates and is usually, but not always, accompanied by foaming action caused by the boiling of the solution. The primary drying period lasts for 1–2 h during which the bulk of heat and mass transfer takes place. The product temperature gradually rises until it reaches the shelf temperature, marking the end of primary drying. The solution solidifies into a foam or a film, and roughly 90% or more of the bulk water is removed by evaporation (Abdul-Fattah et al., 2008; Bronshtein, 2004; Kramer et al., 2002). Secondary drying further reduces the moisture content of the dried product. This step may last longer than that employed in freeze-drying because of the tendency to form a closed-cell structure (i.e., the roof of the foam cake is a continuous layer characterized by lack of pores).

The fact that the foam drying process was developed decades ago but has not been commercially adopted suggests that there are significant challenges to its implementation. Foam drying is an aggressive drying technique that involves several potential stresses on the vaccine. The foaming action involves cavitation that results in cycles of bubbles percolating upward, bursting, and coalescing with neighboring bubbles. Such bubbling action could compromise container-closure integrity because the formulation could splatter to the neck of the vial. In addition, there are significant shear forces at the air–water interface, which could lead to protein denaturation and activity loss. Nevertheless, under optimal formulation conditions, shear stress can be minimized, and excellent recoveries have been reported for air–water interface-sensitive molecules; examples include hGH (Abdul-Fattah et al., 2008), lactate dehydrogenase (Mattern et al., 1997; Miller et al., 1998), an immunoglobulin (Abdul-Fattah et al., 2007a), recombinant human granulocyte colony-stimulating factor (Mattern et al., 1997), live attenuated influenza (Truong-Le and Scherer, 2005), live attenuated human parainfluenza virus (Abdul-Fattah et al., 2007b), live attenuated Ty21a for anthrax PA and shigella vaccine (Chiueh et al., 2007), and Newcastle disease virus (LaSota strain) (Pisal et al., 2006). The cavitation process also results in a variable foam structure with inhomogeneous density, which may cause variability in moisture content within the cake. Another challenge to foam drying is in optimizing the formulation and process parameters to achieve low (<4%) moisture content because increasing the shelf temperature during secondary drying is not always effective, especially once the closed-cell structure has formed. Foam cake structures are variable and present difficulty in establishing release specifications in product appearance as is routinely performed for freeze-dried products.

10.3.4 Formulation and Solid-State Stability

As mentioned previously, the mechanisms of biopreservation in the dry state are complex and dependent not only on the formulation (or stabilizer), but also on the drying process and the solid-state properties of the resultant solids. Ideally, the stabilizer is inert and remain in the same amorphous phase as the biological material. Stabilization mechanisms involved in the dried state have been summarized in two theories (Carpenter et al., 1997; Chang et al., 2005; Franks et al., 1991; Pikal, 2004): water replacement and vitrification. The water replacement hypothesis suggests that thermodynamic destabilization and activity loss during drying are due to the removal of the protein-bound water that occurs during the final stages of drying. This desiccation-induced loss is prevented by hydrogen bonding of a stabilizer with the protein surface, leading to the preservation of protein native structure. The net effect is that the stabilizer acts to preserve the protein conformation by increasing the free energy of unfolding. In the vitrification theory, the biological materials are kinetically immobilized in a rigid, glassy matrix in the dried form in a manner in which the global (α-relaxations because of translational and/or rotational motions) and local molecular motions of the glass and the encased proteins or vaccines (β-relaxations) are suppressed. These two theories are not mutually exclusive, and thus molecular stabilization could come about by both mechanisms.

Through the controlled removal of water, both the chemical and physical stability of biomaterials can be improved by molecular immobilization (Franks et al., 1991). The physical stability of the glassy solid is ensured by storing the sample below its glass transition temperature (T_g) and avoiding contact with water, which tends to decrease the T_g by a process known as *plasticization*. High T_g, however, is not the only requirement to ensure chemical and physical stability, as evidenced by the similarity in protection afforded to a spray-dried IgG by sorbitol (T_g=−10°C) and trehalose (T_g=120°C) (Maury et al., 2005). The stabilization mechanism, in this case, is explained by the water replacement theory, as described above. The extent of molecular mobility depends on the difference between the glass transition and the storage temperatures. It is generally assumed that if the difference between the two temperatures exceeds 50°C, the shelf life of a glassy solid is likely to exceed 2 years; a glassy solid with a T_g > 75°C should remain stable at room temperature and may be transiently exposed to elevated temperatures during shipping.

A great deal of interest has been generated around understanding the role of water in a formulation because water can act as a plasticizer that will decrease both chemical (i.e., bioactive ingredient degradation) and physical (i.e., particle fusion, cake collapse, crystallization) stability. The degree of dryness needed depends on the glass transition of the formulation, the storage condition, and the hydration limit of the formulation, below which molecular motion is minimized, favoring long-term stability (Lechuga-Ballesteros et al., 2002). Interactions of the glassy matrix with water, as well as its potential interactions with the biomolecule, need to be considered. The overall mobility of the glassy matrix may or may not dictate the availability of water to act as a solvent or reactant. Chemical reactions have been observed to occur below the glassy solid's T_g, with the reaction rate increasing with rise in relative humidity (RH) and temperature. In addition, the extent of reaction below the formulation's T_g depends on the "molecular fit" between reactant and glassy solid, with denser glasses (i.e., with lower free volume) being more protective. It has been reported that the addition of small molecular weight stabilizers (also referred to as *plasticizers*, because they depress the glass transition of the glassy matrix) can dampen the local molecular motion, thereby increasing the stability of the glassy matrix (Abdul-Fattah et al., 2007a; Cicerone et al., 2003). Residual moisture can also have an effect on powder rheological characteristics (Maa et al., 1997), which may be of importance if the dry powder is to be processed into a solid dosage form. Sensitivity to moisture may be prevented or reduced by unit dose packaging, as observed for fast dissolving tablets and orally dissolving films. Although low moisture content is desired for improved stability, there is a moisture content threshold below which increased oxidation of amorphous formulations has been observed and may encourage undesired electrostatic charging during powder handling.

Low molecular weight excipients (i.e., nonreducing sugars such as sucrose, trehalose, raffinose, and other polyols such as sorbitol, glycerol, and mannitol) are generally employed to dry biomaterials effectively. In addition to these stabilizers, there are other critical components that are included in the formulation of viruses and bacteria. These include, but are not limited to, buffering components, osmotic agents, adjuvants, surfactants, and proteins (Table 10.2). Buffering components, such as phosphate and HEPES, are included in the formulation to control the pH and the osmolality of the formulation. By controlling the pH of the formulation, the structure (and the aggregation/complexation state) of the labile molecules can be adjusted to confer optimal stability. Furthermore, the kinetics of various degradation mechanisms can be modulated. Osmotic agents, such as sodium chloride, are also included in the formulation to control the osmolality of the formulation and to match the solute concentration at the administration site. Surfactants such as pluronics or polysorbates and proteins such as albumin and gelatin are added to confer protection against interfacial stresses and to inhibit aggregation. Clearly, the specific product has a strong influence on the components and complexity of the formulation; for example, enveloped viruses are more difficult to stabilize against dehydration stress compared to nonenveloped viruses, thus additional components, or a higher concentration of critical components, are required. In contrast, subunits and antigens tend to require a simpler formulation as a result of their greater inherent stability as compared to live vaccines. Interestingly, for the commercial products listed in Table 10.2, the form of the labile material, whether live or inactivated, had less of an impact on the excipients used. Product state, whether lyophilized, frozen, or in liquid form, also dictates the choice of excipients, as the degradation mechanisms differ significantly.

10.3.5 The Impact of Heat-Stable Vaccine Formulation on Delivery Systems

Solid-state stabilization of live virus- and bacteria-based vaccines has enabled the development of nontraditional, solid oral dosage forms for vaccine delivery. One of the most convenient oral dosage formats is a quick dissolving thin film (Cui and Mumper, 2002; Summers, 2007). The thin film is mucoadhesive, dissolves in several seconds, and is designed to deliver pharmaceutical and biological actives into the oral cavity with high efficiency. Patient compliance is expected to be enhanced due to its administration simplicity and quick dissolving characteristic, which would in turn facilitate mass vaccination. In addition to the benefits of the film's portability, compactness and room temperature stability are also expected to benefit the manufacturer, distributor, and the health care provider. The fast dissolving tablet is comparable in dosing configuration and delivery benefits that can be designed to be temperature resistant and, together with the small storage volume, enable stockpiling for mass immunization campaigns. Zydis® (Catalent) technology relies on the *in situ* freeze-drying of a solution of the vaccine and formulation components filled into aluminum blisters. Recently, Zydis technolgy applied to manufacture Grazax® (Alk-Abelló A/S), an allergy vaccine for moderate-to-severe seasonal allergic rhinitis (grass pollen hay fever), has been commercialized in Europe and is currently in Phase III clinical testing to demonstrate its effectiveness in children. Other delivery technologies include transdermal skin patches (Glenn and Kenney, 2006), particulates that can be delivered intradermally using ballistic propulsion (Christie et al., 2006), controlled-release polymer matrices (Gupta et al., 1998), enteric-coated tablets (Wilding et al., 1994), wafers (Rak et al., 2007), and inhalable powders for nasal (Garmise et al., 2007) or pulmonary delivery (Amorij et al., 2007b). Orally delivered virions (e.g., adenovirus) and bacteria (e.g., Ty21a salmonella), as vectors for delivery of other vaccines (e.g., AIDS, flu, anthrax) and gene- or plasmid-based siRNAs for cancer therapy, have also gained attention (Chiueh et al., 2007; Croyle et al., 2001; Evans et al., 2004; Zhang et al., 2007a). Clearly, none of these technologies would find commercial use without the continued development of thermally stabilized vaccines that can withstand the required fabrication, storage, and handling requirements demanded by the modern delivery systems.

10.4 FUTURE OF VACCINE STABILIZATION

Considerable effort has been put forth to improve the stability of vaccines; these include molecular and genetic engineering approaches, but most notably, solid-state formulation and processing approaches. As new and more complex vaccine candidates are created, the need for better stability and convenient delivery systems will become more acute. Currently, most commercial vaccines do not possess long-term stability outside of the cold chain and is administered parenterally, generally using inconvenient delivery systems. Vaccine stability may be increased by optimizing the formulation composition and/or the processing conditions, making use of recent, promising advances in drying technologies to stabilize the vaccine in the solid state. However, there are continuing challenges associated with each technology that need to be overcome, including process stresses on the vaccine, scalability, and optimal dosage form to ensure compatibility with the delivery device. The choice of delivery device/vehicle and potential routes of delivery are constantly expanding. Promising results have been obtained for nasal and pulmonary delivery of vaccines enabled by the production of thermally stable vaccines using advanced stabilization drying technologies. It is now possible to consider the concurrent administration of several multidisease vaccines by physically mixing them prior to inhalation, which eliminates the need for needles, syringes, and sterilization of reconstitution media. The future of vaccine market will be impacted by our ability to better formulate, stabilize, and resolve manufacturing implementation challenges, and thereby enable more convenient delivery.

REFERENCES

Abdul-Fattah AM, Lechuga-Ballesteros D, Kalonia D, Pikal M. The impact of drying method and formulation on the physical properties and stability of methionyl human growth hormone in the amorphous solid state. J Pharm Sci 2008;1:163–184.

Abdul-Fattah AM, Truong-Le V, Yee L, Nguyen L, Kalonia DS, Cicerone MT, Pikal MJ. Drying-induced variations in physico-chemical properties of amorphous pharmaceuticals and their impact on stability (I): Stability of a monoclonal antibody. J Pharm Sci 2007a;96:1983–2008.

Abdul-Fattah AM, Truong-Le V, Yee L, Pan E, Ao Y, Kalonia D, Pikal MJ. Drying-induced variations in physico-chemical properties of amorphous pharmaceuticals and their impact on stability II: stability of a vaccine. Pharm Res 2007b;24:715–727.

Amorij JP, Meulenaar J, Hinrichs WL, Stegmann T, Huckriede A, Coenen F, Frijlink HW. Rational design of an influenza subunit vaccine powder with sugar glass technology: preventing conformational changes of haemagglutinin during freezing and freeze-drying. Vaccine 2007a;25:6447–6457.

Amorij JP, Saluja V, Petersen AH, Hinrichs WL, Huckriede A, Frijlink HW. Pulmonary delivery of an inulin-stabilized influenza subunit vaccine prepared by spray-freeze drying induces systemic, mucosal humoral as well as cell-mediated immune responses in BALB/c mice. Vaccine 2007b;25:8707–8717.

Annear DI. The preservation of bacteria by drying in peptone plugs. J Hyg 1956;54:487–508.

Annear DI. Recovery of *Strigomonas oncopelti* after drying from the liquid state. Aust J Exp Biol Med Sci 1961;39:295–304.

Annear DI. Recoveries of bacteria after drying in glutamate and other substances. Aust J Exp Biol Med Sci 1964;42:717–722.

Baras B, Benoit M-A, Poulain-Godefroy O, Schacht A-M, Capron A, Gillard J, Riveau G. Vaccine properties of antigens entrapped in microparticles produced by spray-drying technique and using various polyester polymers. Vaccine 2000;18:1495–1505.

Bennett JV, Fernandez de Castro J, Valdespino-Gomez JL, Garcia-Garcia ML, Islas-Romero R, Echaniz-Aviles G, Jimenez-Corona A, Sepulveda-Amor J. Aerosolized measles and measles–rubella vaccines induce better measles antibody booster responses than injected vaccines: randomized trials in Mexican schoolchildren. Bull World Health Organ 2002;80:806–812.

Bronshtein V. Preservation by foam formation. Pharm Tecnhol 2004;28:86–92.

Burke C, Hsu TA, Volkin DB. Formulation, stability, and delivery of live attenuated vaccines for human use. Crit Rev Ther Drug Carrier Syst 1999;16:1–83.

Carpenter JF, Chang BS, Garzón-Rodríguez W, Randolph TW. Rational design of stable lyophilized protein formulations: theory and practice. Pharm Biotechnol 2002;13:109–133.

Carpenter JF, Pikal MJ, Randolph TW. Rational design of stable lyophilized protein formulations: some practical advice. Pharm Res 1997;14:969–975.

Chang L, Shepherd D, Sun J, Tang X, Pikal MJ. Mechanism of protein stabilization by sugars during freeze-drying and storage: native structure preservation, specific interaction, and/or immobilization in a glassy matrix? J Pharm Sci 2005;94:1427–1444.

Chiueh G, Pham B, Osorio M, Xu DQ, Kopecko D, Patzer E, Truong-Le V. Room temperature stabilization of oral live attenuated Ty21a *Salmonella typhi* vectored vaccines. 4th International Conference on Vaccines for Enteric Diseases; Poster#29; Lisbon, Portugal; 2007

Christie RJ, Findley DJ, Dunfee M, Hansen R, Olsen SC, Grainger DW. Photopolymerized hydrogel carriers for live vaccine ballistic delivery. Vaccine 2006;24:1462–1469.

Cicerone MT, Tellington A, Trost L, Sokolov A. Substantially improved stability of biological agents in dried form. BioProcess Int 2003;1:36–47.

Costantino HR. Excipients for use in lyophilized pharmaceutical peptide, protein, and other bioproducts. In: Pikal MJ, Costantino HR, editors. *Lyophilization of Biomaterials*. AAPS Press; 2004. p 139–228.

Croyle MA, Cheng X, Wilson JM. Development of formulations that enhance physical stability of viral vectors for gene therapy. Gene Ther 2001;8:1281–1290.

Cui Z, Mumper RJ. Buccal transmucosal delivery of calcitonin in rabbits using thin-film composites. Pharm Res 2002;19:1901–1906.

Cui Z, Xu S, Sun D. Microwave-vacuum drying kinetics of carrot slices. J Food Eng 2004;65:157–164.

Desmond C, Ross RP, O'Callaghan E, Fitzgerald G, Stanton C. Improved survival of *Lactobacillus paracasei* NFBC 338 in spray-dried powders containing gum acacia. J Virol Meth 2002;93:1003–1011.

Dey AK, David KB, Klasse PJ, Moore JP. Specific amino acids in the N-terminus of the gp41 ectodomain contribute to the stabilization of a soluble, cleaved gp140 envelope glycoprotein from human immunodeficiency virus type 1. Virology 2006;360:199–208.

Durance TD, Fu J, Yaghmaee P. Apparatus and method for dehydrating biological materials. US Patent 8718113 B2, 2007.

Evans RK, Nawrocki DK, Isopi LA, Williams DM, Casimiro DR, Chin S, Chen M, D-m Z, Shiver JW, Volkin DB. Development of stable liquid formulations for adenovirus-based vaccines. J Pharm Sci 2004;93:2458–2475.

Frank KJ. Monitoring temperature-sensitive vaccines and immunologic drugs, including anthrax vaccine. Am J Health-Syst Pharm 1999;56:2052–2055.

Franks F, Hatley RHM, Mathias SF. Materials science and the production of shelf-stable biologicals. Pharm Technol Int 1991;3:24–34.

Galazka A. Stability of vaccines. Geneva: World Health Organization, 1989 (published online: WHO/EPI/GEN/89.8).

Galazka A, Milstien J, Zaffran M. Thermostability of vaccines. WHO/GPV/98.07. 1998. http://www.who.ch/gpv-documents/

Garcia J, Dumy P, Rosen O, Anglister J. Stabilization of the biologically active conformation of the principal neutralizing determinant of HIV-1(IIIB) containing a cis-proline surrogate: 1H NMR and molecular modeling study. Biochemistry 2006;45:4284–4294.

Garmise RJ, Staats HF, Hickey AJ. 2007. Novel dry powder preparations of whole inactivated influenza virus for nasal vaccination. AAPS PharmSciTech 8, article 81. DOI: 10.1208/pt0804081.

Glenn GM, Kenney RT. Mass vaccination: solutions in the skin. Curr Top Microbiol Immunol 2006;304:247–268.

Grabenstein JD. Vaccines: countering anthrax: vaccines and immunoglobulins. Clin Infect Dis 2008;46:129–136.

Greiff D. Freezing drying microorganisms; 1968 Oct 2–3; Sapporo, Japan. 1969.

Gupta RK, Singh M, O'Hagan DT. Poly(lactide-co-glycolide) microparticles for the development of single-dose controlled-release vaccines. Adv Drug Del Rev 1998;32:225–246.

Johansen P, Men Y, Audran R, Corradin G, Merkle HP, Gander BI. Improving stability and release kinetics of microencapsulated tetanus toxoid by co-encapsulation of additives. Pharm Res 1998;15:1103–1110.

Johnson OL, Jaworowicz W, Cleland JL, Bailey L, Charnis M, Duenas E, Wu C, Shepard D, Magil S, Last T, Jones AJ, Putney SD. The stabilization and encapsulation of human growth hormone into biodegradable microspheres. Pharm Res 1997;14:730–735.

Katkocin DM, Hsieh C-L. Pharmaceutical aspects of combination vaccines. In: Ellis RW, editor. *Combination Vaccines*. Totowa: The Humana Press; 1999.

Kay WW. Spray dried antigenic products. US patent 5616329: MicroTek R&D Ltd. 1997.

Kim SS, Bhowmik SR. Survival of lactic acid bacteria during spray drying of plain yogurt. J Food Sci 1990;55:1008–1011.

Kramer M, Sennhenn B, Lee G. Freeze-drying using vacuum-induced surface freezing. J Pharm Sci 2002;91:433–443.

Lechuga-Ballesteros D, Charan C, Stults CLM, Stevenson CL, Miller DP, Vehring R, Tep V, Kuo M-C. Trileucine improves aerosol performance and stability of spray-dried powders for inhalation. J Pharm Sci 2008;97:287–302.

Lechuga-Ballesteros D, Miller DP, Zhang J. Residual water in amorphous solids, measurement and effects on stability. In: Levine H, editor. *Progress in Amorphous Food and Pharmaceutical Systems*. London: The Royal Society of Chemistry; 2002. p 275–316.

Maa Y-F, Ameri M, Shu C, Payne LG, Chen D. Influenza vaccine powder formulation development spray-freeze-drying and stability evaluation. J Pharm Sci 2004;93:1912–1923.

Maa Y-F, Costantino HR, Nguyen P-A, Hsu CC. The effect of operating and formulation variables on the morphology of spray-dried protein particles. Pharm Dev Technol 1997;2:213–223.

Maa Y, Nguyen PT, Hsu S. Spray-drying of air–liquid interface sensitive recombinant human growth hormone. J Pharm Sci 2000;87:152–159.

Maa Y, Nguyen P, Sweeney T, Shire SJ, Hsu CC. Protein inhalation powders: spray drying vs spray freeze drying. Pharm Res 1999;16:249–254.

Maa Y, Prestrelski SJ. Biopharmaceutical powders: particle formulation and formulation considerations. Curr Pharm Biotechnol 2000;1:283–302.

Mansfeld J, Vriend G, Van den Burg B, Eijsink VG, Ulbrich-Hofmann R. Probing the unfolding region in a thermolysin-like protease by site-specific immobilization. Biochemistry 1999;38:8240–8245.

Mattern M, Winter G, Lee G. Formulation of proteins in vacuum-dried glasses. Part 1. Improved vacuum-drying of sugars using crystallizing amino acids. Eur J Pharm Biopharm 1997;44:177–185.

Maury M, Murphy K, Kumar S, Mauerer A, Lee G. Spray-drying of proteins: effects of sorbitol and trehalose on aggregation and FT-IR amide I spectrum of an immunoglobulin G. Eur J Pharm Biopharm 2005;59:251–261.

Miller DP, Anderson RE, De Pablo JJ. Stabilization of lactate dehydrogenase following freeze thawing and vacuum-drying in the presence of trehalose and borate. Pharm Res 1998;15:1215–1221.

Milstein J, Galazka A, Kartoglu U, Zaffran M. Geneva: World Health Organization, 2006 (published online WHO/IVB/06.10).

Mongpraneet S, Abe T, Tsurusaki T. Far infrared radiation drying of welsh onion under reduced pressure and convection. ASAE Annual Meeting. Paper number 026163; St. Joseph, MI: The American Society of Agricultural and Biological Engineers; 2002.

Mumenthaler M, Hsu CC, Pearlman R. Feasibility study on spray-drying protein pharmaceuticals: recombinant human growth hormone and tissue-type plasminogen activator. Pharm Res 1994;11:12–20.

Nail SL, Jiang S, Chongprasert S, Knopp SA. Fundamentals of freeze-drying. Pharm Biotechnol 2002;14:281–360.

Nakagawa T, Shimizu H, Link K, Koide A, Koide S, Tamura A. Calorimetric dissection of thermal unfolding of OspA, a predominantly beta-sheet protein containing a single-layer beta-sheet. J Mol Biol 2002;323:751–762.

Nastaj JF. Vacuum contact drying of selected biotechnology products. Drying Technol 1994;12:1145–1166.

Nguyen XC, Herberger JD, Burke PA. Protein powders for encapsulation: a comparison of spray-freeze drying and spray-drying of darbepoetin alfa. Pharm Res 2004;21:507–514.

Peixoto C, Sousa MF, Silva AC, Carrondo MJ, Alves PM. Downstream processing of triple layered rotavirus like particles. J Biotechnol 2007;127:452–491.

Pikal MJ. Mechanisms of protein stabilization during freeze-drying and storage: the relative importance of thermodynamic stabilization and glassy state relaxation dynamics. In: Rey L, Christine J, editors. *Drugs and the Pharmaceutical Sciences: Freeze-Drying/Lyophilization of Pharmaceutical and Biological Products*. New York, NY: Marcel Dekker; 2004. p 63–107.

Pisal S, Wawde G, Salvankar S, Lade S, Kadam S. Vacuum foam drying for preservation of LaSota virus: effect of additives. AAPS PharmSciTech 2006;7:60.

Prajapati JB, Shah RK, Dave JM. Survival of *Lactobacillus acidophilus* in blended spray-dried acidophilus preparations. Aust J Dairy Technol 1987;42:17–21.

Privalov PL. Cold denaturation of proteins. Crit Rev Biochem Mol Biol 1990;25:281–305.

Rak S, Yang WH, Pedersen MR, Durham SR. Once-daily sublingual allergen-specific immunotherapy improves quality of life in patients with grass pollen-induced allergic rhinoconjuctivitis: a double-blind, random study. Qual Life Res 2007;16:191–201.

Rambhatla S, Tchessalov S, Pikal MJ. Heat and mass transfer scale-up issues during freeze drying, III: control and characterization of the degree of supercooling. AAPS PharmSciTech, article 39 2006.

Rhian M, Lynch DC. Recovery of bacterial spores and vegetative cells with a miniature spray drier. J Biochem Microbiol Technol Eng 2004;3:87–94.

Santivarangkna C, Kulozik U, Foerst P. Alternative drying processes for the industrial preservation for lactic acid starter cultures. Biotechnol Prog 2007;23:302–315.

Schiffter H. Spray-freeze-drying in the manufacture of pharmaceuticals. Eur Pharm Rev 2007;3:67–71.

Schiffter H, Condliffe J, Vonhoff S. Spray-freeze-drying of nanosuspensions: the manufacture of insulin particles for needle-free ballistic powder delivery. J R Soc Interface 2010;7(Suppl 4):S483–500.

Shah PS, Hom GK, Ross SA, Lassila JK, Crowhurst KA, Mayo SL. Full-sequence computational design and solution structure of a thermostable protein variant. J Mol Biol 2007;372:1–6.

Shalaev EY, Johnson-Elton TD, Chang L, Pikal MJ. Thermophysical properties of pharmaceutically compatible buffers at sub-zero temperatures: Implications for freeze-drying. Pharm Res 2002;19:195–201.

Shank-Retzlaff ML, Zhao Q, Anderson C, Hamm M, High K, Nguyen M, Wang F, Wang N, Wang B, Wang Y, Washabaugh M, Sitrin R, Shi L. Evaluation of the thermal stability of Gardasil. Hum Vaccin 2006;2:147–154.

Shibata H. Vacuum drying of porous solids under supercooling. Drying Technol 2006;24:541–550.

Sonner C, Maa Y, Lee G. Spray freeze-drying for protein powder preparation: particle characterization and a case study with trypsinogen stability. J Pharm Sci 2002;91:2122–2139.

Summers N. 2007. A no-shot vaccine. Newsweek Magazine; May 28, 2007.

Tang X, Pikal MJ. Design of freeze-drying processes for pharmaceuticals: practical advice. Pharm Res 2004;21:191–200.

Truong-Le V. Formulation and intranasal delivery of FluMist live Influenza virus vaccine. IBC Bio-Production Conference; Munich, Germany; 2004.

Truong-Le V. Preservation of bioactive materials by freeze dried foam. US patent 7135180: MedImmune. 2006.

Truong-Le V, Scherer T. High pressure spray-dry of bioactive materials. USPTO Applicaton#: 20060002862: Medimmune Vaccines, Inc. 2005.

Vehring R. Pharmaceutical particle engineering *via* spray drying. Pharm Res 2007;24:411–437.

Vizcarra CL, Mayo SL. Electrostatics in computational protein design. Curr Opin Chem Biol 2005;9:622–626.

Waldman RH, Mann JJ, Small PA Jr. Immunization against influenza. Prevention of illness in man by aerosolized inactivated vaccine. JAMA 1969;207:520–524.

Webb SD, Cleland JL, Carpenter JF, Randolph TW. Effects of annealing lyophilized and spray-lyophilized formulations of recombinant human interferon-gamma. J Pharm Sci 2003;92:715–729.

Weers J, Tarara T, Clark A. Design of particles for pulmonary drug delivery. Expt Opin Drug Deliv 2007;4:297–313.

Wilding IR, Davis SS, O'Hagan DT. Targeting of drugs and vaccines to the gut. Pharmacol Ther 1994;97:124.

Wong Y-L, Sampson S, Germishuizen WA, Goonesekera S, Caponetti G, Sadoff J, Bloom BR, Edwards D. Drying a tuberculosis vaccine without freezing. Proc Natl Acad Sci U S A 2007;104:2591–2595.

Wunderlich M, Martin A, Schmid FX. Stabilization of the cold shock protein CspB from *Bacillus subtilis* by evolutionary optimization of coulombic interactions. J Mol Biol 2005a;347:1063–1076.

Wunderlich M, Martin A, Stabb CA, Schmid FX. Evolutionary protein stabilization in comparison with computational design. J Mol Biol 2005b;351:1160–1168.

Yagi S. Microwave and far infrared drying under reduced pressure. US patent 5859412. 1999.

Yu Z, Johnston K, Williams RO. Spray freezing into liquid versus spray-freeze-drying: influence of atomization on protein aggregation and biological activity. Eur J Pharm Sci 2006;27:9–18.

Zhang L, Gao L, Zhao L, Guo B, Ji K, Tian Y, Wang J, Yu H, Hu J, Kalvakolanu DV, Kopecko DJ, Zhao X, Xu D-Q. Intratumoral delivery and suppression of prostate tumor growth by attenuated *Salmonella enterica* serovar typhimurium carrying plasmid-basedSmall Interfering RNAs. Cancer Res 2007a;67:5859–5864.

Zhang Y, Wang KH, Guo YJ, Lu YM, Yan HL, Song YL, Wang F, Ding FX, Sun SH. Annexin B1 from *Taenia solium* metacestodes is a newly characterized member of the annexin family. Biol Chem 2007b;388:601–610.

11

PRODUCTION AND CHARACTERIZATION OF ALUMINUM-CONTAINING ADJUVANTS

Stanley L. Hem and Cliff T. Johnston
Purdue University, West Lafayette, IN, USA

Aluminum-containing adjuvants play an important role in many vaccines by potentiating the immune response to the antigen. Although first used in 1926 (Glenny et al., 1926), it is only in recent years that they have been extensively studied. These studies have transformed our thinking of them from being mysterious precipitates to well-characterized materials whose properties can be varied by the application of scientific principles. The immunological aspects of aluminum-containing adjuvants have been recently reviewed (Hem and HogenEsch, 2007a; Hem and HogenEsch, 2007b). This chapter focuses on the structure, properties, manufacture, and characterization of aluminum hydroxide adjuvant, aluminum phosphate adjuvant, and alum-precipitated adjuvant.

11.1 STRUCTURE

The names that have been associated with aluminum-containing adjuvants do not accurately describe their structure. For example, alum is the common name for aluminum potassium sulfate. It is a water-soluble compound that is used in many industries as a source of aluminum cation. The chemical formula of aluminum hydroxide

Vaccine Development and Manufacturing, First Edition.
Edited by Emily P. Wen, Ronald Ellis, and Narahari S. Pujar.

is $Al(OH)_3$, and several polymorphic forms are naturally occurring, such as gibbsite and bayerite that have low surface areas. Aluminum phosphate, $AlPO_4$, is used to form cement when mixed with calcium sulfate and sodium silicate.

The application of X-ray diffraction (XRD), Fourier transform infrared (FTIR), and nuclear magnetic resonance (NMR) spectroscopies has allowed the structure of aluminum-containing adjuvants to be understood. The first aluminum-containing adjuvant was prepared by adding base to a solution of alum and antigen (Glenny et al., 1926). Vaccines continue to be prepared using this method. This adjuvant will be referred to as *an alum-precipitated adjuvant*. Commercially prepared adjuvants are known as *aluminum hydroxide* and *aluminum phosphate adjuvants*. Monographs for these adjuvants have been published (Hem et al., 2006a; Hem et al., 2006b).

11.1.1 Aluminum Hydroxide Adjuvant

The XRD pattern of aluminum hydroxide adjuvant distinguishes it from the highly crystalline phases of gibbsite and bayerite (Shirodkar et al., 1990; Fig. 11.1). The XRD pattern of a particular crystalline phase is characterized by a unique set of d-spacings. The d-spacings at 6.46, 3.18, 2.35, 1.86, 1.44, and 1.31 Å identify aluminum hydroxide adjuvant as boehmite, with a structural formula of $AlOOH\text{-}nH_2O$, where n is approximately one. The chemical name for boehmite is aluminum oxyhydroxide. However, two different minerals, boehmite and diaspore, have the same chemical formula, and the term *aluminum oxyhydroxide* is not specific. The crystallite size of boehmite in aluminum hydroxide adjuvant is very small (Wang et al, 2003), and the XRD reflections are broad and distinct from highly crystalline boehmite.

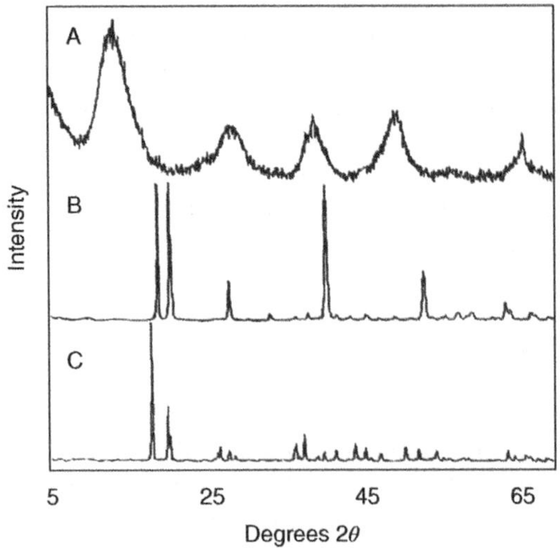

Figure 11.1 X-ray diffraction patterns of (a) aluminum hydroxide adjuvant; (b) bayerite; (c) gibbsite. From Yau et al., 2006. Reproduced with permission from J. Wiley & Sons, Inc., Journal of Pharmaceutical Sciences, 2006.

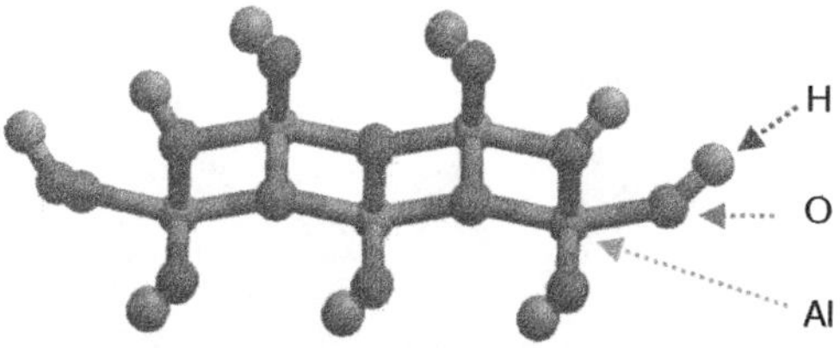

Figure 11.2 Structure of aluminum hydroxide adjuvant showing aluminum in octahedral coordination and surface hydroxyl groups coordinated with aluminum.

The correct term to describe the aluminum oxyhydroxide in aluminum hydroxide adjuvant is *poorly crystalline boehmite*. Poorly crystalline boehmite is used in other industries as an adsorbent and catalyst. The structure of poorly crystalline boehmite is shown in Figure 11.2.

The FTIR spectrum of aluminum hydroxide adjuvant also identifies it as poorly crystalline boehmite. Table 11.1 identifies the bands in the infrared spectrum of aluminum hydroxide adjuvant (Farmer, 1974). The bands at 1065 and 3098 cm^{-1} are associated with structural hydroxyl environments that are unique for poorly crystalline boehmite.

11.1.2 Aluminum Phosphate Adjuvant

Aluminum phosphate adjuvant is amorphous to X-rays, indicating very little long-range order in the structure. However, FTIR and NMR spectroscopies provide diagnostic information about its structure. The FTIR spectrum of aluminum phosphate adjuvant (Shirodkar et al., 1990) is characterized by absorption bands at 3700–2700, 1640, 1100, 640, and 540 cm^{-1}. The strong, broad asymmetric-shaped band in the 3700–2700 cm^{-1} region is assigned to OH-stretching and is due to both structural hydroxyl groups and adsorbed water. When a sample of aluminum phosphate adjuvant was heated to 200°C, the broad band in the 3700–2700 cm^{-1} region decreased, and a prominent band at 3164 cm^{-1} was apparent. This band is evidence of structural hydroxyls. The band at 640 cm^{-1} is associated with the

TABLE 11.1 Infrared Bands Associated With Aluminum Hydroxide Adjuvant (Farmer, 1974)

Band, cm^{-1}	Assignment
3400	Adsorbed water, structural OH
3098	Structural OH
1640	Adsorbed water
1065	Structural OH
765	Al–O stretching
737	Structural OH
623	Al–O stretching
485	Al–O stretching

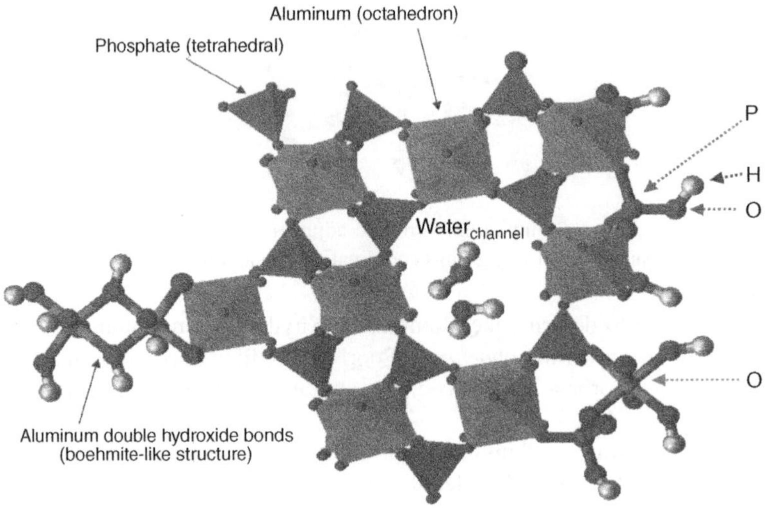

Figure 11.3 Proposed model of aluminum phosphate adjuvant showing aluminum in octahedral coordination, phosphorus in tetrahedral coordination, and surface hydroxyl groups coordinated with aluminum.

bending modes of structural hydroxyls, and that at 1100 cm^{-1} is characteristic of phosphate. The band at 540 cm^{-1} is a P–O-bending band. The band at 1640 cm^{-1} is the OH-bending band of adsorbed water. Although aluminum phosphate adjuvant is amorphous, a model is proposed on the basis of structural concepts found in crystalline aluminum phosphate structures (Fig. 11.3). These structural features are shown in Figure 11.3. The structure comprises aluminum in octahedral coordination, phosphorus in tetrahedral coordination, and surface hydroxyl groups coordinated with aluminum. The structure also shows the presence of channels filled with water molecules, a feature common to crystalline aluminum phosphate structures, such as Wavellite.

In addition to FTIR, NMR provides information about the local structure of aluminum phosphate adjuvant. Nuclear magnetic resonance spectroscopy provides information about the bonding and coordination of both Al and P. A ^{27}Al magic-angle-spinning nuclear magnetic resonance (^{27}Al MAS NMR) spectrum showed that the coordination of aluminum in aluminum phosphate adjuvant is mainly octahedral and is distinct from variscite, a crystalline form of $AlPO_4$ (Klein et al., 2000). Variscite exhibited a chemical shift of −9 ppm consistent with octahedral aluminum having a high number of nearest neighbor phosphorus atoms. In contrast, aluminum phosphate adjuvant exhibited two peaks at chemical shifts corresponding to octahedrally, 0 to −6 ppm, and tetrahedrally, 64–49 ppm, coordinated aluminum. However, the tetrahedral component was very weak, indicating that almost all of the aluminum in aluminum phosphate adjuvant is in octahedral coordination. The position of the Al signal is sensitive to the proximity of both Al and adjacent P atoms. In the case of variscite, each of the oxygen atoms is coordinated with P.

In aluminum phosphate adjuvant, the octahedral peak is shifted upfield as the atomic ratio of Al/P is decreased from that of variscite.

A ^{27}Al MAS NMR study also demonstrated that aluminum phosphate adjuvant is not simply amorphous aluminum hydroxide, $Al(OH)_3$, with phosphate adsorbed at surface sites (Klein et al., 2000). Phosphate solutions were added to a freshly precipitated amorphous aluminum hydroxide suspension. The atomic ratio of Al:P ranged from 6.5 to 0.77. The samples were aged for 24 h and examined using ^{27}Al MAS NMR. The chemical shifts of the octahedral peak were unchanged relative to the amorphous aluminum hydroxide. In contrast, precipitates formed in the presence of phosphate exhibited an upfield shift of the octahedral peak that was directly related to the phosphate content. These results indicate that phosphate is both incorporated into the bulk of aluminum phosphate adjuvant and adsorbed to the surface. The presence of phosphate is important, as it reduces the rate of development of order and interferes with crystallization during aging of the adjuvant. Substitution of phosphate for hydroxyl is believed to sterically inhibit the development of order because phosphate is larger than hydroxyl. Carbonate plays a similar role in stabilizing amorphous aluminum hydroxycarbonate, which is used as an antacid (Serna et al., 1983).

11.1.3 Alum-Precipitated Adjuvant

Alum-precipitated adjuvants are usually prepared by dissolving alum in water and adding a solution of the antigen. The antigen is frequently dissolved in a buffer solution such as phosphate-buffered saline because of solubility and stability factors. The addition of a base such as sodium hydroxide to the alum, antigen, and buffer solution produces an alum-precipitated adjuvant. The structure of the alum-precipitated adjuvant was studied when alum was precipitated in the presence of the following buffers: acetate, carbonate, citrate, and phosphate (Shirodkar et al., 1990). In each case, the precipitate was amorphous when examined using XRD. The infrared spectrum exhibited absorption bands associated with structural hydroxyl, sulfate, and the buffer ion. Thus, alum-precipitated adjuvants are amorphous aluminum hydroxy (buffer ion) sulfate. The structure of alum-precipitated adjuvants is sensitive to the concentrations of aluminum, sulfate, and the buffer ion. Thus, precipitation conditions must be carefully controlled in order to produce alum-precipitated adjuvants having consistent structures.

The location of the antigen in vaccines prepared by *in situ* precipitation of a solution of alum, antigen, and buffer is of interest. The antigen may be adsorbed on the surface of the alum-precipitated adjuvant that was produced by *in situ* precipitation, or the antigen may be occluded within the alum-precipitated adjuvant. A study attempted to answer this question by comparing the elution of lysozyme from a vaccine made by adsorbing lysozyme to a preformed aluminum phosphate adjuvant or a vaccine prepared by *in situ* precipitation (Hem et al., 1996). Sodium dodecyl sulfate completely eluted all of the lysozyme, regardless of the method of preparation of the vaccine. Thus, it was concluded that the antigen was in contact with the liquid phase in both vaccines and that *in situ* precipitation involves two separate processes: the precipitation of amorphous aluminum hydroxy(buffer ion) sulfate and the adsorption of the antigen by the adjuvant.

In summary, aluminum hydroxide adjuvant is chemically aluminum oxyhydroxide, $AlOOH\text{-}nH_2O$. It is a crystalline, stoichiometric compound. Aluminum phosphate adjuvant is amorphous aluminum hydroxyphosphate. It is not a stoichiometric compound, and its composition depends on the precipitation recipe and conditions. The atomic ratio of Al:P is 1.10–1.15:1.0 for commercial aluminum phosphate adjuvant (Hem et al., 2006b). Alum-precipitated adjuvants are amorphous aluminum hydroxy (buffer ion) sulfate. They are similar to aluminum phosphate adjuvant, especially when a phosphate buffer is used.

11.2 PROPERTIES

The properties of aluminum hydroxide and aluminum phosphate adjuvants are different. Many of the properties of each adjuvant can be related to their structures as presented previously.

11.2.1 Surface Groups

Each surface aluminum is coordinated with a hydroxyl in aluminum hydroxide adjuvant (Fig. 11.2). Hydroxyls that are coordinated with a metal ion, such as aluminum, have special properties and are termed *metallic hydroxyls* (Stumm, 1992). As shown in Equation 11.1, metallic hydroxyls have a pH-dependent surface charge. They may accept a proton and exhibit a positive surface charge or donate a proton and exhibit a negative surface charge.

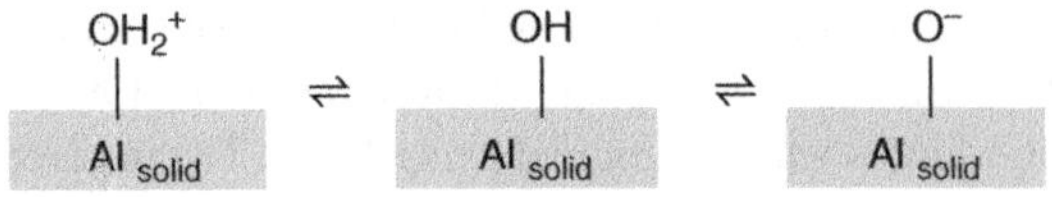

(11.1)

The surface groups in aluminum phosphate adjuvant include phosphates and hydroxyls that are coordinated with surface aluminums (Fig. 11.3). The metallic hydroxyls in aluminum phosphate adjuvant also produce a pH-dependent surface charge.

Understanding the surface groups in both adjuvants gives insight into the potential mechanisms by which antigens may be adsorbed. Electrostatic adsorption may occur with both adjuvants, as both have a pH-dependent surface charge (Seeber et al., 1991). Ligand exchange adsorption of phosphorylated antigens may occur with either adjuvant, as both have surface hydroxyl groups (Shi et al., 2002). The potential for adsorption by ligand exchange is greater for aluminum hydroxide adjuvant, as all of the surface aluminums are coordinated with a hydroxyl that may undergo ligand exchange. However, there are fewer surface hydroxyls in aluminum phosphate adjuvant and, thus, less potential for adsorption by ligand exchange. The potential for ligand exchange adsorption by aluminum phosphate adjuvant is inversely related to the degree of substitution of phosphate for hydroxyl in the adjuvant.

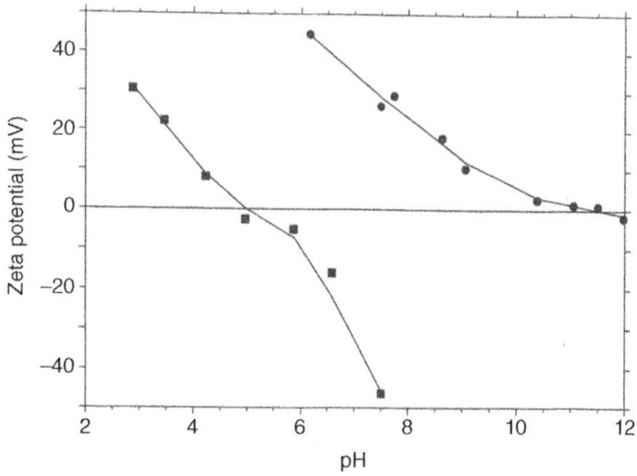

Figure 11.4 Isoelectric point of aluminum hydroxide adjuvant (•) and aluminum phosphate adjuvant (■). From Rinella et al., 1998. Reproduced with permission from Elsevier, Journal of Colloid and Interface Science, 1998.

11.2.2 Isoelectric Point

The pH at which the net surface charge is zero is termed *the point of zero charge* by colloid chemists and *the isoelectric point* (iep) by protein chemists. The terms are equivalent, and iep is used in this chapter. The iep of aluminum hydroxide adjuvant is 11.4 (Fig. 11.4). This is the same value as that reported for poorly crystalline boehmite. The iep of aluminum hydroxide adjuvant may be reduced to approximately 4 by pretreatment with phosphate (Iyer et al., 2003). Thus, aluminum hydroxide adjuvant is positively charged at pH 7.4, but pretreatment with phosphate may reverse the surface charge. Ligand exchange with other anions such as carbonate or sulfate will also reduce the iep of aluminum hydroxide adjuvant.

The iep of aluminum hydroxide, $Al(OH)_3$, is 9.6 (Parks, 1965). Substitution of phosphate for hydroxyl can lower the iep to 4.0 (Jiang et al., 2003). Thus, the iep of aluminum phosphate adjuvant may range from 9.6 to 4.0 depending on the degree of phosphate substitution for hydroxyl. However, commercial aluminum phosphate adjuvants have an iep of approximately 5 and are negatively charged at pH 7.4 (Hem et al., 2006b). Ligand exchange with other anions such as carbonate or sulfate will also reduce the iep of aluminum phosphate adjuvant.

11.2.3 Microenvironment pH

The Guoy-Chapman Double Layer theory of colloid chemistry teaches that charged particles in an aqueous media are surrounded by a region of water that is rich in counterions, that is, ions of the opposite charge as the particle. The double layer surrounding a negatively charged particle will be rich in cations, including protons; similarly, that surrounding a positively charged particle will be rich in anions, including hydroxyls. Thus, an antigen adsorbed to a negatively charged adjuvant will be exposed to a higher concentration of protons at the solid–water interface than in the bulk. An antigen adsorbed to a positively charged adjuvant will be exposed to a more basic than the bulk. The difference between the microenvironment and the bulk pH may be as much as two pH units (Wittayanukulluk et al., 2004). This property is important because adsorbed antigens will undergo pH-dependent reactions such as deamidation, hydrolysis, or oxidation at a rate associated with the pH encountered at the surface rather than the bulk pH.

11.2.4 Morphology

Aluminum-containing adjuvants are composed of primary particles having dimensions on the order of nanometers (Shirodkar et al., 1990). The primary particles form aggregates that are the functioning units in the adjuvants. The primary particles of aluminum hydroxide adjuvant (Fig. 11.5A) are fibers having average dimensions of $4.5 \times 2.2 \times 10$ nm (Wang et al., 2003). They form irregular aggregates having diameters of approximately 1–20 μm. This unusual morphology explains why a crystalline solid can have a very high protein adsorptive capacity.

The primary particles of aluminum phosphate adjuvant are platy having a diameter of approximately 50 nm (Fig. 11.5B). They form irregular aggregates ranging from 1 to 20 μm.

The aggregates of aluminum hydroxide and aluminum phosphate adjuvants are formed by weak interparticle forces. The aggregates readily deaggregate and reaggregate on mixing (Morefield et al., 2004). This property leads to uniform distribution of small doses of antigen during the manufacture of vaccines.

11.2.5 Rheology

The rheology of aluminum-containing adjuvants is related to their morphology. The fibrous primary particles of aluminum hydroxide adjuvant produce thixotropic properties. Undiluted commercial aluminum hydroxide adjuvant containing 2% equivalent Al_2O_3 forms a semisolid when undisturbed but is fluid when shaken. Sedimentation is not observed in the undiluted adjuvant owing to gel formation. The thixotropic properties are reduced as the adjuvant is diluted. The platy primary particles of aluminum phosphate adjuvant exhibit sedimentation without thixotropy on standing.

11.2.6 Surface Area

The surface area of aluminum hydroxide adjuvant is approximately 500 m^2/g (Wang et al., 2003). A surface area this high is unusual for a crystalline solid and approaches the 600–800 m^2/g values reported for expandable clay minerals. The techniques used to measure the surface area of aluminum hydroxide adjuvant cannot be applied to aluminum phosphate adjuvant. However, the small primary particles seen in Figure 11.5B suggest a very high surface area.

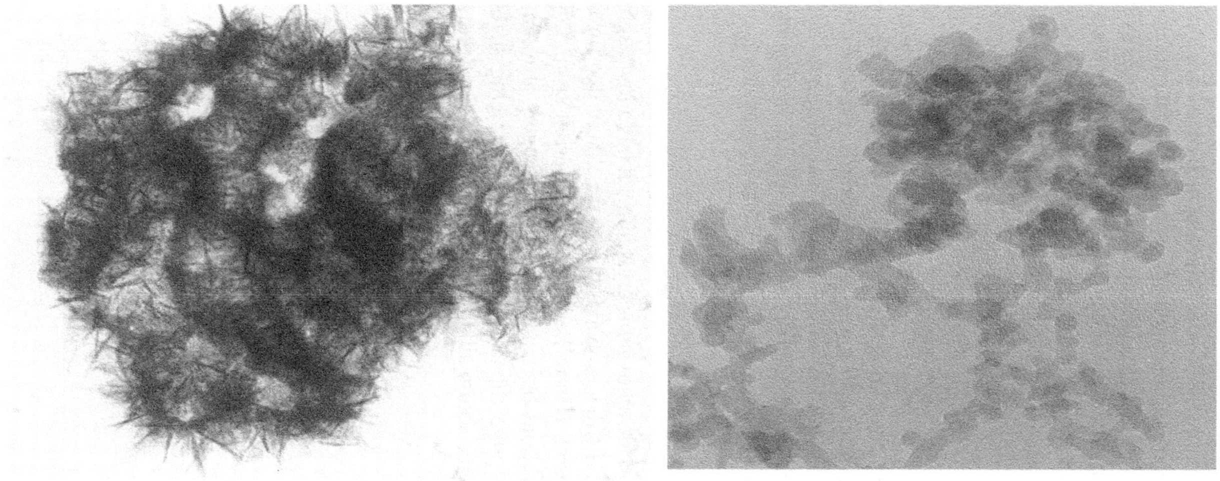

(a) (b)

Figure 11.5 Transmission electron photomicrograph of aluminum hydroxide adjuvant (a) and aluminum phosphate adjuvant (b) at a magnification of 100,000×. From Romero Mendez et al., 2007. Reproduced with permission from Elsevier, Vaccine, 2007.

11.2.7 Detoxification of Endotoxin

Aluminum hydroxide adjuvant has the desirable property of detoxifying endotoxin (Shi et al., 2001). The lipid A portion of endotoxin contains two phosphate groups that adsorb strongly to aluminum hydroxide adjuvant by ligand exchange. The limited number of surface hydroxyls in aluminum phosphate adjuvant reduces the potential for ligand exchange. A 15-μg/kg subcutaneous dose of endotoxin solution or endotoxin mixed with aluminum phosphate adjuvant in Sprague-Dawley rats produced tumor necrosis factor-alpha and interleukin-6. No tumor necrosis factor-alpha or interleukin-6 was detected in rats that received the same dose of endotoxin mixed with aluminum hydroxide adjuvant.

11.2.8 Solubility

The solubility of aluminum-containing adjuvants is pH dependent. The pH-solubility profile of the two adjuvants after a 45-min exposure period is presented in Figure 11.6. Comparison of the two pH-solubility profiles reveals that aluminum hydroxide adjuvant is less soluble than aluminum phosphate adjuvant. This behavior is consistent with the crystalline and amorphous structures of the two adjuvants.

11.2.9 Stability

Although aluminum hydroxide adjuvant is crystalline, it has a low degree of order as demonstrated by its broad diffraction bands. Thus, it is likely that further order will develop during aging. Burrell (Burrell et al., 2001a; Burrell et al., 2001b) demonstrated that the XRD reflections become sharper during aging at room temperature. The pH and protein adsorptive capacity decreased during aging at room temperature. For example, the bovine serum albumin adsorptive capacity decreased from 2.9

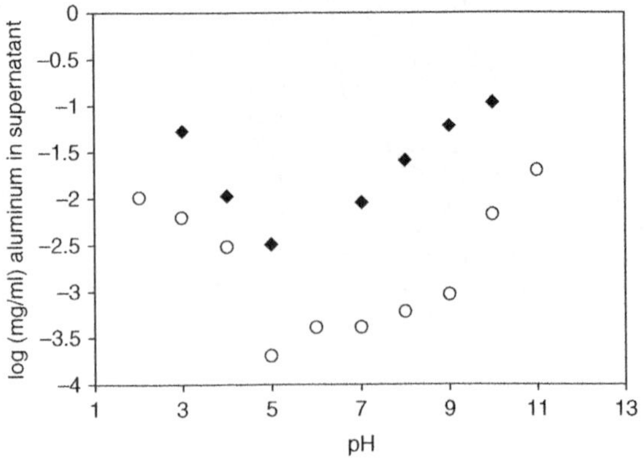

Figure 11.6 Effect of pH on the solubility of aluminum hydroxide adjuvant (◆) and aluminum phosphate adjuvant (O) after a 45-min exposure period. From Rinella et al., 1998. Reproduced with permission from Elsevier, Journal of Colloid and Interface Science, 1998.

to 2.6 mg/mg Al during a 15-month period. These changes are consistent with the development of order.

The amorphous nature of aluminum phosphate adjuvant makes it likely to develop order during aging. This expectation was confirmed by a 15-month stability study at room temperature (Burrell et al., 2001a; Burrell et al., 2001b). The pH and protein adsorptive capacity decreased during aging, indicating the development of order. The adjuvant remained amorphous to X-rays. However, the lysozyme adsorptive capacity decreased from 0.80 to 0.54 mg/mg Al during the aging period.

Because both aluminum hydroxide and aluminum phosphate adjuvants develop order during aging, it is advisable to store each at 4°C and use the adjuvant as soon after manufacture as possible.

Order also develops when the adjuvants are exposed to heat and pressure during autoclaving (Burrell et al., 1999). Autoclaving aluminum hydroxide adjuvant at 121°C and 15.4 psi for 30 min caused the XRD reflections to become sharper. The pH, viscosity, and bovine serum albumin adsorptive capacity also decreased. The decrease in adsorptive capacity was not large enough to be statistically significant. However, a decrease in protein adsorptive capacity indicates a lower surface area and is consistent with the decrease in pH and sharper XRD pattern. The viscosity of suspensions is inversely related to particle size. Thus, the decrease in surface area also affected the viscosity.

Aluminum phosphate adjuvant exhibited a decrease in pH, lysozyme adsorptive capacity, iep, and the rate of acid neutralization at pH 2.5 when autoclaved at 121°C and 15.4 psi. The lysozyme adsorptive capacity deceased from 1.6 to 1.3 mg/mg Al during 60 min of autoclaving. The iep decreased because of the reduced surface area of the adjuvant after autoclaving. The elevated temperature of autoclaving caused desorption of some phosphate ions. The decreased concentration of phosphate at the surface accelerated the development of order and a lower surface area. When the aluminum phosphate adjuvant returned to room temperature, the desorbed phosphate was readsorbed. Because the surface area was lower, the concentration of phosphate at the surface was greater and resulted in a lower iep. The rate of acid neutralization at pH 2.5 is also related to the surface area of the adjuvant. The decreased rate of acid neutralization is further evidence that the surface area decreased as a result of autoclaving.

The study by Burrell (Burrell et al., 1999) indicates that both aluminum hydroxide and aluminum phosphate adjuvants develop order during autoclaving that results in a decreased surface area. Autoclaving procedures that minimize exposure time to elevated temperatures, such as rotating the container to produce more uniform heating, can be used to minimize the effect of autoclaving (Block, 1991). Procedures requiring repeated autoclaving should be avoided.

11.3 PRODUCTION

The first aluminum-containing adjuvants were prepared by *in situ* precipitation of the adjuvant, and vaccines continue to be produced using *in situ* precipitation.

However, preformed aluminum hydroxide or aluminum phosphate adjuvants are frequently used today. The preformed adjuvants offer the advantage of being able to be characterized and standardized before the antigen is added. Erik Lindblad (Lindblad, 2004) has provided an excellent history of the key steps in the evolution of preformed aluminum-containing adjuvants. This section discusses the manufacture of aluminum hydroxide and aluminum phosphate adjuvants. Many of the factors affecting the manufacture of aluminum phosphate adjuvant can be applied to *in situ* precipitation.

11.3.1 Aluminum Hydroxide Adjuvant

The current understanding that aluminum oxyhydroxide is formed by the dehydration of amorphous aluminum hydroxide, $Al(OH)_3$, as shown in Equation 11.2, can be traced to the studies of the mineralogists Pa Ho Hsu (Hsu, 1967) and Tettenhorst and Hofmann (Tettenhorst and Hofmann, 1980). The dehydration is facilitated by the presence of salts such as sodium chloride and/or heat.

$$Al(OH)_3 \text{ amorphous} \rightarrow AlOOH + H_2O \qquad (11.2)$$

Hsu found that bayerite, a crystalline form of $Al(OH)_3$, was produced when 0.1 M NaOH containing up to 0.6 M NaCl was added to 0.2 M $AlCl_3$. A mixture of bayerite and aluminum oxyhydroxide was produced when the sodium chloride concentration was between 0.6 and 2.0 M. Pure aluminum oxyhydroxide was formed when the sodium chloride concentration was greater than 2.0 M. Tettenhorst and Hofmann followed Hsu's method and used 4 M NaCl. However, they exposed the precipitate to heat treatments up to 300°C. Hydrothermal pressure vessels were used for temperatures above 80°C. Higher temperatures and increased heating times produced sharper XRD bands, indicating more highly ordered aluminum oxyhydroxide.

It is important to completely dehydrate the amorphous aluminum hydroxide in order to produce stable aluminum hydroxide adjuvant. Dandashli (Dandashli et al., 2002) exposed amorphous aluminum hydroxide to six thermal treatments ranging from 40°C for 18 h to 105°C for 17 h. All of the samples initially exhibited the XRD bands associated with poorly crystalline boehmite. During aging at room temperature, the samples that were prepared by exposure to lower temperatures or shorter treatment times exhibited a decrease in bovine serum albumin adsorptive capacity. The samples heated at 40°C for 18 h or 80°C for 4 h developed additional XRD bands after aging at room temperature for 6 or 12 months, respectively, which indicated the formation of gibbsite, a crystalline aluminum hydroxide polymorph. Analysis of the initial precipitate by differential centrifugal sedimentation indicated the presence of poorly crystalline boehmite and amorphous aluminum hydroxide in all the samples. The percentage of amorphous aluminum hydroxide was inversely related to the thermal treatment conditions. A sample of amorphous aluminum hydroxide heated at 120°C for 24 h contained only poorly crystalline boehmite. Thus, stable aluminum hydroxide adjuvant can be produced only if all of the amorphous aluminum hydroxide are converted to aluminum oxyhydroxide during production.

Yau (Yau et al., 2006) recently studied the production of aluminum hydroxide adjuvant under conditions of constant reactant concentration. Their study confirmed that high sodium chloride concentration and high temperature facilitated the formation of aluminum oxyhydroxide. They found that either 3 M NaCl or hydrothermal treatment at 110°C for 4 h was required to stabilize the aluminum hydroxide adjuvant.

11.3.2 Aluminum Phosphate Adjuvant

Amorphous aluminum hydroxyphosphate is produced by the precipitation of aluminum cation by base in the presence of phosphate anion. The source of aluminum cation is usually aluminum chloride or alum. The base is frequently sodium hydroxide. For example, five amorphous aluminum hydroxyphosphates were precipitated by dissolving alum, sodium dihydrogen phosphate, disodium hydrogen phosphate, and sodium chloride in water (Jiang et al., 2003). Enough 1 M NaOH was added to bring the pH to 7.1. The precipitate was washed to remove sodium, potassium, and sulfate ions. The concentration of phosphate was different for each precipitation. The P/Al molar ratio of the solid phase of the five adjuvants was directly related to the concentration of phosphate in the precipitation recipe. Thus, aluminum phosphate adjuvant containing any desired degree of phosphate substitution for hydroxyl can be obtained by selecting the appropriate concentration of phosphate for the precipitation recipe. This method of precipitation will be referred to as *the batch method*.

The concentrations of aluminum, hydroxyl, and phosphate ions in solution vary during the course of the batch precipitation of aluminum hydroxyphosphate. Initially, all of the aluminum and phosphate ions are in solution, but the hydroxyl ion concentration is low because the initial pH is approximately 2.5. As the precipitation proceeds with the addition of sodium hydroxide, the concentrations of aluminum and phosphate in solution decrease as solid phase forms and the hydroxyl ion concentration increases. Klein (Klein et al., 2000) studied the batch precipitation method in detail by adding the base in increments and determining the aluminum and phosphate concentrations of the supernatant and solid. Figure 11.7 shows the pH and cumulative percentages of aluminum and phosphate precipitated after each increment of sodium hydroxide was added. The pH increased steadily throughout the precipitation until the buffering capacity was exhausted. The rate of aluminum precipitation was relatively constant for the first 80% of the reaction. However, all of the phosphate had been precipitated when the reaction was approximately 50% complete. The solid phase that formed after all the phosphate was precipitated was composed of only aluminum and hydroxyl. Thus, the composition of the precipitate varied during the precipitation. This is seen more dramatically in Figure 11.8 where the ratio of phosphate to aluminum in the solid phase and in solution at different points in the precipitation is presented. The molar ratio of phosphate to aluminum in the solid phase during the first 40% of the precipitation was approximately 0.8. However, once the phosphate in solution was exhausted, no additional phosphate entered the solid phase, and the phosphate to aluminum molar ratio decreased to approximately 0.3, the theoretical ratio. It appears that the batch precipitation technique for aluminum

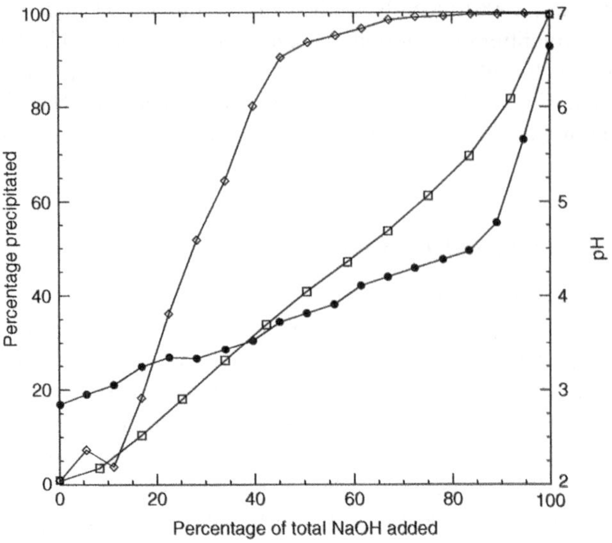

Figure 11.7 Suspension pH and extent of aluminum and phosphate precipitation during the incremental precipitation of aluminum phosphate adjuvant. Key: •, pH; ◇, percentage of total phosphate precipitated; □, percentage of total aluminum precipitated. From Klein et al., 2000. Reproduced with permission from J. Wiley & Sons, Inc., Journal of Pharmaceutical Sciences, 2000.

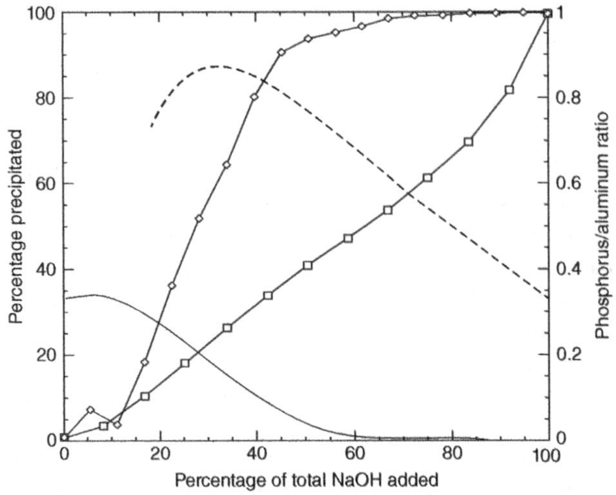

Figure 11.8 Ratio of phosphate to aluminum in the solid phase and in solution during precipitation of aluminum phosphate adjuvant. Key: dashed line, ratio of phosphate to aluminum in the solid phase; solid line, ratio of phosphate to aluminum in solution; ◇, percentage of total phosphate precipitated; □, percentage of total aluminum precipitated. From Klein et al., 2000. Reproduced with permission from J. Wiley & Sons, Inc., Journal of Pharmaceutical Sciences, 2000.

phosphate adjuvant produces a solid phase that is composed of a mixture of aluminum hydroxyphosphates of various phosphate to aluminum ratios, as well as some aluminum hydroxide, $Al(OH)_3$. Such a complicated precipitation reaction requires careful control of all factors in order to produce a consistent aluminum phosphate adjuvant.

A precipitation procedure for aluminum phosphate adjuvant has been proposed, which maintains constant concentrations of the three reactants (Burrell et al., 2001a; Burrell et al., 2001b). An aqueous solution composed of aluminum chloride and sodium dihydrogen phosphate was pumped into a reaction vessel at a constant rate. A second pump infused a sodium hydroxide solution at the rate required to maintain the desired pH. Precipitations were performed between pH 3.0 and 7.5 at intervals of 0.5 pH units. The precipitates were analyzed for composition and properties. A continuum of amorphous aluminum hydroxyphosphates were produced having composition and properties that changed with the precipitation pH. The phosphate content decreased as the pH of precipitation increased, reflecting the increased hydroxyl ion concentration. At higher pH values, the higher concentration of hydroxyl ions competed more effectively with phosphate for coordination sites on aluminum and relatively more Al–OH bonds formed than $Al-PO_4$ bonds. The opposite was true when the pH of precipitation was low.

A characteristic of aluminum phosphate adjuvants precipitated by the batch method is a downward drift in pH during aging (Burrell et al., 2001b). This is due to the production of a range of aluminum hydroxyphosphates and equilibration of the concentration of phosphate at the surface of the particles. In contrast, all of the adjuvants that were precipitated under constant reactant conditions maintained the pH at which they were precipitated for a 3-month aging period at room temperature. This behavior confirms that precipitation under constant reactant conditions produces one aluminum hydroxyphosphate with a specific phosphate to aluminum molar ratio.

11.4 CHARACTERIZATION

The ability to produce vaccines with consistent physical and immunological properties depends in part on the availability of an adjuvant with consistent properties. It is fortunate that at least 12 tests have been described that may be used to characterize aluminum-containing adjuvants. Table 11.2 lists these tests and indicates if they may be applied to aluminum hydroxide or aluminum phosphate adjuvant. The tests that are applicable to aluminum phosphate adjuvant may also be applied to alum-precipitated adjuvants. These tests should provide the basis for specifications that will ensure consistent performance of each batch of aluminum-containing adjuvant.

A useful framework to understand the various means of adjuvant characterization is to consider the scale of information associated with each technique. Each experimental method has a time and a length scale associated with it. An overview of the principal techniques used to characterize aluminum-containing adjuvants is shown in Figure 11.9, and the approximate length scales are listed in Table 11.3. In broad terms, the spectroscopic methods provide atomic and molecular scale information about the

TABLE 11.2 Tests That May Be Used to Characterize Aluminum-Containing Adjuvants

Test	Aluminum Hydroxide Adjuvant	Aluminum Phosphate Adjuvant
Adsorption isotherm	X	X
Chemical composition	X	X
Electron microscopy	X	X
FTIR	X	X
Isoelectric point	X	X
Particle size	X	X
pH	X	X
Phosphilicity	X	X
Rate of acid neutralization		X
Surface area	X	
Thermal analysis	X	X
XRD	X	

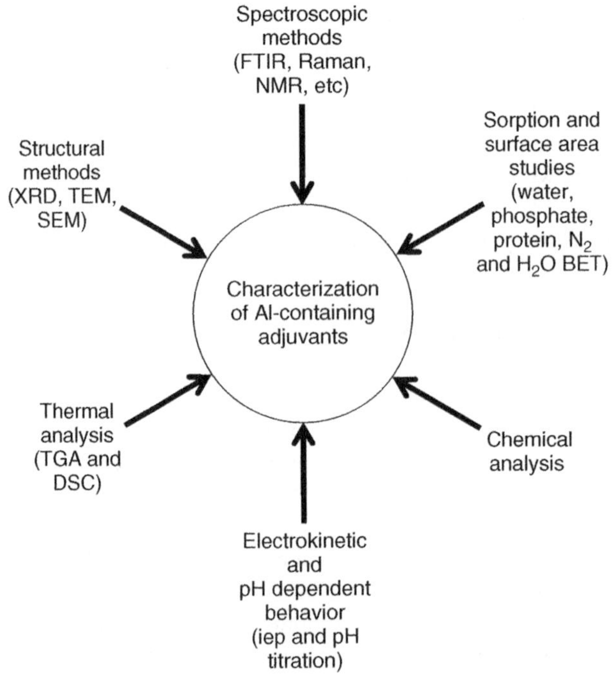

Figure 11.9 Techniques used to characterize aluminum-containing adjuvants.

TABLE 11.3 Scale of Information Associated With Characterization Techniques

Scale	Type of Information
Atomic scale, 0.1–10 nm	^{27}Al and ^{31}P NMR studies of Al and P coordination
Molecular scale, 0.1–10 nm	Fourier transform infared and Raman studies of Al–O, P–O, and O–H bonds
Primary particle scale, 1–100 nm	Powder XRD of crystalline structure and short range order
Aggregate particle scale, 1–100 μm	Transmission and scanning electron microscopy of Al-containing adjuvants
Bulk chemical analysis	Stoichiometry of overall chemical composition
Particle behavior 1: sorption	Surface area measurement using gravimetric/FTIR method, phosphate and protein sorption
Particle behavior 2: acid–base	Surface charge characterization and electrophoretic mobility, acid–base titration

coordination of aluminum and the nature of chemical bonds present with a scale from Angstroms (10^{-10} m) to a few nanometers (10^{-9} m). Powder XRD provides information about the crystalline structure of these adjuvants. Electron microscopy reveals what these particles look like on a scale of 0.01–10 μm. Chemical analysis of the adjuvants is a bulk property of the overall chemical composition. Finally, the behavior of these particles may be examined using two different types of experimental methods. The first examines how water molecules are sorbed on the surface of the adjuvant using a gravimetric/FTIR method that determines the surface area. Phosphate and protein sorption also provide valuable information about the surface chemistry of the adjuvants in suspension. Finally, electrophoretic mobility and pH-titration methods provide information about the surface of the adjuvants at different pH values.

11.4.1 Composition

The chemical composition of aluminum hydroxide adjuvant is that of poorly crystalline boehmite, $AlOOH\text{-}nH_2O$. Approximately one water molecule per AlOOH formula unit is intercalated between layers of AlOOH. The aluminum content is usually determined after dissolution of the adjuvant and is frequently expressed as the concentration of equivalent Al_2O_3. The amount of water is determined using the thermogravimetric analysis (TGA).

Anions such as phosphate, carbonate, sulfate, or borate can undergo ligand exchange with the surface hydroxyls of aluminum hydroxide adjuvant. The substitution of sulfate for some surface hydroxyls is likely to occur if alum, $AlK(SO_4)_2$, is used as the source of aluminum cations in the production of aluminum hydroxide adjuvant. The main effect of the substitution of sulfate or other anions for surface hydroxyls is to lower the iep of the adjuvant. The magnitude of the effect is directly related to the degree of substitution and the valence of the substituting anion.

Defining the composition of aluminum phosphate adjuvant is important, as aluminum hydroxyphosphate is not a stoichiometric compound. The composition of a sample of aluminum phosphate adjuvant is established by dissolving the adjuvant and determining the aluminum and phosphorus concentrations. The combined hydroxyl-water content is determined using TGA.

11.4.2 Powder X-Ray Diffraction

X-ray diffraction is useful for characterizing aluminum hydroxide adjuvant because of its crystalline structure but is not useful for amorphous aluminum phosphate adjuvant. An adjuvant can be identified as poorly crystalline boehmite by the position of the reflections at 6.46, 3.18, 2.35, 1.86, 1.44, and 1.31 Å. The degree of order in the adjuvant can be assessed by measuring the width at half height of the major reflection (020 band at 6.46 Å). This parameter is termed *the full-width-at-half-maximum* (FWHM), and the units are °2θ. Broad diffraction bands indicate a low degree of order. The diffraction bands become sharper as the number of repeating units increase, which reinforces the X-ray reflections. The diffraction bands are typically characterized by their position and FWHM. The sharpness of a given X-ray reflection can be related to the degree of order through the Debye-Scherer equation (Wang et al., 2003). In the case of aluminum hydroxide adjuvant, the XRD reflections are broad, indicating that the primary particles are very small and that the material is poorly crystalline. A direct linear relationship has been found between the albumin adsorptive capacity and the FWHM for five aluminum hydroxide adjuvants (Masood et al., 1994).

11.4.3 Fourier Transform Infrared Spectroscopy

The FTIR spectrum can be used to identify aluminum hydroxide and aluminum phosphate adjuvants as described previously in the Structure section. Insight can be gained into the relative proportion of accessible hydroxyl groups by exposing the sample to deuterium oxide (D_2O) vapor and examining changes in the FTIR spectrum. Deuterium is heavier than hydrogen. Therefore, when any accessible hydroxyls exchange with deuterium, the infrared band positions will shift from the 3700–2700 cm^{-1} region for OH-stretching to the 2700–2200 cm^{-1} region for OD-stretching. The ratio of the area under the OD-stretching region to the total area of the OH- and OD-stretching regions is a measure of the proportion of hydroxyl groups that is accessible to D_2O vapor. A sample of aluminum hydroxide adjuvant exhibited hydroxyl-stretching bands at 3663, 3564, 3445, 3300, and 3098 cm^{-1}. After the sample was exposed to D_2O vapor, these bands shifted to 2702, 2621, 2552, 2466, and 2330 cm^{-1}. Using the areas under the OH- and OD-stretching regions, it was calculated that approximately 75% of the total hydroxyls in this sample of aluminum hydroxide adjuvant was accessible to D_2O. The fraction of accessible hydroxyls can be used to compare different samples of aluminum hydroxide adjuvant, as well as to detect the development of order during aging, as the hydroxyl groups will become less accessible as the adjuvant becomes more highly ordered.

Selective deuteration FTIR measurements can also be used to characterize the accessible hydroxyl groups in aluminum phosphate adjuvant (Burrell et al., 2001a).

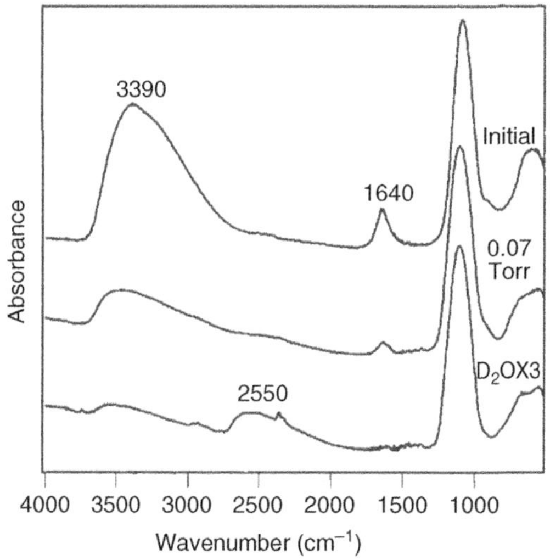

Figure 11.10 FTIR spectrum of aluminum phosphate adjuvant before and after exposure to deuterium oxide vapor. Key: top, initial; middle, after vacuum; bottom, after exposure to deuterium oxide vapor. From Burrell et al., 2001a. Reproduced with permission from Elsevier, Vaccine, 2000.

Figure 11.10 shows that the OH-stretching region from 3700 to 2700 cm^{-1} and the H-O-H bending region from 1660 to 1600 cm^{-1} were greatly reduced when the sample was examined under vacuum. This indicates that the sample contained a large proportion of adsorbed water. The OH-stretching region further decreased on exposure to deuterium oxide vapor, and bands appeared in the OD-stretching region. Figure 11.10 indicates that most the hydroxyl groups in the sample were accessible to D_2O vapor.

11.4.4 Thermal Analysis

Thermogravimetric analysis of aluminum-containing adjuvants provides information about the overall water and hydroxyl content of the sample. In this method, a known amount of sample is placed in a sensitive balance and heated at a constant rate from ambient temperature to a specified temperature of generally between 1000 and 1100°C. The extent of mass loss and the temperature range over which this loss of mass occurs provide useful information about the sample. The mass loss during TGA of aluminum hydroxide and aluminum phosphate adjuvants is shown in Figure 11.11. In the case of the aluminum hydroxide adjuvant, the mass loss occurs in three regions. The first is from ambient temperature to approximately 200°C and represents the loss of water. In the second region, 200–560°C, structural hydroxyls are lost. This sample contained approximately 18% water and 14% structural hydroxyls. A small mass loss occurs from 560 to 1000°C that may reflect some type of phase change. For aluminum phosphate adjuvant, a single mass loss occurs between ambient and approximately 300°C that is due to the loss of water. This sample contained approximately 25% water.

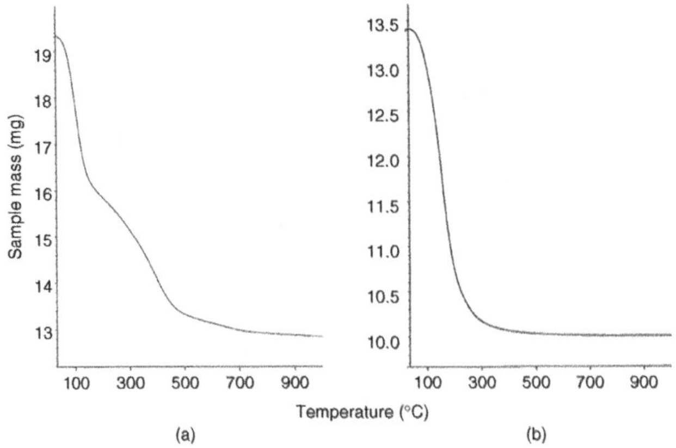

Figure 11.11 Thermogravimetric analysis of aluminum hydroxide adjuvant (a) and aluminum phosphate adjuvant (b).

11.4.5 Transmission Electron Microscopy and Energy Dispersive Spectroscopy

Transmission electron microscopy can provide valuable information about the production of aluminum hydroxide adjuvant. One method of preparing aluminum hydroxide adjuvant is to dehydrate amorphous aluminum hydroxide, $Al(OH)_3$, by heat treatment. Amorphous aluminum hydroxide has a platy morphology. Yau (Yau et al., 2006) showed that when amorphous aluminum hydroxide was exposed to hydrothermal treatment at 110°C for 16 h, the platy morphology changed to the fibrous morphology that is characteristic of aluminum hydroxide adjuvant. The XRD pattern confirmed that $Al(OH)_3$ had dehydrated to form AlOOH.

Transmission electron microscopy was also able to give direct evidence for the physical basis for the unusually low protein adsorptive capacity of a batch of aluminum hydroxide adjuvant (Yau et al., 2006). The batch exhibited the fibrous primary particles associated with aluminum hydroxide adjuvant, but the fibers were larger in each dimension than usually seen in aluminum hydroxide adjuvant.

The energy dispersive spectrum (EDS) can usually be obtained at the same time that a sample is examined using transmission electron microscopy. The EDS displays peaks that correspond to elements that are heavier than oxygen. A pure sample of aluminum hydroxide adjuvant will show only the presence of aluminum, whereas aluminum phosphate adjuvant will exhibit peaks corresponding to aluminum and phosphorus.

11.4.6 pH

The pH is useful because hydroxyaluminum compounds develop order by the sequential deprotonation and dehydration reactions shown in the following section

(Hem and White, 1984).

$$Al(OH_2)_6^{+3} \rightarrow Al(OH)(OH_2)_5^{+2} + H^+ \quad (11.3)$$

$$2Al(OH)(OH_2)_5^{+2} \rightarrow Al_2(OH)_2(OH_2)_8^{+4} + 2H_2O \quad (11.4)$$

This sequence of reactions joins two aluminum atoms by a double hydroxide bridge and releases two protons. Thus, the development of order in either aluminum hydroxide adjuvant or aluminum phosphate adjuvant is associated with a decrease in pH. Burrell (Burrell et al., 2000) demonstrated that the pH, FWHM, and bovine serum albumin adsorptive capacity of aluminum hydroxide adjuvant decreased during aging at room temperature. Likewise, the pH and lysozyme adsorptive capacity of aluminum phosphate adjuvant decreased during aging at room temperature. All these changes are associated with an increase in order.

11.4.7 Surface Area

The morphology of the aluminum-containing adjuvants makes surface area measurement using any method that requires removal of all water from the sample invalid. This includes the standard nitrogen BET (Brunauer–Emmett–Teller) method. Complete removal of water irreversibly agglomerates the primary particles and aggregates, resulting in an erroneously low value for surface area. Fortunately, there are two methods for determining surface area that can be applied to aluminum hydroxide adjuvant. Unfortunately, neither of these methods may be used to determine the surface area of aluminum phosphate adjuvant.

Mathematical analysis of the XRD pattern can yield the dimensions of the smallest repeating unit or primary crystallite. The FWHM of the (020), (200), and (002) XRD bands (Fig. 11.12) is related to the size of the primary crystallite according to the Scherrer equation (Wang et al., 2003). The calculated mean crystallite dimensions of the fibrous aluminum hydroxide adjuvant primary particle are $4.5 \times 2.2 \times 10$ nm. On the basis of these dimensions and the density of aluminum oxyhydroxide, 3.05 g cm^{-3}, the calculated surface area of this sample was 509 m^2/g.

The surface area of aluminum hydroxide adjuvant can also be determined using a gravimetric/FTIR method that measures the water adsorptive capacity (Wang et al., 2003). This technique does not require complete drying of the adjuvant, but requires specialized equipment. This method yielded a surface area of 514 m^2/g for the same aluminum hydroxide adjuvant whose size was determined using its XRD pattern. The two methods were in excellent agreement.

Because aluminum phosphate adjuvant is amorphous, XRD cannot be used to measure its surface area. The gravimetric/FTIR water adsorption method also cannot be applied to aluminum phosphate adjuvant as amorphous aluminum hydroxyphosphate contains water-filled channels (Fig. 11.3). To date, no reliable surface area measurements of aluminum phosphate adjuvant are available, although the 50-nm primary particles indicate that the surface area approaches that of aluminum hydroxide adjuvant.

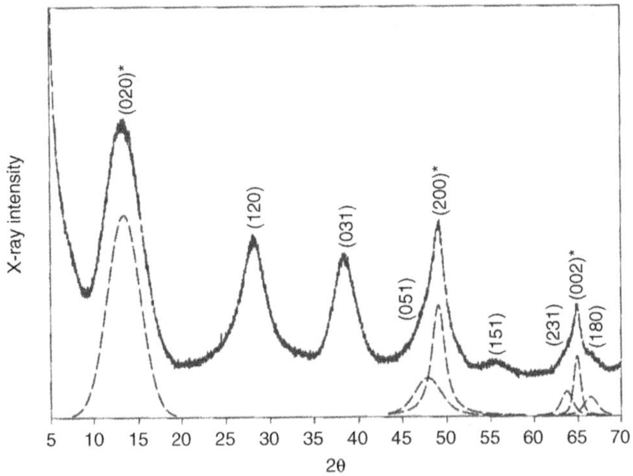

Figure 11.12 X-ray diffraction pattern of aluminum hydroxide adjuvant in the range of 5–70 °2θ. The reflections that were used to calculate the crystallite dimensions are marked *. The dashed lines show the curve-fitting results of these reflections. From Wang et al., 2003. Reproduced with permission from Elsevier, Journal of Colloid and Interface Science, 2003.

11.4.8 Particle Size

The morphology of aluminum-containing adjuvants must be considered when measuring their particle size. The primary particles, which have nanometer dimensions, may be visualized and sized by transmission electron microscopy (Fig. 11.5). Aggregates of primary particles are the functioning unit of the adjuvant suspensions. However, the aggregates are sensitive to shear and deaggregate and reaggregate during mixing (Morefield et al., 2004). Thus, the shear that an adjuvant is exposed to during sample preparation and particle size measurement must be considered when interpreting the resulting particle size distribution. The maximum size of the aggregates may be determined by photographing a sample that has been allowed to equilibrate after sample preparation. Image analysis techniques will yield a size distribution of the aggregates. The aggregates are likely to be affected by the composition of the liquid phase. Thus, dilution, if necessary, should be made with supernatant of the adjuvant that was harvested by centrifuging a separate sample of the adjuvant.

11.4.9 Isoelectric Point

It is important to characterize the iep of aluminum-containing adjuvants because electrostatic attraction is an important adsorption mechanism for many antigens. The iep can be conveniently measured by determining the zeta potential of an adjuvant suspension that has been adjusted to various pH values as shown in Figure 11.4. A buffer should not be used to adjust the pH, as the buffer anions may adsorb to the adjuvant and change the iep. Good practice is to measure the pH of the adjuvant suspension just before the zeta potential measurement is made and again immediately after the measurement is completed. If the pH values are different, the average pH value should be used to express the pH. The pH may be adjusted by the dropwise addition of acid or base. Care must be taken if dilution of the adjuvant is necessary to measure the zeta potential. It is important not to change the composition of the aqueous phase. For this reason, dilution can be made with supernatant of the suspension obtained by centrifuging a separate sample of the adjuvant.

11.4.10 Adsorption Isotherm

A goal of many vaccine formulations is to adsorb the antigen onto the aluminum-containing adjuvant. Valuable information related to this formulation approach can be obtained from an adsorption isotherm (Jendrek et al., 2003). An adsorption isotherm is prepared by dividing the adjuvant suspension into portions and adding different concentrations of antigen solution to each portion. The system is mixed until equilibrium is reached. The concentration of antigen in solution at equilibrium, C, is determined and plotted on the X-axis. The amount of antigen that was adsorbed, *x*, is determined by difference. The amount of antigen adsorbed per mass of adjuvant, *x*/*m*, is plotted on the Y-axis. The adsorption isotherm for anthrax recombinant protective antigen, rPA, and aluminum hydroxide adjuvant in either water at pH 7.4 or Dulbeccos phosphate buffered saline is shown in Figure 11.13. In water, the adsorption of rPA increased as the equilibrium concentration of rPA in solution increased up to 52 μg/ml. In the second region, the amount of rPA adsorbed remained constant as C increased from 52 to 79 μg/ml. Finally, the amount of rPA adsorbed increased as C increased from 79 to 123 μg/ml.

The rate of increase in rPA adsorption in the first phase is related to the strength of the adsorption force, which is termed *the adsorptive coefficient*. The plateau in the

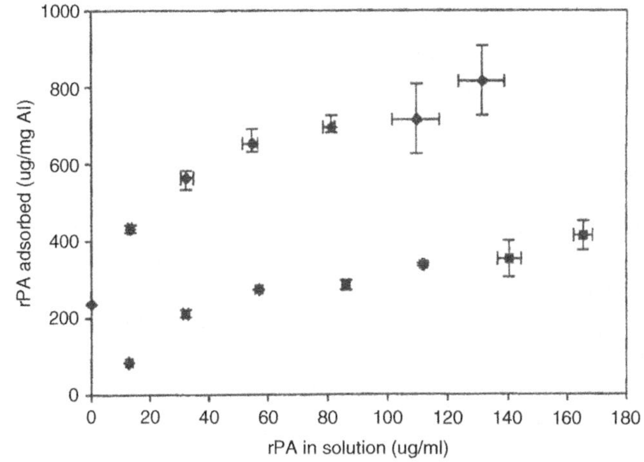

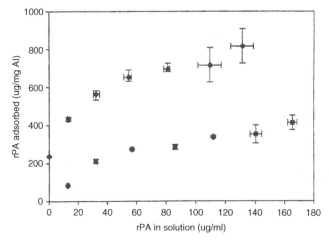

Figure 11.13 Adsorption isotherms of anthrax recombinant protective antigen onto aluminum hydroxide adjuvant. Key: ◆, water; ■, Dulbeccos phosphate buffered saline. From Jendrek et al., 2003. Reproduced with permission from Elsevier, Vaccine, 2003.

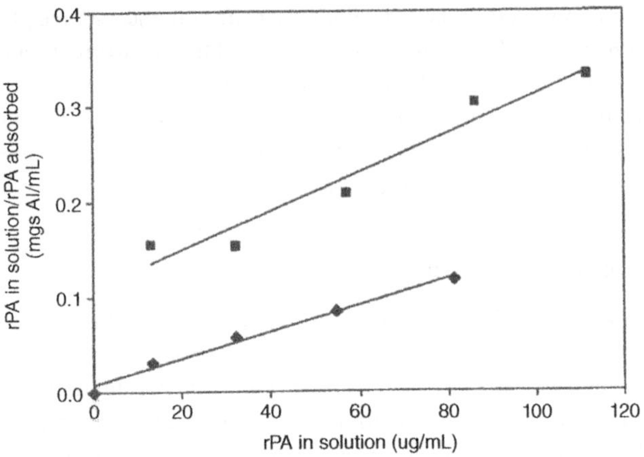

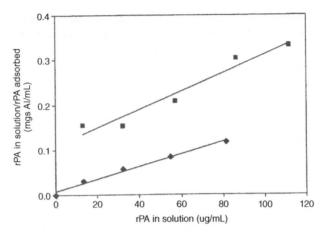

Figure 11.14 Linear Langmuir plots for the adsorption of anthrax recombinant protective a1ntigen onto aluminum hydroxide adjuvant. Key: ◆, water; ■, Dulbeccos phosphate buffered saline. From Jendrek et al., 2003. Reproduced with permission from Elsevier, Vaccine, 2003.

second phase indicates that rPA has formed a complete monolayer, as no additional rPA was adsorbed as the concentration of rPA in the supernatant increased from 52 to 79 μg/ml. The amount of solute adsorbed as a complete monolayer is known as *the adsorptive capacity*. At high concentrations of rPA in solution, the additional rPA adsorbed onto the monolayer of rPA to produce multilayer adsorption. When the data in Figure 11.13 were plotted by the linear form of the Langmuir equation (Fig. 11.14), straight lines resulted. The adsorptive capacity is the reciprocal of the slope of the linear Langmuir graph, and the adsorptive coefficient is equal to the slope divided by the intercept. The data in Figures 11.13 and 11.14 show that the use of Dulbeccos phosphate buffered saline reduced the adsorptive capacity from 0.73 to 0.50 mg rPA/mg Al in comparison to water. The adsorptive coefficient was reduced from 100 to 5 ml/mg by the use of Dulbeccos phosphate buffered saline.

11.4.11 pH-stat

The rate of acid neutralization at pH 3.0 of aluminum hydroxycarbonate, the form of aluminum hydroxide that is used as an antacid, is widely used by the antacid industry as a characterization parameter (Kerkhof et al., 1977). This test has been adapted for aluminum phosphate adjuvant, although the pH had to be lowered to 2.25 in order for the rate of acid neutralization to be conveniently measured (Burrell et al., 2001a; Burrell et al., 2001b; Jiang et al., 2003). Acid neutralization of aluminum hydroxyphosphate is described by the following two reactions.

$$AlPO_4(s) + 3HCl \rightarrow Al^{+3} + 3Cl^- + H_3PO_4 \quad (11.5)$$

$$Al(OH)_3(s) + 3HCl \rightarrow Al^{+3} + 3Cl^- + H_2O \quad (11.6)$$

The logarithms of the equilibrium constants for the aforementioned equations at 25°C are 0.5 and 9.66, respectively, indicating that the aluminum to phosphate bond is more resistant to attack by a proton than the aluminum to hydroxyl bond. Thus, the rate of acid neutralization is inversely related to the degree of substitution of phosphate for hydroxyl in aluminum phosphate adjuvant. The rate of acid neutralization at pH 2.25, 25°C is also sensitive to the degree of order. The rate of acid neutralization decreases as the aluminum phosphate adjuvant ages. The test is frequently referred to as *a pH-stat test*, as the rate of acid neutralization is measured at a constant pH by use of an automated titrator.

Unfortunately, the rate of reaction with protons of aluminum hydroxide adjuvant, even at low pH conditions, is too slow to allow the use of the rate of acid neutralization as a characterization test.

11.4.12 Phosphophilicity

Zhao and Sitrin (Zhao and Sitrin, 2001) have developed a test that measures the affinity of an aluminum-containing adjuvant to adsorb a fluorogenic phosphate compound by ligand exchange. They introduced the term *phosphophilicity* for this characteristic. The test basically detects surface hydroxyls of the adjuvant. It measures the rate of hydrolysis of the adsorbed fluorogenic substrate, 6, 8-difluoro-4-methylumbelliferyl phosphate (DiFMUP). Hydrolysis of DiFMUP releases 6,8-difluoro-4-methylumbelliferyl (DiFMU), which is fluorescent. The phosphophilicity of amorphous aluminum hydroxyphosphate sulfate adjuvants prepared using different processes exhibited different phosphilicity values. Phosphilicity values decreased when the adjuvant was heated, suggesting that this test may be useful to monitor the development of order during the aging of an aluminum-containing adjuvant. Although it was only tested on aluminum hydroxyphosphate sulfate adjuvant, it is expected to be useful for characterizing both aluminum hydroxide and aluminum phosphate adjuvants.

11.5 SUMMARY

This chapter has highlighted a number of key ideas related to the production and characterization of aluminum-containing adjuvants. Progress in improving aluminum-containing adjuvants has been hindered by incorrect information about their structure. It is now accepted that aluminum hydroxide adjuvant is a crystalline compound of known chemical structure. In contrast, aluminum phosphate adjuvant is an amorphous, nonstoichiometric material (Shirodkar et al., 1990). Thus, care must be taken in order to produce equivalent batches of aluminum phosphate adjuvant. This chapter highlighted a precipitation procedure that maintains a constant concentration of the reactants during the entire precipitation as a new approach to produce consistent batches of aluminum phosphate adjuvant (Burrell et al., 2001a; Burrell et al., 2001b).

The surface groups of the adjuvants affect their adsorptive properties. Metallic hydroxyls produce a pH-dependent surface charge that is characterized by the iep. Surface hydroxyls also provide sites for adsorption of phosphorylated antigens by the strongest adsorption mechanism: ligand exchange. Both aluminum hydroxide and aluminum phosphate adjuvants have pH-dependent surface charges, and both may adsorb phosphorylated antigens by ligand exchange, although aluminum hydroxide adjuvant has more surface hydroxyls and a greater potential for ligand exchange than aluminum phosphate adjuvant. This may affect the efficacy of a vaccine, as antigen processing and presentation to T-cells is impaired when the antigen is adsorbed too strongly (Hansen et al., 2007).

The surface groups are also important, as they affect the surface charge of the adjuvant. The pH at the surface of the adjuvant is related to the surface charge and may be different than the bulk pH. When the stability of the antigen is pH dependent, the surface charge of the aluminum-containing adjuvant should be modified to produce the optimum pH for stability of the antigen at the surface rather than in the bulk (Wittayanukulluk et al., 2004).

There are many tests that may be used to characterize aluminum-containing adjuvants. The rate of acid neutralization by aluminum phosphate adjuvant is a relatively new test (Jiang et al., 2003) that has the potential to give information about the number of Al–OH and Al–PO_4 bonds, as well as the development of order during aging.

Although aluminum-containing adjuvants are complex materials, recent advances have revealed their structure and properties. More importantly, this information is critical to obtain the best performance from aluminum-containing adjuvants, as they are currently the only adjuvant licensed for use in human vaccines by the United States Food and Drug Administration.

REFERENCES

Block SS. *Disinfection, Sterilization, and Preservation*. 4th ed. Philadelphia: Lea & Febiger; 1991. p 512.

Burrell LS, Lindblad EB, White JL, Hem SL. Stability of aluminum-containing adjuvants to autoclaving. Vaccine 1999;17:2599–2603.

Burrell LS, Johnston CT, Schulze D, Klein J, White JL, Hem SL. Aluminum phosphate adjuvants prepared by precipitation at constant pH. Part I: composition and structure. Vaccine 2001a;19:275–281.

Burrell LS, Johnston CT, Schulze D, Klein J, White JL, Hem SL. Aluminum phosphate adjuvants prepared by precipitation at constant pH. Part II: physicochemical properties. Vaccine 2001b;19:282–287.

Burrell LS, White JL, Hem SL. Stability of aluminum-containing adjuvants during aging at room temperature. Vaccine 2000;18:2188–2192.

Dandashli EA, Zhao Q, Yitta S, Morefield GL, White JL, Hem SL. Effect of thermal treatment during the preparation of aluminum hydroxide adjuvant on the protein adsorption capacity during aging. Pharm Dev Technol 2002;7:401–406.

Farmer VC. *The Infrared Spectra of Minerals*. London: Mineralogical Society; 1974. p 137–182.

Glenny AT, Pope CG, Waddington H, Wallace U. Antigenic value of toxoid precipitated by potassium alum. J Pathol Bacteriol 1926;29:31–40.

Hansen B, Sokolovska A, HogenEsch H, Hem SL. Relationship between the strength of anitgen adsorption to an aluminum-conatining adjuvant and the immune response. Vaccine 2007;25:6618–6624.

Hem KJ, Dandashli EA, White JL, Hem SL. Accessibility of antigen in vaccines produced by in situ alum precipitation. Vaccine Res 1996;5:187–191.

Hem SL, HogenEsch H. Aluminum-containing adjuvants: properties, formulation, and use. In: Singh M, editor. *Vaccine Adjuvants and Delivery Systems*. Hoboken, NJ: Wiley-Interscience; 2007a. p 81–114.

Hem SL, HogenEsch H. Relationship between physical and chemical properties of aluminum-containing adjuvants and immunopotentiation. Expert Rev Vaccines 2007b;6: 685–698.

Hem SL, Klepak PB, Lindblad EB. Aluminum hytdroxide adjuvant. In: Rowe RC, Sheskey PJ, Owen SC, editors. *Handbook of Pharmaceutical Excipients*. London: Pharmaceutical Press; 2006a. p 36–37.

Hem SL, Klepak PB, Lindblad EB. Aluminum phosphate adjuvant. In: Rowe RC, Sheskey PJ, Owen SC, editors. *Handbook of Pharmaceutical Excipients*. London: Pharmaceutical press; 2006b. p 40–41.

Hem SL, White JL. Characterization of aluminum hydroxide for use as an adjuvant in parenteral vaccines. J Parent Sci Technol 1984;38:2–10.

Hsu PH. Effect of salts on the formation of bayerite versus pseudo-boehmite. Soil Sci 1967;103:101–110.

Iyer S, HogenEsch H, Hem SL. Effect of the degree of phosphate substitution in aluminum hydroxide adjuvant on the adsorption of phosphorylated proteins. Pharm Dev Technol 2003;8:81–86.

Jendrek S, Little SF, Hem S, Mitra G, Giardina S. Evaluation of the compatibility of a second generation recombinant anthrax vaccine with aluminum-containing adjuvants. Vaccine 2003;21:3011–3018.

Jiang D, Johnston CT, Hem SL. Using rate of acid neutralization to characterize aluminum phosphate adjuvant. Pharm Dev Technol 2003;8:349–356.

Kerkhof NJ, Vanderlaan RK, White JL, Hem SL. pH-stat titration of aluminum hydroxide gel. J Pharm Sci 1977;66:1528–1533.

Klein J, Ushio M, Burrell LS, Wenslow B, Hem SL. Analysis of aluminum hydroxyphosphate vaccine adjuvants by ^{27}Al MAS NMR. J Pharm Sci 2000;89:311–321.

Lindblad EB. Aluminum adjuvants-in retrospect and prospect. Vaccine 2004;22:3658–3668.

Masood H, White JL, Hem SL. Relationship between protein adsorptive capacity and the X-ray diffraction pattern of aluminum hydroxide adjuvants. Vaccine 1994;12:187–189.

Morefield GL, HogenEsch H, Robinson JP, Hem SL. Distribution of adsorbed antigen in mono-valent and combination vaccines. Vaccine 2004;22:1973–1984.

Parks GA. The isoelectric points of solid oxides, solid hydroxides, and aqueous hydroxo complex systems. Chem Rev 1965;65:177–198.

Rinella JV Jr, White JL, Hem SL. Effect of pH on the elution of model antigens from aluminum-containing adjuvants. J Colloid Interface Sci 1998;205:161–165.

Romero Mendez IZ, Shi Y, HogenEsch H, Hem SL. Potentiation of the immune response to non-adsorbed antigens by aluminum-containing adjuvants. Vaccine 2007;25:825–833.

Seeber SJ, White JL, Hem SL. Predicting the adsorption of proteins by aluminum-containing adjuvants. Vaccine 1991;9:201–203.

Serna CJ, Lyons JC, White JL, Hem SL. Stabilization of aluminum hydroxide gel by specifically adsorbed carbonate. J Pharm Sci 1983;72:769–771.

Shi Y, HogenEsch H, Hem SL. Change in the degree of adsorption of proteins by aluminum-containing adjuvants following exposure to interstitial fluid: freshly prepared and aged model vaccines. Vacccine 2002;20:80–85.

Shi Y, HogenEsch H, Regnier FE, Hem SL. Detoxification of endotoxin by aluminum hydroxide adjuvant. Vaccine 2001;19:1747–1752.

Shirodkar S, Hutchinson RL, Perry DL, White JL, Hem SL. Aluminum compounds used as adjuvants in vaccines. Pharm Res 1990;7:1282–1288.

Stumm W. *Chemistry of the Solid–Water Interface*. New York: John Wiley & Sons; 1992. p 13–38.

Tettenhorst R, Hofmann DA. Crystal chemistry of boehmite. Clays Clay Miner 1980;28: 373–380.

Wang S-L, Johnston CT, Bish DL, White JL, Hem SL. Water-vapor adsorption and surface area measurement of poorly crystalline boehmite. J Colloid Interface Sci 2003;260:26–35.

Wittayanukulluk A, Jiang D, Regnier FE, Hem SL. Effect of microenvironment pH of aluminum hydroxide adjuvant on the chemical stability of adsorbed antigen. Vaccine 2004;22:1172–1176.

Yau KP, Schulze DG, Johnston CT, Hem SL. Aluminum hydroxide adjuvant produced under constant reactant concentration. J Pharm Sci 2006;95:1822–1833.

Zhao Q, Sitrin R. Surface phosphophilicity of aluminum-containing adjuvants probed by their efficiency for catalyzing the P-O bond cleavage with chromogenic and fluorogenic substrates. Anal Biochem 2001;295:76–81.

12

THE BIOLOGICS LICENSE APPLICATION (BLA) IN COMMON TECHNICAL DOCUMENT (CTD) FORMAT

R.S. Robin Robinett
Merck & Co., Inc., West Point, PA, USA

12.1 INTRODUCTION

The purpose of a biological license application (BLA) is to submit documentation that demonstrates the safety and efficacy of the biologic for which a marketing application is being sought (Section 505 of the Federal Food, Drug, and Cosmetic Act; Part 314 of Title 21 in the Code of Federal Regulations (CFR)). In addition to safety and efficacy data, information regarding the chemistry, manufacturing, and control (CMC) is also submitted. Sources of data for the BLA include information from the original Investigation New Drug Application (IND; e.g., toxicology studies), IND information amendments (e.g., data on drug product formulation, Phase-1 study reports, carcinogenicity study reports, and assay description), and documents created solely for the BLA (e.g., labeling, manufacturing process descriptions, assay validations, and stability data). Vaccine, blood, and gene therapy products are submitted to the Center for Biologics Evaluation and Research (CBER). Other biologics are reviewed by Center for Drug Evaluation and Research (CDER). Guidelines and guidance documents with CBER- and CDER-related regulations can be found on the Food and Drug Administration (FDA) websites at: www.fda.gov/cder/guidance/index.html and www.fda.gov/cber/guidance/index.html.

Vaccine Development and Manufacturing, First Edition.
Edited by Emily P. Wen, Ronald Ellis, and Narahari S. Pujar.

BLAs are submitted in a format known as the Common Technical Document (CTD). This format is used for the registration of all new pharmaceuticals for human use, including vaccines. Submission in the CTD format is mandatory in Japan and the European Union and is "highly recommended" in the United States and Canada. Exceptions in the United States and Canada must be agreed upon at a pre-BLA meeting. The FDA accepts an electronic version of the CTD called the electronic Common Technical Document (eCTD).

The CTD format is a harmonized table of content (TOC) for a marketing application that is the result of an International Conference of Harmonization (ICH) committee. The ICH undertook the harmonization of technical requirements between Japan, Europe, and the United States to avoid the necessity of generating completely different dossiers in these regions (Guidance for Industry—M4: Organization of the CTD). The CTD guidance documents address format only. Scientific and technical content and requirements are covered by the ICH Technical Guidelines (Q, S, and E). The ICH Guidance Documents include the following:

M4: Organization of the CTD
M4Q: Quality (CMC information)
M4S: Safety (nonclinical information)
M4E: Efficacy (clinical information).

They are the basis of the content discussions in this chapter.

The CTD format not only streamlines the preparation process for the applicant, but also helps the regulatory agency reviewers because the location of information is now consistent across all companies.

12.2 ORGANIZATION OF THE BIOLOGICS LICENSING APPLICATION

The CTD is organized into five modules. Module 1 is country or region specific and contains the information that is unique to a region. Module 2 contains summary documents for Modules 3–5. Module 2 is similar to the Expert Report for those who are familiar with the old format used in Europe. Module 3 is called *the Quality Module* and contains all of the CMC information for the new product. Nonclinical data are found in Module 4, and clinical data are presented in Module 5.

Arabic numbers have been assigned to designate the specific sections that should be included in the dossier. The Arabic numbering system described in the Industry Guidance Documents should be used during the assembly of the dossier (General Consideration for Submitting Marketing Applications According to the ICH/CTD format). In the event that more than one drug substance, drug product, or indication is submitted, the numbering system should be repeated for each section. To avoid confusion, if there are multiple drug substances, drug products, or indications, the sections should be clearly labeled with the drug substance, drug product, or indication name. This information should also be in the header on each page.

The organization of the BLA and the type (paper vs electronic) should be agreed on with the FDA at the pre-BLA meeting. If the product has multiple drug substances, multiple formulations, a reconstituting diluent, or multiple indications, the organization and designation of these sections should be included in the discussions.

12.2.1 Module 1: Administrative Information and Prescribing Information

Module 1 contains documents that are specific for each region. Information that is required in a U.S. submission includes the following:

- FDA form 356h
- Comprehensive table of contents indexing the application documents
- Administrative documents
  - Patent information and certification
  - Debarment certification
  - User fee cover sheet
  - Financial disclosure/certification information
  - Letters of authorization for reference
  - Environmental assessment or request for exclusion
  - Statements of claimed exclusivity
  - Waiver requests
- Proposed labeling
  - Draft labeling in new package insert format
  - Annotated package insert
  - Container labeling

For more information about Module 1, see Guidance for Industry, *General Considerations for Submitting Marketing Applications According to the ICH/CTD format*, August 2001.

12.2.2 Module 2: Common Technical Document Summaries

Module 2 is organized into seven sections that contain summaries of the quality, nonclinical, and clinical modules and is the CTD equivalent of the old expert report for the European Authority. The Module 2 documents contain summaries of Modules 3–5 and should not contain any new information. This restriction includes the use of references.

References found in Module 2 must also be used in the corresponding sections (Module 3, 4, or 5). There is a page limit for most sections of Module 2.

12.2.2.1 CTD Table of Contents The TOC in section 2.1 should contain a listing of the sections with their corresponding volume. This TOC is essentially a summary of the TOCs from Module 1, 3, 4, and 5 and should have only the major section numbering outlined by the ICH guideline to the fifth level (e.g., 3.2.S.1.1).

12.2.2.2 CTD Introduction The CTD introduction should include a general introduction to the biologic with information, including the pharmacologic class, the mode of action, and the proposed clinical use. This information should be limited to one page.

12.2.2.3 Quality Overall Summary The quality overall summary (QOS) is a summary of the body of data found in Module 3. Sufficient information should be provided so that the quality reviewer has a good overview of Module 3 content. Discussions in the QOS should include critical key parameters, deviations from guidance documents (if applicable), and an integration of key information from Module 4 or 5 (if applicable).

The QOS should parallel the organization and scope of the body of data found in Module 3. All information, data, or justifications in the QOS must be included in Module 3 or in another part of the dossier. Tables and figures are generally the same as those reported in Module 3. In some cases, new tables may be introduced that summarize information from Module 3.

Since vaccines are biotechnology products, the page limit for the QOS is 80 pages. This limit does not include figures or tables. Summarizing Module 3 in 80 pages or less, which can be hundreds of pages, may seem impossible. A good strategy for writing the QOS is to leverage summary tables and figures that are not included in the page count. Some strategies for summarizing data that have been shown to be successful are briefly outlined.

For manufacturing data (2.3.S.2.3 or 2.3.P.3.3), a quick overview (a few short paragraphs) of the process can be provided followed by detailed flow charts for each part of the process. These flow charts should include starting materials, intermediates, process steps with conditions, critical parameters, testing locations, and assays performed. The detailed flow charts should be the same as those included in Module 3 where the detailed discussion of each manufacturing step is provided.

While a table is a typical format for displaying specifications, batch analyses, and justification of specifications, tables can also be used for assay details and validation data. For assay descriptions (2.3.S.4.2 or 2.3.P.5.2), a table can include test samples, controls, animals or cell lines, brief assay description, expected results, and conformance to guidelines. When evaluating conformance to guidelines for vaccines, World Health Organization (WHO) and ICH guidelines should be considered in addition to the *United States Pharmacopeia* (*USP*). Validation summary tables (2.3.S.4.3 or 2.3.P.5.3) should list the validation parameter studied (preferably as defined in the USP for assay validation), the acceptance criteria, and the actual result from the study. If a qualification is performed, the acceptance criteria and actual results from that study can also be listed. If assays are compared to compendia, those results can also be tabulated by listing the guideline (CFR, ICH, USP, WHO, etc.), the name of the actual guidance document, and the status of the comparison (meets all requirements, etc.). These tables can also be provided in the associated Module 3 sections as an introduction to that assay or validation discussion. If the tables are all organized with the same structure, the FDA reviewer will be able to easily get a "snapshot" of the data and will be able to quickly retrieve a needed detail about an assay or validation while doing their in-depth review.

Reference standard information (2.3.S.5 and 2.3.P.6) can also be provided in a tabular format. Information of interest in the summary includes the reference standard, their source, the assay name, assay where that the reference standard is used, and a list of tests that are used to characterize the standard. A tabular format can also be used to summarize the packaging components, their specifications, testing, and compendial compliance in the container closure system sections (2.3.S.6 and 2.3.P.7).

For more information about the expected content of individual Module 2.3 sections, see the Guidance for Industry, *M4Q: Quality (CMC Information)*.

12.2.2.4 Nonclinical Overview The Nonclinical Overview should provide a comprehensive, factual synopsis of the nonclinical data found in Module 4, as well as an integrated and critical assessment of the pharmacologic, pharmacokinetic, and toxicologic evaluation of the product. This overview includes an evaluation of the pharmacokinetic effects, the mode of action, and potential effects. A discussion of the relevance of the analytical methods, the pharmacokinetic models, and the derived parameters should be included. In addition, an evaluation of the toxic effect with respect to onset, severity, duration, dose dependency, degree of reversibility, and species- or gender-related differences should be provided; also, there should be a discussion of the nonclinical testing strategy, including a justification and the good laboratory practices (GLP) status of the studies. If there is any association between nonclinical findings and either quality characteristics of the test vaccine, clinical studies, or effects with other related products, that information should also be presented. For biotechnology products, an assessment of impurities and degradants is not needed. The page limit for this section is 30 pages. For more information about Module 2.4 content and structural format, see Guidance for Industry, *M4S: Safety (Nonclinical Information)*.

12.2.2.5 Clinical Overview The clinical overview should provide a critical analysis of the clinical data found in Module 5, as well as a brief discussion and interpretation of the results and the conclusions and implications of the data. The content of this section includes a product development rationale, an evaluation of the program (strengths and weaknesses), and study results; overviews of biopharmaceutics, clinical pharmacology, efficacy, and safety; a discussion of the benefits and risks with respect to the intended use of the product; and a discussion of the relevance of the data to the package insert. Regulatory agencies intend to use this section to aid their review of the clinical section and a useful reference regarding the overall clinical results for the quality and nonclinical reviewers. For more information about Module 2.5 content and structural format, see Guidance for Industry, *M4E: Efficacy (Clinical Information)*.

12.2.2.6 Nonclinical Written and Tabulated Summaries The nonclinical written and tabulated summaries section includes an introduction to the pharmaceutical and its proposed clinical uses, a pharmacology written summary, the pharmacology tabulated summaries, a pharmacokinetics written summary, the pharmacokinetics tabulated summary, a toxicology written summary, and the toxicology tabulated summary. There is a prescribed order for the types of studies. If multiple studies of the same type were performed, the summary should be organized by specie, route, and then duration. It is recommended that a 100–150 page limit be observed for the nonclinical written summaries. For more information about Module 2.6 content and organization, see Guidance for Industry, *M4S: Safety (Nonclinical Information).*

12.2.2.7 Clinical Summary The clinical summary section includes summaries of biopharmaceutic studies and their associated analytical methods, clinical pharmacology studies, clinical efficacy and safety studies, and synopses of individual studies. Also included in this section are summaries of any cross-study or meta-analysis performed and reported in Module 5, as well as any available postmarketing data from product marketed in other regions. This section typically ranges from 50 to 400 pages (excluding tables). If the Integrated Summary of Safety (ISS) and Integrated Summary of Efficacy (ISE) would be longer than 400 pages, the complete text of those documents can be put into Section 5.3.5.3, with just a summary included in 2.7. For more information about Module 2.7 contents, see Guidance for Industry, *M4E: Efficacy (Clinical Information).*

12.2.3 Module 3: Quality

Module 3 describes the CMC used during the preparation and release of the proposed vaccine. The development of the drug substance(s) and drug product(s), their characterization, and stability are included in specified sections. Also required is a detailed description of raw materials, testing, compendial compliance of material and assays, and container closure. There are three sections for Module 3 as follows:

3.1 Table of Contents
3.2 Body of Data
3.3 Literature References.

A brief discussion about the content for the Quality Module is provided in the following sections. For additional information about Module 3 contents, see Guidance for Industry, *M4Q: Quality (CMC Information)*, ICH guidelines Q6A for New Chemical Entities (NCE), and Q6B for Biotechnology products. Another very useful document that answers questions about interpretations of the M4Q document is Guidance for Industry *M4: The CTD—Quality Questions and Answers/Location Issues.* Additional ICH guidance documents that can be referred to include the following:

Q1A (R2) *Stability Testing of New Drug Substances and Products* (February 2003)
Q1B *Photostability Testing of New Drug Substances and Products* (November 1996)

Q1D *Bracketing and Matrixing Designs for Stability Testing of New Drug Substances and Products* (February 2002)

Q1E *Evaluation for Stability Data* (February 2003)

Q2 (R1) Validation of Analytical Procedures: Text and Methodology (October 1994/November 1996)

Q3A (R2) *Impurities in New Drug Substances* (October 2006)

Q3B (R2) *Impurities in New Drug Products* (June 2006)

Q3C (R5) *Impurities: Guideline for Residual Solvents* (February 2011)

Q5A (R1) *Viral Safety Evaluation of Biotechnology Products Derived From Cell Lines of Human or Animal Origin* (September 1999)

Q5B *Quality of Biotechnological Products: Analysis of the Expression Construct in Cells Used for Production of r-DNA Derived Protein Products* (November 1995)

Q5C *Quality of Biotechnological Products: Stability Testing of Biotechnological/Biological Products* (November 1995)

Q5D *Derivation and characterization of Cell Substrates Used for Production of Biotechnological/Biological Products* (July 1997)

Q6A *Specifications: Test Procedures and Acceptance Criteria for New Drug Substances and New Drug Products: Chemical Substances* (October 1999)

Q6B *Test Procedures and Acceptance Criteria for Biotechnological/Biological Products* (March 1999)

12.2.3.1 Table of Contents The TOC in Section 3.1 should have only the major section numbering outlined by the ICH guideline to the fifth level (e.g., 3.2.S.1.1). Although it is permissible to add additional subsection to the ICH-defined levels to facilitate organization of the information, the listing of those additional subsections should not be included in the 3.1 TOC. The 3.1 TOC should be used for the Module 3 section of the 2.1 TOC.

12.2.3.2 Body of Data The body of data is divided into drug substance, drug product, appendix, and regional sections. Drug substance sections (3.2.S) should be provided for each active ingredient, and drug product sections (3.2.P) should be provided for each formulation. In some cases when the manufacture and testing of all the active ingredients is very similar, a single drug substance section can be used; however, the differences in the processes and testing need to be clearly indicated. When multiple drug substance or drug product sections are needed, the numbering system is repeated, with the drug substance or drug product clearly indicated in the page header. There are three appendices available. Appendix 1 contains information about all the facilities and equipment that are used to manufacture drug substances and formulate, package, and label drug products. If the drug substance or drug product contains materials of human animal origin, the adventitious agent safety evaluation information is provided in Appendix 2. If novel excipients are used in the formulation, information is provided in Appendix 3. Appendix 2 and 3 are provided only if materials of animal origin or novel excipients are used. The addition of other appendices or changing of the content of the three appendices is not allowed within the CTD format.

3.2.S Drug Substance Sections The information that describes the characterization, manufacture, testing, and stability of the drug substance is organized into seven major sections. If more than one drug substance is combined for the formulation of the drug product, each drug substance must have each of these seven sections.

3.2.S.1 General Information The information in the general information section provides an overview of the drug substance and is further divided into three subsections. The first subsection (3.2.S.1.1) contains information on the nomenclature and should include a discussion of all names that are used to refer to the drug substance, including trademarks where applicable.

Information on the structure is provided in the second subsection (3.2.S.1.2). The actual information provided in this section will be dependent on the type of vaccine. Viral-based vaccines should include information concerning virus state (live or inactivated) and the viral type and family. Protein or polypeptide vaccines should include information about the amino acid sequence and the type and location of any post-translational modifications. Nucleic-acid-based vaccines should include information on the protein coded for the vector and the nucleic acid of the inserted sequence. Polysaccharide-based vaccines should include information on the structure, any modifications, and the source. Gene therapy vaccines should include information about the vector and inserted gene sequence. For all biotechnology products, the method and degree of purification should be discussed. If the product is highly purified, a schematic of the structure with the antigenic sites is useful. If the product is a more crude preparation and is not "highly purified," the major cell components that are present should be discussed.

The final subsection (3.2.S.1.3) describes the general properties of the product and includes any physiochemical and other relevant properties used to describe the vaccine. The actual information should be appropriate for the type of material that is used for the vaccine.

3.2.S.2 Manufacture The information in the manufacture section provides details of the drug substance manufacture, including the manufacturing and package site, the raw materials, the manufacturing process, process controls, process validation, and process development. This section is divided into six subsections. The first subsection (3.2.S.2.1) contains the name and address and responsibility for each proposed manufacturing site.

The detailed description of the manufacturing process is found in the second subsection (3.2.S.2.2). This description represents the applicant's commitment for the manufacturing process and the process controls that will be implemented. The details should include the batch scale and the batch numbering system, whether pooling of materials is allowable, a flow diagram for each part of the process (e.g., the manufacturing of the original inoculums, the cell culture materials, reagents, buffers, intermediates), details of the processing steps, process parameters (e.g., pH, time, temperature), major equipment, sampling locations for in-process testing, and testing performed on samples. A detailed description of the process should accompany the flow diagrams. The information in the flow diagram and the process description should match and be independent (i.e., a flow diagram should not be needed to understand the description or vice versa). If reprocessing of intermediates is permitted, reprocessing procedures with criteria should be included.

Information about all materials (e.g., raw materials, starting materials, solvents, reagents, and catalysts) used in the manufacture of drug substance is found in subsection three (3.2.S.2.3). Each material should be listed with the process step indicated, as well as a discussion of the material's quality and control. For biotechnology products, this specifically includes source and starting materials of biological origin; source, history, and generation of cell substrates; and cell banking systems, characterization, and testing. Information on the suitability of the material for its intended use should also be provided.

Details about testing and acceptance criteria performed at critical steps are provided in the fourth subsection (3.2.S.2.4). This information is used to demonstrate that proper process controls are in place. Experimental data used to justify the acceptance criteria should be included. This subsection also contains quality and control information for intermediates that are isolated during the manufacturing process. For biotechnology products, stability data supporting storage conditions should be included.

The fifth subsection (3.2.S.2.5) provides details on the process validation or evaluation of the drug substance manufacturing process, including aseptic processing and sterilization. The information provided in this subsection should include the validation study plan, results from implementing the validation plan, analysis of the results, and conclusions drawn from the validation study. The study should be designed so that sufficient details can be provided to demonstrate that the manufacturing process will produce material that is suitable for its intended use, that the selection of the critical process controls was appropriate, and that limits established for the critical manufacturing steps were valid. A cross-reference to the location of the analytical procedure and validation sections should be included for each assay used. If validation-specific tests are performed, the details about those analytical procedures and validations should be provided as part of the justification of the selection of critical process controls and acceptance criteria. If reprocessing steps for intermediates are allowed, reprocessing must be included in the validation program.

The manufacturing process development is described in the sixth subsection (3.2.S.2.6) and should include descriptions of changes made to the manufacture of the drug substance batches that are used to support the marketing application (nonclinical or clinical). Changes to the process or to critical equipment should be listed with the reason for the change. Details about the drug substance batches manufactured during the various points in development (i.e., batch number, manufacturing scale, and use) should be provided. Changes should be assessed for their potential impact on an intermediate or the drug substance. Comparative data from analytical testing on relevant drug substance batches should be provided for manufacturing changes that are considered potentially significant. A discussion of the comparative data, the selection of the analytical procedures, and the assessment of the results should also be included. If clinical or nonclinical data are available to support the impact of manufacturing process changes, that data should also be cross-referenced.

3.2.S.3 Characterization The characterization section provides information on the elucidation of the drug substance structure, drug substance characterization, and a discussion of impurities found in the drug substance. This section is further divided into two subsections. The first subsection (3.2.S.3.1) contains the details on the elucidation of the structure and the characterization of the drug substance. Details provided for viral-based vaccines should include structure, biological activity, immunochemical and physiochemical properties, and electron microscopy images. Protein or polypeptide vaccines should include details concerning the primary, secondary, and higher order structures, post-translational modifications, biological activity, purity, and immunochemical and physiochemical properties. Nucleic-acid-based vaccines should include information on the sequence, higher ordered structure, biological activity, and immunochemical and physiochemical properties. Details provided for polysaccharide-based vaccines should include structure, biological activity, and immunochemical and physiochemical properties. If a drug substance is a combination of biotechnology types, the characterization of each component should be addressed.

Information on the impurities should be provided in the second subsection (3.2.S.3.2). Impurities include process-related impurities and contaminants, product-related impurities, and degradation products. For each impurity, a description of the impurity source and the analytical procedures used to test for the impurity should be included. If the analytical procedure is described in 3.2.S.4.2, the method can be referenced, and the detailed information does not need to be repeated in this section. Impurity clearance data should also be provided. Spiking studies, testing, and process validation are all possible sources of impurity clearance data.

3.2.S.4 Control of Drug Substance The information in the control of drug substance section provides the drug substance specifications, analytical procedures used for testing, the associated analytical procedure validations, the specification justifications, and batch analysis data. This section is divided into five subsections. The first subsection (3.2.S.4.1) lists the specification and assay procedures used for the drug substance, intermediates, and in-process samples. Testing should include but not limited to potency, purity, identity, and appearance. The descriptions of these analytical procedures are found in the second subsection (3.2.S.4.2). Test samples, references and controls, test animals or cell lines, a description of the actual procedure, and conformance to guidelines should be discussed for each analytical procedure. Validation of the analytical procedures, with experimental data, is found in the third subsection (3.2.S.4.3) and includes the performance characteristic tested (e.g., accuracy, linearity, limit of detection, limit of quantitation, precision, range, repeatability, ruggedness, and specificity), the target criteria, and the actual validation results. If an assay qualification is performed, the validation data from the original validation, regardless of the test material, can be included along with the qualification protocol and qualification data from the material relevant for the dossier being prepared. The fifth subsection (3.2.S.4.5) is the location for the justification of the specifications.

Descriptions of the relevant lots of drug substance with the results from the lot release testing (batch analysis) are provided in the fourth subsection (3.2.S.4.4). Lots to be considered for inclusion in this section are those used for pivotal clinical trials, bridging studies, clinical consistency trials, manufacturing consistency trials, stability studies, and any other lots that are described in the dossier. Batch analysis for the bulks that were used to formulate the drug product lots that have batch analysis provided in 3.2.P.5.4 should be considered for inclusion here.

3.2.S.5 Reference Standards or Materials The information in this section describes reference standards or reference materials that are used for testing the drug substance and includes the method of manufacture, characterization studies, stability data, and qualification for new standards. Where available, historical data or bridging to clinical trials data can also be included. For convenience, subsections can be added for each reference material (i.e., 3.2.S.5.1, 3.2.S.5.2).

3.2.S.6 Container Closure System The information in this section provides a description of the container closure system used to store the drug substance. For primary packaging (packaging that comes into contact with the material), the identity of the materials and the specifications should be provided for each packaging component. If appropriate, the specifications should include critical dimensions and drawings. Methods used to test the container closure system should be listed with the results. If the methods are noncompendial, validation data should also be included. The discussion should also contain information regarding the suitability of the choice of material with respect to any light or moisture protection that is needed, the compatibility of the drug substance with the container material, possible sorption to the container or leached materials from the container, and safety of the material. If nonfunctional secondary packaging is used, only a brief description is required.

3.2.S.7 Stability The information in the stability section provides an overview of the stability program, including the testing schemes, analytical procedures, and results that were used to establish the drug substance shelf life. This section is further divided into three subsections. The first subsection (3.2.S.7.1) contains a summary of the stability program and includes the types of studies performed, the protocols that were followed, the results of the studies, and all conclusions concerning storage conditions, shelf life, and retest dates (if applicable). The stability studies described should include long-term, accelerated or stressed, and forced-degradation study types. The post-approval stability protocol and stability commitments are provided in the second subsection (3.2.S.7.2). The results from all of the stability studies are provided in the third subsection (3.2.S.7.3). A graphic, tabular, narrative, or a combination of these formats can be used as appropriate for the data being discussed. This subsection should also discuss any analytical procedures used to generate the data and the methods used to validate those assays. If the analytical procedures and the validations have already been described in 3.2.S.4, a reference to the location of the discussion can be provided.

3.2.P Drug Product Sections The information that describes the characterization, manufacture, testing, and stability of the drug product is organized into eight major sections. If more than one drug product formulation is being filed or if there is a reconstituting diluent, each drug product must have each of these eight sections.

3.2.P.1 Description and Composition of the Drug Product The information in this section provides a description of the drug product, including the dosage form and its composition. Included with the list of components should be the amount of component found on a per unit basis (with overages if applicable), the function of the component, and a reference to the compendial monographs or manufacturer's specifications. Also discussed in this section is the type of container used for the drug product. If the drug product requires a reconstituting diluent, a discussion of the composition of the diluents and the container closure system for the diluents should also be provided.

3.2.P.2 Pharmaceutical Development The information in the pharmaceutical development section should describe the development studies conducted to establish that the dosage form, the formulation, the manufacturing process, the container closure system, the microbiological attributes, and the usage instructions are appropriate for the purposes specified in the application. This section is further divided into six subsections. The first subsection (3.2.P.2.1) contains information about the compatibility of the drug substance with the excipients. If there are key physiochemical characteristics of the drug substance that can influence the performance of the drug product, those should be discussed as well. Characteristics of the excipients that can influence the drug product should also be discussed along with an explanation of why the excipients were chosen and how their concentrations were established. If the drug product contains multiple drug substances (a combination product), the compatibility of the drug substances with each other should also be addressed.

The second subsection (3.2.P.2.2) includes discussions of formulation development, overages, and physicochemical and biological properties. The formulation development section should include a brief summary of the studies used to develop the proposed dosage formulation and route of administration. Also included in this section are discussions of differences between clinical material and the final formulation for which licensure is sought and results from comparisons of *in vivo* and *in vitro* studies (if appropriate). If overages in the formulation are defined in 3.2.P.1, a justification should be provided in the overages sections. Any physiochemical or biological property that is relevant to the performance of the drug product is addressed in the physicochemical and biological properties section. These properties include, but are not limited to, pH, ionic strength, dissolution, redispersion, reconstitution, particle size distribution, aggregation, polymorphism, rheological properties, biological activity or potency, and immunological activity.

Manufacturing process development (3.2.P.2.3), the third subsection, includes information on the selection and optimization of the manufacturing process used to prepare the drug product. The critical aspects of this development should be included. In addition, if sterilization is needed, the sterilization method should be discussed and justified. Difference in the manufacturing process used to make pivotal clinical material and the final process for which licensure is sought should be discussed, particularly if the process changes influence the performance of the product.

The suitability of the container closure system used for the drug product is discussed in the fourth subsection (3.2.P.2.4). The information discussed includes the suitability for drug product storage, transportation, and use. Parameters that should be included are choice of material, protection from light and moisture, compatibility of construction material with the dosage form, and material safety. If the device is presented as part of the drug product, the reproducibility of the delivery system should also be discussed.

Microbiological attributes is the subject of the fifth subsection (3.2.P.2.5). For non-sterile products, this section should include information about the rationale for not performing microbial limits testing. For products containing antimicrobial preservatives, the selection and effectiveness of preservative systems should be discussed. For sterile products, this section should include a discussion of the integrity of the container closure system for the prevention of microbial contamination.

The sixth subsection, compatibility (3.2.P.2.6), includes a discussion of the compatibility of the drug product with a reconstituting diluents or a dosage device. The information provided should be appropriate to support labeling.

3.2.P.3 Manufacture The information in this section provides details of the manufacture of the drug product, including the manufacturing and package site, the manufacturing process, process controls, process validation, in-process testing, and process development. This section is divided into five subsections. The first subsection (3.2.P.3.1) contains the name, address, and responsibility for each proposed manufacturing and testing site. A batch formula is found in the second subsection (3.2.P.3.2). A list of all dosage form components, their amount (per unit basis) including overages, and the quality standard reference should be included in the batch formula.

The detailed description of the manufacturing process is found in the third subsection (3.2.P.3.3). A flow diagram should be included that details where materials enter the process; the process steps; process parameters (e.g., pH, time, temperature); major equipment (including type and working capacity where relevant); critical steps; sampling locations for in-process, intermediate, and final product testing; and testing performed on samples. A detailed description of the process, including scale, should accompany the flow diagrams. Greater detail should be provided for novel process or packaging operations that may affect product quality. The information in the flow diagram and the process description should match and should be independent (i.e., a flow diagram should not be needed to understand the description or vice versa). Environmental conditions (e.g., low humidity) should be addressed if critical for the integrity of the product. Critical parameters may be given as expected ranges. If reprocessing of materials is allowed, the proposal for the reprocessing should be provided along with a justification.

Details about the analytical procedures performed at critical steps, their associated acceptance criteria, and the justifications for the expected ranges for the critical parameter are provided in the fourth subsection (3.2.P.3.4). This information is used to demonstrate that proper process controls are in place for the manufacture of the drug product and filled material. Experimental data to justify the acceptance criteria should be included. This subsection also contains quality and control information for intermediates that are isolated during the manufacturing process.

The fifth subsection (3.2.P.3.5) provides details on the process validation or evaluation of the drug product manufacturing process, including aseptic processing and sterilization. The information provided in this subsection should include the validation study plan, results from implementing the validation plan, analysis of the results, and conclusions drawn from the validation study. The study should be designed so that sufficient details can be provided to demonstrate that the manufacturing process will produce material that is suitable for its intended use, that the selection of the critical process controls was appropriate, and that limits established for the critical manufacturing steps were valid. A cross-reference to the location of the analytical procedure and validation sections should be included for each assay used. If a validation-specific test is used, the details about the analytical procedure and validation should be provided as part of the justification of the selection of critical process controls and acceptance criteria. If reprocessing steps for intermediates are allowed, reprocessing must be included in the validation program.

3.2.P.4 Control of Excipients The information in the control of excipients section provides the excipient specifications, analytical procedure used to release the excipients, the associated analytical validation, and the justification of specifications. Also included in this section is a discussion of excipients of human or animal origin and novel excipients. This section is divided into six subsections. The first subsection (3.2.P.4.1) lists the specifications and assay procedures used to test excipients that are used to formulate the drug product. A discussion about the compliance to compendial requirements is also required. The description of these analytical procedures is found in the second subsection (3.2.P.4.2). Compendial compliance for the analytical procedure should be included in this discussion. For noncompendial analytical procedures, more detail concerning how the assay is performed should be included, as well as the assay validation information. Validation information, including the experimental data is located in the third subsection (3.2.P.4.3). Justification of specification should be provided for all analytical procedures and should be included in the fourth subsection (3.2.P.4.4). Information about excipients of human or animal origin is located in the fifth subsection (3.2.P.4.5) and includes details about adventitious agent sources, testing, specifications, and viral safety data. The final subsection (3.2.P.4.6) provides details for excipients that have not been previously used in a drug product formulation or that are used in a new route of administration. Details should include the manufacture, characterization, testing including specifications, and a cross-reference to nonclinical or clinical safety data.

3.2.P.5 Control of Drug Product The information in the control of drug product section provides the specifications, analytical procedure used to release the drug product, the associated analytical validation, the justification of specifications, and batch analysis data. This section is divided into six subsections. The first subsection (3.2.P.5.1) lists the specifications and assay procedures used for the drug product in the final formulated bulk, filled container, and marketed container configurations. The description of these analytical procedures is found in the second subsection (3.2.P.5.2). If the analytical procedure is identical to that used for a drug substance test, a reference to the appropriate drug substance section (3.2.S.4.2) can be provided. If the testing was not used for any drug substance testing, similar information should be provided for these procedures as was described for the drug substance analytical procedures. This is also the case for the analytical procedure validations found in the third subsection (3.2.P.5.3) where a reference can be made if the validation was described in the drug substance section (3.2.S.4.3). The details that should be provided for a new assay are the same as that described for the drug substance sections. The sixth subsection (3.2.P.5.6) is the location for the justification of the specifications.

Descriptions of relevant lots of drug product with the results from that lot release testing (batch analysis) are provided in the fourth subsection (3.2.P.5.4). Lots to be considered for inclusion in this section are those used for pivotal clinical trials, bridging studies, clinical consistency trials, manufacturing consistency trials, stability studies, and any other lots that are described in the dossier.

The fifth subsection (3.2.P.5.5) contains information on the characterization of impurities. Information on impurities that are introduced from the drug substance should have been discussed in 3.2.S.3.2, and a cross-reference to that section can be provided here. If there are additional impurities as a result of the drug product formulation, that material should be included in this section.

3.2.P.6 Reference Standards or Materials The information in this section describes reference standards or reference materials that are used for testing the drug product. If the materials have already been described in the drug substance sections, a reference can be made to the appropriate section in 3.2.S.5. If there are new materials, the details provided should be the same as those described for the other materials. For convenience, subsections can be added for each reference material (i.e., 3.2.P.6.1, 3.2.P.6.2).

3.2.P.7 Container Closure System The information in this container closure system section provides a description of the container closure system used to store the drug product. For primary packaging (packaging that comes into contact with the material), the identity of the materials and their specifications should be provided for each packaging component. If appropriate, the specifications should include critical dimensions and drawings. Methods used to test the container closure system should be listed with the results. If the methods are noncompendial, validation data should also be included. The discussion should also contain information regarding the suitability of the choice of material with respect to any light or moisture protection that is needed, the compatibility of the drug product with the material, possible sorption to the container or leached materials from the container, and safety of the material. If nonfunctional secondary packaging is used, only a brief description is required; however, additional information should be provided for functional secondary packaging.

3.2.P.8 Stability The information in this stability section provides an overview of the stability program, including the testing schemes, assays, and results, that was used to establish the shelf life and in-use storage conditions (if applicable) for the drug product, including the formulated bulk, the filled material, and the marketed product. This section is further divided into three subsections. The first subsection (3.2.P.8.1) contains a summary of the stability program and includes the types of studies performed, the protocols that were followed, the results of the studies, and all conclusions concerning storage conditions, shelf life, and in-use storage conditions (if applicable). The stability studies described should include long-term, accelerated or stressed, and forced-degradation study types. The post-approval stability protocol and stability commitments are provided in the second subsection (3.2.P.8.2), and the results from all of the stability studies are provided in the third subsection (3.2.P.8.3). A graphic, tabular, narrative, or a combination of these formats can be used as appropriate for the data being discussed. This subsection should also discuss any analytical procedures used to generate the data and the methods used to validate those assays. If the assays and the validations have already been described in 3.2.P.5, a reference to the location of that discussion can be provided.

3.2.A.1 Facilities Appendix The information in the facilities appendix includes flow of personnel, raw materials, intermediates, and waste within the manufacturing facility; details about developmental or approved product that are manipulated or manufactured within the same facility; equipment and material preparation, cleaning, sterilization, and storage; and procedures and design features that prevent contamination or cross-contamination of areas and equipment. The information about equipment should include product contact and whether the equipment is dedicated or multiuse. In addition, information concerning rooms adjacent to the manufacturing areas should be presented if there is concern that activities in these areas may impact the integrity of the product.

3.2.A.2 Adventitious Agents The information in this section provides an assessment of risk of potential contamination from adventitious agents. Information from evaluation steps for the manufacturing steps intended to remove or inactivate viral contaminants should be provided in this section.

Nonviral adventitious agents include transmissible spongiform encephalopathy agents, bacteria, mycoplasma, and fungi. This section should include details for the avoidance and control of these types of agents. Certification and/or testing of raw materials and excipients are an example of information that can be provided. Another example is the control of the production process with respect to material, process, or agents.

Viral agent evaluation study data should be included in this section. The purpose of viral evaluation studies is to demonstrate that the approaches used to test, evaluate, and eliminate the potential risks are suitable and that the materials used in the manufacture are considered safe. For cell banks, viral cell bank qualification should be included in addition to information about the selection, testing, and assessment of cells for potential viral contamination. Detail of the virological tests (e.g., test type, sensitivity, specificity, frequency) and justification of the test selection should be provided. Results of unprocessed bulks testing, manufactured material testing, and viral clearance studies should also be provided.

3.2.A.3 Novel Excipients If a novel excipient is used in the formulation of the product, details about manufacturing, testing, and characterization may be provided in this section. Details should be sufficient for a thorough evaluation by the FDA for the appropriateness of this new excipient in this particular formulation.

3.2.R Regional Information Regional specific information regarding the drug substance or drug product belongs in this section. Examples of additional information requested by the FDA include executed batch records, method validation package, and comparability protocols.

New Information Required in the CTD Format When developing a new vaccine product, it is important to keep in mind that there are several types of information that are expected with the CTD-formatted dossiers. This "new information" includes details about drug substance manufacturing development (3.2.S.2.6), the container closure system for the drug substance (3.2.S.6), excipient details including the analytical procedures used to test the materials and the assay validation results (3.2.P.4), and a discussion of the control of critical steps and intermediates (3.2.S.2.4 and 3.2.P.3.4). For older products, minimal information may be available for some of these items. Data may need to be generated if an "older" excipient or drug substance is used for the new product being registered.

12.2.3.3 Literature References The literature reference section contains copies of all literature references that are cited in the body of the data.

12.2.4 Module 4: Nonclinical Study Reports

Module 4 provides safety data for the proposed vaccine and includes nonclinical pharmacology and toxicology study reports. There are three sections for Module 4 as follows:

4.1 Table of Contents
4.2 Nonclinical Study Reports
4.3 Literature References.

A brief discussion about the content for the Nonclinical Module is provided in the following sections and is based on information about Module 4 found in Guidance for Industry, *M4S: Safety (Nonclinical Information)*. Additional ICH guidance documents that can be referred to include the following:

M3: *Nonclinical Safety Studies for the Conduct of Human Clinical Trials for Pharmaceuticals* (November 1997)

S1C (R2): *Dose Selection for Carcinogenicity Studies of Pharmaceuticals* (September 2008)

S7A: *Safety Pharmacology Studies for Human Pharmaceuticals* (July 2001)

12.2.4.1 Table of Contents A TOC listing all of the data presented in Section 4.1 should be provided. If data are not being provided for all types of possible reports, there are two options. Either list all of the possible subsections and indicate that no data are provided or skip the numbers that are not used. Note that when certain study reports are not included in the application and numbers are skipped, the numbering system should not be changed or adjusted for missing numbers. The number is associated with the type of report. The 4.1 TOC should be used for the Module 4 section of the 2.1 TOC.

12.2.4.2 Nonclinical Study Reports The order in which the nonclinical study reports in Module 4 are provided is pharmacology (4.2.1), pharmacokinetics (4.2.2), and toxicology (4.2.3). Pharmacology study reports may include primary pharmacodynamics (4.2.1.1), secondary pharmacodynamics (4.2.1.2), safety pharmacology (4.2.1.3), and pharmacodynamic drug interactions with other drugs (4.2.1.4). Primary study reports contain data that demonstrate the effects that are related to the therapeutic indication and include pharmacodynamic ED_{50} in dose-ranging studies and mechanism of action if known. Secondary pharmacodynamics studies should be listed in order of clinical importance with respect to adverse effects or ancillary therapeutic effects. If data have been provided in a previous section, they do not have to be repeated but can be referenced.

Pharmacokinetics sections include analytical methods and validation reports (4.2.2.1), absorption (4.2.2.2), distribution (4.2.2.3), metabolism (4.2.2.4), excretion (4.2.2.5), pharmacokinetic drug interactions (nonclinical) (4.2.2.6), and other pharmacokinetic studies (4.2.2.7). Toxicology sections include single-dose toxicity in order by species and by route of administration (4.2.3.1), repeat-dose toxicity (4.2.3.2), *in vitro* and *in vivo* genotoxicity (4.2.3.3), carcinogenicity (4.2.3.4), reproductive and developmental toxicity for fertility and early embryonic development, embryo-fetal development, and prenatal and postnatal development (4.2.3.5), local tolerance (4.2.3.6), and other toxicity studies (4.2.3.7). Toxicology data are to be presented in a specified animal order (mouse, rat, hamster, other rodents, rabbit, dog, monkey, other nonrodent mammal(s), and nonmammals). The order of route of administration is the same within each animal (intended route of administration in male and then female animals, oral, intravenous, intramuscular, intraperitoneal, subcutaneous, inhalation topical, other *in vivo, in vitro*).

The following points should be considered while writing Module 4. All chemical names and structural formulas for drug substance, metabolites, and reference compounds should be clearly identified. All animal suppliers and strains should be specified. Good laboratory practices statements should be included in the safety reports (314.50(d)(2)(v) and 21 CFR Part 58).

12.2.4.3 Literature References The literature reference section contains copies of all literature references that are cited in the pharmacology and toxicology study reports.

12.2.5 Module 5: Clinical Study Reports

Module 5 provides efficacy data for the proposed vaccine and includes a tabular listing of all clinical studies, clinical study reports, and related information. There are four sections for Module 5:

5.1 Table of Contents for Clinical Study Reports and Related Information
5.2 Tabular Listing of all Clinical Studies
5.3 Clinical Study Reports and Related Information
5.4 Literature References.

A brief discussion about the content for the Clinical Module is provided in the following sections and is based on information about Module 5 found in Guidance for Industry, *M4E: Efficacy (Clinical Information)* and Guidance for Industry, *M-4: CTD—Efficacy Questions and Answers* (December 2004). Additional ICH guidance documents that can be referred to include:

E1A: *The Extent of Population Exposure to Assess Clinical Safety: For Drugs Intended for Long-Term Treatment of Non-Life-Threatening Conditions* (March 1995)
E2A: *Clinical Safety Data Management: Definitions and Standards for Expedited Reporting* (March 1995)
E3: *Structure and Content of Clinical Study Reports* (July 1996)
E4: *Dose–response Information to Support Drug Registration* (November 1994)
E5: *Ethnic Factors in the Acceptability of Foreign Clinical Data* (June 1998)
E7: *Studies in Support of Special Populations: Geriatrics* (August 1994)
E9: *Statistical Principles for Clinical Trials* (September 1998)
E10: *Choice of Control Group and Related Issues in Clinical Trials* (May 2000)
E11: *Clinical Investigation of Medicinal Products in the Pediatric Population* (December 2000).

12.2.5.1 Table of Contents A TOC listing all of the data presented in Section 5.1 should be provided. As discussed for Module 4, if data are not being provided for all types of reports, the option is to list all of the sections and indicate that no data is provided or to just skip those numbers where data were not generated. Sections should not be renumbered. The 5.1 TOC should be used for the Module 5 section of the 2.1 TOC.

12.2.5.2 Tabular Listing of all Clinical Studies A tabular listing of all clinical studies should be provided. For each clinical study, the information in the table should include the type of study, the study identifier, the location of the study report, study objective(s), study design and type of control, test product(s), dosage regimen, route of administration, number of participants, healthy patients or diagnosis of patients, duration of treatment, study status, and type of report.

12.2.5.3 Clinical Study Reports and Related Information The order in which the clinical study reports in Module 5 are provided is biopharmaceutic studies (5.3.1), studies pertinent to pharmacokinetics using human biomaterials (5.3.2), human pharmacokinetic studies (5.3.3), human pharmacodynamic studies (5.3.4), efficacy and safety studies (5.3.5), postmarketing experience (5.3.6), and case report forms (CRFs) and individual patient listings (5.3.7). The efficacy and safety studies section should contain study reports of controlled clinical studies pertinent to the claimed indication, study reports of uncontrolled clinical studies, and reports of analyses of data from more than one study (e.g., formal integrated analyses, meta-analyses, and bridging analyses).

The data analysis reports from more than one study include many types of analyses. If the ISE and ISS are longer than 400 pages, the full text may be placed in Section 5.3.5.3, with a shorter summary in Module 2.7. Items that may be included in the ISE include a summary combining the results of efficacy studies, a table of adequate and well-controlled and uncontrolled studies, a comparison and analysis of results of all controlled trials, results of uncontrolled studies, analyses of dose response information and of responses in subsets of overall population, and evidence of long-term effectiveness. For data from controlled studies, if the results are pooled, the statistical considerations should also be provided. Items that may be included in the ISS include a table of all investigations pertinent to safety, an overall extent of exposure, demographic and other characteristics of the study population, adverse experiences in clinical trials, clinical laboratory evaluations, a summary of adverse events (AEs) from all source, animal data, an analysis of dose response information, drug–drug interactions, drug–demographic and drug–disease interactions, pharmacological properties other than property of principal interest, and long-term and withdrawal effects.

The acceptance of non-US-controlled data is discussed in 21 CFR 314.106. The FDA should be consulted during the IND phase and at the pre-BLA meeting regarding the submission of non-US-generated data in the dossier. Foreign data must be applicable to US populations, and the data from the studies must reflect US medical practice. (Guidance for Industry, Acceptance of Foreign Clinical Studies, March 2001). There is also an ICH Guideline on the ethnic factors in the acceptability of foreign clinical data issued in 1998 that describes strategies for acceptance of foreign data using bridging studies and intrinsic and extrinsic ethnic differences.

In the initial submission, CRFs should be submitted for each patient who died during the clinical studies and for all patients who dropped out of the clinical study because of an AE. For the patients who dropped out because of AEs, the CRF should be provided even if the patient received a comparative drug or placebo. The FDA may request other CRFs during the review.

12.2.5.4 Literature References The literature reference section contains copies of all published articles, a copy of FDA meeting minutes, and other advice or guidance from regulatory agencies.

12.3 HINTS FOR PREPARING THE BIOLOGICAL LICENSING APPLICATION

While preparing dossiers for review by regulatory agencies, a useful philosophy is to prepare reviewer-friendly dossiers. A reviewer-friendly dossier can speed up the review of a document. Dossiers that are difficult to review are frequently set aside for another time. The bottom line is that the better written and more understandable a dossier is, the quicker the review, the faster the approval, and the sooner the product can get onto the market.

The following factors include a number of areas for consideration when compiling a dossier. These suggestions are based on experience from preparing dossiers that were received favorably by the FDA and that resulted in an approval of the proposed vaccine.

12.3.1 Dossier Organization

The overall organization of the dossier should *not* be altered. There should be strict adherence to the dossier organization as described in the Guidance Documents. Using the described dossier organization, the sponsor knows where the information should be inserted, and the agency reviewer knows where to look for the information. This approach saves time during the preparation and the review processes.

12.3.2 Reduce The "Annoyance Factor"

By submitting a dossier with a minimum of "annoyance factors," the review should go more smoothly. Reviewers may stop reviewing a document when they get frustrated. By reducing factors that annoy reviewers, the review period before they get frustrated may be longer, which can translate into a shorter overall review period. Annoying factors include, but are not limited to the following:

- **Avoid using company jargon.** Company jargon is any term or short-hand phrase/word that is used to describe a process, method, material, and so on. If the term is not used industry wide or cannot be found in a dictionary, change the term to a more generic description.
- **Format and organize tables and figures consistently.** Although it is not possible to have all tables or figures designed exactly the same, it is possible to standardize the look and content of tables and figures. When the same type of information is located in the same place on a table or figure, after reviewing just a couple of tables/figures, a reviewer will be able to quickly find the information.

- **Use proper English.** Avoid the use of fancy, impressive sounding terms. The reviewer will be impressed more by a readable document. For many reviewers, English is their second language. If there is a fancy term they do not know, they will have to stop their review and look up the term in the dictionary. It is a good idea to check a dictionary to make sure that the terms used actually mean what was intended.
- **Make terminology consistent.** The goal of a dossier should be a clear, readable document that accurately describes the vaccine under review. When terms are used consistently, the reviewer can easily follow from one section to another. If different terms are used for the same item or process, the reviewer will not necessarily make the connections that he or she should make without a much larger time investment in the review. While checking for consistency takes time up-front for an editor, it speeds up the review on the other side.
- **Reference guidance documents.** Carefully read the guidance documents and comply with page requirements, margin requirements, font size, and so on. These requirements are provided to ensure that the document is easy for the reviewer to read.
- **Define acronyms and abbreviations.** At a minimum, acronyms and abbreviations should be defined the first time they are used in a module.
- **Reference appropriate style guide.** Preparing a style guide before dossier preparation is highly recommended if your company does not have a company style guide. Having a consistent style provides less distraction for the reviewer.

12.3.3 Common CMC Issues

A number of issues have been reported as common problems found by the FDA during the licensing process. Although this list is not all inclusive, it will provide the types of areas that the FDA looks at closely. This list has been developed on the basis of the experience of numerous sponsors and comes from many marketing applications.

- Insufficient stability data on commercial drug product
- Questionable bioequivalence between clinical trial material and proposed commercial product
- Lack of preapproval inspection (PAI) readiness of sponsor
- Lack of PAI readiness of drug master or biological master file (DMF/BMF) holder
- Lack of adequate methods validation
- DMF/BMF deficiencies
- Impurity profile not properly defined
- Sensitivity of analytical methods
- Process scale-up changes

12.3.4 Some Pros and Cons of Electronic Submissions

When considering whether to file a paper or an electronic BLA, one key fact should be kept in mind—once eCTD, always eCTD. This statement basically means that if the original application is filed in eCTD format, everything filed after that, including response letters, must be filed electronically. For a large company that is committed to an eCTD path, the proper infrastructure needed to file and maintain eCTD dossiers can be set up and maintained. Smaller companies can contract with other companies that produce eCTD dossiers if they do not want to invest in the infrastructure themselves; however, this relationship will have to continue and may be more costly than the small company first realizes. The filing plans (paper or electronic) should be discussed with the project manager at the FDA.

Once a format (CTD vs eCTD) has been decided, it is important to find out the actual requirements for the CTD sections. There are subtle differences in the requirements for the file organization for the CTD and eCTD dossier versions. There can also be specific requirements for table and figure names and references depending on which software is used to produce the eCTD. It is important to find out all of the specific program requirements as soon as possible. Last minute changes to conform to software requirements can mean the difference between filing on the timeline and missing dates because of "fixing" formatting issues.

For more information about eCTD, see ICH guideline M2 EWG: *Electronic Common Technical Document Specifications* (February 2004).

REFERENCES

Web Sites

www.fda.gov/cder/guidance/index.htm

www.fda.gov/cber/guidance/index.htm

Guidance Documents

FDA Guidance for Industry for Quality

M4: *Organization of the CTD* (August 2001)

General Considerations for Submitting Marketing Applications According to the ICH/CTD format (August 2001)

M4Q: Quality (CMC Information) (August 2001)

M4: The CTD—Quality Questions and Answers/Location Issues (June 2004)

ICH Guidelines for Quality

Q1A (R2) *Stability Testing of New Drug Substances and Products* (February 2003)

Q1B *Photostability Testing of New Drug Substances and Products* (November 1996)

Q2 (R1) Validation of Analytical Procedures: Text and Methodology (October 1994/November 1996)

Q3A (R2) *Impurities in New Drug Substances* (October 2006)

Q3B (R2) *Impurities in New Drug Products* (June 2006)

Q3C (R5) *Impurities: Guideline for Residual Solvents* (February 2011)

Q5A (R1) *Viral Safety Evaluation of Biotechnology Products Derived From Cell Lines of Human or Animal Origin* (September 1999)

Q5B *Quality of Biotechnological Products: Analysis of the Expression Construct in Cells Used for Production of r-DNA Derived Protein Products* (November 1995)

Q5C *Quality of Biotechnological Products: Stability Testing of Biotechnological/Biological Products* (November 1995)

Q5D *Derivation and characterization of Cell Substrates Used for Production of Biotechnological/Biological Products* (July 1997)

Q6A *Specifications: Test Procedures and Acceptance Criteria for New Drug Substances and New Drug Products: Chemical Substances* (October 1999)

Q6B *Test Procedures and Acceptance Criteria for Biotechnological/Biological Products* (March 1999)

FDA Guidance for Industry for Safety

M4S: Safety (Nonclinical Information) (August 2001)

ICH Guidelines for Safety

M3: *Nonclinical Safety Studies for the Conduct of Human Clinical Trials for Pharmaceuticals* (November 1997)

S1C (R2): *Dose Selection for Carcinogenicity Studies of Pharmaceuticals* (September 2008)

S7: *Safety Pharmacology Studies for Human Pharmaceuticals* (August 2000)

FDA Guidance for Industry for Efficacy

M4E: Efficacy (Clinical Information), (August 2001)

ICH Guidelines for Efficacy

E1A: *The Extent of Population Exposure to Assess Clinical Safety: For Drugs Intended for Long-Term Treatment of Non-Life-Threatening Conditions* (March 1995)

E2A: *Clinical Safety Data Management: Definitions and Standards for Expedited Reporting* (March 1995)

E3: *Structure and Content of Clinical Study Reports* (July 1996)

E4: *Dose–response Information to Support Drug Registration* (November 1994)

E5: *Ethnic Factors in the Acceptability of Foreign Clinical Data* (June 1998)

E7: *Studies in Support of Special Populations: Geriatrics* (August 1994)

E9: *Statistical Principles for Clinical Trials* (September 1998)

E10: *Choice of Control Group and Related Issues in Clinical Trials* (May 2000)

E11: *Clinical Investigation of Medicinal Products in the Pediatric Population* (December 2000)

ICH Guidelines for Electronic Submissions

M2 EWG: *Electronic Common Technical Document Specifications* (February 2004)

OTHER USEFUL REFERENCES

Uniform Requirements for Manuscripts Submitted to Biomedical Journals, International Committee of Medical Journal Editors (ICMJE), current edition.

13

THE ORIGINAL NEW DRUG APPLICATION (INVESTIGATIONAL NEW DRUG)

R.S. Robin Robinett
Merck & Co., Inc., West Point, PA, USA

13.1 INTRODUCTION

Pharmaceutical product development has three phases: discovery, development, and commercialization. In the discovery phase, basic research is conducted on the molecule of interest, and those study materials are tested in preclinical studies in animals. Once the safety of the study material has been sufficiently demonstrated in animals, the program moves on to the development phase where the study material (clinical material or clinical supplies) is tested in humans. Finally, when the safety and efficacy have been established in human, the program moves on to the commercialization phase where a marketing application is submitted, and material is launched once approval is obtained.

The purpose of an investigational new drug (IND) application (21 Code of Federal Register (CFR) 312) is to seek permission from the Food and Drug Administration (FDA) to test a new pharmaceutical, vaccine, or biologic in the development stage in humans. Investigational new drugs must be submitted whenever clinical studies are initiated on a new vaccine in the United States, when a new indication is being investigated, or when a different route of administration for an already approved vaccine is desired. Data are required to support the start of a clinical trial in humans. Sources for this data include nonclinical animal studies and clinical studies conducted in earlier developmental phases, in other countries, and for other indications.

Vaccine Development and Manufacturing, First Edition.
Edited by Emily P. Wen, Ronald Ellis, and Narahari S. Pujar.

There are three clinical phases in the development stage. Phase 1 clinical trials are the first-time dosing conducted in humans. The purpose of Phase 1 clinical trials is to determine safety and dosage, and it uses a test population of 20–100 healthy volunteers. Phase 2 clinical trials are the first controlled studies in patients. The purpose of Phase 2 clinical trials is to evaluate the effectiveness of the drug and to monitor it for potential side effects. A test population of 100–200 patient volunteers is used. Phase 2 clinical trials can be divided into Phase 2A and Phase 2B. In Phase 2A clinical trials, patients are first exposed to the drug, and the response in those patients is monitored. The dose-response study completion and the initial efficacy and safety determination in patients are the purposes of the Phase 2B clinical trials. Phase 3 clinical trials include expanded controlled and uncontrolled studies in patients (pivotal trials); pharmacokinetic studies looking at absorption, distribution, metabolism, and excretion; and bioavailability and bioequivalence studies that are intended to show very similar blood levels of an active drug from different formulations.

Clinical studies typically begin with Phase 1. As the development of the potential drug continues and the program moves from Phase 1 to Phase 3, more information about the test material becomes available, and changes in the manufacturing and testing occur as the process develops. The level of detail required for each phase reflects the type of data that should be available for the product at that point in development.

The information that is required for inclusion in an IND is mandated by the FDA IND guidelines, and the requirements are found in 21 CFR. The requirements are product specific and can vary with FDA reviewing division and the clinical indication. Other guidelines and guidance documents with the Center for Biological Evaluation and Review (CBER)-related and the Center for Drug Evaluation and Review (CDER)-related regulations can be found on the FDA websites at: www.fda.gov/cder/guidance/index.html and www.fda.gov/cber/guidance/index.htm. A list of FDA guidelines can be found in Appendix 1 at http://www.fda.gov/cber/pubinfo/roboguide.pdf.

13.2 FORMAT FOR SUBMITTING AN IND

Investigational new drugs are submitted in a format known as the Common Technical Document (CTD). The CTD format was originally developed for marketing applications and is a harmonized table of content (TOC) that is the result of an International Conference of Harmonization (ICH) committee. The ICH undertook the harmonization of technical requirements between Japan, Europe, and the United States to avoid the necessity of generating completely different dossiers in these regions. The CTD guidance documents address format only. Scientific and technical content and requirements are covered by the ICH Technical Guidelines (Q, S, and E). ICH Guidance Documents include the following:

M4: Organization of the CTD

M4Q: Quality (chemistry, manufacturing, and control (CMC) Information)

M4S: Safety (Nonclinical Information)

M4E: Efficacy (Clinical Information).

Information in the CTD format is organized as follows:

Module 1	Regional Administrative Information.
Module 2.1	CTD Table of Contents.
Module 2.2	CTD Introduction.
Module 2.3	Quality Overall Summary.
Module 2.4	Nonclinical Overview.
Module 2.5	Clinical Overview.
Module 2.6	Nonclinical Written and Tabulated Summary.
Module 2.7	Clinical Summary.
Module 3	Quality (Chemistry, Manufacturing, and Control).
Module 4	Nonclinical Study Reports.
Module 5	Clinical Study Reports.

The CTD format has been adapted for IND submissions. Because much of the information required for a marketing application is generated during the IND phase, some sections of the CTD may have minimal or no information. If a section does not apply to the IND phase, it either can be kept with a note that information is not available at this time or can be skipped. If a section is skipped, it is important that the section numbering not be changed to eliminate a "skip" in the numbering system. The numbering system is associated with the information that is found in that section. This numbering scheme is an advantage to the applicant because it streamlines preparation of the dossier and the dossier review by the FDA. Since the location of information is specified, the FDA reviewers can easily find the information they need because the location of information is consistent across all companies.

13.3 DETAILED DISCUSSION OF INFORMATION REQUIRED IN THE CHEMISTRY MANUFACTURING AND CONTROL SECTIONS

The CMC section of the IND application discusses the materials that are used in the manufacture of the study vaccine (clinical supplies), how the material is made, and what testing is performed on the material. This is a very important section and is looked at closely by the FDA. The FDA wants assurance that the study material is manufactured in a manner that produces a quality product that is safe.

For clinical studies that include a placebo or a comparator arm, information about the composition, manufacture, packaging, labels, testing, and stability of that placebo/comparator must be included. If a diluent is required to reconstitute a lyophilized vaccine, similar information for that diluent must also be included. The investigational labeling for these materials must also be provided in the application.

An environmental assessment is required by 21 CFR Part 25. Investigational new drugs are usually categorically excluded from the environmental assessment requirements on the basis of low environmental burden. Although INDs typically qualify for the exclusion, the sponsor must request the exclusion.

13.3.1 MODULE 3: CHEMISTRY, MANUFACTURING, AND CONTROL IN COMMON TECHNICAL DOCUMENT FORMAT

The CTD format makes it easy to organize the CMC material because this format has specific locations for all types of information. The detailed outline of the quality information provided in Module 3 is organized as follows:

Module 3.1	**Table of Contents**
Module 3.2.S	**Drug Substance**
Module 3.2.S.1	General Information
Module 3.2.S.2	Manufacture
Module 3.2.S.3	Characterization
Module 3.2.S.4	Control of Drug Substance
Module 3.2.S.5	Reference Standards or Materials
Module 3.2.S.6	Container Closure System
Module 3.2.S.7	Stability
Module 3.2.P	**Drug Product**
Module 3.2.P.1	Description and Composition of Drug Product
Module 3.2.P.2	Pharmaceutical Development
Module 3.2.P.3	Manufacture
Module 3.2.P.4	Control of Excipients
Module 3.2.P.5	Control of Drug Product
Module 3.2.P.6	Reference Standards or Materials
Module 3.2.P.7	Container Closure System
Module 3.2.P.8	Stability
Module 3.2.A	**Appendices**
Module 3.2.A.1	Facilities and Equipment
Module 3.2.A.2	Adventitious Agents Safety Evaluation
Module 3.2.A.3	Novel Excipients
Module 3.3	**References**

The type of information that should be included in the IND sections is based on the phase of the clinical trial. A discussion of level of detail for each of these items is found later in this chapter. If information is not available or not relevant for a particular product, those sections are not included. The numbering system does not change even when one or more sections are not needed.

13.3.2 Level of Investigational New Drug Detail For Different Clinical Phases

Guidelines are available that describe the information that should be provided in an IND. The level of detail is dependent on the Phase (1, 2, or 3) of the clinical trial. For more information about information required in the CMC section, see the following FDA Guidance for Industry documents:

- *Content and Format of Investigational New Drug Applications (INDs) for Phase 1 Studies of Drug* (November 1995)

- *INDs for Phase 2 and 3 Studies, Chemistry, Manufacturing and Controls Information* (May 2003)
- *Guideline on Submitting Documentation for the Manufacture of and Controls for Drug Products* (February 1987)
- *Guideline on the Preparation of Investigational New Drug Products* (1991) http://www.fda.gov/downloads/Drugs/GuidanceComplianceRegulatory Information/Guidances/ucm070315.pdf
- *CGMP for Phase 1 Investigational Drugs* (July 2008)
- *Drug Product Chemistry, Manufacturing and Controls Information* (January 2001).

Also useful are the ICH Guidelines:

Q1A (R2) *Stability Testing of New Drug Substances and Products* (February 2003)

Q1B *Photostability Testing of New Drug Substances and Products* (November 1996)

Q1D *Bracketing and Matrixing Designs for Stability Testing of New Drug Substances and Products* (February 2002)

Q1E *Evaluation for Stability Data* (February 2003)

Q2 (R1) Validation of Analytical Procedures: Text and Methodology (October 1994/November 1996)

Q3A (R2) *Impurities in New Drug Substances* (October 2006)

Q3B (R2) *Impurities in New Drug Products* (June 2006)

Q3C (R5) *Impurities: Guideline for Residual Solvents* (February 2011)

Q5A (R1) *Viral Safety Evaluation of Biotechnology Products Derived From Cell Lines of Human or Animal Origin* (September 1999)

Q5B *Quality of Biotechnological Products: Analysis of the Expression Construct in Cells Used for Production of r-DNA Derived Protein Products* (November 1995)

Q5C *Quality of Biotechnological Products: Stability Testing of Biotechnological/Biological Products* (November 1995)

Q5D *Derivation and characterization of Cell Substrates Used for Production of Biotechnological/Biological Products* (July 1997)

Q6A *Specifications: Test Procedures and Acceptance Criteria for New Drug Substances and New Drug Products: Chemical Substances* (October 1999)

Q6B *Test Procedures and Acceptance Criteria for Biotechnological/Biological Products* (March 1999)

Q7 *Good Manufacturing Practice Guide for Active Pharmaceutical Ingredients* (November 2000).

The CFR describes requirements for the IND, and a copy is available at: http://www.gpoaccess.gov/cfr/index.html. Most of the information in the CFR relevant to drugs and biologicals for human health are found in Parts 200–299 and Parts 600–699. The following excerpt from the Title 21 index provides locations for specific information. The shaded areas may be of particular interest when writing the IND.

Title 21 Food and Drugs

Title 21 Food and Drugs	
Chapter I—Food and Drug Administration, Department of Health and Human Services	
Part	
200	General
201	Labeling
202	Prescription drug advertising
203	Prescription drug marketing
205	Guidelines for State licensing of wholesale prescription drug distributors
206	Imprinting of solid oral dosage form drug products for human use
207	Registration of producers of drugs and listing of drugs in commercial distribution
208	Medication Guides for prescription drug products
209	Requirement for authorized dispensers and pharmacies to distribute a side effects statement
210	Current good manufacturing practice in manufacturing, processing, packing, or holding of drugs; general
211	Current good manufacturing practice for finished pharmaceuticals
216	Pharmacy compounding
225	Current good manufacturing practice for medicated feeds
226	Current good manufacturing practice for Type A medicated articles
250	Special requirements for specific human drugs
290	Controlled drugs
299	Drugs; official names and established names
600	Biological Products: general
601	Licensing
606	Current good manufacturing practice for blood and blood components
607	Establishment registration and product listing for manufacturers of human blood and blood products
610	General biological products standards
640	Additional standards for human blood and blood products
660	Additional standards for diagnostic substances for laboratory tests
680	Additional standards for miscellaneous products

A detailed description of the information required for the CMC section of the IND is provided.

13.3.2.1 Introduction (3.1) The introduction includes information concerning the chemistry and manufacturing differences between the drug product intended for clinical use and the materials that were used in the toxicology studies. This discussion should also include the potential effects that the process changes may have on drug product safety. For Phase 2 and 3 INDs, differences between the material used in the previous and current phases should be included. It is also recommended that a summary of changes since the previous submission be included. Finally, if any information from the previous submission has changed, that information needs to be updated.

13.3.2.2 Drug Substances (3.2.S)

General Information (3.2.S.1) All names used to describe the drug substance including generic, compendial, company, or other nonproprietary names are provided in the general information section. For biological-based pharmaceuticals or vaccines, the biological activity should be discussed, as well as information relevant to the type of biologic that is being used and the method of structural elucidation. Viral-based vaccines should include information concerning virus state (live or inactivated) and the viral type and family. Protein- or polypeptide-based vaccines should include information about the amino acid sequence and the type and location of any post-translational modifications. Nucleic-acid-based vaccines should include information on the protein coded for, the vector, and the nucleic acid of the inserted sequence. Polysaccharide-based vaccines should include information on the structure, any modifications, and the source. Gene therapy vaccines should include information about the vector and inserted gene sequence. Reference standard preparation and characterization data should also be included for all reference standards. For both Phase 2 and 3 INDs, any additional information about the active molecule that has been determined since the previous submission should be added.

Manufacture (3.2.S.2) For biologic-based products such as vaccines, the process is usually an integral part of the definition of the product. The biological process typically starts with fermentation or cell culture, and this process produces either cell-associated (pellet is the source of the drug substance molecule, some type of cell disruption is needed) or secreted molecules (supernatant is the source of the drug substance molecule). Purification steps may be necessary to remove medium components (e.g., BSA), processing materials (e.g., protease, detergents, chemical agents to disrupt membranes), cellular by-products (e.g., DNA, RNA, lipids, proteins), or post-translational modification reagents. The materials and processes used to manufacture the study material are described in this section.

Manufacturer (3.2.S.2.1) The name and address of the manufacturing and testing (quality control or QC) sites for the drug substance are provided in this subsection. If a contract manufacturing organization (CMO) was used to make any part of the drug substance, their name, addresses, and function should be explained. Changes in any site should be reported in the Phase 2 or 3 IND. For Phase 3 material, it is recommended that the intended commercial manufacturing sites be used if possible.

If this is not possible, additional work may be required to demonstrate equivalency of material produced between the different sites.

Description of Manufacturing Process and Process Controls (3.2.S.2.2) For biologic-based products, the manufacturing process section includes descriptions of the cell banks, seeds, culture media, additives, and manipulations used in the processes. A written process description including appropriate parameters, sequence of steps, and equipment should be provided for the harvests, purification processes, modification reactions, filling, storage, and shipping activities. The batch size and scale of manufacture should also be included. If pooling at any step is allowed, the requirements for pooling should be detailed. A flow diagram with the material inputs, critical steps, and process controls is a useful tool for the reviewer.

For a Phase 2 IND, the process description provided at Phase 1 should be updated with more details, including acceptance criteria for critical process steps and complex materials. Flow diagrams should also be updated with the additional information. If required, update the section with reprocessing information for virus/impurity clearance.

Flow diagrams in a Phase 3 IND should include batch size ranges, ratios of reagents, process control procedures, critical step identity, intermediate controls, and literature references. The step-by-step process description, including the reprocessing description, should be updated with detailed information. If there are changes in the drug substance sterilization process (e.g., terminal to aseptic processing), those changes should also be detailed. It is recommended at Phase 3 that the processes used to make material for the clinical studies is as close to the intended commercial process as possible but can be manufactured using a minimum scale. The validation of aseptic processes does not need to be submitted for an IND.

Control of Material (3.2.S.2.3) The control of materials section includes information on the starting materials; a list of the origin and source of viruses, bacteria, fermentation, and cell culture materials; and compendial grade or testing performed for all materials. For materials of human or animal origin, details about the source, manufacturer, and characterization should be provided. In Phase 2, specifications for the starting materials should be available and included in the IND. The Phase 3 IND should include updates on starting material specifications, reference quality standard for each material, and tests performed on receipt for all starting materials. In addition, information on the origin of the fermentation product or natural substances should be provided if not previously submitted.

Control of Critical Steps (3.2.S.2.4) Key process steps are typically not identified until later in process development. In Phase 3, the tentative key process steps should be identified and listed in the IND. If assay descriptions for process monitoring are not provided in 3.2.S.4, they should be provided in this section.

Process Validation (3.2.S.2.5) There is no process validation requirement listed for Phase 1, 2, or 3 INDs. For Phase 3, plans for the process validation may be included.

Development (3.2.S.2.6) Drug substance process development performed since the manufacture of the previous material should be summarized. In addition to text describing the changes, a table or figure highlighting the changes is recommended as a reviewer aid. For Phase 1 INDs, this discussion would include manufacturing development and process changes since the manufacture of the safety assessment material. For Phase 2 and 3 INDs, manufacturing changes since the manufacture of the previous phase material should also be included.

Characterization (3.2.S.3) The characterization section includes information about structure, activity, characterization, and impurities.

Elucidation of Structure and Other Characteristics (3.2.S.3.1) A discussion of the elucidation details of the drug substance structure and characterization is provided in this subsection. Characterization information may include biological activity, sequence or structure (primary and higher order), and physiological and immunochemical properties. The actual type of information provided dependents on the class of biological from which the active ingredient is composed. Information for protein- or polypeptide-based vaccines includes post-translational modification and purity, whereas nucleic-acid-based vaccines would include the DNA or RNA sequence. Viral-based vaccines would include whether the virus was active, inactive, or attenuated. For Phase 2, any updated characterization information is provided. A summary of the reference standard characterization data should also be provided. Analytical procedures used to characterize primary reference standards should be provided at Phase 3.

Impurities (3.2.S.3.2) Information on process-related impurities and contaminants should be included with the Phase 1 IND. As changes are made to the manufacturing processes for Phase 2 and 3, this subsection should be updated to include the additional impurities identification and qualification data. If additional data on product-related impurities and degradation products are available, that information should also be added.

Control of Drug Substance (3.2.S.4) The control of drug substance section lists the release specifications, specification justification, and assay procedures used for testing the drug substance, intermediates, and in-process samples. Compendial compliance information for the assay procedures should also be included.

Specifications (3.2.S.4.1) Proposed acceptance limits for test intermediates, drug substance, and in-process samples are provided in this subsection. For the Phase 2 IND, updated specifications should be provided. In Phase 3, a detailed listing of specifications should be available.

Analytical Procedures (3.2.S.4.2) Descriptions of the analytical methods used to test intermediates, drug substance, and in-process samples are provided in this subsection. The compendial compliance of these methods should also be described. For Phase 2 and 3 INDs, information on changes to analytical procedures and descriptions of additional testing should be included.

Validation of Analytical Procedures (3.2.S.4.3) Submission of method validation reports is not required for Phase 1 or 2 INDs. The method validation data should be included with the Phase 3 IND, especially for potency assays.

Batch Analyses (3.2.S.4.4) For Phase 1, 2, or 3 INDs, batch analysis data should be included for all drug substance lots used to manufacture the drug product lots reported in the drug product stability section (3.2.P.8). These lots would include the drug product materials that will be used in the clinical trial and lots used to establish stability.

Justification of Specifications (3.2.S.4.5) Information on setting specifications should be provided as it becomes available.

Reference Standards and Materials (3.2.S.5) Details about the reference standards used for potency testing should be provided, including details about material preparation and purification. In Phase 2, the expectation is that progress is being made toward establishing a well-characterized primary standard (if not already available). If a primary standard is not yet available, a working standard relative to typical drug substance batch should be qualified, and that data should be submitted. In Phase 3, the information to establish primary standards should be provided if not submitted yet. In addition, if not already provided, a description of the preparation and purification of the primary and working standards should be submitted in addition to a description of the methods used to qualify the primary and working standards.

Container Closure Systems (3.2.S.6) A description of the container closure system used to store the drug substance should be discussed. For Phase 2 and 3, a summary of container closure system should be included if not already provided. If the data have been provided previously, updated information should be included if changes were made to container closure system. In Phase 3, methods to ensure container closure integrity should be included, as well as extractable data from the container surfaces. In addition, a summary of studies performed to support choice of packaging should be included.

Stability (3.2.S.7) Stability studies are performed to establish that the material being studied in clinical trials will be stable from the beginning of the manufacturing process through the end of the clinical trial. This section should include material storage conditions, stability study protocols, and stability study results for all relevant stability studies. Information on analytical procedures used to generate the data should also be provided if not already described in Section 3.2.S.4.

In Phase 2, a detailed stability plan (i.e., tests performed, acceptance criteria, test stations, storage conditions, and study duration) should be provided. Updated stability data tables for Phase 1 clinical trials supplies should also be included.

For Phase 3, updated stability data tables and summary information for development batches evaluated to date should be provided in addition to any additional information from stress and/or accelerated stability studies. The sponsor should also consider submitting the stability protocols for stability studies that will be used to support the BLA.

13.3.2.3 Drug Product (3.2.P) Recommendations for drug product sections cover information to be submitted for drug product, placebo, product-specific diluent, and reference products (comparators) that will be used in the proposed clinical studies.

Description and Composition of the Drug Product (3.2.P.1) The components and quantitative composition for dosage form(s) should be provided in this section. These details include a list of the drug substances (i.e., active ingredient (AI), the excipients used in the formulation, the quantity of all components per unit (e.g., per tablet, per capsule, per milliliter), and the quantity of each component in each batch. The quality (e.g., USP/NF) should be included for each component. If the product requires a reconstituting diluent or if there is a placebo or comparator for the clinical trial, the composition of those materials should also be provided. Diluent, placebo, and/or comparators should have complete but separate drug product sections. For Phase 2 and 3 INDs, changes made to the formulation and updated formulation and composition (per unit quantity) information should be included. If the drug product formulation is delivered by devices (e.g., MDIs, DPIs), ensure that the devices are comparable to the intended commercial product. This is especially important for Phase 2 dose-ranging studies and Phase 3 clinical trials.

Pharmaceutical Development (3.2.P.2) Drug product manufacturing process and formulation development performed since the manufacture of the previous material should be summarized. In addition to text describing the changes, a table or figure highlighting the changes is recommended as a reviewer aid. For Phase 1 INDs, this discussion would include manufacturing development, process changes, and formulation updates since the manufacture of the safety assessment materials. For Phase 2 and 3 INDs, manufacturing, process, and formulation changes since the manufacture of the previous phase material should also be included.

Manufacturing Process and Controls (3.2.P.3) The materials and processes used to formulate and fill the study material (including the manufacturing, packaging, and labeling site information) are described in this section. This information would also need to be included for a diluent (for lyophilized products), placebo, or comparator if applicable.

Manufacturer (3.2.P.3.1) The name and address of the manufacturer, the contract packager or labeler, and any contract QC laboratories should be listed. If there are changes to the manufacturing or QC testing site for Phase 2 or 3 clinical supplies, the updated information should be submitted with the Phase 2 or 3 IND. In addition to the manufacturing and QC testing sites, packaging and stability sample storage site information should be included with the Phase 3 IND.

Batch Formula (3.2.P.3.2) A quantitative composition including reasonable ranges should be provided in the batch formula subsection. For Phase 2, a representative batch formula including ingredients should be provided. If manufacturing flexibility is desired, a representative range in batch sizes may be shown. In Phase 3, batch formula for all strengths to be used in the clinical trials, including the diluent, placebo, and/or comparator should be provided. In addition, if there is any additional information that can support the Phase 2 or 3 studies, that information should be included as well.

Manufacturing Process/Process Controls (3.2.P.3.3) A brief written process description should be provided along with a process flow diagram in this subsection. Manufacturing details for the drug product formulation, filling, and packaging must be included. These details should include the equipment used, the process steps, any provisions for reprocessing (if allowed), and packaging details (e.g., bottle size, material). The description for the Phase 2 IND should include step-by-step unit operation process descriptions, including appropriate parameters, sequence of steps, packaging, and scale. If there are process changes for the manufacture of Phase 2 clinical supplies, an updated flow diagram with material inputs, critical steps, and process controls and description should be included. In addition to updated flow diagrams and process descriptions for the Phase 3 IND, a brief description of packaging and labeling operations and an update with any changes to the sterilization process (if applicable) should be added.

Control of Critical Steps (3.2.P.3.4) Key process steps are typically not identified until later in process development. In Phase 3, the tentative key process steps should be identified and listed in the IND. If assay descriptions for process monitoring are not provided in 3.2.S.4 or 3.2.P.5, they should be provided in this section.

Process Validation (3.2.P.3.5) There is no process validation requirement listed for Phase 1, 2, or 3 INDs; however, sterility assurance validation is required but the data are not submitted. For Phase 3, plans for the process validation may be included.

Control of Excipients (3.2.P.4) Although there are no requirements listed, if an excipient is noncompendial, the control information (Certificate of Analysis) is typically included. If a novel excipient is used in the drug product formulation, the details should be provided.

In Phase 2, a list of testing and specifications for noncompendial excipients should be submitted if not previously provided. If a novel excipient is used, information should be provided, which is consistent with level of detail typically submitted for drug substance. For the Phase 3 INDs, testing performed beyond those specified in a compendium should be described if applicable.

Control of Manufactured Material (3.2.P.5) The control of manufactured material section lists the release specifications, specification justification, and assay procedures used for testing intermediates and drug product. This information would also need to be included for a diluent (for lyophilized products), placebo, or comparator if applicable. Compendial compliance information for the assay procedures should also be included.

Specifications (3.2.P.5.1) Proposed acceptance limits for intermediates, drug product, and placebo are provided in this subsection. In addition, for sterile parenteral drug product, data demonstrating sterility and apyrogenicity should be included to address these safety issues. For the Phase 2 IND, updated specifications should be provided. In Phase 3, a detailed listing of specifications should be available.

Analytical Procedures (3.2.P.5.2) Descriptions of the analytical methods used to test intermediates, drug product, and placebo are provided in the subsection. The compendial compliance of these methods should also be commented on. For Phase 2 and 3 INDs, information on changes to analytical procedures and descriptions of additional testing should be included.

Validation of Analytical Procedures (3.2.P.5.3) Submission of method validation reports is not required for Phase 1 or 2 INDs. The method validation data should be included with the Phase 3 IND, especially for potency assays.

Batch Analyses (3.2.P.5.4) Batch analysis data to support specification and stability and batch analysis for lots that are associated with the clinical supplies should be included with Phase 1, 2, or 3 INDs.

Justification of Specifications (3.2.P.5.5) Details concerning setting specifications should be provided as it becomes available.

Impurities Characterization (3.2.P.5.6) Information on impurities introduced as a result of the DP formulation is discussed in this subsection. For Phase 2 and 3 INDs, updates with results of studies on impurities/degradation products characterization should be included. For Phase 2, impurity qualification should be discussed with the data being provided in the Phase 3 IND. In Phase 3, specifications and validation of impurities method(s) should also be provided. The material used in pivotal clinical studies should be representative of the purity of the intended commercial material.

Reference Standards (3.2.P.6) For a Phase 1 IND, there is no requirement for information. For Phase 2 and 3 INDs, information should be provided on the reference standards if there are reference standards in addition to those described in the drug substance section (3.2.S.5).

Container Closure System (3.2.P.7) Although there are no requirements to provide information in a Phase 1 IND, it is recommended that a description and the initial specification of the container used to fill the material should be included in this subsection. The specifications should contain the components, material of construction, and the dimensions. For a Phase 2 IND, a brief description of the container closure system should be provided if it was not included in the Phase 1 IND. For Phase 2 and 3 INDs, specifications should be updated if additional information is available or if any component of the container closure system has changed. If a special delivery system will be used for the drug product, the delivery device should match intended commercial container closure in Phase 3.

Stability (3.2.P.8) Stability studies are performed to establish that the material being studied in clinical trials will be stable through the end of the clinical trial. The storage conditions for the drug product should be listed, as well as a brief description of stability study and assay procedures. For a Phase 1 IND, the data typically provided includes 1-month long-term stability and some accelerated stability data. Data may only be available for one batch.

In Phase 2, a detailed stability plan (i.e., tests performed, acceptance criteria, test stations, storage conditions, and study duration) should be provided. The studies should minimally cover the clinical study duration. If the expiry dating for the drug product is update on the basis of stability data, that new dating should be reported. If applicable, stability data for reconstituted drug product should also be included. If administration aids are used, data as appropriate to demonstrate compatibility with those administration aids should be provided.

For Phase 3, specifications and methods should be updated. Stability data from development batches should be provided, as well as summary information for drug product batches evaluated in stability studies. The study duration should minimally cover the clinical study duration. For a new formulation, site of manufacture or packaging configuration provides at least 3 months of stability data from a representative batch. If the drug product expiry dating is updated on the basis of stability data, the new dating should be reported. Updated data for reconstituted drug product and compatibility with administration aids as applicable should also be provided. The sponsor should also consider submitting ICH stability protocol and overall plan to support the New Drug Application (NDA) or Biologics License Application (BLA) for FDA review and comment.

13.3.2.4 Appendices (3.2.A)

Facilities and Equipment (3.2.A.1) Information on facility and equipment should be included for biotechnology products. This information will change for Phase 2 and 3 if the facilities to manufacture the material are changed with scale-up.

Adventitious Agents (3.2.A.2) If raw materials of human or animal origin were used in the manufacture of the drug substance or the drug product, information about viral testing of these materials should be provided in this section. Additional information can be added to Phase 2 and 3 INDs as it becomes available.

Novel Excipients (3.2.A.3) If novel excipients are used in the formulation of drug product, information about that material is provided in this section.

13.4 GENERAL OVERVIEW OF INFORMATION REQUIRED IN THE REGIONAL, NONCLINICAL, AND CLINICAL ITEMS

Formatting IND information in the CTD format started in around 2005. If there are any questions about where reviewing groups expect to find specific information, discuss this issue with the FDA project manager. The following recommendations for placement of information into the CTD format is based on logical placement of the information based on the descriptions of these sections for a marketing application.

13.4.1 Module 1: Regional Information

The cover letter and Form FDA 1571 are included in Module 1. A Form FDA 1571 is required for all IND submissions, including the original IND and is required to make the contract with the FDA legal. Information on Form FDA 1571 includes sponsor name, address, and telephone number; IND number; name of vaccine and the indication; the phase of clinical investigation covered by the IND; a list of all IND and product license applications associated with the drug; the IND serial number; the type of submission (original IND or amendment type); contents of the application; the name and title of the person responsible for monitoring the conduct and progress of the clinical investigation; the name(s) and title of the person responsible for review and evaluation of information relevant to the safety of the drug; and the name, address, and phone number of the name of the sponsor or sponsor authorized representative.

Environmental assessment and categorical exclusion information and labeling information are provided in Module 1. A copy of the official FDA pre-IND meeting minutes should also be included. If any information provided in the IND has been translated to English from another language, Module 1 is the location where the details about that translation, including the translation certification, should be placed. In addition, if there is radiolabeling of the product, that information would also be located in Module 1.

13.4.2 Module 2: Common Technical Document Summaries

13.4.2.1 Table of Contents The TOC is a useful tool for the FDA reviewer. It gives an overview of the information found in the dossier, as well as insight into the dossier organization. To facilitate the review, the TOC should be clear, concise, and reviewer friendly. The level of details should be sufficient so that the reviewers can easily find the information they are looking for.

13.4.2.2 Introductory Statement The information in the introductory statement is very important because this may be the reviewer's first experience with the drug being considered for a clinical trial. The general information to be included in this section includes the name of the drug, the active pharmaceutical ingredient(s), the pharmacological class, the structural formula, the formulation, the dosage, and the route of administration. In addition, there should be a discussion of the broad objectives and the planned duration for the proposed clinical studies. If the active ingredient or product formulation was previously studied in humans outside the United States, a brief summary of those studies should be included. If there were other United States studies using a different formulation or for a different indication, a reference to those INDs, NDA, or BLA should be provided. Finally, if any non-U.S. regulatory actions are associated with the drug or any safety concerns are known, that information should be included.

13.4.3 Module 4: Nonclinical Pharmacology and Toxicology

The first section should be a summary of animal pharmacological, pharmacokinetics, and toxicological studies that support the clinical development of the compound. The identification and qualifications of individuals who evaluated animal safety data should be appended to the written summary. The signature on the written summary attests to the accuracy of the data and the safe passage in man. Individual study reports should follow the written summary.

The pharmacology section should include a description of the pharmacological effects, the mechanisms of action, primary and secondary pharmacodynamics, and results from safety pharmacology studies. Include data from all studies (*in vitro* and *in vivo*) that have been performed, even data from "uncontrolled" laboratory studies. The potential relevance of this data to humans should be explored.

The animal pharmacokinetics section should include absorption, distribution, metabolism, and excretion information for the animal models. Information on the analytical methods used to quantify systemic levels of parent compounds and metabolites should be provided. If applicable, oral bioavailability before initiating toxicity studies, topical absorption data, and drug–drug interaction data should be discussed. Finally, the section should contain a review of all nonclinical pharmacokinetic data.

The toxicology section includes study reports and a discussion of the various types of toxicology studies performed (e.g., acute, subacute, special studies, chronic, genotoxicity, carcinogenicity, reproduction, and toxicokinetic). The toxicology report includes a description of the trial design, the dates when the studies were conducted, the location where the studies were performed and where the records are kept, a GLP-compliance statement, a systematic presentation of findings from the animal toxicology and toxicokinetic studies, and full data tabulations for each toxicology study that is intended to support safety of the proposed clinical trial.

There are eight potential types of toxicology data that may be included in an IND. An acute toxicity study includes one or more doses administered over a period until 24 hours, subacute or subchronic studies are designed to reflect the intended clinical use and typically have a duration of up to 3 months, and chronic studies in rodents are conducted for 6 or 9 months. Special studies include hemolysis studies for intravenous (IV) or intramuscular (IM) administration, venous irritation studies for IV administration, dermal irritation studies for topical clinical applications, and corneal abrasion studies for ophthalmic administration. Genotoxicity testing includes a battery of *in vivo* and *in vitro* tests that are designed to detect compounds that induce genetic damage and is used primarily for predicting carcinogenicity. Carcinogenicity studies are 24-month studies in rats and are required for licensing if the duration of the clinical administration will be 3–6 months or longer. Reproduction toxicology studies have three segments (fertility, conception to embryotoxicity, and prenatal and postnatal development) and may be required by the FDA before starting IND clinical trials if the FDA suspects that there is a potential reproduction impact. Toxicokinetic studies are designed to generate pharmacokinetic data as a component of nonclinical toxicity studies to assess nonclinical systemic exposure for interpretation, as it may relate to the clinical safety of the product.

For more information about information required in the nonclinical section, refer to the following ICH Guidelines:

- S7A: *Safety Pharmacology Studies for Human Pharmaceuticals* (July 2001)
- S7B: *Safety Pharmacology Studies for Assessing the Potential for Delayed Ventricular Repolarization (QT Interval prolongation) by Human Pharmaceuticals* (October 2005)
- *Toxicokinetics—Guidance on the Assessment of Systematic Exposure in Toxicity Studies* (March 1995)
- *Single Dose Acute Toxicity Testing for Pharmaceuticals* (August 1996)
- *Guidance on Genotoxicity Testing And Data Interpretation For Pharmaceuticals Intended For Human Use* (November 2011)
- *Need for Long-Term Rodent Carcinogenicity Studies of Pharmaceuticals* (March 1996)
- *Detection of Toxicity to Reproduction for Medicinal Products* (September 1994)
- *Detection of Toxicity to Reproduction for Medicinal Products Addendum: Toxicity to Male Fertility* (April 1996)
- S5(R2): *Detection Of Toxicity to Reproduction for Medicinal Products & Toxicity to Male Fertility* (1994)
- S3A: *Toxicokinetics: The Assessment of Systemic Exposure in Toxicity Studies* (March 1995)

The following FDA guidance for industry documents also provide information on nonclinical issues:

- *Content and Format of INDs for Phase 1 Studies of Drugs, Including Well-Characterized Therapeutics Biotechnology-Derived Products* (November 1995)
- *Investigators, and Reviewers: Exploratory IND Studies* (January 2006)
- *Nonclinical Safety Evaluation of Pediatric Products* (February 2006)
- *Immunotoxicology Evaluation of Investigational New Drugs* (October 2002)
- *Reproductive and Developmental Toxicities—Integrating Study Results to Assess Concerns* (September 2011)

13.4.4 Module 5: Clinical Study Reports

13.4.4.1 General Investigation Plan The general investigation plan should include the rationale for selecting the clinical supplies, the proposed indication, and the clinical research to be performed. The discussion about the general approach should include the number of doses, administration route, and study length. If a series of studies will be performed, the proposed types of clinical trials to be conducted in the following year should be outlined. If the study results are needed to make decisions about a follow-up study design, the process of making study decisions should be outlined. Finally, if anticipated risks are known either from nonclinical data or from previous human experience, including information from related drugs, information about those risks should be included.

13.4.4.2 Investigator's Brochure The investigator's brochure (IB) is one of the most important sections of the IND. The information contained within the IB is the only information from the IND to which the clinical investigator has access. Therefore, the information contained in this document is used by the clinical trial investigators to help them decide whether they will participate in the clinical trial.

Some of the information is also provided in other sections of the IND, so it is important to make sure that this information is consistent between sections. General information also found in other sections includes a summary of all data known to the sponsor (clinical and nonclinical), a summary of significant information relevant to clinical development for the current stage, and possible side effects or risks based on previous experience with this or related drug. The nonclinical section is typically the most detailed part of the IB, especially for early Phase 1 clinical trials. For the clinical section, a good summary of data from all previous clinical trials should be provided. Any previous clinical data will provide a good guide for decisions about whether a clinical trial should be executed. In addition, previous clinical data can be used to develop a list of adverse events (AE). The AE list should be as complete as possible in the IB because any event not listed in the IB must be reported as "unexpected" and a safety report may need to be filed.

Also included in this document is the labeling for the test drug, a TOC for the IB, an introduction, any guidance for investigators that the sponsor has based on their experience with the drug, and any precautions or special monitoring of which the clinical monitor should be aware. As with the TOC for the IND, the TOC for the investigator's brochure should be clear, detailed, and easy to follow.

For more information about information required in an IB, see 21 CFR 312.23(a)(5) and ICH GCP Guideline E6.

13.4.4.3 Study Protocols The protocol for the clinical study that is the subject of the IND is included in this section. Because much of this information is also included in the IB, the protocol should be carefully reviewed against the IB to ensure consistency of data between the two items. The investigator information included in the protocol is a signed FDA Form 1572 for all principal investigators, facilities data and Institutional Review Board (IRB) data for all sites (foreign and domestic), a copy of each principal investigator's Curriculum Vitae, and a financial disclosure form for foreign investigators if the trial is run under an IND. Information about the study in itself includes a protocol cover sheet with the protocol number; a protocol synopsis; background information; and clinical trial objectives, purposes, and design. There should also be a discussion of the selection inclusion and exclusion criteria and withdrawal and the treatment of the patients (e.g., number of visits, what happens at each visit, and type of data gathered). An assessment of efficacy and safety is provided, as well as a full statistic section with a complete analysis plan and details of quality control and quality assurance should be provided. It is also important to include informed consent and IRB approval documents for each site.

13.4.4.4 Previous Human Experience This section primarily contains information about human experience with the drug for which the FDA does not have access. Integrated summaries from non-U.S. clinical trials should be provided with their corresponding study reports if available. If the drug is marketed in other countries, the non-U.S. marketing experience and a list of countries where the drug is marketed outside United States should be included. If significant regulatory actions have arisen either from non-U.S. clinical trials or from non-U.S. marketing experience, this information should also be included. The other possible source of data is from published clinical experience, including pharmacologically related drugs. If this data exist, an integrated summary of the data should be provided with copies of the reprints.

For more information about information required in the previous human experience section, the following FDA guidance for industry documents can be referenced:

- FDA Final Rule: *INDs and NDAs Requiring presentation of efficacy and safety data for important demographic subgroups* (February 1998).
- *Providing Clinical Evidence of Effectiveness for Human Drug and Biological Products* (May 1998).

In addition, the following ICH document can be used:

- E3: *Structure and Content of Clinical Study Reports* (July 1996).

REFERENCES

Guidance Documents

Biological Related Guidelines—ICH (relevant for Phase I through Marketing Applications)

CBER—Blood, Vaccines, Tissue, Allergenic Based Products (contents of CMC section for Phase II and III, draft)—http://www.fda.gov/cber/gdlns/indbiodft.pdf

CDER—Biological Therapeutic Products—http://www.fda.gov/cder/biologics/default.htm

21 CFR 312.23(a)(5)

Guidance for Industry Investigational New Drug Applications (INDs)—Determining Whether Human Research Studies Can Be Conducted Without an IND (Draft Guidance October 2010)

ICH Guidelines

Q5A (R1): *Viral Safety Evaluation of Biotechnology Products Derived from Cell Lines of Human or Animal Origin* (September 1999)

Q5B: *Quality of Biotechnological Products: Analysis of the Expression Construct in Cells Used for Production of r-DNA Derived Protein Products* (November 1995)

Q5C: *Quality of Biotechnological Products: Stability Testing of Biotechnological/Biological Products* (November 1995)

Q5D: *Derivation and Characterization of Cell Substrates Used for Production of Biotechnological/Biological Products* (July 1997)

Q6B: *Specifications: Test Procedures and Acceptance Criteria for Biotechnological/Biological Products* (March 1999)

E6: *Good Clinical Practice: Consolidated Guidance* (May 1996)

14

FACILITY DESIGN FOR VACCINE MANUFACTURING—REGULATORY, BUSINESS, AND TECHNICAL CONSIDERATIONS AND A RISK-BASED DESIGN APPROACH

Anand Ekambaram

Merck & Co., Inc., West Point, PA, USA

Abraham Shamir

Shamir Biologics LLC, Ft. Washington, PA, USA

14.1 INTRODUCTION

The dramatic changes in the public health, business, and public policy areas in the last two decades have created significant new challenges and opportunities for suppliers of vaccines. In the public health arena, the efforts of bodies such as the Bill and Melinda Gates Foundation, PATH, WHO, and countless others have helped to bring about an awareness of the opportunities that vaccines represent and the challenges that still exist in bringing the benefits of vaccines to the people who most desperately need them. The WHO estimates that over 22 million children remain unvaccinated every year (WHO, 2014), and over 2 million, about half of them younger than 5 years, die every year because of diseases that are preventable by vaccines that are available today. In the business world, vaccines such as PREVNAR® and GARDASIL® have demonstrated (largely untapped) commercial opportunities for new and innovative vaccines and the immense public health benefits associated

Vaccine Development and Manufacturing, First Edition.
Edited by Emily P. Wen, Ronald Ellis, and Narahari S. Pujar.

with them. The high profile acquisitions of vaccine companies by pharmaceutical giants Pfizer and Astra-Zeneca illustrate the importance that large pharmaceutical companies now accord to vaccines; the $15 billion acquisition of Medimmune by Astra-Zeneca is the largest in the history of the vaccine business. In the political arena, the public debates following the influenza vaccine shortages and SARS epidemic earlier this decade helped create an awareness of the global nature of infectious issues and the fragile nature of the current vaccine supply chain.

The manufacture of vaccines requires highly specialized facilities. The cost of ownership of such facilities has become a critically important consideration because it is a significant component of the cost of the product. Most of the 26 million children who go unvaccinated live in the developing world and subsist on less than $2 a day. Even in more affluent societies, the cost of medicines is often the subject of intense public scrutiny and debate. Misinterpretation of the current Good Manufacturing Practice (cGMP) requirements and the pressures of obtaining timely regulatory approval have favored more conservative (and expensive) design solutions. Proper design solutions require scientific understanding of the product and the process and a risk-based analysis. Furthermore, correct approaches to containing costs and achieving better returns on assets need to focus on the total cost of ownership over the lifetime of the asset.

The lead times for design, construction, qualification, and approval will continue to challenge the creativity of facility designers. Shorter lead times allow the expenditure to occur later in the product development cycle when the risk of product failure is lower.

Reliability of supply is important for medicines in general. It is all the more important for vaccines because alternative products are often not available owing to the limited number of vaccine manufacturers and the long lead times for new facilities. After the public debate that followed influenza vaccine shortages in 2004, policy initiatives for improving the reliability of vaccine supply included encouragement to the industry, under the "Current Good Manufacturing Practice for the 21st Century" initiative, to adopt the use of quality systems and risk-based approaches that build quality into the manufacturing process (Goodman, 2005). Designers of vaccine manufacturing facilities should be aware that regulators assessing their facilities will be assessing the overall reliability of the facility and will likely apply the same quality system and risk-based approaches mentioned earlier during facility inspection and approval.

The purpose of this chapter is to provide the reader with a general understanding of the design of bulk (drug substance) vaccine manufacturing facilities. The manufacture of vaccine drug product is not covered in this chapter because the aseptic processing technology used for formulation, filling, and packaging of vaccines is not significantly different from that used for other classes of sterile drug products.

Sections 14.2 and 14.3 discuss the regulatory and business considerations that influence the design of bulk vaccine manufacturing facilities. The remaining sections describe the modules typically present in a vaccine facility, design concepts, and a risk-based methodology application of these design concepts. This chapter is not intended to be a comprehensive source of detailed design information for vaccines because of the fact that information is readily available elsewhere. Baseline engineering guides published by the International Society of Pharmaceutical Engineering (ISPE) are an excellent source of that level of detail. Volume 6 of the ISPE series (ISPE, 2013) covers the design of biopharmaceutical facilities. The design concepts and standards presented in volume 6 are applicable, for the most part, to vaccines as well.

There are frequent references in this chapter to "conventional medicinal products" (meaning those that are, in general, manufactured using chemical and physical methods) that are extremely well characterized. The references are provided to orient the average reader who likely has a general understanding of the pharmaceutical industry but no specific experience with biologics or vaccines. Although vaccines and other biologics have registered impressive growth over the last decade, conventional medicinal products are still the dominant group and form the experience base of the vast majority of manufacturing professionals currently in the pharmaceutical industry.

14.2 REGULATORY CONSIDERATIONS

Conventional medicinal products are, in general, used for the treatment of acute or chronic conditions. In comparison, vaccines are usually given to healthy patients, the vast majority being in the pediatric age group. This explains, at least in part, why vaccines, of all medicinal products, are often subjected to the highest level of regulatory oversight and public scrutiny.

In the United States, vaccines are regulated under Section 351 of the Public Health Service Act (PHS Act). However, because vaccines also meet the definition of "drugs" under Section 201 (g) (1) of the Federal Food, Drug, and Cosmetic Act (FD&C Act), they are also subject to regulation under the FD&C Act. Vaccines are subject to provisions of both acts as well as the cGMP regulations, which are found under Title 21 of the Code of Federal Regulations, Parts 210 and 211, as well as the biologics regulations in 21 CFR Part 600–680. Additional guidance for the manufacture of vaccines may be found in US Food and Drug Administration (FDA's) "Compliance Program Guides" (US Food and Drug Administration (FDA), 2014; US Food and Drug Administration (FDA), 2008), which are used to train their inspectors.

The federal FDA has charged one of its centers, the Center for Biologics Evaluation and Research (CBER) with the task of regulating vaccines. CBER's approach to oversight of vaccines is best illustrated by these quotes from their Website:

> *"In contrast to most drugs that are chemically synthesized and their structure is known, most biologics are complex mixtures that are not easily identified or characterized. Biological products, including those manufactured by biotechnology, tend to be heat sensitive and susceptible to microbial contamination. "In CBER's view," the consistency, safety, efficacy and stability of these products, especially vaccines, are dependent on clearly defining and adhering to the processes described in an application, because the important structural features of the final product cannot be defined and there is an increased risk of the introduction of adventitious agents."*
>
> (US Food and Drug Administration (FDA), 2008).

In Europe, Directive 2003/94/EC, of October 8, 2003, lays down the principles and guidelines for good manufacturing practice for medicinal products for human use. Detailed guidelines in accordance with the principles in these directives are described in the Guide to Good Manufacturing Practice, which is the basis for review of applications for manufacturing authorizations and also for inspections of facilities. The guide consists of two parts—Part I covers basic requirements and Part II GMP for Active Pharmaceutical Ingredients (API). The Guide also contains a series of annexes providing additional detail for specific areas. The principles and specific requirements for biological products, including vaccines, are described in Annex 2.

European agencies expect vaccine manufacturing to comply with the requirements in Part I and II and any annexes that might apply. For example, a vaccine produced using recombinant methods and aseptic downstream processing would need to comply with the principles and specific requirements in Part I, Part II, as well as Annex I (Sterile Medicinal Products) and Annex II (Biological Medicinal Products for Human Use).

Annex 2 describes the principles the European Union (EU) adopted in regulating vaccines, and these are very similar to the expectations articulated by CBER. Annex 2 states:

> *"Unlike conventional medicinal products, which are reproduced using chemical and physical techniques capable of a high degree of consistency, the production of biological medicinal products involves biological processes and materials, such as cultivation of cells or extraction of material from living organisms. These biological processes may display inherent variability, so that the range and nature of by-products are variable. Moreover, the materials used in these cultivation processes provide good substrates for growth of microbial contaminants. Control of biological medicinal products usually involves biological analytical techniques which have a greater degree of variability than physicochemical determinations. In-process controls therefore take on a great importance in the manufacture of biological medicinal products."*
>
> Rules and Guidance for Pharmaceutical Manufacturers and Distributors, 2014.

The regulatory agencies approach to vaccines is based on the view that, for vaccines, the method (which includes facility, equipment, and processing parameters) used for manufacture is an inseparable component of product definition. This view is often summarized as "process = product." The facility is one of the critical control elements for ensuring that the vaccine is produced in a consistent manner and is free of contamination. It therefore follows that the design, qualification, and operation of the facility are also critical for controlling product attributes and quality.

The conditions that are used for production of vaccines (i.e., temperature and carbon source) are conducive to the proliferation of microbial contaminants or what is called *bioburden*. Methods for prevention and control for microbial contamination are important design objectives and receive a high level of scrutiny during regulatory review. The methods used to prevent or control microbial contamination or what is called *bioburden control* (i.e., closed-system process, steam sanitization of empty vessels, and medium sterilization using filters or heat) are often the same as those required for aseptic processing (i.e., processing after the final sterilization step).

This has sometimes resulted in the blurring of distinctions between the two. Clearly, there are vaccine manufacturing steps that require aseptic processing. However, aseptic processing standards are not automatically required for all vaccine manufacturing steps. The design process must clearly identify the point at which aseptic processing begins and the "sterile envelope," which is the boundary within which aseptic processing conditions are required. The culture of applying aseptic process standards to upstream areas where they are not required is one of the common instances of "over-engineering." US Food and Drug Administration (FDA) (2008) states "*Biological products are manufactured in a controlled environment. The entire process does not have to be performed under aseptic conditions, but the firm should have established the point at which aseptic controls begin. Products should be maintained in a controlled environment throughout the process and have specified in-process bioburden action and alert limits for which the firm can provide a meaningful rationale.*"

Regulatory literature from the FDA, European Medicines agency (EMEA), and other agencies point to a few consistent themes. Although there are some aspects of cGMPs that are applicable to all medicinal products, chemical, or biological, there are safeguards and cGMP expectations that apply specifically to vaccine manufacturing as summarized in Table 14.1 with the implications for facility design.

14.3 THE BUSINESS CONTEXT

Developing a new medicinal product carries significant risk of failure, and vaccines are no exceptions to this general rule. However, there are significant differences in the business models for vaccines when compared to other medicinal products, and these affect the timing and the size of the initial investment and the lifetime of the facility.

The construction of a new vaccine manufacturing facility represents a significant capital investment. The capital investment can range from $50 MM for a small-scale facility that leverages existing infrastructure to about $300 MM for a large facility with significant infrastructure requirements. Vaccine facilities tend to be specialized because of the diversity in the bulk technology platforms used for vaccine manufacture. They also tend to be very capital intensive, require longer lead times, and have lower return on investment (ROI) compared to pharmaceutical facilities.

Once a facility is licensed, the user can expect a longer payback period compared to pharmaceuticals. Many of the vaccines currently in the market were first introduced over 25 years ago. The barriers to entry for follow-on products have traditionally been quite high because of the specialized nature of the technology used in manufacturing and the difficulty in characterizing the product. In the United States, vaccines are not included in the scope of the Hatch-Waxman Act (Drug Price Competition and Patent Term Restoration Act of 1984), which allows the use of bioequivalence studies for the approval of generic versions of conventional medicinal products.

Early investment may result in a facility that is idle because product failed in later stages of clinical testing. A facility constructed for one vaccine is not always a good

TABLE 14.1 Regulatory Themes and Their Implications for Vaccine Manufacturing

Theme	Implication for Vaccine Facility Design
Compared to conventional medicinal products the materials used in biological processes are often good substrates for the growth of microbial contaminants. Time and temperature are key factors during processing.	Controls should specifically address contamination risks, particularly bioburden and endotoxin contamination. Bioburden control is a significant issue. Controls include measures such as closed-system processing, controlled "clean" manufacturing areas, defined processing times, temperature controls, and so on.
Analytical methods for characterization of biologics are often less precise than those used for conventional medicinal products. In-process controls to ensure consistent operation are of great importance. This view is often expressed as "process = product."	For new products, this creates a strong driver for Phase III (clinical consistency and pivotal efficacy) supplies to be produced in the launch facility using the process intended for commercial production. This requires investment in the launch facility earlier in the product development cycle.
	Design should facilitate consistent operation of the manufacturing process, minimizing opportunities for lot-to-lot variability. Straight-through processing (i.e., without any hold steps) often offers the best opportunity for consistent manufacturing. Intermediate hold points and conditions must be selected carefully and validated to ensure that no product degradation occurs during the hold steps. Facility design must ensure that product and materials flow in a logical pattern that precludes potential cross contamination, for errors and mix-ups.
	Any changes after initial licensure will likely be subject to regulatory scrutiny. Therefore, it is important for processes to be well developed before they are installed in the facility. Site and scale changes are considered to be major changes by regulatory agencies requiring, in some cases, clinical data as a condition for approval. As a result, vaccine processes are significantly less "portable" compared to other medicinal products. Capacity planning must be performed carefully because the lead time for bringing new facilities on line is in the range of 4–6 yr.

fit for the next vaccine in the research pipeline owing to the specialized nature of the technology platforms used in bulk production. At the same time, delaying the investment in a commercial manufacturing facility, which has a lead time of 4–6 years, could result in launch delays, loss of "first-to-market" advantage, and millions of dollars in lost revenue. Many vaccines have significant public health benefits and address diseases that have no alternative therapies. The delay in availability of such a vaccine may affect how the company is perceived by the public.

On the positive side, historically, vaccines have demonstrated a higher probability of success (POS) at the preclinical stage, when compared to small-molecule pharmaceuticals. The POS for the vaccine preclinical candidate is typically about 25% (Struck, 1996) compared to about less than 10% for small-molecule pharmaceuticals (Kola and Landis, 2004). Preclinical candidates for vaccines are typically far fewer in number.

For the reasons as outlined previously, it is important for designers of vaccine facilities to understand the role that the facility will play in the supply strategy and the clinical development strategy for the product. A discussion of modular design methods and grouping facilities by technology platforms is provided in Section 14.4, following the description of modules in a typical vaccine manufacturing facility. These approaches are helpful in mitigating the risk of early investment in a facility for novel vaccine products.

In the world of traditional (small-molecule) pharmaceuticals, multiproduct launch facilities are often used to minimize capital outlay early in the product development cycle. This type of facility is typically capable of supplying clinical trials and the first few years of commercial production for a wide variety of compounds. If the product is successful, it is then moved to a long-term supply facility. The launch facility is then reused for the next product in the pipeline. The advantage of this flow-through approach is that it defers the need for investment in a new facility by a few years, to a time when there is significantly more information available on the viability of the product. This "flow-through" approach works well for small-molecule pharmaceuticals because they are well characterized; source changes have typically much shorter lead times, and any product changes on transfer to a new manufacturing facility can be easily detected and corrected. In addition, the technology platforms used for small-molecule pharmaceuticals are, in general, not as diverse as they are for vaccines, and the retrofit for the next product in the pipeline is typically much easier.

This strategy is not widely used for the commercial manufacture of vaccines (modular, multiproduct facilities are in use for early stage clinical trials). Vaccine manufacturing processes are significantly less portable for the reasons discussed previously in Section 14.2. Although it is not uncommon for manufacturers to build a small-scale facility to supply Phase III and launch supplies, these facilities are not the kind of "flow-through" facilities used by small-molecule medicinal products. Table 14.2 shows how the stage of development of the product and the supply strategy could influence design strategy.

TABLE 14.2 Influence on Design Strategy by the Stage of Product Development and Supply Strategy

Type of Facility	Key Design Drivers	Level of Automation	Buffer and Media Manufacture
Clinical supplies for early stage clinical testing	Primary design objective is for the flexibility of a wide range of products, multiproduct use, with emphasis on segregation and ease of changeover. Campaigns are usually very short, ranging from a week to several months.	Automation level is typically low because a high level of process automation can impede rapid changeovers.	Buffer and media manufacturing is typically outsourced. Buffers are often supplied in large bags.
Phase III and launch	Design emphasis is on speed and capital conservation because decisions are often made at risk at early stage of product development. This launch facility is typically used for supplying key efficacy or clinical consistency studies.	Facilities are typically designed with a low level of process automation. Facility construction starts when manufacturing process is not fully defined at the time the equipment is being ordered. Lower level of automation allows faster response to process development changes.	Buffer and media manufacturing is typically outsourced.
Long-term supply, after launch	Emphasis is on achieving lowest possible unit cost through economies of scale and efficiency. Facility design is performed at a time when there is good assurance of commercial success. Decision to build these new facilities is often tied to launch in new territories and to expansion of the initial indications.	Facilities are designed with a high level of process automation to facilitate efficient operations. Companies will often consider investing in process analytical technology (PAT) and data collection systems.	Buffer and media manufacturing modules are typically part of the facility. A make-and-use approach is commonly used. Buffers are prepared and stored for short periods in large tanks several thousand liters at a time and piped to points of use.

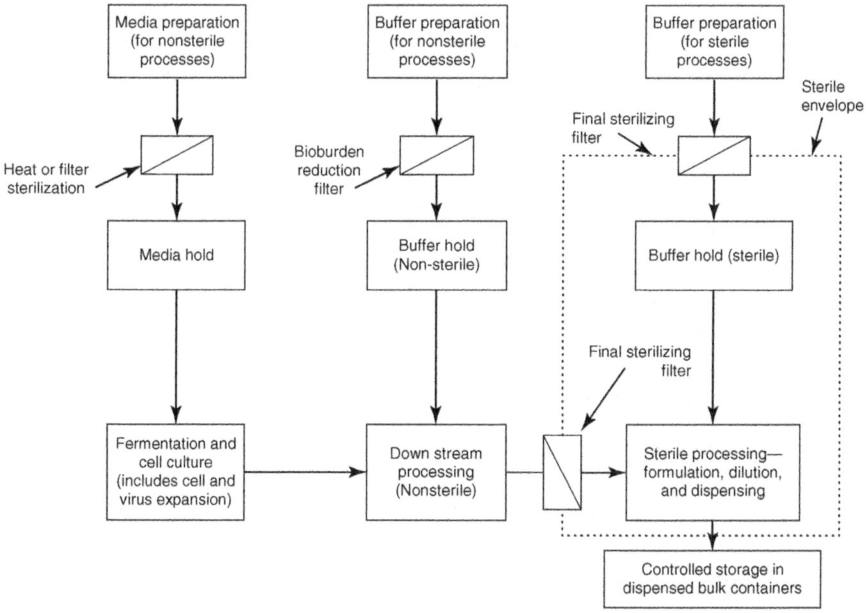

Figure 14.1 Modules typically present in a bulk vaccine manufacturing facility.

14.4 VACCINE MANUFACTURING FACILITY—OVERVIEW

A schematic of a typical vaccine manufacturing facility as it relates to bulk vaccine manufacturing is provided in the following section (Fig. 14.1). The schematic is intended to illustrate the typical modules that may be present in a vaccine manufacturing facility and their primary design objectives and possibilities for the modular design. It is not intended to suggest that every vaccine manufacturing facility must have these modules. Their presence in a facility is dependent on the overall objectives of the facility and the operational philosophy. For example, facility operators may choose to purchase ready-made buffers from an external supplier (an option that is quite feasible if the volumes required are on the order of a few hundred liters), in which case the buffer manufacturing infrastructure is not needed. Descriptions of the modules are provided in the following sections:

14.4.1 Fermentation and Cell Culture

This module houses the steps used for the propagation/growth of the active ingredient under controlled conditions by microbial or cell culture, including those based on recombinant DNA technology. For these processes, the primary design objective is to ensure culture purity (i.e., that only the desired organism is present). Fermentation and cell culture processes are at risk for culture purity failures because conditions during processing (i.e., growth promoting media, temperatures, aeration, and long incubation periods) are conducive to rapid proliferation of contaminant organisms. If contamination occurs, it is usually easily detected and results in the termination of fermentation followed by the cleaning and sterilization of equipment. Fermentation and cell culture processes are typically performed in closed systems, although open processing may sometimes be used in the early stages (e.g., seed development in shake flasks). The media used in fermentors are typically heat or filter sterilized; however, the purpose of sterilization, in general, is to ensure culture purity of the fermentation process.

In some cases, the purified product is not amenable to filter sterilization. In those cases, the maintenance of aseptic processing conditions in all stages of manufacturing becomes the design objective.

14.4.2 Downstream Processing

This includes pooling of the harvested cells, separation of the active ingredient from the cells, and purification. The primary design driver for downstream processing is bioburden control (to prevent product degradation and endotoxin failures).

14.4.3 Sterile Envelope

The aseptic envelope refers to all the steps carried out during and after the final sterilizing filter until completion of processing (i.e., when the product is dispensed into bulk containers). These steps may include formulation, addition of excipients, and dilution to achieve target potency. For bulk biological products that cannot be sterile filtered (e.g., live virus vaccines and alum adsorbed vaccines), the sterile envelope includes all parts of the bulk process that employ closed-system sterile processing. The sterile envelope may include in-process or holding tanks used for short-term storage of sterile buffers. The primary design objectives for this process module are maintenance of sterility and prevention of leaks. The sterile envelope is not required if the product is terminally sterilized or if there is a sterile filtration step downstream, before filling.

The design of equipment and processes within the sterile envelope requires the highest level of attention to detail and a thorough understanding of all the aspects of aseptic manufacturing. Even a minor breach in the integrity of the system could pose a risk to the patient and will usually result in discard of the lot.

14.4.4 Media and Buffer Preparation

The preparation of buffers and media includes the addition of liquid components as well as dissolving powders and salts in water. Solutions are filtered through sterilizing grade filters or heat sterilized after preparation. Buffers may be held in hold tanks for several weeks before use. Sterility is a requirement only for those buffers that are used downstream of the final product sterilization step. For other nonsterile media or buffers, the purpose of filter or heat sterilization is to control bioburden during the hold period that typically follows preparation. The primary design objective for the media area is control of bioburden, endotoxin, and external particulate contamination.

14.4.5 GMP Support Areas

Most vaccine facilities contain areas that are used for preparation of equipment and components that are used in production. The equipment processed through these support areas are typically of a smaller scale such as chromatography columns, valve assemblies, and filter housings. Large equipment is usually cleaned and sterilized in place. Most vaccine facilities also make extensive use of disposable components. These are usually prepared for use in the process support area. Process support areas have clean rooms designated for receipt, cleaning, assembly, and sterilization of equipment.

14.4.6 GMP Storage Areas

The areas are designed for storage of raw materials, intermediates, and final product. Since most are temperature sensitive, the typical GMP storage area in a vaccine facility is controlled and monitored for temperature and humidity.

14.4.7 Utility Areas

A typical vaccine manufacturing facility's utility systems may include the following systems, which are located outside the classified process areas or "clean rooms":

- Water purification, storage, and distribution systems
- Clean steam generators and distribution
- Equipment for clean-in-place (CIP) operations of process equipment
- Waste inactivation (for biohazards) and waste treatment systems
- Compressed air generators
- Vacuum systems
- Emergency power
- Process heating/cooling
- Inert gas generators
- HVAC (heating, ventilation, and air conditioning)
- Sanitary sewer.

The utilities in a vaccine manufacturing facility are categorized on the basis of product contact. ISPE's Biopharmaceutical Manufacturing Facilities Guide recommends, for example, categorizing the utilities as "direct impact systems" and "indirect or no impact systems" (International Society for Pharmaceutical Engineering (ISPE), 2001). Direct impact systems, as the name implies, are utilities that come in contact with product or product-contact surfaces. Pharmaceutical grade water systems, CIP and SIP (Steam-in-place) systems, are examples of direct impact systems. A glycol-chiller and the associated distribution pipes are examples of "indirect impact systems." The chilled glycol is used to maintain the contents at 5°C. Cooling is achieved by circulating chilled glycol through the cooling jackets of tanks or through heat exchangers. Although direct impact systems may be located outside the classified process space, they are held to the same GMP standards as process equipment for design, construction, qualification, and routine operation. Indirect impact systems are commissioned in accordance with local codes and standards. GMP standards, if applied, are used very selectively. Good Engineering Practice (GEP), as defined in ISPE's Baseline Guide on Commissioning and Qualification, is the standard typically applied to indirect impact systems.

14.4.8 Non-GMP Support Areas

These include office areas for personnel involved in supporting the production operations, documentation storage rooms, control rooms housing the automation hardware, pilot laboratories used for process trouble shooting (note that laboratory areas used for conducting release and in-process are considered GMP areas), and training rooms. The importance of well-designed non-GMP support areas is often underestimated. Vaccine processes are among the most complex in the pharmaceutical industry, and reliable supply requires a well-knit team of operations, quality, engineering, and scientific staff. Colocation of these groups in the same office area can make a significant difference to the overall reliability of the process and the response time when problems arise.

14.4.9 Modular Design

In Section 14.3, a discussion of the business considerations that drive facility design, particularly the need to minimize the risk to investment for new products, is provided. These investments occur when the clinical and commercial success of the product is not assured. Modular design is one of the ways in which the impact of clinical and commercial setbacks can be minimized.

Although the technology platforms for vaccine manufacture are indeed diverse, that diversity is seen only in fermentation/cell culture and downstream purification. Qualified utilities, equipment preparation areas, and buffer and media manufacturing areas are not significantly different across technology platforms. With the appropriate segregation and controls, it is possible, for example, to design a buffer and media preparation area to serve the needs of more than one product. This type of a modular approach can help improve asset usage and minimize the impact of failure of one product. Clearly, it requires a site that that holds multiple manufacturing facilities. Similarly, when constructing qualified utilities, it is common to design the utility module to serve more than one facility. Even in areas such as fermentation and purification, a modular design approach is possible but can be used only by other products that use the same technology platform.

A modular design approach requires an understanding of the pipeline of products in development and the company's long-term vision for that manufacturing site. Initial costs for modular design are typically higher because of the additional controls needed to ensure suitability for multiple products. The payoff comes in the form of reduced risk to the investment.

14.5 EXPECTATIONS FOR DESIGN OF VACCINE FACILITIES

Before reviewing the methods used in the design found in vaccine facilities, it is useful to have an understanding of some key expectations. First and foremost, a vaccine facility must serve the purpose intended (i.e., it should be suited to house the unit operations required for the product in a logical and orderly manner), meet building codes, safety requirements, and manufacturability and ergonomic considerations. These are all important in their own right, and they are no different from design considerations that would apply to any manufacturing facility, not just to vaccines.

However, there are expectations beyond the ones of process fit and intended purpose that apply uniquely to vaccines. These are also the perspectives that regulatory agencies apply during the evaluation of a facility. The purpose of this section is to introduce these concepts.

1. Segregation

   A basic level of segregation is an expectation for manufacture of all medicinal products. For vaccine facilities, segregation methods receive a heightened level of scrutiny because live agents are often used for the manufacture of vaccines and the ability to quantify the impact of such contamination is often limited. Opportunities for cross-contamination and mix up should be evaluated during the design process. These opportunities may be present during transport of clean and used equipment, between raw materials or buffers that are being staged for use in the production area, between upstream and downstream steps of manufacture, and between two different products.

   The control of live agents requires special design and procedural safeguards if the organisms pose a risk to humans. The guidelines for design of facilities that handle infectious agents are well established (National Institutes of Health (NIH), 2013).

2. Suite hygiene

   Suite hygiene describes the level of control over particulate and microbial contamination in the area housing a biological process. The level of control required for a process depends on the nature of processing (open or closed), the frequency and duration of open operations, and the impact of contamination. Open operations during manufacture of buffer solutions pose a very different risk to the process when compared to that used in aseptic processing (i.e., downstream of the final sterilizing filter).

   The levers that can be used to control overall suite hygiene include air-exchanges, periodic cleaning and disinfection of the manufacturing area, gowning levels of personnel entering the area, closed-system processing (particularly when live agents are being processed), and decontamination of incoming materials. Air-exchanges help maintain suite hygiene by flushing out airborne contamination, particulate, and microbial. Effective control of suite hygiene requires knowledge of the potential sources of contamination. For example, increasing the number of air-exchanges by itself will not improve suite hygiene if the main source of contamination resides on the surface of equipment brought into the manufacturing area.

3. Primary and secondary controls

   Primary controls are those that are designed to directly address the risk identified during the design process. Secondary controls should be designed as a measure of redundancy to anticipate realistic deviations of the primary controls from ideal design conditions.

   For a fermentation process, closed-system processing is usually the primary control to prevent contamination. A controlled environment in the area housing the fermentor is typically selected as the secondary control. The secondary control is used because of the recognition that even the most robust closed-system processing may develop leaks.

   The transfer of a buffer from a storage tank to a receiving tank using a closed transfer line is another instance for the application of the primary and secondary control concepts. The closed transfer line is the primary control for the prevention of bioburden and particulate contamination during the transfer of the buffer. However, transfer lines, particularly those that have valves or triclover connections, will occasionally develop leaks. Most leaks are usually detected by preoperational checks such as pressure testing. However, sometimes, leaks develop after the preoperational checks. A point of using a 0.2-μm filter at the receiving tank as a secondary control measure ensures that such leaks, if they occur, will not have bioburden or particulate impact on the contents of the receiving tank.

   A secondary control is not needed for every primary control. The need for secondary controls should be assessed as part of the design process. The reliability of the primary control and the impact of its failure determine the need for a secondary control.

4. Preference for engineering controls over procedural controls

   Once a risk is identified, designers have the option of addressing the risk using engineering or procedural controls. Engineering control refers to equipment or facility design features that eliminate the source of the risk. Procedural control refers to options that do not eliminate the root cause of the risk; they prevent the realization of the risk by relying on operator compliance with specific procedures.

   Eliminating the root cause through design or engineering changes may not always be possible. However, engineering controls should be the preferred solution wherever technically feasible and commercially available because they are inherently more reliable than procedural controls. Relying solely on procedural controls may result in an adverse regulatory review, particularly, if the risk could have been addressed through an engineering control.

14.6 RISK-BASED PRINCIPLES FOR DESIGN OF VACCINE FACILITIES

In the preceding sections, the business and regulatory drivers for vaccines were discussed, and the modules and the design elements that are most commonly used for the design of a vaccine manufacturing facility were described. The risk-based methodology described in this section helps integrate these concepts and show how they may be applied for the design of a vaccine manufacturing facility.

The pharmaceutical industry, in general, has lagged behind other industries in applying and realizing the benefits of risk management techniques. In the past, facility design was influenced significantly by the aseptic processing mindset. Standards that were developed and relevant for aseptic processing were applied to upstream (nonaseptic) portions of bulk manufacturing, with little consideration to the specific quality risks that may exist and whether the controls chosen addressed those specific risks. Design features, such as area classification and airlocks, were often selected without a complete understanding of the intended purpose (fermentation, purification, buffer preparation, etc.), the type of equipment (open vs closed), in-process controls, and operational philosophy (single vs multiproduct).

This section presents two concepts:

1. Risk management as applied to design of vaccine manufacturing facilities.
2. Design elements in vaccine manufacturing facilities and the specific benefits they provide for contamination control.

1. Application of risk management to facility design

   The risk management principles presented in this chapter are similar to the ones described in ICH Q9 "Quality Risk Management" for pharmaceutical quality, including manufacturing. The two key principles articulated in ICH Q9 are as follows:

   (a) the evaluation of the risk to quality should be based on scientific knowledge and ultimately link with the protection of the patient; and
   (b) the level of effort, formality, and documentation of the quality risk management process should be commensurate with the level of risk.

   At its core, risk management, as applied to facility design, consists of three elements—risk assessment, risk reduction, and communication. Risk assessment is the process by which risk is identified, analyzed, and evaluated and consists of asking the following questions:

   (a) What are the potential sources or opportunities for contamination and cross contamination at this step? What are the opportunities for inconsistent operation or lot-to-lot variability? (Identification)
   (b) What is the probability of occurrence? Are there any process-specific conditions that amplify or mitigate the risk? Will the failure be obvious; are the analytical tools designed to detect this failure? (analysis)
   (c) What is the impact should such a failure occur? (evaluation)

   Risk reduction allows facility designers to select controls that address the specific contamination risk. Controls can be facility design features, equipment design, procedural controls, or a combination of these.

   Risk communication is the process of documenting and sharing the information about risks and the rationale for selecting certain controls over others. It brings transparency to the decision-making process for that facility. This document can serve the basis of discussions during regulatory inspections and also serve as the basis for review of risks when new products are introduced into the facility or when modifications are made to the existing facility. ISPE Baseline Guide for Biopharmaceutical Manufacturing Facilities recommends authoring a Product Protection Control Strategy (PCCS) document to provide a comprehensive review of the facility, process, and procedural controls.

Although there are a number of formal risk management tools available [(Annex I of ICH Q9 Quality Risk Management, 2006) is a good source for a summary of these tools and their specific applications], it is not necessary to use these tools for every design project. Informal risk management tools can be just as effective. What is important is that the designers go through the process of risk assessment, risk reduction, and communication and that they document and address findings.

2. Design elements in vaccine manufacturing facilities

   This section describes design elements that are commonly used in vaccine facilities and the specific benefit or protection that they provide. These are as follows:

   (a) Closed system processing and suite hygiene
   (b) Controlled spaces, HVAC, and area classification
   (c) Personnel gowning
   (d) Airlocks
   (e) Layouts and flow patterns for materials, product, people, and waste
   (f) Wall/floor finishes.

1. Closed system processing and suite hygiene—a closed-system design allows physical segregation of the product from the surrounding environment and is, by far, the most effective way of preventing contamination from the surrounding environment (including personnel). Transfers into and out of the system occur through sterilizing grade filters or equivalent methods. Although there is no universally accepted definition of a closed system, the following features are typically present:
   (a) Validated methods such as media hold tests or microbial ingress tests are used to prove that, under normal processing conditions, the system will not allow bioburden in the surrounding environment to contaminate product.
   (b) Validated sterilization methods are used to sterilize the vessel and its contents (if needed) before the start of processing.
   (c) Systems are leak-tested using pressure hold tests.
   (d) Use of welded connections is maximized because they offer the best assurance of long-term leak-proof conditions.
   (e) Transfers into and out of the system are performed through sterilizing grade filters.
2. Controlled spaces, HVAC, and area classification—these are used to control the quality of the environment surrounding the manufacturing operations. The quality is typically assessed in terms of the viable and nonviable particulates

that are present at rest and under dynamic conditions in the room environment. Manufacturing steps for vaccines should, at a minimum, be housed in controlled areas at a minimum.

The microbial and particulate levels in the environment are controlled by maintaining a steady flow of clean, filtered air through the room, disinfecting of materials entering the room, periodic sanitization of the walls and floors, entry/exit airlocks, and operator gowning. The airflow should be sufficient to maintain a differential pressure between the clean room and the surrounding space. Recirculation of exit air is allowed unless there are special conditions such as flammable gases or biohazards present in the room.

The controlled spaces range from controlled nonclassified, which does not have any viable or nonviable particulate specifications, to Grade A (also known as Class 100 or ISO 5), which is the highest grade applied in the pharmaceutical industry and has the most stringent specifications. The grade specified depends on the type of operations and the level of closed system processing employed. Closed system operations are not susceptible to contamination by the surrounding environment, and controlled nonclassified spaces are usually sufficient. Aseptic processes that have open operations require Grade A conditions with unidirectional airflow. Table 14.3 provides guidance on the selection of classified spaces for the facility modules shown in Figure 14.1.

3. Personnel gowning—the microorganisms present on the skin and clothes are a significant source of bioburden in the clean room. Gowning ensures that bioburden present on the skin and garments of the operator are retained to varying degrees and not exposed to the room environment. Recommended gowning levels shown in are calibrated to the grade level of the clean room.
4. Airlocks—these are spaces that separate a clean space from the surrounding area. Airlocks also serve as spaces for operators to gown or degown before entering or exiting the clean room. They can also be used for the disinfection of incoming equipment. Airlocks are expected to meet the at-rest conditions of the clean room that they lead to.
5. Layout and flow patterns for materials, product, people, and waste—a layout that allows a logical and orderly placement of unit operations is a basic GMP expectation. The layout should be designed to minimize opportunities for cross contamination and mix-ups. Cross-contamination is a particularly significant concern when live agents are being processed because these can be transmitted through the movement of personnel in the facility. Even if live agents are not involved, the potential for mix-ups between upstream and downstream portions of the same process, between used and unused equipment, and between the various buffers must be considered when developing the layout. The controls are the most reliable when they are embedded in the design of the facility. Controls that rely solely on operator compliance with procedures are the least desirable and should be used only when other options have been exhausted.
6. Wall and floor finishes—the basic requirement for wall and floor finishes is that (a) they must not shed particulate matter or cause contamination in the

TABLE 14.3 Area Classification and Gowning Standards Used for Vaccine Manufacturing

Type of Operation	Closed/Open Processing	Room Classification Recommended	Gowning Levels
Fermentation and purification	Closed—for example, when bioreactors are used.	Controlled Unclassified.	Company issued uniform covered by smock. Hair, beard and shoe covers, and gloves.
	Open—for example, early fermentation steps conducted in shake flasks.	Grade C or equivalent—if the operations are conducted under a Grade A type Laminar Flow Hood.	Company issued uniform covered by one or two piece jump suit gathered at wrists and ankles; hair, beard, and shoe covers. Sterile gloves and sleeves should be used when manipulating the shake flasks.
		Grade D or equivalent—if the operations are conducted in an isolator or glove box.	Same as that for controlled unclassified.
Preparation of buffer solutions and media	Open—buffer and media preparation typically requires charging powders	Grade C or equivalent—if the solutions are intended to be sterile.	Company issued uniform covered by one or two piece jump suit gathered at wrists and ankles; hair, beard, and shoe covers.
		Grade D or equivalent—if the solutions are for use in steps upstream of the final sterilizing filter.	Same as that for controlled unclassified.
Operations downstream of the final sterilizing filter	Closed	Grade C or equivalent	Company issued uniform covered by one or two piece jump suit gathered at wrists and ankles; hair, beard, and shoe covers.
	Open	Grade B or equivalent surrounding a Grade A or equivalent area. Unidirectional airflow such as that provided by a laminar flow hood is required in the Grade A area.	Company issued uniform covered by one or two piece jump suit gathered at wrists and ankles; hair, beard, and shoe covers.

clean room; (b) they must permit routine cleaning and disinfection; (c) they do not provide crevices or spaces, which allow for accumulation of dirt or sustain microbial growth.

Typically, all controlled areas are constructed with smooth surface walls. Ceilings are expected to be monolithic, and false ceilings must not be used. Floors are expected to be nonporous, with no joints or seams that might support microbial growth. Floor/wall junctions should be integral with the floor system.

14.7 CONCLUSIONS

This chapter aims to present an overview of the regulatory and business issues that influence the design of a bulk vaccine manufacturing facility. The chapter also explains the design concepts and a risk-based approach for the application of these concepts. There are many interesting scientific developments in the area of vaccines, and new applications that are in development target applications outside the traditional realm of infectious diseases, in areas such as cancer. While the vaccine production techniques may change, the risk-based design methods explained in this section will continue to be applicable.

REFERENCES

The Drug Price Competition and Patent Term Restoration Act of 1984, usually referred to as the Hatch-Waxman Act, established the legislative framework that allows the FDA to approve generic medicinal products on the basis of bioequivalence studies.

Goodman, JL. 2005. Influenza vaccine: current status, lessons learned and preparing for the future. Available at http://www.hhs.gov/asl/testify/t050210a.html. Accessed 2014 Aug 14.

ICH Q9 Quality Risk Management. Annex 1. Methods and tools-Basic risk management facilitation methods. 2006.

Medicines and Healthcare Products Regulatory Agency (MHRA). *Rules and Guidance for Pharmaceutical Manufacturers and Distributors*. Pharmaceutical Press; 2014.

International Society for Pharmaceutical Engineering (ISPE). *Baseline Pharmaceutical Engineering Guide for New and Renovated Facilities*. Commissioning and Qualification. Vol. 5. ISPE, Tampa, Florida. 2001.

International Society for Pharmaceutical Engineering (ISPE). *Baseline Pharmaceutical Engineering Guide for New and Renovated Facilities*. Biopharmaceutical Manufacturing Facilities. Vol. 6. 2013. p 119.

Kola I, Landis J. Estimate based on success rates from first-in-humans to registration. Nat Rev Drug Discov 2004;3:711–716.

National Institutes of Health (NIH). *Guidelines for Research Involving Recombinant DNA Molecules*. Appendix G 2013. Published online at http://osp.od.nih.gov/office-biotechnology-activities/biosafety/nih-guidelines.

Struck M-M. Vaccine R&D success rates and development times. Nat Biotechnol 1996; 14:591–593.

US Food and Drug Administration (FDA). *Compliance Program Guidance Manual.* Chapter 56, Drug quality assurance, Inspections of licensed biological therapeutic drug products. Program 7356.002M. Center for Biologics and Evaluation and Research (CBER); 2006.

US Food and Drug Administration (FDA). 2014. Center for Biologics Evaluation and Research. Frequently Asked Questions. Available at http://www.fda.gov/AboutFDA/CentersOffices/OfficeofMedicalProductsandTobacco/CBER/ucm125684.html. Accessed 2014 Aug 14.

US Food and Drug Administration (FDA). *Compliance Program Guidance Manual.* Chapter 45, Inspection of biological drug products. Program 7345.848:55. Center for Biologics and Evaluation and Research (CBER); 2008.

World Health Organization. 2014. Progress towards global immunization goals-2013, summary presentation of key indicators, based on children who did not receive DTP3; Available at http://www.who.int/entity/immunization_monitoring/data/SlidesGlobalImmunizationData.pdf. Accessed 2014 Aug 12.

15

VACCINE PRODUCTION ECONOMICS

ANDREW SINCLAIR
Biopharm Services US, Maynard, MA, USA
PETER LATHAM
Latham Biopharm Group, Maynard, MA, USA

15.1 INTRODUCTION

Over the last 10 years, the need to understand and control manufacturing costs has become more relevant to the biopharmaceutical industry. This need for cost controls is no more apparent than for vaccines where the margins are lower compared to that of the rest of the pharmaceutical industry (Prifti, 2010). Although dosing is generally low for vaccines, the price that can be charged, particularly in less developed countries, is dramatically lower than for traditional biologics. As such, it becomes important to look at costs beyond the manufacture of bulk product and to consider the implications of formulating, filling, packaging, and shipping when evaluating the total cost and economic viability of a vaccine product.

Fortunately, the techniques for modeling and evaluating the cost drivers in bulk production can be extended to those for the "secondary" activities necessary to get vaccines to the patient. Nevertheless, the system must be analyzed as a whole. For example, when looking at economies of scale associated with large, centralized manufacturing capacity, one must also consider the costs of shipping and the potential benefits of a more distributed manufacturing approach.

When evaluating manufacturing cost, one must also consider decisions within the context of the global project timeline, as risk and delays can often have a greater impact on the economic viability of a product than the absolute costs themselves.

Vaccine Development and Manufacturing, First Edition.
Edited by Emily P. Wen, Ronald Ellis, and Narahari S. Pujar.

This chapter reviews the interplay between these elements and outlines the techniques often used to evaluate the cost implications of manufacturing decisions. Case studies are also presented to demonstrate these techniques in actual practice.

15.2 VACCINE MANUFACTURING, HISTORY, AND DRIVERS

The history of vaccines dates back over 200 years ago to the development of a smallpox vaccine by Edward Jenner in 1798. Developments in vaccination have advanced sufficiently to protect humans and animals from most life-threatening diseases, with large focus applied to these preventative steps during the 1930s, the 1970s, and again today. The invention of antibiotics took the focus away from vaccines during the Second World War, and it was not returned until 1970, when research was revived. The mapping of the human genome coupled with advancements in the understanding of molecular genetics has brought about new interest and techniques for discovery. Today's challenges lie with the prevention of cancer, HIV, and hepatitis. There are two broad types of vaccine used today, each with their own cost structure.

15.2.1 Traditional

Attenuated—the virulent organism is weakened by unnatural host conditions or special modification, with the resultant effect of a scaled down immune response.

Inactivated—the virus is treated with an agent that destroys its replicative function.

Hepatitis B plasma derived—the first cancer vaccination was derived from the blood serum of a patient with hepatitis B. The sample was purified and attached to an alum adjuvant, resulting in a safe and effective entity. However, the complex downstream processing and concerns over the safety of human blood serums meant that this solution was only short-lived.

15.2.2 Modern

These vaccines have been developed following developments in molecular genetics and are based on modern processes manufactured in state-of-the-art facilities. They differ from traditional vaccines in that they are highly purified and well characterized.

Recombinant yeast and Escherichia coli derivatives—recombinant techniques have been used to introduce antigens into bacteria and yeasts. The purified antigens are used to mediate an immune response, ideally resulting in an effective vaccination against the target disease. The early yeast experiments fell short, with very large amounts of antigen required to mediate a response. *E. coli* methods started to show more promise; however, they manufacture nonglycosylated proteins that can sometimes limit the effectiveness of the vaccination.

Recombinant viral vaccines—this has traditionally been very similar to attenuated/inactivated methods, although recently more work has been undertaken in developing effective viral vectors (see gene therapy example). Progression had been limited because of safety concerns over using the vaccinia virus; however, new hosts are showing potential.

Attenuated bacterial vectors—the use of a bacterium that is delivered orally stimulates mucosal immunity that helps to maximize antigenicity. These tackle Salmonella and Calmet-Guerin.

Nucleic acid—there is a lot of interest in using nucleic acids to mimic the action of a pathogen within the host cell. This method is ideal for creating an immune response; however, there are concerns over the potential integration of viral DNA into the human genome.

Peptide—synthetic antigens that are recognized by antibodies provide a good alternative to using a virus that contains actual DNA. The largest challenge in this area is the presentation of the synthetic antigen in manner such that it sufficiently mimics the antigen epitope in order to elicit an efficacious immune response.

15.3 THE IMPORTANCE OF CAPITAL IN BIOLOGIC MANUFACTURING

In the last 10 years, there has been substantial investment in vaccine manufacturing capacity. To better understand the capital structure of the industry, it is useful to compare the level of capital intensity in the biopharmaceutical industry relative to other sectors. Capital intensity, calculated as a percentage, is capital expenditure divided by total revenue for a given period. Morgan Stanley has published comparative data for the pharmaceutical sector (Elmasry, 2004), and the U.S. Department of Commerce carried out an assessment for the biotechnology sector in 2001 (US Department of Commerce, 2003).

By comparing the two sets of data (Fig. 15.1), it is clear that the biopharmaceutical sector has a much greater capital intensity at 12.4% compared to general pharmaceuticals at 9%. This does not bode well for an industry where there is pressure to reduce prices. If process manufacturing capital requirements do not change, then the capital intensity value will increase further as health care providers, competitive products, and generics start to put increasing pressure on biopharmaceutical and vaccine pricing.

The high capital intensity partially explains high drug manufacturing costs; however, it also presents the industry with a challenge that must be taken seriously—reducing the cost of manufacture. Another factor in drug pricing is the cost of development and time taken to develop drugs (currently about 7 years; Tufts Center for the Study of Drug Development, 2005). There is much discussion on reducing development times, but much of this is focused on the clinical trials (the critical path in the product life cycle) where the industry will look to accelerate drug

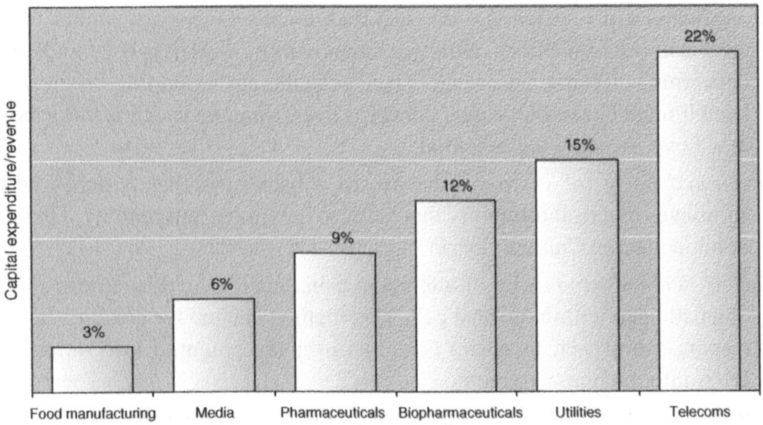

Figure 15.1 Capital intensity for different industries.

development through expanded use of information technologies in clinical trials management (Tufts Center for the Study of Drug Development, 2007). However, the trends for the cost and duration of development are increasing.

Given this background, the emphasis is on developing cost-effective, robust, and compliant processes where process development will not feature on the critical path. This is made more difficult by the increasing costs and the duration of product development. There are three ways to approach this challenge:

- Develop better processes
- Apply novel/new manufacturing technologies
- Operate facilities more effectively.

Fortunately, all of these approaches can be modeled to determine, in advance, their relative impact on the economics of a vaccine product. This chapter considers these cost modeling techniques that can be used to support the achievement of cost-effective processes. With the appropriate use of modeling tools, one can gain insight and knowledge on the best ways to design manufacturing processes, thereby managing the capital and operating costs.

15.4 PROCESS DESIGN AND OPTIMIZATION

High capital costs, complex processes, and long product development cycles result in high manufacturing costs in the biopharmaceutical industry. There is pressure to reduce these costs, and this can be achieved by considering the whole product life cycle and understanding what modeling tools can be used to help gain insight and guide decision making. The key benefits of the modeling techniques are to develop processes that are as follows:

- simple, robust, and compliant
- able to employ the most effective technology
- able to operate effectively in an actual manufacturing facility
- account for the economics of the entire process
- account for time and risk in addition to cost.

In addition, the focus is on tools that can manage change within existing facilities so that they can be used to support process and operational improvements and the introduction of new products.

A product starts off in research and if successful is manufactured for use in the clinic. During the life cycle of the product, opportunities to reduce the cost of manufacture become scarcer as the product matures. By breaking the product life cycle down into discrete stages (Table 15.1), cost objectives can be identified and modeling tools/techniques that support the objectives can be implemented.

Process development can be defined as the start of the product life cycle, and it is at this stage that the manufacturing process is defined in terms of unit operations (discrete manufacturing operations). There are significant pressures on the process development to be rapid (not on the critical path of a clinical program) and to reduce the cost of development. The cost pressures are related to clinical risk insofar that a product entering clinical trials (Pavlou and Reichert, 2004) has a high probability of not reaching approved status (there is a high attrition rate). Consequently, there is little incentive to put a lot of effort into developing an efficient process early on. Often, a second-generation process is developed once product success is assured.

It is a goal of modeling, together with automated and rapid process development techniques, to remove the necessity for first- and second-generation processes by developing the optimum process first time round, within the constraints of the clinical program. As a product moves from research into manufacturing, the opportunities for improving the cost effectiveness of the manufactured product diminish. The later

TABLE 15.1 Modeling Requirements

Stage	Objectives	Tools
Process development early phase	Rapid development Minimal development effort	MAb "platform" process Cost models
Process development late phase (for manufacturing)	Cost-effective robust process Optimum process Optimal process conditions Best manufacturing technology Good manufacturing fit Manufacturing strategy	Cost models Process unit operation models Process/facility simulations
Facility design (for a new or existing operation)	Minimize impact on facility Minimize capital	Process/facility simulations
Facility operation	Best operational performance Manage change	Cost models Process/facility simulation Operational effectiveness

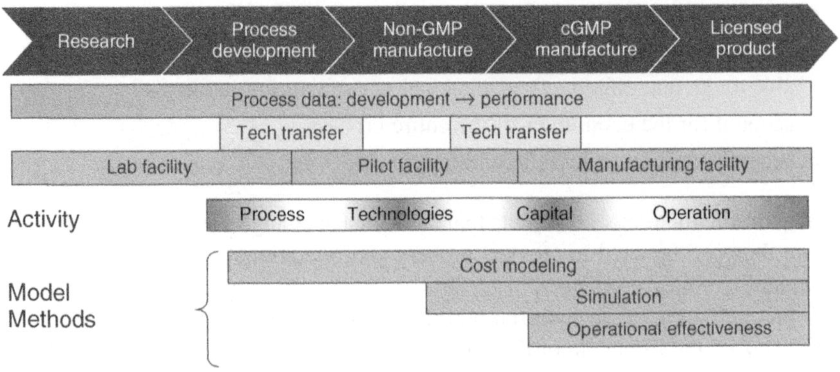

Figure 15.2 Product life cycle modeling approaches.

stages of the life cycle are more about efficient operation of facilities. As such, optimizing processes with the help of cost modeling are often most effective when performed as early as possible in the process.

To illustrate this point, Figure 15.2 shows the relationships between process information and facilities superimposed on the typical product life cycle. Process information links all the modeling tools with the facility required for manufacture.

15.5 PROCESS DEVELOPMENT KNOWLEDGE MANAGEMENT—CAPTURING THE DATA

One of the key elements to economic modeling is the concept of "garbage in—garbage out." For a model to accurately predict future costs, it must be fed with accurate data, much of which comes from process development. As such, a key to maximizing the benefits of process development is knowledge management within and between products (Hill and Sinclair, 2007). Currently, there is no consistency in the approaches to managing and using process information. To mature to the efficiency levels of other industries, vaccine manufacturers must consider moving to a consistent, standard terminology for representing bioprocesses. This is essential in order to create a data model that can be applied broadly.

Such a general model for batch manufacturing already exists and is defined by the Instrumentation, Systems, and Automation Society—the ISA-88 Standard for Batch Control point. It is widely used for control systems and automation (American National Standards Institute/Instrumentation, Systems, and Automation Society (ANSI/ISA), 1995; American National Standards Institute/Instrumentation, Systems, and Automation Society (ANSI/ISA), 2003). Two aspects of ISA-88 are especially useful for defining a bioprocess model: a separation of process requirements from equipment capability and a modular design approach. The concept of defining a process in dimensionless terms is inherent to scale-up and facility-fit assessments, and the practice of defining bioprocesses as a sequence of unit operations is essentially a modular design.

Ultimately, the goal of a knowledge management model is to enable feedback from manufacturing performance to guide process development and create a model that supports continuous improvement and better process understanding. Various modeling tools are commonly used in the industry to gain a better view of the effect of process development decisions on manufacturability, and the knowledge management model should support more effective use of these modeling tools. By enabling assumptions and relationships defined in the model to be compared to historical process data, modeling tools can be refined and improved continually. For example, cost models can assess the impact of process development decisions on manufacturing costs, and simulation models can assess facility fit and overall manufacturing performance and resource usage.

15.6 MODELING APPROACHES

15.6.1 Cost Modeling for Vaccine Manufacture

Cost models, in the broadest sense, can be widely applied as tools to analyze processes and manufacturing options and support decision making. They have been used in our industry to:

- assess the cost of outsourcing,
- evaluate and screen process development options,
- help develop capacity and expansion strategies,
- compare existing and novel processing/manufacturing technologies,
- assess the economic viability of a vaccine or therapeutic.

In this section, the different approaches to cost modeling are considered, and the merits of each approach are described and compared.

15.6.1.1 Basic Accounting Principles Most cost models draw on the principles of financial and management accounting to assess the cost impact of different investment and operating decisions. In traditional financial accounting, the impact of manufacturing changes is seen primarily in three of the four basic financial statements: the balance sheet and the income and the cash flow statements.

The balance sheet shows the balance between the company's assets and its liabilities and equity at a given point in time. Manufacturing-related activities such as equipment purchases and increases in inventory levels will be apparent on the asset side of the balance sheet, as well as the corresponding decrease in cash or increase in debt/equity financing required to support these assets.

In contrast to the "snapshot" view offered by the balance sheet, the income and the cash flow statements show the flow of money in and out of the company over a period. The income statement, also referred to as *a Profit and Loss (P&L) statement*, shows the translation of revenue into net profit for the company after expenses are taken out for a given financial period. Because the income statement is often based on accrual accounting methodologies, the revenue and expenses shown in the income statement do not correspond directly to the actual cash received and spent by the company during the same period. This information is instead shown in the cash flow statement, which is often used to assess the short-term financial stability of a company. Cash flows are especially important for cost models, as the timing of cash flows related to a specific project is commonly used for financial models such as net present value (NPV) and internal rate of return (IRR).

For manufacturing, the most significant line item on the income statement is the cost of producing goods for sale (referred to as *cost of goods sold or cost of sales*), which is often reported directly below net sales revenue. Subtracting the cost of goods sold from the sales revenue results in a company's gross profit, which is an important measure of operating performance. The cost of goods sold is also related to inventory valuation, as the basic equation for calculating the book value of inventory is (Remer and Idrove, 1991) as follows:

$$\text{Beginning inventory} + \text{net purchases} - \text{cost of goods sold} = \text{ending inventory}$$

By separating the direct costs involved in producing goods for sale from other expenses, such as selling, general, and administrative (SG&A) and research and development (R&D) expenses, interest, and taxes, it is possible to evaluate manufacturing performance as a distinct measure that contributes to overall business performance. This distinction is particularly important from an executive management perspective because improvements in manufacturing performance that result in increased gross margin are made visible, although the bottom line may remain unchanged or even fall because of increased expenses elsewhere in the company.

Unfortunately, traditional cost of goods sold calculations do not accurately account for the time and risk elements involved in manufacturing products. Nevertheless, the components of the cost of goods calculation that include labor, materials, and overheads are relevant to any analysis and are considered in detail in the following section.

A robust, well-structured cost model enables managers to have a better insight into the key cost drivers of the manufacturing process, as well as the sensitivity of overall cost of goods to changes in these key parameters. These models enable the cost impact of implementing different technologies to be evaluated, as well as the effect of process changes such as increasing product titers and yields, and these can be validated with financial accounting data.

It is worth noting that some management accounting techniques such as life cycle cost analysis and activity-based costing are also incorporated into manufacturing cost models in recognition of the significant effect manufacturing efficiency has on the average cost of goods. Particularly, the number of successful production runs per year and the cost of facility downtime and batch failure often have a much greater effect on overall manufacturing costs than changes in raw material or labor costs.

15.6.1.2 Project Appraisal Some of the typical methods for evaluating projects are NPV, IRR, and return on investment (ROI). All of these provide useful tools for decision making, particularly for capital investment and project approval. Net present value and IRR are particularly popular for evaluating potential long-term projects because they account for the upfront investment required, as well as the timing of future cash flows and the risk and/or opportunity cost of the project.

The basic calculations for NPV and IRR are the following (Rouf et al., 2001; Shanklin et al., 2001):

$$\text{NPV} = \text{Initial investment} + \sum_{t=1}^{N} \frac{C_t}{(1+r)^t},$$

$$\text{Initial investment} = \sum_{t=1}^{N} \frac{(C_t)}{(1+\text{IRR})^t}$$

where initial investment is the cash invested at the beginning of the project ($t=0$), t is the unit of time (measured in years), N is the lifetime of the project in years, C_t is the net cash flow for each year of the project, and r is the discount rate, also referred to as *rate of return, interest rate, hurdle rate, or cost of capital* (COC).

For NPV calculations, one of the most crucial considerations is the discount rate. The rate at which future cash flows are discounted to represent their present value is generally based on a required rate of return, which for financial planning purposes is typically the rate that would be expected from an investment of comparable risk. Many companies choose to use their weighted average cost of capital (WACC) as the discount rate for all project appraisals, as this value reflects the company's financing structure and risk profile, whereas others choose to use higher discount rates for riskier projects. For biotechnology investments, the required rate of return is often quoted at 21% or higher to reflect the high risk and uncertainty associated with positive cash flows in this business sector. One indicator of this higher risk is illustrated in Figure 15.3 where the sales price of a specific biologics manufacturing facility fluctuated dramatically over time.

When interpreting NPV, the accepted logic is that projects that have a positive NPV will add value to the company and should be undertaken, whereas those with a negative NPV should be rejected. If a project's NPV is zero, then the company should be indifferent to the project, as it will neither add to nor subtract from the value of the company. The decision to go ahead with the project should therefore be based on other criteria such as strategic benefits, which are not captured in the NPV analysis.

Internal rate of return analysis offers an alternative view to the same series of project-related cash flows. In financial terms, IRR is the annualized compound rate of return from the initial investment, and in mathematical terms, the IRR is the discount rate that results in a NPV of zero for a given series of cash flows. In general, if a project's IRR is greater than the company's acceptable COC for the project, then the project will add value and should be accepted.

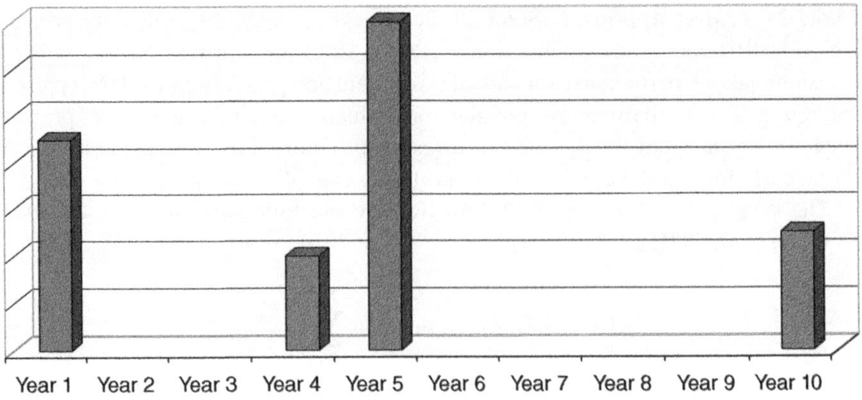

Figure 15.3 Construction cost and sales price of a biologics manufacturing facility (sold three times in 10 years).

Although both NPV and IRR are based on the same financial principle, there is some debate about which measure is most appropriate for evaluating long-term projects. Academics tend to prefer NPV, as it directly measures incremental value to the company, whereas many executives prefer IRR, as it indicates a percentage rate of return. Both measures are powerful tools, but should be used with caution. As investment decision tools, IRR is best used to evaluate a single project rather than to compare alternative projects, whereas the discount rate chosen should be considered carefully when using NPV to evaluate a single project.

Another method of evaluating expected return is ROI, which is useful for a variety of considerations such as short-term projects. In simple terms, ROI is the ratio of money gained or lost as a result of an investment to the money invested. For example, if a \$500 million capital investment resulted in an incremental revenue of \$150 million and incremental expenses of \$100 million in the first year, the ROI would be (\$150 M − \$100 M)/\$500 M = 10% ROI. Return on investment may be based on cash flows or net income/loss and on a single point in time or may account for the present value of gains/losses.

Some pharmaceutical companies use options pricing theory models to evaluate future products. The concept is that pursuing a development program is effectively buying an option to continue with the program or drop it at a defined point before commercial launch. Although this provides a technically rigorous way of evaluating projects, the mathematics can become quite complex, particularly when looking at multiphase projects (options to buy options or compounded options pricing). Typically, the assumptions driving the analysis are less accurate than the level provided by this cumbersome modeling approach.

Of the methodologies described in the following sections, cost of goods (CoG) is by far the most commonly used. Although not the most rigorous, it does have the merit that most people in the industry understand this approach. Cost of goods should not be used where there is a need to understand the interplay between the expenditures and project risk. Net present value is the best technique to analyze alternative technologies and manufacturing strategies, as it can account for the impact of delays in expenditures and properly account for the time value of money. It is not commonly used but is rigorous and can be used to support decision making.

Finally, it should be noted that the one virtual certainty about any cost model is that the absolute output will be wrong. As such, it is important to use modeling approaches and techniques that allow for the rapid generation of sensitivity analyses. These provide a picture of the dependency of the output on the assumptions driving the model and are critical in identifying the key drivers that determine the outcome of the analysis. Sometimes, it is more important to know the parameters that drive manufacturing cost than the absolute cost itself.

15.6.1.3 Manufacturing Cost Models (CoG) To illustrate the CoG approach, a spreadsheet-based and modular approach initiated at BioPharm Services that has been adopted for the implementation of over 50 models of actual manufacturing processes is examined. The cost model is configured as modules (i.e., capital, materials, consumables, and labor) using the worksheets in a Microsoft Excel workbook. Figure 15.4 shows the relationship between the various worksheets and the cost components that constitute the overall manufacturing cost. The spreadsheet methodology has the advantage that it is scalable, flexible, user-friendly, and transparent. As such, the structure and methodologies shown in the following section could be used in any calculation-based modeling structure to determine the CoGs and sensitivities for virtually any vaccine manufacturing process.

The use of CoG is a fairer comparison than capital cost because it accounts for all differences in facility throughput, material costs, labor costs, etc. The indirect (fixed) cost consists of the capital charges, insurance, and taxes, whereas the direct (variable) costs include the consumables, materials, and labor. Figure 15.4 shows the component items that contribute each of the cost categories for bulk vaccine manufacture, for example, the consumables class includes the column gel, filters, and single-use bags.

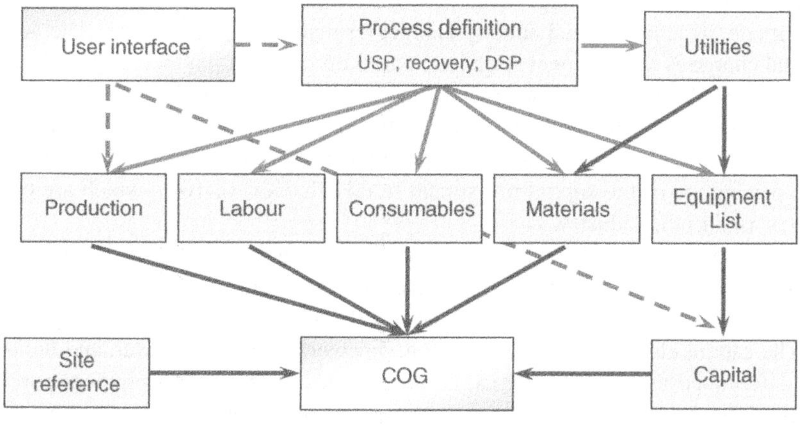

Figure 15.4 Structure of the CoG model.

A brief description of the key modules is provided in this section, including details of the user inputs that form the basis of the model and the calculation method.

User Interface. The user interface enables rapid assessment of the impact of predefined key model input parameters for what-if analyses. Examples include changing the production scale and switching between different manufacturing options. Such an interface enables changes in the underlying data to run sensitivity analyses that can be reviewed rapidly and conveniently.

Process Definition. The operating costs are determined by the process definition (e.g., upstream cell culture, recovery, downstream purification operations, formulation, and fill), which forms the core of the cost model. A detailed breakdown of each unit operation into subunit steps is captured. Key parameters include the type and total quantity of solutions/utilities used, the number of preparation/hold operations, the volume of vessel/bag used, the operating time, the elapsed time, the labor headcount for each substep, and the manual hours needed to carry out the operation.

Production. The user-defined parameters in this module consist of the campaign length, maintenance duration, and validation time. These parameters are used to compute the total available operating time. The limiting step per batch for each area (e.g., cell culture, recovery, and purification) is calculated. This figure is then used to calculate the process bottleneck and the annual number of production batches generated, given the particular operating constraints.

Equipment List. The objective of this module function is to generate a priced equipment list and a total purchase cost estimate for the major and supporting equipment items in the manufacturing option. If the cost of a piece of equipment is unknown, a cost estimate can be deduced from a known cost for that type of equipment and the ratio of the capacities raised to an index value (Adamson, 2006).

Capital Charge. The charge on the total fixed capital investment is factored into the cost model as an amortized annuity charge, termed *the capital charge*. The annuity capital charge is the payment for a loan based on constant payments and a constant interest rate. In the model, the capital charge is calculated on the basis of an 8-year period, a value of 12% for the COC (the interest rate for the capital investment), and a future value (the residual value attained after the last payment is made, expressed as a percentage of the capital investment in this chapter) of 10%, which are typical values used in the industry.

Table 15.2 shows the capital factors that constitute the total capital investment. This provides a time- and risk-weighted estimate for the cost of the manufacturing capital and allows for adjustments in the risk (COC) on the basis of the project.

The capital elements (e.g., installation, pipework, electrical power, and building) are determined as using benchmarked percentages of the total equipment purchase costs. Discount factors have been incorporated into certain capital estimates to account for the use of disposables.

TABLE 15.2 Capital Estimation

Category	Description
A. Fixed equipment costs	Total equipment purchase costs
B. Capital estimates	
Installation	α% of A
Pipework[a]	β% of A
HVAC[a]	χ% of A
Instrumentation and Control[a]	δ% of A
Electrical Power	ϵ% of A
Process Utilities	ϕ% of A
Building[a]	γ% of A
—Fit-out	η% of A
C. Total cost of works	A + B
D. Others	
Validation	λ% of C
Fee	μ% of C
E. Total capital investment (TCI)	C + D
F. Annuity charge (capital charge)	PMT (Cost of capital, period, E, future value[a] E)

[a]Discount factors included for disposable.

Materials. Process materials include media, buffer solutions, and cleaning chemicals (i.e., caustic and acid), which are made-up from solid ingredients using purified water (PW) or water for injection (WFI). The process equipment for cleaning includes the preparation and hold vessels, bioreactors, housings, and skids. The molecular weight, pack size, pack unit, and cost per pack for the raw chemicals are user-defined variables, which are used to determine the unit cost per liter for the solutions. The costs are obtained from vendors or suppliers. The compositions of each solution are indicated by specifying the composition of each of the chemicals in the solution. The total volume per batch for each type of solution and cleaning chemical is reported. The amount used is multiplied by the unit cost to calculate the total cost per batch.

Consumables. The user-defined consumables costs include filters, chromatography resins, chromatography membrane devices, and the disposable preparation and hold bags. The total consumption of consumables per batch is determined. For disposable consumables, the costs per batch are calculated by multiplying the number of each type of consumable used and the unit cost. In the case of reusable consumables, the cycle limit and cycles per batch are used in the calculation.

Labor. Labor headcount is estimated for each unit operation within the cost model. The assignation of labor costs to a manufacturing batch is based on the allocated time that the direct operation staff spent in production on a particular batch. The number of manual hours required per batch is calculated for the following categories.

- Production—the direct production operators and supervisors required in the main process and supporting activities such as buffer preparation and cleaning. The labor hours for the direct production operators is used to estimate the manual hours required for supervisors by applying a benchmarked percentage.
- Quality—the staff required in validation, quality assurance (QA), and quality control (QC). These are estimated using a function of the direct production labor using figures from benchmarking studies.
- Others—logistics and general management. The labor requirement is calculated using a function of the direct production personnel.

The different categories of personnel, their annual salaries, and overheads are user input parameters. The wage per hour for each personnel category is calculated using the annual salary, operating weeks per year, operator hours per week, and overheads. The number of manual hours and the hourly wage are then used to determine the total labor costs per batch.

Utilities. The cost model collates all process uses of PW and WFI to provide minimum estimates of the capacities of the PW and WFI generators and the volume of the storage vessels. The input parameters required for the estimation include effective usage, still blowdown, and fill time for storage tanks. The costs of the utility systems are added as fixed costs to the total equipment purchase costs.

Site. Other running costs for the manufacturing process include the following:

- Insurance and others—estimated as a function of the total fixed capital investment.
- Engineering and spares—determined as a function of the direct production labor.
- Utilities—calculated as a function of the total fixed capital investment.

The factors used in the estimation can be obtained from benchmarking studies of biomanufacturing facility operations at a comparable scale.

Outputs CoG. The key cost components (i.e., capital charge, materials, consumables, labor, and other applicable costs) can be summarized as in Table 15.3, constituting the estimation of CoG. The cost of operation should take into account the impact of facility throughput, material costs, labor costs, etc., to provide a better approximation of the total operating costs of the manufacturing process.

15.7 COST MODELS IN PRACTICE

The cost modeling structure detailed previously represents a powerful approach to understanding and evaluating the cost implications of a vaccine manufacturing

TABLE 15.3 Cost of Goods Estimation

Category	Description
A. Capital charge	From Table 15.2
B. Materials	
1. Process media	Cell culture media
2. Process buffers	Process solutions
3. Cleaning materials	Caustic (i.e., NaOH) and acids (i.e., H3PO4) for cleaning
C. Consumables	
1. Column resins	Protein A, ion exchange matrices
2. Disposable bags	Single-use plastic bags
3. Filters	Depth, ultrafiltration, viral, and sterile filters
D. Labor	
1. Process	Direct production labor costs
2. Quality	υ% of D1
3. Others (e.g., logistics)	ω% of D1
E. Others	
1. Insurance	ρ% of TCI
2. Engineering and spares	σ% of D1
3. Utilities	τ% of TCI
Total	A + B + C + D + E

process. Additional techniques common in the industry include simulation-based modeling and NPV analysis as described in section 15.5. To better illustrate the use of these models, CoGs and NPV-based case studies are discussed in the following sections:

15.7.1 Manufacturing Technologies—Single-Use Systems

Disposable technologies have been used in the industry for the last 15 years; however, it is only within the last 7 years that they have gained widespread acceptance. The main application is solutions handling, where most companies now use disposable containers for holding buffers, media, and products up to the maximum commercially available bag size (3000 l). Emerging areas that are gradually gaining acceptance include the following:

- Disposable bioreactors (up to 2000 l). Disposable bioreactors are now used in GMP (Good Manufacturing Practice) production, especially for seed preparation. Their use is expected to become more widespread within the next 5 years.
- Disposable mixing systems. The business case for disposable mixers is yet to be developed because of technical issues and high costs. Therefore, although there are already products in the market, they are yet to gain widespread acceptance.

- Membrane chromatography (low capacity). This method is finding significant acceptance for the removal of impurities in flow-through mode for the purification of monoclonal antibodies (mAbs). It is predicted that it will find more widespread use in these areas over the next 2–5 years.
- Membrane chromatography (high capacity). High capacity membrane chromatography does not exist as yet, and technical challenges remain, although some companies are preparing capture columns in disposable formats. Cost is likely to be an issue in this case.
- Ultrafiltration systems. Currently, these are available only for small-scale use, and there are technical problems to do with scale-up, so the widespread use for medium- to large-scale processing is not envisaged.

The emerging field of disposable technologies has the potential to reduce initial start-up capital costs and plant complexity significantly, and may play an increasing role in biomanufacturing operations—perhaps more efficiently than their reusable counterparts—without sacrificing on product quality. The traditional stainless steel equipment would be replaced by presterilized disposable components, incurring minimal cleaning costs. In addition, such technologies offer greater process flexibility, simplify material and personnel flow, eliminate cleaning validation costs, and reduce the risk of cross-contamination between batches in multiproduct facilities. Disposable-based engineering could be implemented throughout the production plant (Hodge, 2014), such as the use of single-use membrane chromatography devices, disposable prepacked chromatography columns, and single-use bags for fluid handling. A detailed study of the design concept for a facility based around single-use systems and the potential benefits of such a layout has been carried out (Sinclair and Monge, 2004; Sinclair and Monge, 2005).

15.7.1.1 Impact of Disposables on Product and Solution Handling—Bulk Manufacturing The process used for the assessment as given in the following section is based on the production process for a typical mAb (Table 15.4). Although there can be substantial differences between vaccine and mAb production processes, the techniques for evaluating the impact of disposables as shown in the following section can be applied to virtually any biologics process. The process examined consists of the inoculation of the seed fermenter through to bulk-purified sterile-filtered product.

To assess the impact of disposable solution handling technologies, Biopharm Services prepared a cost model on the basis of a facility operated at 2 × 5000 l production scale reactors with a product titer of 2 g/l. Two options were evaluated with the main difference between them being that one uses stainless steel vessels and the other implements the use of disposable bags for fluid handling. The process steps and all the associated major equipment are similar in the two cost scenarios modeled. The estimates for the cost parameters are drawn from data contained in BioPharm Services' proprietary cost databases consisting of benchmarking information from over 10 biomanufacturing operations.

TABLE 15.4 Process Sequence

No	Category	Unit Operation	Yield (%)	Product Conc. (g/L)	Volume (L)	Mass (g)
1	Cell culture	50-l Seed Bioreactor				
2	Cell culture	500-l Seed Bioreactor				
3	Cell culture	500-l Production Bioreactor		2.00	5,000	10,000
4	Recovery	Centrifugation	85%	2.00	4250	8500
5	Recovery	Depth Filtration	85%	1.70	4250	7225
6	Purification	UF/DF # 1	95%	16.15	425	6864
7	Purification	Affinity Chromatography	90%	3.28	1885	6177
8	Purification	Virus inactivation	98%	3.15	1923	6054
9	Purification	Ion exchange chromatography	95%	6.10	942	5751
10	Purification	Polishing chromatography	95%	5.80	942	5.464
11	Purification	Viral filtration	98%	5.68	942	5354
12	Purification	UF/DF#2	98%	27.84	188	5247
13	Purification	Sterile filtration	98%	27.28	188	5142
Overall downstream process yield			51%			

The vessels and bag containers are classified according to specific duty in the facility:

- Product hold
- Media preparation
- Media hold
- Buffer preparation
- Buffer hold

The cleaning of vessels is a major user of quality utilities in the biotechnology facility. Cleaning is required after every vessel use. In the disposable option, single-use bag systems are used to prepare and store media, buffers, and products before further processing within the facility. The bag systems are provided pre-assembled, sterile, and ready for process use. Vessel liners are used to hold the bag for solution preparation. Where the solution volume exceeds the maximum bag size, a stainless steel vessel of the next available size is selected. The limitations of the bag technology in the facility are the following:

- Maximum single-use hold bag volume of 3000 l
- Solution preparation in disposable bags up to 2000 l

Each solution prepared in-house is passed through a 0.2-μm filter before storage in a hold tank. The disposable hold bag comes with a sterile filter. The cost analysis in this section identifies differences (i.e., water usage, capital requirements, and fixed and variable operating costs) in the performance of the disposable bag production line when compared to the conventional stainless steel vessel facility.

Results. There was a 26% reduction in capital for the disposables-based facility where the capital fell from $67 million to $49 million. To gain insight into the impact of disposables, the CoG was analyzed by comparing the impact of this technology on capital charges, materials, consumables, and labor.

A summary of the CoG breakdown is provided in Figure 15.5. As expected, the costs of some categories (e.g., cell culture media, process buffers, and column resins) are the same for both options, as the manufacturing strategies differ only in the preparation and holding of fluids. The key outcomes are as follows:

- The capital charge is the highest cost-saving category. The reduction in the process equipment minimizes the extent of the design and installation, which significantly reduces the capital requirements.
- The labor category contributes about 3% to the total cost savings. This is attributed to the reduction in vessel cleaning activities.
- Material savings of 1% are gained by reducing the consumption of caustics and acids used for cleaning.
- There is an overall 4% increase in the consumables category towing to the use of plastic disposable bags.

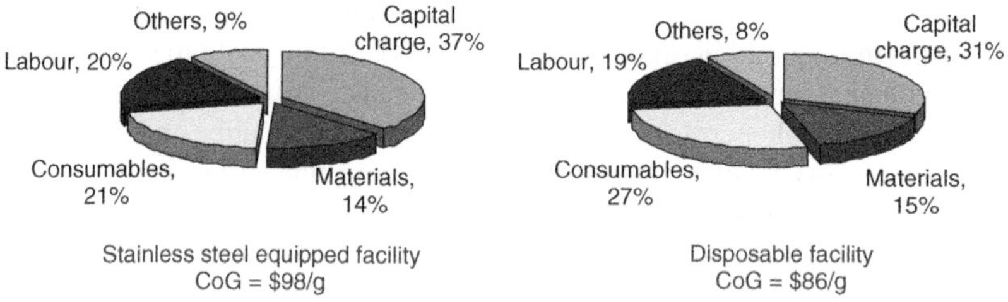

Figure 15.5 Breakdown of CoG for the two manufacturing options.

- The cost benefits provided by reduced process equipment, materials consumption, and labor more than compensate for the increased consumables costs, translating to an overall CoG saving of about 12% in the running costs per gram for the disposable option.

By considering all aspects of operation, including capital investment, materials, consumables, and labor, the key cost benefits of single-use technology can be identified as follows:

- Disposables switch fixed capital costs to variable consumables costs that are only applicable when the facility is operational.
- Overall operating costs for the disposable option are reduced despite the increase in consumable costs.
- Other disposable benefits such as the simplification of materials and personnel flow, the streamlining of process development, and the elimination of cleaning validation cannot be easily quantified. These benefits increase the attractiveness of this technology.

15.7.1.2 Aseptic Filling The aforementioned model presents an analysis of the cost tradeoffs of using new technology (disposables) in bulk drug manufacture. As mentioned earlier, however, the key cost drivers for vaccines manufacture/delivery often lie in the other manufacturing activities. For this reason, when evaluating the total costs of vaccine manufacturing, it is important to look at cost contributors such as aseptic filling. The following analysis looks at the economic comparison for the filling of a vaccine in two delivery options—vial (single-dose) and syringe.

A spreadsheet-based cost model, comprising several linked worksheets, was developed to evaluate the cost effectiveness of these two filling techniques. Start-up capital costs were identified separately from routine operating costs. The model consisted of a breakdown of individual cost categories—capital charge, materials, consumables, labor, and others.

The annual capital charge is the payment for a loan based on constant payments and a constant interest rate. Applying a COC accounts for the interest that must be paid on loans that were taken out to purchase the equipment and finance the build. The material costs include the costs of the bulk active substance and utilities (i.e., WFI, PW, and steam) incurred in running the process and cleaning activities. The consumables costs include the costs of disposable bags, vials, syringes, stoppers, overseals, and plungers. The labor costs consist of direct production, quality, and indirect labor. The others category include the insurance, taxes, and engineering spares.

The comparison was based on equivalent manufacturing capacity, that is, same number of doses, in the two filling facilities. The case study assumed the following:

- There are 40 batches per year, and 5 million doses of vaccine are produced.
- In both facilities, disposable bags are used to hold the bulk drug substances before being filled in vials/syringes.
- In the vial-filling facility, the stoppers would arrive loose and nonsterile. They would be loaded into a washing machine to be washed, siliconized, and sterilized. The vials are washed and passed through a depyrogenation tunnel before the filling process.
- In the syringe-filling facility, the syringes, plungers, and stoppers would arrive presterilized.

Results. The cost of goods breakdown for the comparison is illustrated in Figure 15.6. There was an overall cost savings of about 20% for the syringe-filling facility relative to the vial-filling option. The bulk of the cost savings was derived from the capital charge (22%). The additional equipment costs for the stopper and vial washers and depyrogenation tunnel contributed to the increased in capital cost requirements.

15.7.2 The Impact of Time and Risk

The CoG models described previously provide a good overview of the cost tradeoffs for the use of disposables and different filling options. Nevertheless, these models

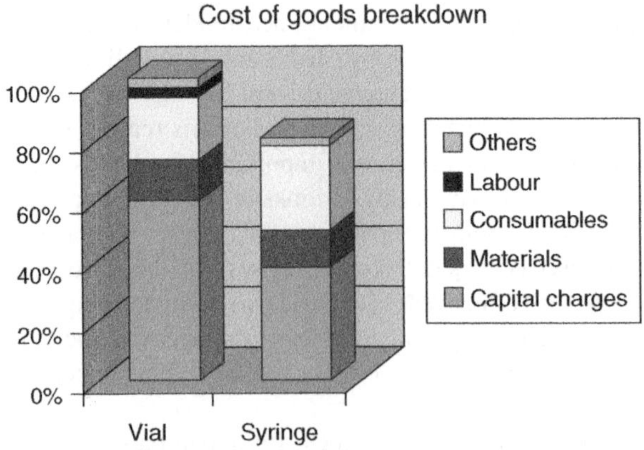

Figure 15.6 Cost comparison for aseptic filling of different containers using different sterilization techniques.

make assumptions about the timing and risk of the project that are not always accurate depictions of the vaccine environment. To better understand the implications of time and risk, NPV- or IRR-based models are considered. One such model examines the impact of reducing the time it takes to build and validate a facility.

Typical facilities can take 4 years or longer to build and validate. Assuming that a facility must be ready by market launch, this implies that the capital commitment must be made when the product is still fairly early-on in clinical trials. As a result, the risk carried by these capital outlays can be quite large. If one could delay the start of the facility build, by pursuing a modular facility concept for example, one could hold off on committing the capital until the risk profile is substantially lower.

In an effort to model/quantify the value of this approach, the build and operation of a biologics facility running 2×2000 l production bioreactors are considered. In this case, the facility cash flows over time on the basis of two scenarios were mapped as follows: (1) the facility takes 4 years to build and validate, and (2) the facility takes 2 years to build and validate. The cash flows because of capital spend were estimated over the timeline to build and validate, and the facility operating cost was estimated in a manner similar to the CoG analyses shown previously (not including the upfront and capital elements).

For each of the two scenarios stated previously, however, there is a wide variety of possible outcomes that the product: underperforms commercially, fails in phase II trials, fails in phase III trials, is a success, etc. To fully understand the value of time against these risks, one must therefore consider all of these potential outcomes.

This is where NPV models are particularly powerful. When cash flows are translated into NPV terms, they can then be compared on equal footing. For example, if one discounts the cash flows of the scenario that a product fails in phase II back to today's dollars, one can then apply a probability to that outcome and compare it directly to the probability adjusted, discounted cash flows of the scenario in which a product is successful. Adding up the probability adjusted NPVs of every potential outcome, one can then compare the two scenarios directly.

In doing so, it was found that the ability to compress the facility build time from 4 to 2 years cuts the weighted NPV of manufacturing roughly to half. This demonstrates the significant impact that time and risk can have on the vaccine industry and provides a strong argument for using NPV- or IRR-based analysis when these elements come into play.

Finally, as mentioned previously, modeling is most powerful when it enables sensitivity analyses that identify the importance of the various assumptions and inputs. In the example stated previously, the sensitivities were run to such parameters as the potential resale value of the facility (in the scenario in which the facility is almost completed when the product fails) to the COC. Although all of the inputs had an impact on the analysis, the benefits of compressing build time remained significant in almost all scenarios. As a result, we were not only able to show that the analysis was robust, but also to identify areas of threat and the areas most likely to be drivers of the benefit.

15.8 CONCLUSIONS

As pricing pressures drive the need for better manufacturing economics, there will be a greater call for the understanding and reduction of costs. This will be most evident in vaccines where the margins are already lower, and the costs of "secondary" manufacturing operations such as filling and packaging play a greater role. Against this backdrop, companies are using increasingly sophisticated modeling tools to define their processes and identify areas for savings. Tools that consider technology alternatives while taking into account the time and risk elements of the vaccine marketplace are particularly relevant. It is also important to note that the use of a variety of tools and sensitivity analyses is critical to gaining a sound picture of the cost tradeoff to manufacturing decisions. Drawing from NPV, IRR, ROI, and CoG analysis, a company can better understand their costs and optimize their processes to meet the challenges of a more price-conscious market.

ACKNOWLEDGMENTS

The authors acknowledge the support and help given by their colleagues at Biopharm Services and, in particular, Claire Hill and Dr. Janice Lim.

REFERENCES

Adamson R. (2006). A new era in biotechnology. Presentation at: Disposables for Biopharmaceutical Manufacturing; 2004 Oct 24–26; Dublin, ROI.

American National Standards Institute/Instrumentation, Systems, and Automation Society (ANSI/ISA). *ANSI/ISA-88.01–1995 Batch Control Part 1: Models and Terminology*. Research Triangle Park, NC; 1995.

American National Standards Institute/Instrumentation, Systems, and Automation Society (ANSI/ISA). *ANSI/ISA-88.00.03–2003 Batch Control Part 3: General and Site Recipe Models and Representation*. Research Triangle Park, NC; 2003.

Elmasry H. Capital Intensity and Stock Returns. Morgan Stanley Investment Management, Winter 2004.

Hill C, Sinclair A. Process development: maximizing process data from development to manufacturing. Biopharm Int 2007;21(7):38–43.

Hodge G. Disposable components enable a new approach to biopharmaceutical manufacturing. BioProcess Int 2014;17(3):38–49.

Lim JAC, Sinclair A, Kim DS, Gottschalk U. Economic benefits of single-use membrane chromatography in polishing—a cost of goods model. BioProcess Int 2007;5(2):48–56.

Pavlou A, Reichert J. Recombinant protein therapeutics—success rates, market trends and values to 2010. Nat Biotechnol 2004;22(12):1513–1519.

Prifti, C. 2010 Vaccine Industry, an Overview, University of Pennsylvania Center for Bioethics. Available at: http://www.vaccineethics.org/issue_briefs/industry.php.

Remer DS, Idrove HJ. Cost estimating factors for biopharmaceutical process equipment. Pharm Technol Int 1991;3(9):36–42.

Rouf SA, Douglas PL, Moo-Young M, Scharer JM. Computer simulation for large scale bioprocess design. Biochem Eng J 2001;8(3):229–234.

Shanklin T, Roper K, Yegneswaran PK, Marten MR. Selection of bioprocess simulation software for industrial applications. Biotechnol Bioeng 2001;72(4):483–489.

Sinclair A, Monge M. Biomanufacturing for the 21st century. Designing a concept facility based on single-use systems. BioProcess Int 2004;2(9):26–31.

Sinclair A, Monge M. Concept facility based on single-use systems, part 2—leading the way for biomanufacturing in the 21st century. BioProcess Int 2005;3(6):51–55.

Tufts Center for the Study of Drug Development. *Outlook 2005*. 2005.

Tufts Center for the Study of Drug Development. *Outlook 2007*. 2007.

US Department of Commerce. *A Survey of the Use of Biotechnology in US Industry*. US Department of Commerce Technology Administration Bureau of Industry and Security; 2003.

INDEX

Vaccine Development and Manufacturing, First Edition.
Edited by Emily P. Wen, Ronald Ellis, and Narahari S. Pujar.